Lifetime Fitness and Wellness

Melvin H. Williams

Old Dominion University

Lifetime Fitness and Wellness

fourth edition

a

personal

choice

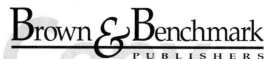

Brown & Benchmark
PUBLISHERS

Madison, WI Dubuque Guilford, CT Chicago Toronto London
Mexico City Caracas Buenos Aires Madrid Bogotá Sydney

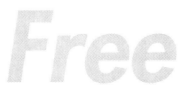

Book Team

Publisher *Bevan O'Callaghan*
Managing Editor *Ed Bartell*
Developmental Editor *Megan Rundel*
Production Editor *Jane C. Morgan*
Proofreading Coordinator *Carrie Barker*
Designer *Katherine Farmer*
Art Editor *Tina Flanagan*
Photo Editor *Rose Deluhery*
Production Manager *Beth Kundert*
Production/Costing Manager *Sherry Padden*
Production/Imaging and Media Development Manager *Linda Meehan Avenarius*
Marketing Manager *Pamela S. Cooper*

Basal Text *10/12 Times Roman*
Display Type *Frutiger*
Typesetting System *Macintosh™ QuarkXPress™*
Paper Stock *50# Mirror Matte*

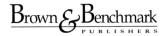

Vice President of Production and New Media Development *Vickie Putman*
Vice President of Sales and Marketing *Bob McLaughlin*
Vice President of Business Development *Russ Domeyer*
Director of Marketing *John Finn*

 A Times Mirror Company

Consulting Editor: Eileen Lockhart

The credits section for this book begins on page 408 and is considered an extension of the copyright page.

Cover illustration by Zita Asbaghi

Copyedited and proofread by Rose R. Kramer

Printed in the United States of America by Times Mirror Higher Education Group, Inc., 2460 Kerper Boulevard, Dubuque, IA 52001

10 9 8 7 6 5 4 3 2 1

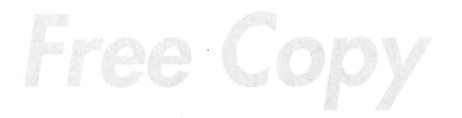

Contents

v

8

Stress-Reduction Techniques *175*

9

Health Effects of High-Risk Behaviors *191*

10

Exercise and Nutrition Concerns for Women *222*

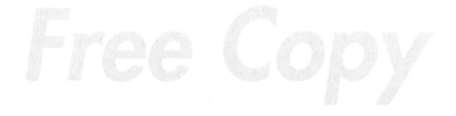

Laboratory Inventories

Preface

*H*appiness! We all want it and tend to seek it in a variety of ways. However, Bertrand Russell, the venerable philosopher, noted that man is an animal whose happiness depends on his physiology more than he likes to think. Unfortunately, many Americans have abused their own natural physiology, the wonderful functioning of the human body that gives us life, so much that the quality of life, or happiness, as well as the quantity of life, or longevity, may be significantly diminished.

Fortunately, the United States is in the midst of a health and fitness boom that has endured for over a decade and continues to grow, with millions of Americans changing their life-styles by initiating exercise programs, shifting to a more natural healthful diet, maintaining an ideal body weight, breaking the smoking habit, decreasing alcohol consumption, recognizing the importance of safe sex practices, and using various stress-reduction techniques, all in order to look and feel better. This movement is a positive one, for these life-style changes may provide us with the immediate health benefits we desire now, and may also help us prevent many of the degenerative diseases that plague our modern society and decrease the quality and quantity of life in later years. Collectively, these healthful changes characterize a Positive Health Life-style, and they are in accord with and based on the health promotion objectives documented in the Public Health Service report, *Healthy People 2000: National Health Promotion and Disease Prevention Objectives.*

The health and fitness boom originated among individuals in their thirties and forties; however, increasing numbers of college-aged students have adopted changes and characteristics of a Positive Health Life-style after being exposed to these concepts in college courses with titles similar to "Personal Wellness" or "Health through Exercise." This textbook is designed to be used in conjunction with such courses, but the presentation of the materials is also suitable for students to use on an individual basis. It provides contemporary information concerning the beneficial effects of a Positive Health Life-style and how to implement and live such a life-style. With proper knowledge and guidance, the student can design and implement his or her own Positive Health Life-style, one that can last a lifetime. This effort is facilitated by the presence on the campuses of many colleges and universities of Wellness Centers.

This book is organized into twelve chapters. Key concepts and key terms are highlighted at the beginning of each chapter; numerous figures and tables are included to help explain the major concepts. Contemporary research findings that support the chapter content are documented at the end of each chapter, grouped as books that provide broad overviews, reviews that synthesize and interpret current research, and specific studies that focus on a particular topic of interest.

Chapter 1 establishes the basis for adopting a Positive Health Life-style. Chapter 2 presents an overview of human energy systems and basic principles of designing and implementing an individualized exercise program and other life-style changes.

The heart of the textbook, chapters 3 through 9, offers specific guidelines for adopting a Positive Health Life-style. Chapter 3 covers aerobic exercise programs; chapter 4 focuses upon resistance-training programs for muscular strength and endurance; chapter 5 deals with the development of flexibility; chapter 6 provides the basis for healthy nutrition; chapter 7 integrates the roles of diet, exercise, and behavior modification in weight control; chapter 8 explores stress reduction techniques; and chapter 9 discusses the potential health consequences associated with various high-risk behaviors, such as substance abuse (particularly cigarette smoking and alcohol intake) and unsafe sex practices.

Chapter 10 covers several health issues of particular interest to females, while chapter 11 stresses a Positive Health Life-style as a lifelong program of contributing to healthful aging. This chapter emphasizes the impact of a Positive Health Life-style upon a number of major degenerative diseases in our society today, such as cardiovascular diseases, metabolic disorders, and musculoskeletal problems. Finally, chapter 12 provides a brief discussion of adherence, or maximizing the ability to stay with the Positive Health Life-style for a lifetime.

Other features include Laboratory Inventories, which help assess an individual's current health life-style and provide guidelines for modifications; a glossary of terms; and five appendices—the Food Lists of the American Dietetic Association and the American Diabetes Association; scoring charts for Dr. Kenneth Cooper's aerobic fitness tests; caloric expenditure for a variety of physical activities; calories, fat, and cholesterol in products sold in common fast-food restaurants; and energy expenditure in METS for a variety of daily activities. Parts of this text, particularly nutrition components in chapters 6 and 7, have been excerpted from *Nutrition for Fitness and Sport,* Fourth Edition, by Melvin H. Williams and also published by Brown & Benchmark

This text asks the individual to think about the possible consequences of his or her current life-style, not only for now but for the future. More importantly, it provides a mechanism for change by actively involving the student in a number of laboratory inventories designed to help implement a Positive Health Life-style. There are thirty-four Laboratory Inventories that will, among other things, help you evaluate your current life-style related to various health behaviors, determine which life-style changes you may be able to undertake successfully, evaluate your fitness level and plan an appropriate exercise program, assess the quality of your diet, determine you healthy body weight, survey factors that may increase your level of stress, and give you an idea of your predisposition to substance abuse. We learn best by doing, so taking the appropriate laboratory inventory and initiating appropriate life-style changes may help you implement a life-style that will become lifelong.

Overall, this text will provide you with the essential knowledge necessary to implement and maintain a Positive Health Life-style. However, since it covers so much territory, the amount of information offered is somewhat limited. If you develop an interest in a specific area covered in this text, such as nutrition, exercise, or stress management, check with your university or college catalogue, or with your advisor, to see if an advanced course, such as a basic course in nutrition, will work into your degree program of study.

Additionally, there are numerous professional employment opportunities in the health sciences and health education areas. As you most likely know, health care reform is a major focus of governmental activity to help reduce the financial burden associated with health care in the United States. One effective way to decrease health care costs is through health promotion, and professionals are needed to help educate the American public regarding the various components of the Positive Health Life-style, and to help them implement such life-style changes. Such career opportunities should increase in the 1990s and beyond, particularly as the population of our nation becomes increasingly older.

I would like to acknowledge the late Mr. Ed Jaffe, editor for Wm. C. Brown Publishers, who encouraged me to write this textbook. I would also like to thank my current editors at Brown & Benchmark Publishers, Scott Spoolman and Megan Rundel, and my production editor, Jane Morgan, for their invaluable assistance throughout the various stages of development.

The contributions reviewers made to the development of this text are greatly acknowledged. They have made many useful recommendations relative to its reorganization and content. The reviewers were Scott Armstrong (Malone College), W. Dianne Hall (University of South Florida), Kim D. Hansen (North Central College), Gary D. Reinholtz (Gustavus Adolphus College), and Jill E. White-Welkley (Emory University).

Finally, I extend my sincere appreciation to Jeanne J. Kruger for her assistance in the preparation of the final manuscript.

Melvin H. Williams
Virginia Beach, VA

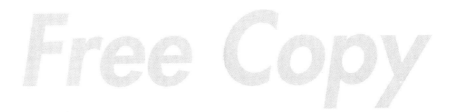

1

A POSITIVE HEALTH LIFE-STYLE

Key Terms

behavior modification	experimental research	health risk appraisal (HRA)	prudent health behavior
chronic diseases	functional age	personal choice	relative risk (RR)
chronological age	health promotion practices	Positive Health Life-style	risk factor
disuse phenomena	health protection services	preventive services	self-efficacy
epidemiological research			

Key Concepts

- Of the three major classes of health objectives developed for the nation by the Public Health Service, health promotion practices are primarily under the control of the individual.

- Chronological aging is inevitable, and although the catabolic effects usually associated with the chronological aging process also appear to be inevitable, you may maintain a younger functional age by following a Positive Health Life-style.

- Four major components of a Positive Health Life-style are a properly planned exercise program, a balanced nutrition program, appropriate methods to enhance mental health, and the avoidance of substance abuse.

- Personal health promotion and preventive medicine encourage personal choices of positive health behaviors that will help counteract key risk factors. Self-responsibility is a key to personal health promotion.

- Key preventable risk factors associated with the onset of chronic diseases include physical inactivity; excess body weight; a diet high in fat, cholesterol, and salt; high blood pressure; excessive stress; smoking habits; and excessive alcohol intake.

- Health risk appraisals, educational tools designed to analyze your current health life-style, offer a general idea of areas in your life that may pose a health risk.

- A Positive Health Life-style is not solely concerned with the prevention of chronic diseases; it is also concerned with helping you achieve the healthiest body and mind possible, within natural limitations.

- Although the development of a Positive Health Life-style should be encouraged as early in life as possible, the benefits of adopting such a life-style may be achieved at almost any age.

- A Positive Health Life-style helps you meet the short-term goals of looking better physically and feeling better mentally, and also helps you to meet long-range goals of preventing the onset of chronic diseases.

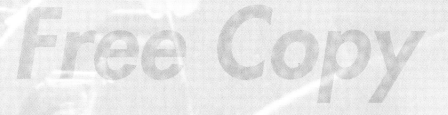

INTRODUCTION

Health is often defined as the general condition of the body and mind. Good health is normally associated with vigor and vitality, while poor health is identified with disease or other ailments. The two major factors that impact on your health status are your genetic background and your personal environment, respectively often referred to as nature and nurture. In relation to diseases, some are caused purely by genetics (e.g., sickle cell anemia), others are caused purely by environment (e.g., lead poisoning), while most are caused by the interaction of genetics and environment (e.g., heart disease). Although in the future genetic engineering research may enable scientists to repair faulty genes and prevent the development of certain genetic disorders, at the present time we can do little regarding our genetic predisposition to various diseases. However, for most of us, environmental factors exert the most significant effects on our health status, either directly or by interacting with our genetic predisposition, and we can do much to influence these environmental effects by making healthy choices throughout life. Healthy choices in various aspects of your life, which we shall designate as the **Positive Health Life-style,** underlie the concept of wellness.

One factor that influences your perception of your health status is your age. College and university student populations are becoming increasingly diverse, particularly in relation to age. It is not uncommon for a typical college-aged student (one aged eighteen to twenty-four) to take courses, even fitness and wellness courses, along with students in their thirties, forties, and beyond. If you are a young college student, most of your concerns about the quality of your physical and mental health are probably grounded in the present. Basically, you want to look good physically and feel good mentally—*now.* You probably do not spend a great deal of time worrying about the distant future, such as whether or not you will develop heart disease, cancer, or diabetes, how you will take care of yourself during your retirement years, or how long you are going to live. However, such thoughts may have crossed your mind at one time or another. On the other hand, if you are older than the typical college-aged student, these thoughts may have become increasingly important to you.

Regardless of your age, you can make a number of changes in your current life-style that will probably help you to look better physically and to feel better mentally in a relatively short time. Interestingly, these rather simple life-style changes that center around fitness and wellness may not only improve the quality of your life in the present, they will help enhance the quality of life over time and improve longevity. Although genetics plays an important role in your future health, we know more about health promotion and preventive medicine today than our parents and grandparents did in the past, so we may be able to prevent some of the health problems that they experienced. Genetics is an important factor relative to your health, but so too is how you deal with your personal environment. Nature deals you a set of cards, but you play them.

Fitness and *wellness* are two key buzzwords of the 1990s. Just look around. We have best-selling books focusing on nutrition and exercise, popular magazines called *American Health* and *Eating Well,* wellness newsletters by universities and consumer-protection organizations, separate sections in our daily newspapers covering health and fitness, television channels devoted almost exclusively to medicine and health, videotapes by movie stars and television celebrities on how to become physically fit at home, and the increased use of health and fitness to advertise products ranging from breakfast cereals to beer.

In the United States, an increased emphasis on fitness and wellness developed in the 1960s and stimulated considerable research activity regarding the effects of various life-style changes, such as increased exercise participation and low-fat diets, on the development of various diseases. Numerous studies over the past three decades, as shall be documented throughout this book, have provided substantial evidence supporting the manifold health benefits of appropriate life-style modifications, and many individuals have initiated personal fitness and wellness programs designed to enhance their health status. However, recent surveys suggest that Americans, in general, appear to be exercising less, eating less sensibly, and getting fatter.

In order to improve the health status of more Americans, in 1991 the Public Health Service (PHS) of the United States Department of Health and Human Services released a document entitled *Healthy People 2000: National Health Promotion and Disease Prevention Objectives.* This document outlines a national strategy for significantly improving the health of the nation. More than three hundred specific health objectives fall into three major categories: health protection, preventive services, and health promotion. There are also several subclassifications for each major category.

Health protection services are those related to environmental or regulatory measures that confer protection on large segments of the population, such as water fluoridation for prevention of tooth decay and legislation requiring seat belt use. Others generally perform these services to protect our health.

Preventive services include screening, counseling, or other services provided in a clinical setting. Included in this category are screening programs for the early detection of high blood pressure and immunization to prevent the development or spread of certain diseases. Again, others usually provide these services for our health benefit.

Health promotion practices focus upon eight major areas, five of which are most relevant to this text: physical fitness and exercise, nutrition, mental health, smoking and health, and misuse of alcohol and drugs. In contrast to health protection services and preventive services, health promotion practices involve life-style factors basically under the control of the individual. Moreover, health protection and preventive services will not succeed unless personal health promotion practices are observed. For example, legislation to enforce seat belt use will be ineffective if you do not wear your seat belt every time you drive, as will an education program to prevent the development of cancer if you do not practice certain recommendations, such as regular breast or testicular self-examination.

Although many of the health objectives are designed to address immediate health problems, such as avoidance of unintentional injuries, much of the emphasis behind recent governmental support for health promotion and preventive medicine programs is the reduction of the magnitude of future health care costs associated with the "graying of America." For example, individuals born during the baby boom era of the late 1940s, now in their late thirties and early forties, will soon be in their sixties, the time of life when serious health problems begin to become magnified. **Chronic diseases,** such as coronary heart disease, cancer, diabetes, and osteoporosis, generally occur with advancing age, particularly if individuals had unhealthy life-styles during earlier adulthood. Thus, from a financial point of view, it is important for the government to keep people healthy for as long as possible. Research has indicated that health promotion programs focused on the elderly may reduce health-care costs.

On the other hand, many of the specific health objectives for the nation include the young, not only young children and adolescents, but also young adults of college age. If healthy life-styles can be developed early, they may be more likely to persist throughout the years and thus exert a significant impact upon one's health later in life. Consequently, by attempting to educate the young about healthier life-styles, the federal government is looking even further down the road to help reduce health-care costs.

However, many young adults exercise or diet to improve their appearance and to feel good about themselves now, not to prevent later health problems such as coronary heart disease or cancer. Fortunately, with the selection of proper health-related behaviors, both short-term and long-term benefits may be achieved concomitantly.

Although relevant information regarding health protection and preventive services will be discussed, this book focuses upon health promotion practices. It is designed to help you develop a set of health behaviors that constitutes a high energy life-style, known throughout this text as a Positive Health Life-style, a life-style fashioned after the concept of positive health developed in 480 B.C., by Hippocrates, the Greek physician known as the Father of Medicine. Such health behaviors stress responsibility for one's health and should enable you to increase control of your life, to maximize your ability to operate or function at or near your potential, or as a popular advertising phrase goes, to "be all that you can be." A Positive Health Life-style can maximize your ability to work at your potential in the present and will enable you to experience the joys of aging without the handicaps.

As Browning wrote, "Grow old along with me! The best is yet to be." ▪

Aging and Health Risk Factors

Although we age in different ways, we all begin to age from the first day of conception. **Chronological age** represents the passage of time. It is marked by our birthday each year and is relatively easy to determine. **Functional age** represents the capacity of the body to perform certain specific tasks and is usually evaluated in a variety of ways, such as tests of vision and hearing, physiological functioning during exercise, psychomotor ability, and health status.

Some of the changes in the aging process (such as your external appearance) are readily observable, while other internal changes are not as easily detected (fig. 1.1). We can note rather easily such changes as gray hair, impaired hearing and vision, increased body weight, stiff joints, and wrinkled skin; however, clogged arteries, less efficient lungs and heart, and diminished function of certain glands may not readily be noticed.

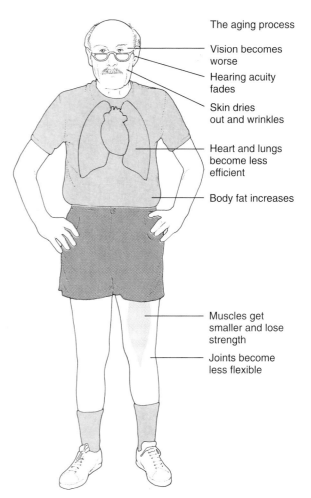

The aging process

Vision becomes worse

Hearing acuity fades

Skin dries out and wrinkles

Heart and lungs become less efficient

Body fat increases

Muscles get smaller and lose strength

Joints become less flexible

Figure 1.1 *Physiological changes associated with the aging process. A number of physiological changes occur during the natural aging process. Some of the changes, such as decreased visual ability, are not too preventable. However, others, such as decreased cardiovascular functions, may be prevented to some degree by a Positive Health Life-style.*

At the present time, chronological aging is inevitable, and many of the changes in body functions that accompany the aging process and increase functional age also appear to be inevitable. However, in an affluent society that places a high value on a youthful appearance, certain technological and medical advances may counteract some of these adverse effects. We can obtain an almost undetectable aid to improve hearing, use soft contact lenses to correct vision, or undergo plastic surgery to smooth facial wrinkles. Some of these applications, however, may be unnecessary. Hearing losses may or may not be preventable, depending on whether hearing loss is a natural occurrence of the aging process or is brought about by exposure to continuous periods of loud noise during younger years. Wrinkling of the skin may be minimized by avoiding prolonged exposure to the sun or excessive use of tanning beds.

Although there exists this close general relationship between chronological and functional ages, there may be marked differences between the two, particularly in relationship to physiological functioning and health status. In other

Table 1.1 Risk Factors and Some Associated Health Problems

Risk Factor	Associated Health Problems
Excessive body weight	Coronary heart disease Diabetes
Low leisure-time physical activity	Coronary heart disease Obesity
Low levels of planned exercise	Coronary heart disease Obesity
Poor diet habits	Cancer Obesity
High fat and cholesterol diet	Atherosclerosis Obesity
High salt diet	High blood pressure Stroke
High blood pressure	Coronary heart disease Stroke
Excessive stress	Coronary heart disease Mental illness
Cigarette smoking	Lung cancer Coronary heart disease
Excessive alcohol consumption	Cirrhosis of the liver Motor vehicle accidents
Poor driving habits	Accidents
Poor physical exam habits	Cancer
Indiscriminate sex habits	Sexually transmitted diseases

words, depending upon your life-style, you may have a younger or older functional age compared to your chronological age. For example, studies from Scandinavia and from the National Institute of Aging revealed that highly physically active individuals in their fifties and sixties were able to reduce the risk of functional decline and had exercise capacities and body fat levels comparable to those of healthy but sedentary twenty-five-year-olds. Conversely, some individuals in their twenties who have abused their health may have the health status of someone in their forties or fifties.

Although some of the genetic effects of aging may be inevitable, many that impact upon your health may be under your control. By identifying and eliminating or minimizing factors in your life-style that may be potentially harmful to your health, you may be able to reduce the rate at which you age functionally. Although you cannot stop the clock chronologically, you can slow down functional aging and maintain the physiological function and health status of a twenty-year-old for years to come.

Since your functional age may be evaluated on the basis of your health status, usually determined by the number of health risks you possess, it is often referred to as your risk age. Over the years, scientists in the field of epidemiology (the study of disease patterns in human populations) have identified a number of life-style factors considered to be health risks; these life-style practices are known as risk factors.

A **risk factor** is a health behavior or personal characteristic that has been associated with a particular disease. A cause-and-effect relationship does not have to be present in order to label a particular factor as a risk to health, but some form of statistical relationship between the risk factor and the presence of the disease in a given population group should be evident.

Table 1.1 presents a broad overview of some major risk factors that may be favorably modified with proper health promotion practices, or the implementation of a Positive Health Life-style. One or two of the possible health problems that may occur is listed with each risk factor.

Life-Style Health Risk Factor Assessment Inventory

There are numerous health assessment inventories available today. Such inventories are often known as **health risk appraisals,** or **HRAs.** Some are very simple and can be completed in less than a minute, giving you a general measurement of your health life-style. Other versions are computerized and may take an hour or so to complete; they offer you an estimate of the probability of developing a particular chronic disease or forecast how many years you will live by determining your functional, or risk, age. Because validity studies of these more extensive inventories are not yet available and the reliability of several widely used HRAs has been reported to be less than desirable, we cannot verify their accuracy and will not duplicate them here. Those who are interested in such an analysis may contact several of the companies or agencies that administer them. A listing can be found in the pamphlet *Health Risk Appraisals: An Inventory,* which may be obtained by writing to the National Health Information Clearinghouse, P.O. Box 1133, Washington, D.C., 20013. Your course instructor may have a source, or you may wish to contact local distributors of computer software to see what programs are available. The major point to keep in mind concerning any of these inventories is that, although they may be effective health-education tools, they are not to be used for diagnosis or for general medical screening purposes.

However, an HRA may alert you to health risks in your present life-style. Moreover, you may use a health risk appraisal to retest yourself after you have implemented behaviors consistent with a Positive Health Life-style. It might be interesting and informative to keep the results of your initial assessment and compare them to a reassessment at the end of this course.

The Health Life-style Assessment Inventory (Laboratory Inventory 1.1) is designed to assess your current health life-style and to give you a general idea of areas in your life that may need to be modified to achieve an optimal Positive Health Life-style. The inventory is educational in nature and will help you get a broad look at your overall health life-style. Several more detailed inventories, presented in later chapters, deal with specific topics such as dietary habits and stress profiles.

Since this inventory is general and educational in nature, it has some limitations. For example, it does not take into account family history of diseases that may exert a significant

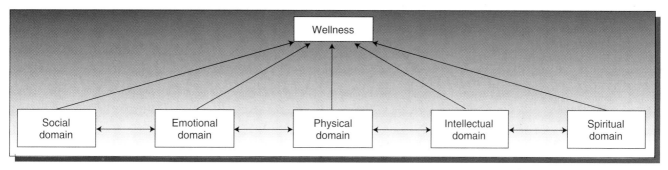

Figure 1.2 *The domains of wellness. Total wellness is dependent upon interactions of the social, emotional, physical, intellectual, and spiritual domains.*

influence on your future health. A number of chronic diseases appear to be related to genetic predisposition and, thus, tend to run in some families. Moreover, it does not look at your personal health history. You may have or have had diabetes, asthma, allergies, rheumatic heart disease, or other disorders, that may influence your health life-style. With these limitations in mind, please complete The Health Life-style Assessment Inventory on page 177 before reading any further.

The Positive Health Life-Style

The health objectives published in *Healthy People 2000* are an extension of a previous endeavor. In 1980 the Public Health Service established a series of health objectives for the nation with the hope of meeting these objectives in the 1990s. In subsequent years, a number of studies conducted by the PHS to evaluate progress toward these objectives found that many had already been met. In most cases, gains were in the areas of health protection services and preventive health services and were the result of legislative action or intensive national programs. For example, many state legislatures have passed laws requiring the use of seat belts; this has resulted in a decrease in motor-accident deaths. In addition, a national campaign has led to the early detection and subsequent treatment of high blood pressure in millions of individuals, resulting in a significant decrease in the incidence of heart disease and stroke.

On the other hand, the PHS has noted that other areas continue to pose challenges, particularly the health promotion area. Little progress has been made in meeting the objectives related to nutrition, body weight, fitness and exercise, and stress control. The development of a Positive Health Life-style is consistent with the health objectives set forth by the PHS in the area of health promotion.

However, a Positive Health Life-style is not concerned solely with preventing the onset of chronic disease later in life; that is only a secondary goal. Its primary goal is to achieve the healthiest body possible within natural limitations; to achieve a style of life characterized by high energy levels and a *joie de vivre;* in other words, to enhance the quality of life by increasing your healthy life expectancy. In order to attain optimal function and optimal health, you must intellectually learn and understand how the human body functions and how to treat it well. You need to develop a life-style that,

according to current medical evidence, provides you with the greatest statistical probability of remaining healthy. Adopting a Positive Health Life-style is not going to guarantee protection against all chronic diseases and health problems, but it may delay the onset of such diseases or reduce the severity of disabling symptoms and enable you to enjoy life to the fullest.

Mind-Body Interrelationships and the Dimensions of Wellness

A Positive Health Life-style is based on a wellness model that views the individual as a whole, such that there is a sense of unity between the mind and body. One model of wellness, depicted in figure 1.2, segments the mind and body into various domains, most notably the social, emotional, physical, intellectual, and spiritual domains, the health implications of which are described briefly below.

- The social domain focuses on the development of meaningful personal relationships with family and friends.
- The emotional domain focuses on the development of self-confidence and a positive self-concept, the ability to handle stress, the ability to express emotions appropriately, and to accept one's own limitations.
- The physical domain focuses on the ability to exercise properly, to eat a healthful diet, and to avoid high-risk behaviors.
- The intellectual domain focuses on the ability to think critically, to identify and solve problems, and to use information to enhance personal development.
- The spiritual domain focuses on the ability to find meaning and purpose in life, to develop faith in nature, religion, or some other higher entity to enhance moral and ethical development.

The specific domains in this model are related to the mind-body concept; the social, emotional, intellectual, and spiritual domains are closely associated with the mind, while the physical domain is associated primarily with the body. However, all of these domains are interrelated so that disease processes or disturbances in one can cause disease in either the mind or the body. In this book, the term psychological health will be used to encompass those health behaviors that influence the mind, while physical health will relate to health

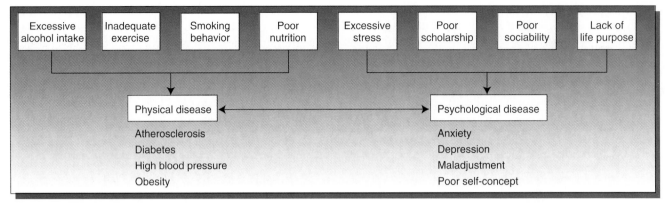

Figure 1.3 *Mind-body interrelationships. Physical disease may lead to psychological disease, and vice versa. Contributing risk factors to each type of disease may be modified by positive health behaviors.*

behaviors that influence the body. Figure 1.3 illustrates the interrelationships between the mind and the body and some possible contributing factors to physical/psychological diseases. For example, disturbances in the physical domain, such as improper exercise habits and diet, may contribute to obesity (a physical disease) which may lead to the development of a poor self-concept and maladjustment (psychological problems). Conversely, poor sociability may lead to depression (psychological disorder), which may contribute to the development of obesity by promoting sedentary behaviors and excessive food intake.

Promotion and Prevention Versus Treatment

Most of us have been exposed to individuals who have developed a chronic disease and are aware of the excellent treatment they have received from our technologically sophisticated medical community. Today, physicians and hospitals are equipped with a wide array of diagnostic tools, advanced surgical techniques, medicines, and drugs to treat some of the major chronic diseases. In many cases, what may have been a fatal disease in the past now has a favorable prognosis for partial or complete recovery. Medical advances have been phenomenal during the first 50 to 60 years of this century and have been instrumental in eradicating many of the previous causes of premature death—tuberculosis, polio, diphtheria, etc. Moreover, medical advances in the past 30 years have been even more phenomenal and are helping to treat the major chronic diseases that are now the main threats to our health. The research and development of these modern medical techniques for treating chronic and other diseases, however, has been extremely costly, with medical care costs expanding at an extremely rapid rate during the past decade. For example, at the time of this writing, a coronary artery bypass operation costs $30,000, while a liver transplant costs $250,000.

This rapid rise in medical care costs and an increasing tendency towards national health care legislation have helped to begin to change the focus of medical care from treatment to prevention. A spokesperson for the American Medical Association has noted that 90 percent of the health problems in the United States are preventable to one degree or another, stressing personal health decisions as the key to preventing disease. In support of these remarks, a study published in the *Journal of the American Medical Association* has revealed that excess deaths from nine major chronic diseases (coronary heart disease, stroke, diabetes, chronic obstructive pulmonary disease, lung cancer, breast cancer, cervical cancer, colorectal cancer, and chronic liver disease) in the United States could be prevented by simple life-style changes, such as stopping cigarette smoking, controlling high blood pressure, eating a healthier diet, reducing body fat, moderating alcohol consumption, becoming physically active, and using available screening techniques for early detection of cancer.

Prudent Health Behaviors

How do we know what effect a particular life-style change will have upon our health? To find answers to specific questions of concern to you, you should rely primarily on the findings derived from scientific research. Since this book presents a number of general recommendations concerning the impact of life-style changes on fitness and wellness, it is important to review briefly the nature and limitations of scientific research with humans that support these recommendations.

Several research techniques have been used to explore the effect of life-style on health, but the two most prevalent have been epidemiological and experimental research. **Epidemiological research** involves studying large populations to find relationships between two or more variables. For example, obesity is a risk factor associated with the development of diabetes in adulthood. Individuals who become obese have a higher statistical probability of developing diabetes than those who remain at a healthy body weight. However, no exact cause (obesity) and effect (diabetes) relationship has yet been determined, although some plausible theories are being studied. Thus, if you become obese you may not develop diabetes, but you will increase your risk of doing so. Researchers often establish a **relative risk (RR)** regarding the association between some health behavior and a disease. An RR of 1.0 means there is neither an increased nor a decreased risk, an RR of 2.0 means individuals may be twice as likely to develop the disease, while an RR of 0.5 indicates individuals are only at half the risk. In some cases, such as the association between cigarette smoking and certain forms of cancer, the RR may be 10 or even much higher.

Epidemiological research is useful in identifying relationships among variables and inferring causality, but **experimental research** is essential to help verify a cause-and-effect relationship. In such studies an independent variable or variables (cause) is manipulated so that changes in a dependent variable or variables (effect) can be studied. With some risk factors, a direct cause-and-effect relationship can be observed. The results of epidemiological research, such as cirrhosis in alcoholics due to chronic excessive alcohol intake, often stimulate experimental research in order to establish a cause-and-effect relationship. For example, experimental studies with humans have shown significant deteriorative effects in liver function tests with the consumption of excessive amounts of alcohol over a short period of time, while experimentation with animals over a longer period of time has shown that excessive alcohol consumption causes cirrhosis of the liver. Experimental research currently is being conducted with many risk factors in order to help establish such cause-and-effect relationships.

However, it is important to realize that the results of one study with humans, even though published in a respected medical journal, do not prove anything. Studies need to be repeated by other scientists and a consensus developed; the experimental evidence should support the epidemiological findings. Unfortunately, such a consensus is often lacking to support recommendations about specific modifications for improved health, for it is very difficult to conduct experimental research with humans regarding the effect of a single life-style change on health. For example, many diseases, such as cancer and heart disease, are caused by the interaction of multiple risk factors and may take many years to develop. It is not an easy task to control all of these risk factors in freely living human beings in order to isolate one independent variable, such as dietary fat, and to study its effect on the development of heart disease over 10 to 20 years.

Nevertheless, a tremendous amount of both epidemiological and experimental research has been conducted regarding the effect specific life-style behaviors may have upon health and wellness. Although in many cases we still do not have absolute proof that a particular health behavior will produce the desired effect, we do have sufficient information to make recommendations that are prudent, meaning that they are likely to do some good and cause no harm. Thus, the recommendations offered in this text should be considered to be **prudent health behaviors;** they are based upon a careful analysis and evaluation of the available scientific literature, including specific studies or comprehensive reviews of the pertinent research by individuals or public and private health organizations. When a sufficient number of research studies is available a meta-analysis, which provides a statistical comparison of the results of all selected studies, may provide one of the most significant means to evaluate specific health behavior recommendations.

What are some recommended prudent behaviors that may have a positive effect on your health, happiness, and general well-being? Several surveys have been conducted to determine whether there are any behaviors that appear to help attain or maintain a state of good health. As a general overview of what is to come in later chapters, a synthesis of these reports suggests that the following behaviors are associated with a healthy life-style.

1. Exercise. Get at least 20 minutes per day of regular, moderate, aerobic exercise at least three to four days a week. Or, do 30 minutes of moderately-intense exercise, such as gardening, stair-climbing, and walking, during your leisure time on most days of the week. Exercise is inexpensive medicine.

2. Nutrition. Eat wholesome, natural foods, including a good breakfast and two other healthy, well-balanced meals per day; avoid unnecessary snacking. Let your food be your medicine.

3. Body weight. Maintain an optimal body weight through a sound exercise and diet program.

4. Rest. Get about 7 to 8 hours of restful sleep each night; use relaxation techniques when necessary.

5. Alcohol. If you do drink, use alcohol in moderation.

6. Smoking. If you do not smoke, do not begin; stop smoking if you currently do smoke.

7. Personal environment. Avoid toxins and pollutants when possible; use care with insecticides and pesticides.

8. Personal injury. Be safety conscious; when driving, use seat belts and avoid excessive speed or use of alcohol or drugs.

9. Stress. Use socially acceptable, yet effective techniques to deal with daily problems and to reduce hostility and anger.

10. Healthy sexuality. Practice safe sex habits.

11. Self-worth. Develop a feeling of personal value, a feeling that you are in control of your personal environment, a feeling that you are able to make personal choices. Do not equate money with success.

12. Intelligence and memory. Exercise your mind. Practice memory techniques.

13. Social ability. Practice social skills. Resolve to be cheerful and helpful. Learn to talk less and listen more.

14. Relationships. Develop friendly relationships within your family and with others at school, work, or other situations.

15. Laughter. Laugh more often. Laugh heartily. Read the comics or watch funny shows. Look for humor in everyday events.

Total health involves a balanced relationship between the mind and the body. To be totally healthy, you should possess an optimal level of both physical and psychological fitness. Both types of fitness are interrelated and very complex. Although our concern in this book is primarily with

Table 1.2 Modifiable Aspects of Aging by Personal Choice of a Positive Health Behavior

Aging Factor	Positive Health Behavior Required
Body weight	Exercise, diet
Cardiovascular functioning	Exercise, diet, nonsmoking
Dental decay	Diet, proper cleaning
Glucose tolerance	Weight control, exercise, diet
Intelligence tests	Training, practice
Memory	Training, practice
Osteoporosis	Weight-bearing exercise, diet
Physical endurance	Exercise, weight control
Physical strength	Exercise
Pulmonary reserve	Exercise, nonsmoking
Reaction time	Training, practice
Serum lipids and cholesterol	Diet, weight control, exercise
Skin aging	Sun avoidance, nonsmoking
Social ability	Practice
Systolic blood pressure	Weight control, salt limitation, exercise

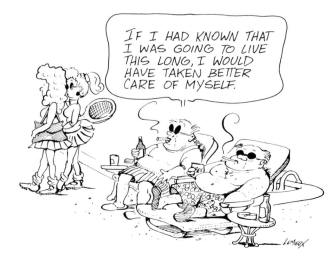

Figure 1.4 *The life-style we lead while young may exert a significant impact on the quality of our lives now and in later years.*

physical fitness, particularly health-related physical fitness, and the factors that may influence it, we shall also emphasize the associated relationships with psychological health.

The prudent key health behaviors addressed in the remainder of this book primarily parallel the major set of health objectives set forth by the Public Health Service in the area of health promotion. They include:

1. Physical fitness and exercise (chapters 2 to 5)
2. Nutrition (chapter 6)
3. Healthy body-weight control (chapter 7)
4. Stress management (chapter 8)
5. Cigarette smoking (chapter 9)
6. Alcohol and drug abuse (chapter 9)
7. Sexually transmitted diseases (chapter 9)
8. Health concerns of females (chapter 10)
9. Risk reduction for chronic diseases (chapter 11)

Benefits of a Positive Health Life-Style

Many individuals do not adopt a Positive Health Life-style because it requires some personal restraint or effort. For example, they might not buckle seat belts because it takes a little effort. Moreover, Americans, in general, expect immediate results and benefits from such personal restraints and efforts. Unfortunately, many of the physiological benefits of sound positive health behaviors are not readily observable. Without medical technology, we cannot see the fall in blood lipids, the change in blood cholesterol, the increased vitality

of the lungs and liver, the alteration in hormones to reduce the stress on the heart, and other such physiological changes that may help to prevent the development of certain chronic diseases. However, there are some clues that prove a Positive Health Life-style program is working. We can see our body weight begin to change, feel our breathing improve, experience less coughing in the morning, measure our slower heart rate, suffer less physical and mental fatigue, and develop a feeling of self-worth.

Although we cannot alter the true aging process at the present time, it appears that the development of positive health behaviors may help to prevent some of the adverse effects that may be due to factors other than the true aging process. One such factor may involve **disuse phenomena,** which, simply translated, means that if we don't use something, we lose it. Physical abilities, intellectual capacity, memory, and social skills may deteriorate if they are not continually utilized. Thus, disuse may add to the deterioration that usually occurs in these processes as a natural consequence of the true aging process.

Numerous research studies have indicated that a proper exercise program and other positive health behaviors can aid in slowing down many physiological aging processes and enhance the quality of life. Table 1.2 presents some aging factors that may be ameliorated by personal choice of a positive health behavior.

As noted in figure 1.4, your preparation for a healthy life in your later years should begin when you are young. Although individuals of all ages, even those in their sixties, seventies, eighties, and nineties, may obtain health benefits from the implementation of a Positive Health Life-style, the benefits will be greater if initiated early in life. As a college-aged student, you are in an enviable position to initiate such a life-style and reap the benefits. Nevertheless, it is never too late to reap some of the benefits resulting from a Positive Health Life-style.

Personal Choice and Health Promotion Behaviors

Personal Choice

The ultimate key to a Positive Health Life-style is an attitude of self-responsibility for your own health status. The concept of **personal choice** in relationship to health behaviors is an important one. An estimated 90 percent of all illnesses may be preventable if individuals would make sound personal health choices based upon current medical knowledge. We all relish our freedom of choice and do not like to see it constrained when it is within the legal and ethical boundaries of society. The structure of American society allows us to make almost all personal decisions relevant to our health. If we so desire, we can smoke, drink excessively, refuse to wear seat belts, eat whatever foods we want, and live a completely sedentary life-style without any exercise. The freedom to make such personal decisions is the crux of our society, although the wisdom of these decisions can be questioned. Personal choices relative to health often pose a dilemma. As one example, you may know the health implications relative to a bout of heavy alcohol consumption but may be pressured by peer approval into believing it is the socially accepted thing to do at a party.

A multitude of factors, both inherited and environmental, influence the development of health-related behaviors, and it is beyond the scope of this text to discuss all these factors as they may impact upon any given individual. However, the decision to adopt a particular health-related behavior is usually one of personal choice. There are healthy choices and there are unhealthy choices. In discussing the ethics of personal choice, Fries and Crapo drew a revealing analogy in their excellent book, *Vitality and Aging*. They suggest that knowingly indulging in a behavior that has a statistical probability of shortening life is similar to attempting suicide. Thus, if you are interested in preserving both the quality and quantity of life, personal health choices should reflect those behaviors associated with a statistical probability of increased vitality and longevity, or in other words, adoption of a Positive Health Life-style.

Personal Health Promotion Behaviors

How can you adopt a Positive Health Life-style? The first step is to develop an awareness of areas in your life that need improvement. The Health Life-style Assessment Inventory (Laboratory Inventory 1.1) should be helpful in this regard. The ultimate goal is to develop a set of permanent health behaviors that, based upon current scientific evidence, should provide you with the greatest opportunity to attain and/or maintain a state of optimal health.

In order to change from an unhealthy behavior to a healthy one, you will need to undertake some form of behavior modification. **Behavior modification** is a term you will see periodically throughout this text. For our purposes, it involves a variety of useful techniques for changing your unhealthful life-style behaviors to healthy ones, so it may also be referred to as life-style modification. Although some life-style changes may be done "cold turkey," such as using your willpower to

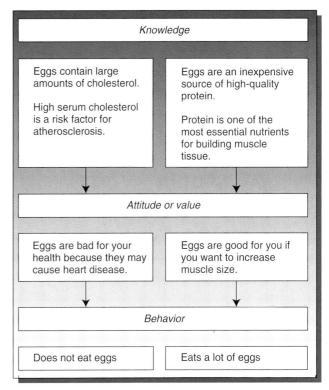

Figure 1.5 *Development of different health behaviors. Knowledge influences attitude development, which leads to actual behavior.*

stop smoking, most behavioral changes are usually accomplished in small steps and are more moderate in nature, gradually evolving into a total Positive Health Life-style. Appropriate guidelines for behavior modification will be presented in relevant chapters, but it is important for you to understand some of the key points of behavior modification, so a general overview will be provided at this point.

A model often used to explain the development of a set of behaviors involves a sequence of acquisition of knowledge, formation of an attitude or set of values, and development of a particular behavior (fig. 1.5). For example, you may acquire the knowledge that eggs are very high in cholesterol, and that high levels of some forms of cholesterol in the blood are associated with the development of atherosclerosis and coronary heart disease. This knowledge, plus other information you possess about coronary heart disease, may help you shape a personal attitude that eggs are bad for your health. This attitude may then be reflected in your actual behavior with the result that you will not eat eggs. On the other hand, you may have learned that eggs are an inexpensive, excellent source of complete protein and are high in nutrient value. This knowledge may help you acquire an attitude that eggs are good for your nutritional health. Your behavior may reflect this attitude, with the result that you eat a lot of eggs. Thus, one of the keys to shaping your health behavior patterns is the knowledge you receive.

In this particular case, there is some truth to both points of view. Eggs are high in cholesterol, but they are also an excellent, inexpensive source of protein. Thus, if you are into bodybuilding but also want to consume a diet that may protect against elevations of serum cholesterol, you may learn that all of the cholesterol and fat are in the yolk. Eating only egg whites will provide you with the protein but will eliminate the cholesterol.

Also inherent in this model is the acquisition of a variety of skills that have important health implications. Learning to exercise properly, to read food labels and select products that conform to guidelines for healthful eating, to induce relaxation through several techniques, and if you drink, to drink sensibly, are several of the skills inherent in a healthful life-style, but may take time to develop.

Accordingly, you may need to establish both long-term and short-term goals. For example, a long-term goal may be to lose 30 pounds in 6 months, but you may have multiple short-term, or intermediate, related goals, such as to lose 5 pounds per month. An even shorter term goal in this case would be to lose 1 pound per week. Both long-term and short-term goals need to be reasonable and attainable. Nothing breeds success like success, so it is extremely important to set short-term goals that may be attainable in a reasonable length of time, so that you may experience multiple successes in pursuit of your long-term goal. As you achieve each short-term goal, you should reward yourself with something appropriate to the occasion, for a reward will provide you with a positive feedback to your commitment to change an unhealthy behavior.

This book may be used for self-instructional purposes and provides you with sufficient information in each chapter to help you modify unhealthy behaviors. However, it has been designed primarily to be used in conjunction with a college or university course, so your instructor will help guide you in the acquisition of appropriate knowledge and skills conducive to the Positive Health Life-style and will also help you in establishing appropriate goals.

Although you may learn the appropriate knowledge and develop the essential skills to initiate healthful behavior changes, all will be for naught if it is only for the purpose of passing this course. If you do not develop a personal health ethic, an attitude, so to speak, that these behavior changes will have a positive effect on your life, you will most likely stop using them at the end of the semester. To help develop this attitude, you should generalize the skills you learn beyond the classroom or exercise room to a variety of other settings and times. For example, if you learn to monitor your heart rate during exercise while doing aerobic dancing, do it also as you incorporate exercise into your weekend with brisk walking or jogging. Probably the most important factor in determining your ability to develop and sustain a healthy behavior is your **self-efficacy,** or your belief in your ability to do so. By doing it, and doing it repeatedly in a variety of situations, you will continually reaffirm your ability to sustain a healthful behavior that will eventually become entrenched as a valued personal health ethic to help guide your health behaviors for a lifetime. As a popular advertising slogan goes, "Just do it!" It might not be a bad idea to use this slogan, or a similar one, as your own personal motto to help reinforce your behavior changes.

Although we have been focusing upon the benefits associated with behavioral changes leading to a Positive Health Life-style, it is important to realize that such changes may not confer equal benefits to everyone. The prudent health behaviors discussed previously are general recommendations believed to be beneficial to the general population. But we are individuals. We all possess biological individuality and thus might react differently to a particular intervention. For example, increased salt in the diet will increase the blood pressure of some individuals, but not of others. Thus, restricting salt consumption may be beneficial for one individual but will have little effect on another.

It is also important to realize that health behavior changes may also involve some risks. For example, you may have been genetically endowed with the ability to be a good runner and thus might find jogging to be easy and pleasant. Thus, you may become overzealous and do too much too soon, predisposing yourself to an overuse injury that will limit your ability to jog until you recover. However, if you plan properly, the risks associated with most health behavior interventions are minimal and are overwhelmingly outweighed by the benefits. Guidelines to minimize risks associated with behavior changes will be presented in each chapter where appropriate.

Often, when individuals initiate a health behavior change, experience the related benefits, and develop a personal health ethic relative to that behavior, they begin to modify other unhealthy behaviors as well. Exercise may be a key health behavior in this regard, for it may spur interest in other health behavior changes, such as a change to a healthier diet or cessation of smoking. However, engaging in one health behavior does not automatically lead to other behavior changes. The more healthful behavior changes you make, the greater the probability of living life to its fullest. The next ten chapters will provide you with the knowledge and skill base to develop a set of specific health behaviors believed to be conducive to such a goal, while the last chapter will supply you with some guidelines for adhering to such a program for a lifetime.

After completing Laboratory Inventory 1.1, Laboratory Inventory 1.2 may help you identify those behaviors that you desire to change most. It provides you with an evaluation of your self-efficacy to modify specific health-related behaviors, and will help you prioritize those behavior changes where your chances of success are maximized because you feel you can effectively control your behavior in these areas. Being successful in one positive health behavior change, such as implementing a moderate walking exercise program, may help you with more difficult behavior changes, such as stopping smoking.

Keep in mind, however, that the Positive Health Life-style is not simply a set of health behaviors. It is more; it is a life-style to be lived daily that is based on the premise of the late Norman Vincent Peale that if you do the best with what you have, you will maximize your individual potential for a healthful, productive life.

References

Books

Bouchard, C., et al., eds. 1994. *Physical activity, fitness, and health.* Champaign, Ill.: Human Kinetics.

Dunn, J. 1961. *High level wellness.* Arlington, Va.: R. W. Beatty.

Feinstein, A., ed. 1992. *Training the body to cure itself.* Emmaus, Pa.: Rodale Press.

Fries, J., and L. Crapo. 1981. *Vitality and aging.* San Francisco: W. H. Freeman.

Hafen, B., et al. 1988. *Behavioral guidelines for health and wellness.* Englewood, Colo.: Morton.

National Research Council. 1989. *Diet and health: Implications for reducing chronic disease risk.* Washington, D.C.: National Academy Press.

Shils, M., et al., eds. 1994. *Modern nutrition in health and disease.* Philadelphia, Pa.: Lea and Febiger.

Tkac, D., ed. 1990. *Lifespan-plus: 900 natural techniques to live longer.* Emmaus, Pa.: Rodale Press.

United States Department of Health and Human Services. Public Health Service. 1981. *Health risk appraisals: An inventory.* Washington, D.C.: National Health Information Clearinghouse.

United States Department of Health and Human Services. Public Health Service. 1991. *Healthy people 2000: National health promotion and disease prevention objectives.* Washington, D.C.: U.S. Government Printing Office.

Winett, R., et al. 1989. *Health psychology and public health.* New York: Pergamon Press.

Reviews

American College of Sports Medicine. 1990. The recommended quantity and quality of exercise for developing and maintaining cardiorespiratory and muscular fitness in healthy adults. *Medicine and Science in Sports and Exercise* 22:265–75.

Astrand, P. O., and G. Grimby. 1986. Physical activity in health and disease. *Acta Medica Scandinavica Supplementum* 711:1–244.

Blair, S. 1993. 1993 C. H. McCloy research lecture: Physical activity, physical fitness, and health. *Research Quarterly for Exercise and Sport* 64:365–76.

Blair, S., et al. 1993. Physical inactivity. *Circulation* 88:1402–5.

Bouchard, C. 1993. Heredity and health-related fitness. *Physical Activity and Fitness Research Digest* November: 1–7.

Bruce, G. 1993. Implementing a university campus wellness model. *AAOHN* 41:120–23.

Cavenee, W. and R. White. 1995. The genetic basis of cancer. *Scientific American* 272 (March): 72–79.

Centers for Disease Control. 1987. Protective effect of exercise on coronary heart disease. *Morbidity and Mortality Weekly Report* 36:426–30.

Conway, T. 1989. Behavioral, psychological and demographic predictors of physical fitness. *Psychological Reports* 65:1123–35.

Dubbert, P. 1992. Exercise in behavioral medicine. *Journal of Consulting Clinical Psychology* 60:613–18.

Farquhar, J. 1993. Keynote address: How health behavior relates to risk factors. *Circulation* 88:1376–80.

Fentem, P. 1992. Exercise in the prevention of disease. *British Medical Bulletin* 48:630–50.

Fletcher, G., et al. 1992. Statement on exercise: Benefits and recommendations for physical activity programs for all Americans. *Circulation* 86:340–44.

Goldberg, L., and D. Elliot, eds. 1985. Symposium on medical aspects of exercise. *Medical Clinics of North America* 69:1–214.

Hagburg, J. 1987. Effect of training on the decline of $\dot{V}O_{2max}$ with aging. *Federation Proceedings* 46:1830–33.

Haskell, W. 1987. Is there an exercise RDA for health? *Western Journal of Medicine* 146:223–24.

Krick, J., and J. Sobal. 1990. Relationships between health protective behaviors. *Journal of Community Health* 15:19–34.

Kuntzleman, C. 1993. Childhood fitness: What is happening? What needs to be done? *Preventive Medicine* 22:520–32.

Lee, I-M. 1995. Physical activity and cancer. *Physical Activity and Fitness Research Digest* 2 (June): 1–8.

Leff, M., ed. 1992. What's lurking on your family tree? *Consumer Reports on Health* 4:65–68.

Levine, G., and G. Balady. 1993. The benefits and risks of exercise training: The exercise prescription. *Advances in Internal Medicine* 38:57–79.

Lundberg, G., ed. 1987. Leads from the MMWR. Sex-, age-, and region-specific prevalence of sedentary lifestyle in selected states in 1985: The Behavioral Risk Factor Surveillance System. *Journal of the American Medical Association* 257:2270–72.

Masoro, E. 1990. Assessment of nutritional components in prolongation of life and health by diet. *Proceedings of the Society for Experimental Biology and Medicine* 193:31–34.

Nickens, H., and R. Petersdorf. 1990. Perspectives on prevention and medical education for the 1990s. *American Journal of Preventive Medicine* 6:1–5.

Nieman, D. 1994. Clinically relevant symposium: Exercise and immunology. *Medicine and Science in Sports and Exercise* 26:125–94.

Paffenbarger, R. 1994. 40 years of progress: Physical activity, health and fitness. In *American College of Sports Medicine—40th Anniversary Lectures.* Indianapolis, Ind.: ACSM, 93–109.

Pate, R., et al. 1995. Physical activities and public health. A recommendation from the Centers for Disease Control and Prevention and the American College of Sports Medicine. *Journal of the American Medical Association* 273:402–7.

Perls, T. 1995. The oldest old. *Scientific American.* 272 (January): 70–75.

Pescatello, L., and L. DiPietro. 1993. Physical activity in older adults. *Sports Medicine* 15:353–64.

Powell, K., and S. Blair. 1994. The public health burdens of sedentary living habits: Theoretical but realistic estimates. *Medicine and Science in Sports and Exercise* 26:851–56.

Rooney, E. 1993. Exercise for older patients: Why it's worth your effort. *Geriatrics* 48:68–77.

Schilke, J. 1991. Slowing the aging process with physical activity. *Journal of Gerontological Nursing* 17:4–8.

Scrimshaw, N. 1990. Nutrition: Prospects for the 1990s. *Annual Reviews in Public Health* 11P:53–68.

Sharkey, B. 1987. Functional versus chronological age. *Medicine and Science in Sports and Exercise* 19:174–78.

Shephard, R. 1993. Exercise and aging: extending independence in older adults. *Geriatrics* 48:61–64.

Simons-Morton, B., et al. 1987. Children and fitness: A public health perspective. *Research Quarterly for Exercise and Sport* 58:295–302.

Sternfeld, B. 1992. Cancer and the protective effect of physical activity: The epidemiological evidence. *Medicine and Science in Sports and Exercise* 24:1195–1209.

U.S. Centers for Disease Control and Prevention and American College of Sports Medicine. 1993. Summary statement—Workshop on physical activity and public health. *Sports Medicine Bulletin* 28:7.

Wachtel, T. 1993. The connection between health promotion and health-care costs: Does it matter? *American Journal of Medicine* 94:451–54.

Wenger, N. 1994. 40 years of progress: Physical activity in the primary and secondary prevention of heart disease. In *American College of Sports Medicine—40th Anniversary Lectures.* Indianapolis, Ind.: ACSM, 41–54.

Specific Studies

Blair, S., et al. 1993. Physical activity, physical fitness, and all-cause mortality in women: Do women need to be active? *Journal of the American College of Nutrition* 12:368–71.

Centers for Disease Control. 1993. Prevalence of sedentary lifestyle—behavioral risk factor surveillance system, United States, 1991. *Morbidity and Mortality Weekly Report* 42:576–79.

Centers for Disease Control. 1993. Public health focus: Physical activity and the prevention of coronary heart disease. *Morbidity and Mortality Weekly Report* 42:669–72.

Hahn, R., et al. 1990. Excess deaths from nine chronic diseases in the United States, 1986. *Journal of the American Medical Association.* 264:2654–59.

Hofstetter, C., et al. 1991. Illness, injury and correlates of aerobic exercise and walking: A community study. *Research Quarterly for Exercise and Sport* 62:1–9.

Kavanagh, T. and R. Shephard. 1990. Can regular sports participation slow the aging process? Data on master athletes. *Physician and Sportsmedicine* 18:94–103.

Kusaka, Y., et al. 1992. Healthy lifestyles are associated with higher natural killer cell activity. *Preventive Medicine* 21:602–15.

Larsson, B., et al. 1984. Health and aging characteristics of highly physically active 65-year-old men. *International Journal of Sports Medicine* 5:336–40.

Ornish, D., et al. 1990. Can lifestyle changes reverse coronary heart disease? The Lifestyle Heart Trial. *Lancet* 336:129–33.

Paffenbarger, R., et al. 1993. The association of changes in physical activity level and other lifestyle characteristics with mortality among men. *New England Journal of Medicine* 328:538–45.

Ross, J., and R. Pate. 1987. The National Children and Youth Fitness Study II. A summary of findings. *Journal of Physical Education, Recreation and Dance* 58 (November–December): 51–56.

Simonsick, E., et al. 1993. Risk due to inactivity in physically capable older adults. *American Journal of Public Health* 83:1443–50.

Smith, K., et al. 1989. The reliability of health risk appraisals: A field trial of four instruments. *American Journal of Public Health* 79:1603–7.

Sobal, J., et al. 1992. Patterns of interrelations among health-promotion behaviors. *American Journal of Preventive Medicine* 8:351–59.

Sytkowski, P., et al. 1990. Changes in risk factors and the decline in mortality from cardiovascular disease. The Framingham Heart Study. *New England Journal of Medicine* 322:1635–41.

2

GENERAL GUIDELINES FOR YOUR PERSONAL EXERCISE PROGRAM

Key Terms

benefit/risk ratio
exercise
exercise duration
exercise frequency
exercise intensity
exercise mode

health-related fitness
metabolic specificity
neuromuscular specificity
overload principle
physical activity
physical fitness

principle of disuse
principle of progression
principle of reversibility
principle of specificity
principle of use

progressive resistance
  exercise (PRE)
structured physical activity
unstructured physical activity
warm-down
warm-up

Key Concepts

■ With proper knowledge of the underlying principles of physical fitness, you should be able to design and implement your own personalized exercise program.

■ Both unstructured and structured physical activity may confer some health benefits, so participation in both types of activities is encouraged when possible.

■ The most important physical fitness components related to personal health include cardiovascular-respiratory fitness, muscular strength and endurance, flexibility, and body composition.

■ The four components of a personalized physical fitness program are assessment, planning, implementation, and evaluation.

■ In planning your personal exercise program, you need to develop both short-term and long-term objectives to help you meet your goals.

■ The major principles of exercise training are the principles of use and disuse and the associated principles of overload, progression, specificity, warm-up and warm-down, recuperation, and reversibility.

■ The major components of the overload principle utilized in the design of any exercise program are intensity, duration, and frequency.

■ The principle of progression indicates that exercise programs should be easy in the beginning and should gradually increase in intensity as the individual becomes more fit.

■ The principle of specificity deals with the mode of exercise to be used. The body adapts to the energy system and neuromuscular patterns involved in a specific exercise mode.

■ The warm-up and warm-down are important components of each individual exercise session.

■ The principle of reversibility is related to the principle of disuse, for health benefits will fade away if exercise training ceases. In essence, use it or lose it!

■ Exercise is lifelong medicine. You must exercise for the remainder of your life in order to receive the optimal benefits from a proper exercise prescription.

INTRODUCTION

As mentioned in the last chapter, exercise may be one of the key health behaviors to a total Positive Health Life-style. But what kind of exercise, and how much? We will try to provide you with some answers to these general questions later, but first let us look at the relationships among several terms, such as physical fitness, health-related fitness, physical activity, and exercise, that we will use in this chapter

Fitness, Physical Activity, and Exercise

In a general sense, **physical fitness** is defined as a set of abilities individuals possess in order to perform specific types of physical activity. In the past, most tests of physical fitness stressed motor skills important in sports, such as power and speed, and were not overly concerned with the measurement of the health-related aspects of fitness. In recent years, the overall concept and definition of physical fitness has been undergoing some important changes, and there now appears to be some consensus on its definition, particularly as it relates to health. Some helpful guidelines are provided in later chapters.

The development of physical fitness is an important concern of the American Alliance for Health, Physical Education, Recreation, and Dance (AAHPERD), which has categorized fitness components into two different categories—health-related and motor skill-related. Motor skill-related physical fitness, although important for participation in athletics, does not appear to emphasize health-related benefits. On the other hand, **health-related fitness** components appear to be related to the development of cardiovascular-respiratory health, maintenance of an optimal body weight, and the development of adequate flexibility and muscular strength and endurance important for various strenuous daily activities and the prevention of low back injury and pain (fig. 2.1). Thus, physical fitness needs to be defined in relationship to its components. For the purpose of this textbook, the definition of physical fitness refers to physical fitness as it is related to functional health, not motor-skill ability. The exercise programs recommended in this textbook are, in general, designed to contribute to the development of health-related physical fitness. Table 2.1 presents the components of both health-related and motor skill-related physical fitness.

In general, **physical activity** involves any bodily movement caused by muscular contraction that results in the expenditure of energy. For purposes of studying its effects on health, epidemiologists have classified physical activity as either unstructured or structured.

Unstructured physical activity includes many of the usual activities of daily life, such as walking, climbing stairs, cycling, dancing, gardening and yard work, various domestic and occupational activities, and games and other childhood pursuits. Although unstructured physical activity, which generally is of low intensity but for a longer duration than planned exercise, may not improve physical fitness, it may provide some protection against the development of certain chronic diseases. Both the American College of Sports Medicine (ACSM) and the American Heart Association (AHA) have recognized the value of unstructured physical activity in their recent reports supporting the role of exercise as a health-promotion behavior. The Public Health Service (PHS), in *Healthy People 2000*, has established several objectives for unstructured physical activity in the section entitled "Physical Activity and Fitness":

Increase to at least 30 percent the proportion of people aged six and older who engage regularly, preferably daily, in light to moderate physical activity for at least 30 minutes per day.

Reduce to no more than 15 percent the proportion of people aged six and older who engage in no leisure-time physical activity

At certain points in this book we shall discuss how to incorporate more unstructured physical activity into your daily life, particularly in chapter 7, which deals with body weight control. In such cases, you may actually be making an unstructured physical activity a structured one.

Structured physical activity, as the name implies, is a planned program of physical activities usually designed to improve physical fitness. For the purpose of this book, we shall refer to structured physical activity as **exercise,** particularly some form of vigorous exercise. The major focus of both the AHA and the ACSM reports, in concert with a statement by the Federation Internationale de Sports Medicine (FISM), stresses the importance of exercise as a means to health-related fitness. Additionally, the PHS has also established several related objectives under "Physical Activity and Fitness":

Increase to at least 20 percent the proportion of people aged eighteen and older and to at least 75 percent the proportion of children and adolescents aged six through seventeen who engage in vigorous physical activity that promotes the development and maintenance of cardiorespiratory fitness three or more days per week for 20 or more minutes per occasion

Increase to at least 40 percent the proportion of people aged six and older who regularly perform physical activities that enhance and maintain muscular strength, muscular endurance, and flexibility

Increase to at least 50 percent the proportion of overweight people aged twelve and over who have adopted sound dietary practices combined with regular physical activity to attain an appropriate body weight

Appropriate exercise programs relative to these health objectives are detailed in later chapters—cardiorespiratory fitness (chapter 3), muscular strength and muscular endurance (chapter 4), flexibility (chapter 5), and weight control (chapter 7).

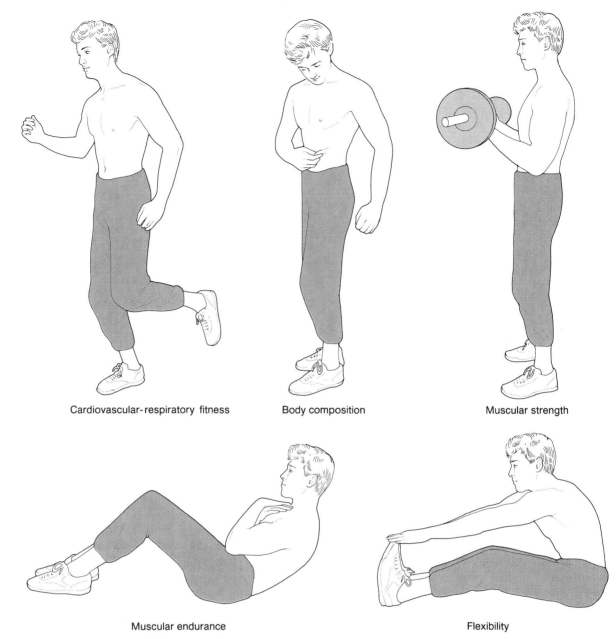

Cardiovascular-respiratory fitness

Body composition

Muscular strength

Muscular endurance

Flexibility

Figure 2.1 *Health-related fitness components. The most important physical-fitness components related to personal health include cardiovascular-respiratory fitness, body composition, muscular strength, muscular endurance, and flexibility.*

Table 2.1 Physical Fitness Categories and Components

Health-Related Fitness Components	Motor Skill-Related Fitness Components
1. Cardiovascular-respiratory function	1. Power
2. Body composition	2. Speed
3. Flexibility	3. Agility
4. Muscular strength	4. Balance
5. Muscular endurance	5. Coordination

Importance of Exercise in Health Promotion

Why is exercise so important to health? The PHS notes that physical inactivity, or lack of exercise, is thought to contribute to a number of health problems, including high blood pressure, chronic fatigue and resulting physical inefficiency, premature aging, poor musculature, and lack of flexibility. Such factors are the major causes of low back pain and injury, mental tension, obesity, and coronary heart disease. Relative to the latter health problem, a recent review of relevant research by the Centers for Disease Control in Atlanta concluded that a causal relationship existed between physical inactivity and coronary heart disease, and that this relationship was similar to that found for other major risk factors for coronary heart disease, such as high serum cholesterol and cigarette smoking. In the *Journal of the American Medical Association,* Lundberg noted that because of the multiple health benefits that can be derived from exercise, the promotion of prudent physical activity should become a national priority for the PHS.

Other medical groups have supported the value of exercise as well. In its *Special Report: Exercise Standards,* the AHA made a number of key points, including the statement that a sedentary life-style is a key independent risk factor for developing cardiovascular disease. Additionally, in the *Statement on Exercise,* the AHA reports that regular exercise can play a role in both primary and secondary prevention of cardiovascular disease. In primary prevention, regular exercise directly improves the physiological function of the heart, while in secondary prevention, exercise reduces other risk factors associated with heart disease, such as unfavorable serum lipid levels, high blood pressure, obesity, and diabetes. The ACSM supports these viewpoints, and also indicates that exercise may protect against other diseases, such as osteoporosis. Other epidemiological research suggests exercise may help prevent certain forms of cancer.

Exercise may not only help in the prevention of various chronic diseases, but it may also be useful in the treatment of patients with cardiovascular disease, high blood pressure, diabetes, asthma, and other health problems. Physicians may prescribe individualized exercise programs that may help patients achieve optimal physical and emotional health.

Relative to mental health and emotional fitness, William P. Morgan summarized the consensus statements generated at a conference conducted by the National Institute of Mental Health. In brief, Morgan noted that exercise and physical fitness are associated positively with mental health and well-being, reduction of stress emotions, and decreased levels of mild to moderate depression and anxiety.

Several reviews indicate that physicians have begun to recognize the beneficial efforts of exercise in a wide variety of disease states. They believe that exercise is a neglected medicine. Bortz even states that there is no product in the *Physician's Desk Reference* that offers such an array of benefits in such a diverse set of pathological conditions as does exercise. Leach notes that physicians should write exercise prescriptions and attempt to persuade their patients to view them in the same light as a drug prescription. The viewpoint is also advanced that an active exercise program may help to retard many of the adverse effects commonly attributed to aging and, thus, that such a program should be a part of daily living patterns at all age levels. For a detailed review of how physical activity can have an impact upon health, the interested reader should refer to the magnificent tome *Physical Activity, Fitness, and Health,* edited by Claude Bouchard and his associates.

The roles that exercise may play in the prevention of some chronic diseases and other risk factors associated with the aging process are discussed throughout this book, particularly in chapter 11. As you shall see, a well-designed exercise program appears to be a key factor in diminishing some of the adverse processes of aging. Some epidemiological evidence, notably the extensive research conducted by esteemed epidemiologist Ralph Paffenbarger, suggests that exercise may also increase your longevity.

You should realize that both moderate unstructured physical activity and moderate structured physical activity as exercise independently convey health benefits. Exercise need not be strenuous to improve health. A joint report by the U.S. Centers for Disease Control and Prevention and the ACSM chaired by Russell Pate, notes that most Americans perceive that they must engage in high-intensity, continuous exercise to reap health benefits, but this report reveals that the available scientific evidence clearly demonstrates that regular, moderate physical activity, a total of about 30 minutes or more on most, preferably all, days of the week, may provide some substantial health rewards. In this regard, William Haskell, a distinguished scientist from the Stanford Center for Research in Disease Prevention, has noted that there currently is a shift from an emphasis on intense exercise training to promote physical fitness to an emphasis on physical activity to promote health. The reason for this shift is that so many Americans are at risk because they are completely sedentary. These totally unfit individuals, as noted above, may benefit healthwise if they become moderately fit by doing as little as 30 minutes of daily moderate physical activity, such as walking part or all of the way to work instead of driving, climbing stairs instead of using the escalator, using a push mower to mow the lawn instead of a power model, and other comparable forms of unstructured activity. Steven Blair, an esteemed epidemiologist at the Cooper Institute for Aerobics Research, has indicated that such a change in daily exercise behavior would reduce health risks comparable to cessation of cigarette smoking. Blair also notes that the activity does not have to be continuous, so that three 10-minute walks during the day may produce health benefits comparable to one 30-minute walk. To promote the concept of moderate physical activity to help get Americans moving, the ACSM has launched a program entitled *Exercise Lite.* You may receive information on this program and the ACSM Fit Society by contacting the ACSM at P.O. Box 1440, Indianapolis, IN 46206–1440.

As noted above, both unstructured physical activity and exercise may independently convey health benefits. Thus, although sedentary individuals may realize some significant health benefits by incorporating daily moderate physical activities into their lives, a structured exercise program may complement these daily activities and provide optimal health benefits. Although many of the authors in *Physical Activity, Fitness, and Health* indicate that additional well-controlled research is necessary to further substantiate some of the health benefits associated with exercise, perusal of this authoritative text reveals that engaging in appropriate levels of physical activity and exercise to enhance physical fitness is a prudent health behavior.

Nevertheless, although a regular exercise program may be a valuable health adjunct, it is not a panacea. Although unusual, it is possible for you to be fit, but not healthy. Thus, exercise should be considered to be only a part of a total Positive Health Life-style, but a very important part, and may be a key to other health behavior changes as well.

Personal Physical Fitness Programs

The design of any physical fitness program is based upon the ultimate purposes or goals that have been established by or for any given individual. In some cases, goals are established for individuals. A physician may design an exercise program for a postcardiac patient entering a rehabilitation program, with the ultimate goal of regaining normal cardiovascular efficiency. Similarly, a coach may design a strenuous training program for a high school athlete with the potential to run a 4-minute mile. Although we may recognize the differences in the health status of the individuals in these two cases, similar principles are used in the design of the two vastly different training programs. Our primary concern in this book is not with rehabilitative exercise for patients or with training of athletes for high levels of competition, but with exercise programs that would improve a normal, healthy individual's physical fitness level. Four components are involved in the design of a personalized physical fitness program: assessment, planning, implementation, and evaluation.

Your Personal Fitness Needs—Assessment

Before you are able to design a comprehensive personal physical fitness program for yourself, you should know your current physical fitness status. In other words, in what kind of shape are you? As mentioned above, physical fitness represents a complex assortment of components that may be grouped as either motor skill-related or health-related. Motor skill-related components include such factors as strength, power, speed, agility, reaction time, and balance. Although important to physical performance, they are more related to athletics than they are to the health of the average individual. On the other hand, cardiovascular-respiratory function, muscular strength and endurance, flexibility, and body composition are important health-related fitness components. Since the thrust of this book is toward health-related physical fitness, personal fitness needs will be addressed only in relation to these components. Thus, you will need to assess your current status in the following areas:

1. cardiovascular-respiratory function
2. muscular strength
3. muscular endurance
4. flexibility
5. body composition

How do you assess your current status and determine what your physical fitness needs are in each of these areas? You will be presented with some guidelines and assessment techniques in chapter 3 for cardiovascular-respiratory function,

in chapter 4 for muscular strength and endurance, in chapter 5 for flexibility, and with some body composition techniques in chapter 7.

Your Personal Fitness Goals and Objectives—The Basis of Planning

The basic short-term goal of the Positive Health Life-style is to become as healthy, both physically and mentally, as you possibly can. The long-term goal is to remain in optimal health by preventing the development of chronic diseases and by improving your longevity. A properly designed exercise program can help you reach these goals, but these goals are somewhat difficult to measure. You need to establish specific, measurable objectives that you can attain in the pursuit of these goals. Once you have assessed your current fitness status relative to each of the five health-related fitness categories, you will be in a better position to establish reasonable objectives for yourself. Overall, these personalized objectives will serve as the basis for planning your fitness program.

When planning your fitness program, ask yourself a series of questions. Some of these questions are addressed briefly at this point, but more specific information will be provided in the succeeding chapters.

What type of exercise should I do? The answer to this question depends primarily upon which fitness objective you have in mind. For example, for strength development you may choose resistance training, but for cardiovascular-respiratory fitness improvement you would choose one of a variety of aerobic exercises. We refer to this as the **exercise mode.** Try to select an exercise mode that you enjoy, but recognize the fact that exercise is not fun all the time. Also, vary your mode of exercise.

How hard should I exercise? This question refers to **exercise intensity,** which may be measured in a variety of ways. For example, in the next chapter you will learn to use your heart rate to measure exercise intensity during aerobic exercises. In general, learn to go slow at first.

How long should I exercise? **Exercise duration,** the amount of time you need to exercise to reap benefits, is another important concept of training; it interacts with exercise intensity. Thus, the amount of time you need to exercise daily may vary depending upon your fitness objective. For example, in weight loss programs, increased duration of exercise is important. You may increase the duration of your exercise as you become more physically fit.

How often should I exercise? This question refers to **exercise frequency,** usually interpreted as how many times you should exercise per week. Again, exercise frequency depends upon your fitness objectives and may vary from three to seven days per week.

How do I determine my health-related fitness objectives, and how long will it take me to achieve them? One of the distinguishing characteristics of the health-related physical fitness components is that they can be improved through a proper training program. Later on in this text you will perform several tests that will provide an assessment of your fitness level in each of the health-related physical fitness components. For each of these areas, you are provided with norms and/or other data to determine your current fitness status. Based upon this information, you will be able to establish specific objectives. You may establish short-term and long-term objectives, but it is important in the initial stages of a training program to establish personal fitness objectives that are attainable. For example, you may set a short-term goal to lose 5 pounds in a month or run a mile nonstop; you may set a long-term goal to lose 40 pounds or complete a 10-kilometer race. Guidelines are presented for each major health-related physical fitness component in the following chapters.

Starting and Staying with the Plan—Implementation and Adherence

How ready are you to begin an exercise program? Laboratory Inventory 2.1 is an adaptation of Project PACE (Physician-based Assessment and Counseling for Exercise) which was developed in conjunction with the Centers for Disease Control and Prevention (CDC), and completion of Part A will help you determine your current physical activity level. Please complete Part A before proceeding and note that completion of Laboratory Inventory 2.2 is recommended before you initiate an exercise program or increase your exercise intensity.

You may know some friends who are precontemplators and you might recommend to them that they complete part B of Laboratory Inventory 2.1. However, you are most likely either a contemplator or an active exercise participant because you are enrolled in this fitness or wellness class or program, or are reading this book independently with the idea of starting an exercise program. If you are a contemplator, completion of Part C of Laboratory Inventory 2.1 will help you in planning the initial stages of your exercise program and show you how to avoid some of the roadblocks. If you are currently physically active, completion of Part D may be important if you plan to expand your exercise program, such as adding a new activity. The points covered in Parts B, C and D will be discussed in more detail in other sections of this text.

You should consider a number of factors before you implement your personal fitness program. At this point, several factors involved in starting and staying with your exercise program will be briefly discussed.

Medical Clearance

Exercise is generally safe for most people, but may be a risk for individuals with predisposing health problems, especially cardiovascular disease.

Of concern is the type of medical clearance you should have before initiating an exercise program or taking an exercise test, particularly one that stresses the cardiovascular system. There appears to be some controversy over who needs to see a physician before initiating or increasing the intensity of an exercise program, particularly when the physical examination includes an exercise ECG stress test. The National Heart, Lung, and Blood Institute (NHLBI), American Heart Association (AHA), and American College of Sports Medicine (ACSM) have all developed guidelines relative to this issue; some differences do exist in their recommendations. No thorough review

of these guidelines is presented here because they are extensive and beyond the scope of this text. However, some practical suggestions that represent a synthesis of these and other viewpoints are offered.

1. If you have concern about any facet of your health, check with your physician before starting an exercise program. Complete Laboratory Inventory 2.2, Revised Physical Activity Readiness Questionnaire (rPAR-Q) prior to taking an exercise test or increasing the amount of physical activity in your life, particularly initiating an exercise program.

2. No matter what your age, if you have any of the coronary heart disease risk factors noted in table 2.2, you should have a physical examination. Additional details on risk factors are presented in chapter 11.

3. If you are young (twenties or early thirties), healthy, and have no risk factors, it is probably safe to initiate an exercise program. As a matter of fact, it is probably more dangerous to your health in the long run not to exercise than it is to remain inactive simply because you have not had a physician's examination.

4. Controversy begins after you reach age thirty-five. If you are physically active and have no risk factors, you may continue with your customary program and even progressively increase the intensity on a gradual basis. If you possess any risk factors, see your physician. If you are sedentary without any risk factors, it would be a good idea to check with your physician, although you may be able to initiate a gradual, sensible exercise program, such as walking, with minimal risk. The older you are, the better the idea to get a medical examination. In fact, it is prudent for men over age forty and women over age fifty to have an examination.

For individuals who do have a physical examination, the physician may recommend an exercise ECG stress test. Although not foolproof in detecting heart disease, an exercise ECG stress test is usually prescribed in suspected cases of coronary heart disease and may serve several useful purposes. It can be used to diagnose the presence of coronary heart disease in most individuals, to prescribe a safe exercise program, and to evaluate the rehabilitative effects of such a program. In essence, the patient exercises on a treadmill under the supervision of trained medical personnel. The ECG is monitored continuously, and the individual exercises to the point of exhaustion or to some other predetermined termination point. You should take an ECG stress test only if it is prescribed by a physician and conducted under proper medical supervision. Some fitness organizations advertise a heart-rate stress test without medical control for a lesser cost, but such tests should not be regarded as a substitute for the ECG test.

Benefit/Risk Ratio

Although exercise training may confer some health benefits, exercise is not without risk. The **benefit/risk ratio** refers to the relationship between the potential benefits you expect to get from your exercise program and the potential risks you

Table 2.2 Major and Predisposing Risk Factors Associated with Coronary Heart Disease

1. High blood pressure
2. Cigarette smoking
3. High blood lipid levels: cholesterol and triglycerides
4. Diabetes
5. Obesity
6. Abnormal resting electrocardiogram (ECG)
7. Family history of coronary heart disease before age fifty

Source: Data from *American College of Sports Medicine.* ACSM's Guidelines for Exercise Testing and Prescription, *5th ed., 1995; and from American Heart Association,* Coronary Risk Factor Statement for the American Public, *1986.*

may encounter in the program. The potential benefits, discussed previously, include less body fat, improved cardiovascular functioning, more strength and, in general, enhanced physical and mental health. Although some forms of exercise may aggravate existing health problems, such as heavy weight lifting with a hernia, most of the potential risks focus upon injuries. The type of injury you may incur is usually specific to the exercise mode you choose. Some sports pose a risk for accidental injury, such as falls in outdoor bicycling. Others pose a problem with overuse injuries, such as sore muscles in the calves of runners or the shoulders of swimmers from exercising too much or too strenuously when not prepared. Although the scope of this book does not allow for a detailed coverage of injury prevention and treatment, some key points will be provided where appropriate. While very rare, the most extreme risk associated with exercise is sudden death, usually by heart attack in those with cardiac abnormalities or those predisposed to cardiovascular disease. This topic will be discussed in chapter 3, but in a recent editorial in the *New England Journal of Medicine,* Curfman noted that although there are risks of heart attack in acute bouts of exercise, these risks are probably overshadowed by the long-term benefits of habitual exercise. There are other risks associated with exercise, including doing too much exercise, and these risks will also be addressed where appropriate.

Skills and Equipment

A high degree of skill is not necessary to reap fitness benefits through exercise. Although elite swimmers and bicyclists have developed highly technical skills in order to succeed in competition, most of us can learn the rudiments of swimming and bicycling that are essential for fitness. Moreover, some of the most effective exercises, such as walking, jogging, and running, are so natural that they require little or no skill training. Because of this and other factors important to the development of a fitness program, these latter types of exercise will be stressed in relation to aerobic fitness.

Although you do not need any special equipment or facilities at all for some types of exercise programs, proper equipment may help to make some activities more enjoyable and may also be important to help minimize the risk of injury. For example, special clothing may help keep you warm while bicycling in cold weather, while an approved helmet will protect your head in case of a fall. In activities such as jogging and running, your major investment will be in a good pair of shoes, but proper clothing may be an important consideration under certain environmental conditions. Depending upon the nature of the exercise activity that you choose and the size of your wallet or purse, you will find a variety of equipment available to help make exercise more enjoyable and safe.

Adherence

Starting an exercise program is the easy part. For many people, staying with it, or adherence, is the hard part. Research has shown that many individuals will stay with an exercise program for approximately six months and then drop out for one reason or another. If you are initiating an exercise program in conjunction with a health-related fitness or wellness course, you most likely will stay with the program at least through the end of the semester, at least if you want a good grade in the course. Whether you continue beyond that time will depend on the personal health ethic you develop toward exercise, as discussed in chapter 1. Since principles of adherence relate to other health behaviors besides exercise, we shall discuss these principles in the last chapter, "Staying with the Positive Health Life-style," after you have been exposed to other health-related behaviors such as healthful nutrition, management of stress, and avoidance of substance abuse.

However, because exercise is such an important component of a total wellness program, a few important points relative to exercise adherence are introduced at this point. Many of these points are discussed in detail at various points throughout this book.

1. You are the key to maintaining your program of exercise. You need to cultivate an attitude that exercise is a significant part of your life-style, akin to brushing your teeth. You need to develop a sense of self-efficacy, that you possess the knowledge, skills, and personal resources to sustain your exercise habit. You need to develop an intrinsic self-motivation that helps you overcome barriers to exercising. Review Laboratory Inventory 1.2 and evaluate your Self-Efficacy Potential for Change score for exercise. Can you improve this score by modifying factors in the scale which affect it favorably—such as planning the time to exercise or associating with individuals who exercise?

2. You need to establish specific objectives and goals. You may establish long-range goals, but you need to establish short-range, achievable objectives in pursuit of these goals.

3. You need to plan an individualized exercise program. Planning involves a number of variables, but the following points are crucial.

   a. Find time in your daily schedule. Practice time management by planning your daily schedule to incorporate exercise, be it early in the morning, at lunch, or sometime after work. Plan three 10-minute brisk walk breaks during the day if your schedule is full.

b. Do exercises that are enjoyable for you. Jogging and running are excellent, practical activities, but not everyone enjoys them. Aerobic dance, among a host of other activities, may be an excellent alternative. Riding a stationary bicycle and watching television may help you combine two activities into one. Associate with other individuals who enjoy your form of exercise. Join a local bicycling, walking, hiking, or running club. Exercising with others with similar exercise interests adds enjoyment to exercise. If you desire to join a commercial fitness club, some guidelines for selecting one are presented in chapter 12.

c. Learn a variety of physical activities. Walking, jogging, aerobic dancing, bicycling, and the use of various exercise machines, such as stationary bicycles, are only a few of the activities that will provide health benefits. Using a variety of these and other activities adds spice to your exercise program. Additionally, if you become injured and cannot perform one type of activity for a while, such as jogging, you may substitute another activity, such as bicycling, and continue to exercise while your injury heals.

d. Go slow at first. You do not need to exercise intensely to benefit from exercise. Exercise at a mild intensity at first as you become accustomed to exercise, and gradually increase your intensity to the moderate level.

e. Keep a record of your progress toward your short-term objectives and your long-range goal. Reestablish new objectives and goals as you achieve them.

f. Reward yourself as you achieve your objectives or goal. Buy yourself some new equipment.

g. Recognize that your regular exercise program may be disrupted by other responsibilities, such as final examinations week, business travel, vacations, or injury. Proper planning may help you to still schedule a daily exercise session during changes in your daily routine, and learning a variety of exercise modes may help you exercise during an injury. However, most individuals do eventually experience interruptions in their regular exercise routine and some guidelines for preventing this occurrence or resuming an exercise program are presented in chapter 12.

Meeting Your Objectives—Evaluation

After you have assessed your needs, set your objectives, planned your program, and implemented it for a period of time, you need to evaluate your progress toward your established objectives. Often, simply doing your daily exercise program serves as an evaluation; for example, one of your short-term objectives may be to run one mile nonstop, which may actually be achieved in one of your daily workouts. Other objectives, such as to lose 10 pounds or to reduce your body fat by 3 percent, may be evaluated by the use of weight scales or appropriate body composition techniques.

In some cases you may not have met your specific fitness objectives, so you will need to give yourself more time. In others, you may have met or exceeded your objectives, and at this point you can either plan to maintain yourself at the attained level or to set your sights a little higher. Evaluation on a periodic basis is important, for it provides information relative to your progress toward or maintenance of a health-related fitness objective or goal.

General Principles of Training

Individuals engage in physical fitness programs for a variety of reasons. Some want to increase strength, power, or speed; others are interested in losing excess body weight and improving appearance; others may want to improve cardiovascular endurance capacity. The major principles underlying the development of any physical training program are the principles of use and disuse. In essence, the **principle of use** indicates that you need to do a specific fitness component to improve it. Unlike machines, which tend to deteriorate with use, the human body possesses the ability to adapt to use and to increase the capacity and efficiency of the body systems being utilized. Conversely, the **principle of disuse** dictates that if you are fit but stop training, your level of fitness will decline. In other words, use it or lose it. Several other principles elaborate on the concepts of the use-disuse principles.

The Overload Principle

The **overload principle** is the most important principle for all conditioning programs. It relates to the principle of use in that your body systems must be stressed beyond their normal levels of activity if they are to improve. The three major components of the overload principle are intensity, duration, and frequency of exercise. All three may be adjusted in order to impose an overload.

The intensity of the exercise is a very important component of the overload principle. Intensity is synonymous with rate of exercise, or tempo, in such activities as running and swimming. In weight lifting, intensity is related to the amount of resistance offered (fig. 2.2). There are a number of ways to express the intensity of an exercise task, such as amount of weight lifted, speed, and heart rate. Heart rate is a commonly used method in many general conditioning programs for cardiovascular fitness. Other methods for determining proper intensity levels for specific exercise programs, including a technique involving psychological perception of exercise intensity (rating of perceived exertion), are also presented in the next chapters.

A second component of the overload principle is duration. An overload may be imposed by simply increasing the length of the exercise period. The intensity of the exercise is generally inversely related to the duration—as intensity increases, duration decreases and vice versa. If duration of exercise is an important concern, the intensity level must be decreased correspondingly.

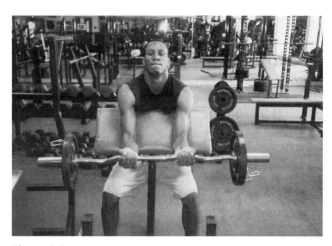

Figure 2.2 *The overload principle in action with resistance training. In order to continue to improve strength, weights must be increased.*

The frequency of training refers to the number of days per week that an individual exercises. For the average individual, three to four days per week are sufficient to elicit a training effect (improvement in physiological functions), but increased frequency may be necessary for weight loss programs or for athletes training for competition.

The Principle of Progression

Associated with the overload principle as applied to a physical conditioning program is the **principle of progression,** often referred to as progressive overload or progressive resistance. In resistance training, this principle is often known as **progressive resistance exercise (PRE).**

All too often individuals will initiate exercise programs with great enthusiasm but with little planning, such as a New Year's resolution. Unfortunately, for one reason or another, these programs usually result in a high rate of dropouts after a relatively short period of time. One reason may be the lack of a plan for progression. For example, an individual may recall that three years ago she was able to run two miles nonstop, so she tries this on her first couple of exercise sessions, develops severe muscle soreness, and terminates the program.

Thus, progression of overload is an important planning concept. The initial stages of the training program, especially for the habitually sedentary individual, should be mild to moderate. As the body begins to adapt to the exercise routine, the intensity, duration, and/or frequency may be increased. However, it is important to progress slowly, as too rapid a progression may contribute to the development of overuse injuries.

The Principle of Specificity

In the next chapter, we will discuss the three human energy systems in the muscles. One of the most important of these for health-related fitness is the oxygen system. The **principle of specificity** indicates that you must train a specific energy system and specific muscle groups in order for them to improve.

Training a specific energy system is often known as **metabolic specificity,** while training a specific muscle group is known as **neuromuscular specificity.**

In relation to the three energy systems, metabolic specificity is critical; a specific energy system must be overloaded if it is to improve. If you want to develop the oxygen system, you must design a training program that primarily utilizes that particular energy system. Physical activities that involve large muscle groups over sustained periods of time depend on the oxygen system and will eventually increase its efficiency and capacity.

Neuromuscular specificity is important in relation to the mode of exercise that you use to develop the oxygen system. Three common exercise modes for conditioning the oxygen system are running, swimming, and cycling. Appropriate conditioning programs in each activity increase the capacity of the oxygen system in general, but the improvement in performance level is greatest for that activity in which the individual trains. One person training via a running program and another via a swimming program may make equal gains in utilization of oxygen. However, the swimmer will perform better in a swimming test, while the runner will do better in a running test. This indicates that specific neuromuscular involvement is extremely important if one is training for increased performance in a given activity. The particular muscles, including the neuromuscular pattern, involved in any given activity in which improvement is desired should be included in the conditioning program.

The Warm-Up Principle

A properly designed exercise session will include three components—a warm-up, a stimulus period, and a warm-down. The stimulus period, the heart of your exercise program, applies the overload principle to improve your fitness. **Warm-up** is a term used to describe activities used to prepare your body for the more strenuous exercise in the stimulus period. Although there are a variety of ways to do a warm-up, the usual technique involves the use of less intense levels of the actual exercise you will do during the stimulus period, followed by some gentle stretching exercises. The **warm-down,** often called active cool-down, is done immediately after the conclusion of the stimulus period. Like the warm-up, it involves milder exercises than those used during the stimulus period. Stretching is very important during the warm-down. At this time your muscles are warm from the body heat produced during the exercise bout, and they are more flexible and less likely to be overstretched or torn.

Both the warm-up and warm-down may be important in the prevention of several problems associated with more strenuous exercise, such as muscle soreness and injury. They may also help in the prevention of excessive strain on the heart. Research has shown that engaging in sudden strenuous exercise may lead to an abnormal heart rhythm that could be dangerous to someone with hidden heart problems. A warm-up will gradually increase the circulation and will help to eliminate this effect. Furthermore, if you suddenly stop exercising (for instance, if you abruptly stop running), there is a tendency for the blood to pool in the legs; this decreases the blood's return to the heart. This may also stress the heart and lead to abnormal rhythms in some individuals. A warm-down, a gradual tapering of your exercise, such as walking or jogging easily at the completion of more strenuous running, will help to maintain blood flow to your heart and will help prevent this potential problem. An adequate warm-down is probably more important than the warm-up.

The Principle of Recuperation

As noted above, exercise places a stress on the body during active exercise and for a short time afterwards. During your recovery period over the following day or so, your body systems will adapt to this stress and become stronger and more efficient. Thus, a period of rest or recuperation is essential if you wish to benefit from your exercise program. In most individuals, a day or two is adequate. Inadequate recuperation time may lead to injuries associated with excessive exercise, often known as overuse injuries. On the other hand, extended periods of rest may lead to deterioration in fitness.

The Principle of Reversibility

The **principle of reversibility** is another way of stating the principle of disuse. If one of your energy systems is not utilized, it deteriorates to a level congruent with your level of activity. For example, research has shown that bedridden individuals experience tremendous decreases in the oxygen energy system in relatively short periods of time, as do highly conditioned endurance athletes who go through a period of detraining. Thus, in order to maintain a desired level of fitness, you need to continue to provide an exercise overload. Unfortunately, we cannot "bank" fitness.

Exercise As a Prescription

Your personal fitness goals and specific fitness objectives to meet these goals are the major determinants of your exercise prescription. Exercise may be used to improve your performance in all five health-related fitness components—cardiovascular endurance, muscular strength, muscular endurance, flexibility, and body composition.

As related to a Positive Health Life-style, exercise may also be effective in the prevention or treatment of a variety of health disorders, including coronary heart disease, high blood pressure, diabetes, obesity, and low back problems. Some epidemiological evidence even indicates that exercise, particularly early in life, may help in the prevention of cancer. In this sense, exercise may be thought of as medication; it can exert its effect upon the body in a number of ways. Exercise can increase the efficiency of the cardiovascular system, oxidize body fats, expend energy, strengthen muscle tissues, and increase flexibility, to name but a few of its implications for health. However, just as a physician must prescribe an appropriate dose of a specific medication for a given disease, so too must a specific type of exercise and appropriate dosage be

prescribed for different fitness goals. The principle of specificity deals with the type of exercise to be prescribed; the overload principle relates to the dosage.

When we have a serious medical problem we need to consult a physician, who will diagnose our condition and prescribe some form of treatment, which in many cases may involve prescription drugs. However, for minor ailments such as colds and headaches, we may do our own diagnosis and prescribe our own over-the-counter medication, such as taking several aspirin. Although some individuals, particularly those at high risk for cardiovascular disease, may need an exercise prescription from a physician, most of us may be able to prescribe our own exercise regimen if we have adequate information.

In the succeeding chapters, you will learn the details for prescribing your own exercise program. In chapter 3 you will learn the specific types of exercises that may be used to train the cardiovascular system and the appropriate guidelines for the dosage of intensity, duration, and frequency. Chapter 4 will focus upon exercise programs designed to improve muscular strength and endurance. Chapter 5 will help you improve flexibility. Chapter 7 explains the role of exercise, combined with dieting, as a means to increase muscle mass or lose excess body fat. Finally, chapter 8 indicates how exercise may be used to help reduce stress.

Some therapies are effective in a single dose; a shot of penicillin may help cure an infection somewhere in the body. Other drugs need to be taken repeatedly for only a certain period of time; aspirin may be used for several weeks to help treat a persistent inflammation in a muscle tendon. Still others must be taken for a lifetime; insulin must be administered daily in some diabetic patients. As an analogy to medication, exercise falls into this last category. A single dose elicits some physiological effects in the body, but does not produce any long-lasting changes in body structure or function. On the other hand, the body adapts to repeated doses of exercise, and, if the exercise is appropriate, many of these adaptations have beneficial health effects. However, these beneficial bodily adaptations revert to normal if exercise is discontinued. For example, a study on blood pressure presented at an American Heart Association meeting revealed that moderate exercise three days a week helped to reduce blood pressure and reverse heart damage, but that beneficial effects disappeared if the exercise was not continued. In general, exercise must be done on a regular basis or some key health benefits may be lost. The beneficial effects of an acute exercise bout on certain blood lipids and blood pressure may begin to dissipate after 24–48 hours; this research finding is sometimes referred to as the last-bout effect, indicating some health gains from exercise are fairly transient. Other health gains from exercise may last somewhat longer, but will eventually deteriorate with complete cessation of exercise.

Thus, for a Positive Health Life-style, exercise is a lifelong prescription. Combined with proper nutrition and relaxation techniques, you will maximize your opportunity to feel and be healthy, both physically and mentally.

References

Books

American Alliance for Health, Physical Education, Recreation, and Dance. 1980. *Lifetime health-related physical fitness.* Reston, Va: AAHPERD.

Blair, S. 1991. *Living with exercise.* Dallas: American Health Publishing Company.

Bouchard, C., et al., eds. 1994. *Physical activity, fitness, and health.* Champaign, Ill: Human Kinetics.

Heyward, V. 1991. *Advanced fitness assessment and exercise prescription.* Champaign, Ill: Human Kinetics.

McArdle, W., F. Katch, and V. Katch. 1991. *Exercise physiology.* Philadelphia: Lea and Febiger.

Stamford, B., and P. Shimer. 1990. *Fitness without exercise.* New York: Warner Books.

United States Department of Health and Human Services. Public Health Service. 1991. *Healthy people 2000: National health promotion and disease prevention objectives.* Washington, D.C.: U.S. Government Printing Office.

Williams, M. 1995. *Nutrition for fitness and sport.* Dubuque: Brown & Benchmark Publishers.

Reviews

American College of Sports Medicine. 1990. ACSM position stand: The recommended quantity and quality of exercise for developing and maintaining cardiorespiratory and muscular fitness in healthy adults. *Medicine and Science in Sports and Exercise* 22:265–74.

American College of Sports Medicine. 1994. ACSM position stand: Exercise for patients with coronary artery disease. *Medicine and Science in Sports and Exercise* 26 (3): i–v.

American Heart Association. 1990. AHA medical/scientific statement. Special report: Exercise standards. *Circulation* 82:2286–2322.

American Heart Association. 1992. Statement on exercise: Benefits and recommendations for physical activity programs for all Americans. *Circulation* 86:340–44.

Armstrong, L., et al. 1993. Symptomatic hyponatremia during prolonged exercise in heat. *Medicine and Science in Sports and Exercise* 25:543–49.

Blair, S. 1991. Rigidity or adaptability in exercise science and clinical practice. *Sports Medicine Bulletin* 26:5.

Blair, S. 1993. 1993 C. H. McCloy research lecture: Physical activity, physical fitness, and health. *Research Quarterly for Exercise and Sport* 64:365–76.

Bortz, W. 1980. Effect of exercise on aging—Effect of aging on exercise. *Journal of the American Geriatric Society* 28:49–51.

Casaburi, R. 1992. Principles of exercise training. *Chest* 101 (5 Suppl): 263S–267S.

Centers for Disease Control. 1987. Protective effect of exercise on coronary heart disease. *Morbidity and Mortality Weekly Report* 36:426–30.

Corbin, C., and B. Pangrazi. 1993. The health benefits of physical activity. *Physical Activity and Fitness Research Digest* 1 (1): 1–6.

Curfman, G. 1993. Health benefits of exercise. *New England Journal of Medicine* 328:574–76.

DeBenedette, V. 1990. Are your patients exercising too much? *Physician and Sportsmedicine* 18 (August): 119–22.

Dyment, P. 1993. Frustrated by chronic fatigue? *Physician and Sportsmedicine* 21 (November): 47–54.

Eichner, R. 1987. Exercise, lymphokines, calories, and cancer. *Physician and Sportsmedicine* 15 (June): 109–18.

Franklin, B. 1994. Giving your body a 'road test'. *Physician and Sportsmedicine* 22 (March): 127–28.

Franklin, B., et al. 1994. Exercise and cardiac complications: Do the benefits outweigh the risks? *Physician and Sportsmedicine* 22 (February): 56–68.

Friedewald, V., and D. Spence. 1990. Sudden cardiac death associated with exercise: The risk-benefit issue. *American Journal of Cardiology* 66:183–88.

Gauthier, M. 1986. Can exercise reduce the risk of cancer. *Physician and Sportsmedicine* 14 (October): 171–78.

Gong, H. Jr., 1992. Breathing easy: Exercise despite asthma. *Physician and Sportsmedicine* 20 (March): 159–67.

Haskell, W. 1994. Health consequences of physical activity: Understanding and challenges regarding dose-response. *Medicine and Science in Sports and Exercise* 26:649–60.

Herbert, W., and V. Froelicher. 1991. Exercise tests for coronary and asymptomatic patients. *Physician and Sportsmedicine* 19 (March): 129–33.

International Federation of Sports Medicine. 1990. Physical exercise: An important factor for health. *Physician and Sportsmedicine* 18 (March): 155–56.

Kenney, M., and D. Seals. 1993. Postexercise hypotension. Key features, mechanisms, and clinical significance. *Hypertension* 22:653–64.

Kibler, B., et al. 1992. Musculoskeletal adaptations and injuries due to overtraining. *Exercise and Sport Sciences Reviews* 20:99–126.

Kohl, H., and K. Powell. 1994. What is exertion-related sudden cardiac death? *Sports Medicine* 17:209–12.

Lavie, C., et al. 1992. Exercise and the heart. Good, benign, or evil. *Postgraduate Medicine* 91:130–34, 143–50.

Leach, R. 1981. Rx exercise: Effects and side effects. *Hospital Practice* 16:72A–72W.

Leff, M., ed. 1994. Which exercise is best for you? *Consumer Reports on Health* 6:37–40.

Levin, S. 1993. Does exercise enhance sexuality? *Physician and Sportsmedicine* 21 (March): 199–203.

Lundberg, G., ed. 1987. Leads from the MMWR. Sex-, age-, and region-specific prevalence of sedentary lifestyle in selected states in 1985: The Behavioral Risk Factor Surveillance System. *Journal of the American Medical Association* 257:2270–72.

Morgan, W. 1984. Coping with mental stress: The potential and limits of exercise intervention. (Final report). Bethesda: National Institute of Mental Health.

Paffenbarger, R., et al. 1994. Physical activity and physical fitness as determinants of health and longevity. In *Physical activity, fitness, and health,* eds. C. Bouchard, et al. Champaign, Ill: Human Kinetics.

Pate, R., et al. 1995. Physical activity and public health. A recommendation from the Centers for Disease Control and Prevention and the American College of Sports Medicine. *Journal of the American Medical Association* 273:402–7.

Redland, A., and A. Stuifbergen. Strategies for maintenance of health-promoting behaviors. *Nursing Clinics of North America* 28:427–42.

Serfass, R. and S. Gerberich. 1987. Exercise for optimal health: Strategies and motivational considerations. *Preventive Medicine* 13:79–99.

Sharp, N., and Y. Koutedakis. 1992. Sport and the overtraining syndrome: Immunological aspects. *British Medical Bulletin* 48:518–33.

Shephard, R. 1994. Readiness for physical activity. *Physical Activity and Fitness Research Digest* 1 (February): 1–6.

Stamford, B. 1987. Warming up. *Physician and Sportsmedicine* 15 (November): 168.

U.S. Centers for Disease Control and Prevention and American College of Sports Medicine. 1993. Summary statement—Workshop on physical activity and public health. *Sports Medicine Bulletin* 28(4):7.

Vorhies, D., and B. Riley. 1993. Deconditioning. *Clinics in Geriatric Medicine* 9:745–63.

Wichmann, S., and D. Martin. 1992. Exercise excess: Treating patients addicted to fitness. *Physician and Sportsmedicine* 20 (May): 193–200.

Specific Studies

Blair, S., et al. 1989. Physical fitness and all-cause mortality. A prospective study of healthy men and women. *Journal of the American Medical Association* 262:2395–2401.

Bouchard, C., et al. 1980. Training of submaximal working capacity: Frequency, intensity, duration, and their interactions. *Journal of Sports Medicine and Physical Fitness* 20:29–40.

Browne, R., and C. Gillespie. 1993. Sickle cell trait. A risk factor for life-threatening rhabdomyolysis? *Physician and Sportsmedicine* 21 (June): 80–88.

DeBusk, R., et al. 1990. Training effects of long versus short bouts of exercise in healthy subjects. *American Journal of Cardiology* 65:1010–13.

Ekelund, L., et al. 1988. Physical fitness as a predictor of cardiovascular mortality in asymptomatic North American men: The Lipid Research Clinics mortality follow-up study. *The New England Journal of Medicine* 319:1379–84.

Morris, J., et al. 1990. Exercise in leisure time: Coronary attack and death rates. *British Heart Journal* 63:325–34.

Schwartz, R. 1987. The independent effects of dietary weight loss and aerobic training on high density lipoproteins and apolipoprotein A-1 concentrations in obese men. *Metabolism.* 36:165–71.

Tucker, L. 1990. Television viewing and physical fitness in adults. *Research Quarterly for Exercise and Sport* 61:315–20.

Young, D., and M. Steinhardt. 1993. The importance of physical fitness versus physical activity for coronary artery disease risk factors: A cross-sectional analysis. *Research Quarterly for Exercise and Sport* 64:377–84.

3

AEROBIC EXERCISE

Key Terms

aerobic dancing
aerobic fitness
aerobic walking
anaerobic threshold
ATP
ATP-PC system
Calorie
circuit aerobics

cross-training
energy
fatigue
interval training
lactic acid system
maximal heart rate reserve
   (HR_{MAX} reserve)

maximal oxygen
   consumption ($\dot{V}O_{2MAX}$)
megajoule (MJ)
MET
oxygen debt
oxygen system
rating of perceived exertion
   (RPE)

steady-state threshold
stimulus period
target heart rate range
   (target HR)
threshold stimulus

Key Concepts

■ The human body has three basic systems to produce energy for exercise: the ATP-PC system, the lactic acid system, and the oxygen system.

■ Two common methods used to express energy expenditure are measuring Calories and measuring oxygen consumption; other methods include the MET and the megajoule (MJ).

■ Aerobic fitness (cardiovascular-respiratory efficiency) is the single most important health component of physical fitness.

■ Aerobic fitness involves the interaction of four physiological functions—respiration, central circulation, peripheral circulation, and muscle metabolism.

■ Maximal oxygen uptake ($\dot{V}O_{2MAX}$), expressed in ml O_2/kg body weight/minute, is one important measure of aerobic fitness. Another important measure is the ability to sustain exercise at a high percentage of $\dot{V}O_{2MAX}$.

■ Indirect tests such as walking, distance running, swimming, and bicycling are the most practical means available to evaluate aerobic fitness. Step tests are valuable in demonstrating the adaptation of the heart to aerobic training.

■ In general, most healthy young adults do not need an exercise stress test prior to starting an aerobic exercise program, but if you have concern about any facet of your health, check with your physician.

■ The four key components of an aerobic program are mode, intensity, duration, and frequency of exercise.

■ Exercise intensity is the most important component of an aerobic exercise prescription. Measurement of the threshold (target) heart rate is a valuable method of assessing exercise intensity, but the use of the rating of perceived exertion (RPE) is also a practical method and is increasingly popular.

■ Aerobic exercise programs must involve large muscle groups. Although a number of different modes of exercise may be used to achieve aerobic fitness, a walk-jog-run program is probably the most practical one available.

■ According to the American College of Sports Medicine (ACSM), the minimum amount of exercise for aerobic fitness is an intensity level of 50 to 85 percent of the heart rate reserve (or 60–90 percent of the maximal heart rate), for a duration of 15 to 60 minutes, at a frequency of three to five times per week.

■ It is important to take it easy when beginning an aerobic exercise program. Aerobic walking is a recommended approach, particularly for those who are habitually sedentary. The intensity of the exercise should gradually be increased over weeks to months.

■ Unstructured physical activity may provide some health benefits for completely sedentary individuals, but an optimal program involves structured aerobic exercise. An exercise equivalent of about 2,000 Calories per week appears to be a reasonable goal.

■ Although there are some risks associated with any aerobic exercise program, the benefits to your health appear to outweigh them, particularly if you are aware of potential problems and take precautions to avoid them.

■ A warm or hot environmental temperature is one serious problem that confronts the normal individual who exercises. You must be aware of means to avoid heat illnesses when exercising under hot and/or humid conditions.

INTRODUCTION

Of all of the different types of exercise programs available, those that stress aerobic exercise appear to possess the greatest potential for improving your health. As noted in chapter 2, aerobic exercise by itself is obviously not a panacea for all diseases, but available research data support its use as a treatment for various medical conditions and its value in an overall program of health promotion. In this latter regard, aerobic exercise also may serve as a catalyst to other Positive Health Life-style changes, such as nutrition, weight control, and smoking. In a sense, then, aerobic exercise is medicine. It has tremendous potential to elicit substantial benefits for physical and mental health, as documented extensively in *Physical Activity, Fitness, and Health,* the proceedings of an international consensus conference edited by Claude Bouchard and his associates.

But how much aerobic exercise do you need to reap health benefits? Although there is no simple answer to this question for each individual, research has provided us with some very reasonable guidelines. Literally thousands of epidemiological and experimental studies have been conducted over the past decade to explore the medical aspects of physical activity and exercise, and many of these studies have looked at the intensity, duration, frequency, and mode of aerobic exercise and how these variables affect risk factors associated with certain diseases.

The effectiveness of any given medicine may be related to its dosage. In order to achieve some benefit, a minimum dose must be given, and increasing benefits may accrue to some maximum dose. However, an overdose may actually be harmful, not helpful. The amount of exercise you need may be compared to medical dosages. For example, there is some evidence to suggest that even a minimum threshold dose of exercise, such as simply increasing your exercise energy expenditure through unstructured physical activity like walking or yard work, or participating in recreational sports such as golf and bowling in your leisure time, may confer some significant health benefits, particularly for those who have been habitually sedentary. Research also indicates a dose-response relationship, suggestive of increased health benefits with higher dosages of exercise, at least up to some maximal level. No additional benefits appear to accrue beyond this maximal level, and if exercise becomes excessive (overdosage), health risks, instead of benefits, may increase.

Based upon a synthesis of the prevailing research, the purpose of this chapter is to discuss the basic principles underlying the development and implementation of your personalized aerobic exercise program ∎

Human Energy

Before discussing the principles of exercise training, it is important to provide an overview of the human energy processes, for these processes serve as the basis for all exercise training programs. Knowledge of energy storage and production in the human body is also essential background for weight control, a topic detailed in chapter 7. Exercise demands energy. In this section, we shall cover how energy is stored in the human body and how the body uses three different energy systems to produce muscular energy at various

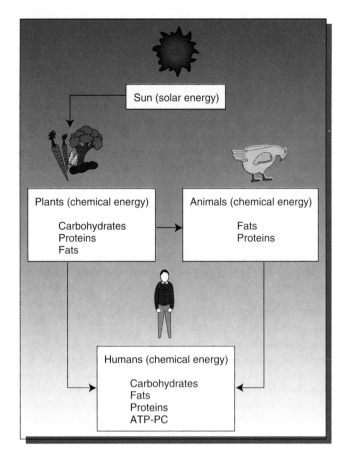

Figure 3.1 *Through photosynthesis, plants utilize solar energy from the sun and convert it to chemical energy in the form of carbohydrates, fats, or proteins. Animals eat plants and convert the chemical energy into their own stores of chemical energy—primarily fat and protein. Humans ingest food from both plant and animal sources and convert the chemical energy for their own stores and use.*

rates. We shall also introduce you to the concept of energy equivalents, for when you read scientific literature you may see energy expressed in ways other than Calories.

Energy Forms in the Body

Energy is the capacity to do work and, although energy may exist in six different forms, our concern is primarily with chemical energy, mechanical energy, and thermal energy. One of the major characteristics of energy is that one form may be transformed into another. For example, the chemical energy that is stored in a gallon of gas can be converted into thermal energy in an automobile engine and then into mechanical energy to drive the pistons and move the car.

The sun is the ultimate source of energy. Solar energy is harnessed by plants, through photosynthesis, to produce either plant carbohydrates, fats, or proteins, all forms of stored chemical energy. When humans consume plant and animal products, the carbohydrates, fats, and proteins undergo a series of metabolic changes and are utilized to develop body structure, to regulate body processes, or to provide a storage form of chemical energy (fig. 3.1). Chemical energy may be stored in a variety of forms in the human body. Carbohydrate may be found in the blood as glucose, a simple sugar. Carbohydrate

Table 3.1 Characteristics of Human Energy Systems

Characteristic	ATP-PC	Lactic Acid	Oxygen
Aerobic/anaerobic	Anaerobic	Anaerobic	Aerobic
Rate of ATP production	Fastest	Fast	Slow
Time limits of maximal exercise	4–5 seconds	1–2 minutes	Hours
Capacity for ATP production	Lowest	Low	High
Lactic acid production	No	Yes	No
Fatigability	Highest	High	Low
Energy source	ATP-PC	Carbohydrate	Carbohydrate, fat
Track event	100 meters	400–800 meters	10 kilometers
Expected time for elite athlete	(0:09)	(0:45–1:45)	(27:00)

may also be stored in the muscle or liver as glycogen, a combination of glucose molecules. Fat may be stored as triglycerides, primarily in the blood, muscle tissue, and adipose tissue. Although protein is not usually a major source of human energy, it may be under certain conditions, such as starvation. Most of the soft tissue of the body, such as the muscles, consists of protein. Although chemical energy may be stored as carbohydrate, fat, or protein, the body cannot use them as an immediate source of energy for such functions as muscle contraction. They must be converted into **ATP** (adenosine triphosphate), another form of chemical energy in the human body. ATP, a high-energy compound, is the immediate source of energy in humans. Another compound, PC (phosphocreatine; also called creatine phosphate), also formed in the body, serves to replace ATP very rapidly as it is used up.

In order to do mechanical work (exercise), ATP must be utilized. The faster you work, the more ATP your body needs. However, since the ATP available in the muscle is sufficient for only about one second of maximal work, it must be restored rapidly if work is to continue. The faster or harder you work, the more rapidly the ATP must be replenished.

Exercise is classified as being aerobic or anaerobic. Aerobic ATP production utilizes oxygen in the body. Carbohydrates and fats combine with oxygen in a series of complex metabolic reactions to produce ATP. Anaerobic ATP production occurs in the absence of oxygen by one of two processes. ATP itself may provide energy anaerobically and be resynthesized by the utilization of PC. Or, ATP may be formed anaerobically when carbohydrate (muscle glycogen), in the absence of adequate oxygen, breaks down into lactic acid. Note that carbohydrate may be a source of ATP production under both aerobic and anaerobic conditions.

Human Energy Systems

There are three major classifications of energy systems in the human body. The major characteristics of these systems are presented in table 3.1. All three systems are designed to replenish ATP. Although all systems appear to operate under a wide variety of exercise intensities, one system usually predominates. In sprinting activities lasting less than 10 seconds, the **ATP-PC system** predominates. In maximal exercise of

about 1 to 2 minutes duration, such as running a fast 400- or 800-meter race, the **lactic acid system** predominates. In low levels of activity, such as rest and long slow-distance running, the **oxygen system** predominates. Thus, the ATP-PC and lactic acid system can produce ATP rapidly, while the oxygen system produces ATP at a slower rate but can sustain production for a longer time. It is important to keep in mind that, in most exercises, all of the energy systems are used to one degree or another. The lactic acid system may predominate in a fast 400- to 800-meter run, but it is not the exclusive energy system; the oxygen system also contributes some portion of the energy demand.

An important distinction between the oxygen (aerobic) energy system and the anaerobic energy systems is the rate of fatigue. **Fatigue** is a complex phenomenon that may have a variety of causes. For our purposes here, it is important to note that the anaerobic processes involving the lactic acid system result in fatigue within a relatively short period of time largely due to the accumulation of lactic acid in the muscle cell, which may disrupt normal functioning. On the other hand, aerobic exercise does not lead to lactic acid accumulation and may be continued for longer periods of time, although fatigue may also occur due to other factors, such as fuel depletion or dehydration.

A summary of the three human energy systems is presented in figure 3.2.

Energy Equivalents

The oxygen system is utilized as the main energy source during rest and at low levels of exercise. It may also be the major energy source for high levels of sustained aerobic activity. For the time being, however, we are concerned about the relationship of oxygen to energy expenditure.

Increasing oxygen consumption results in an increased caloric expenditure, which can have considerable value in a weight control program. In order for the oxygen to be utilized, it must be transported from the atmospheric air to the muscle tissues. This is the major function of the cardiovascular-respiratory system—the heart, lungs, and blood. Exercise programs designed to stress the oxygen system concomitantly benefit the cardiovascular-respiratory system and hence are known as aerobic exercises.

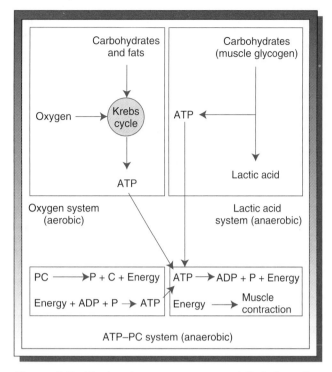

Figure 3.2   *The three human energy systems. ATP, the immediate source of energy for most processes in the human body, needs to be replenished.*

The oxygen system. *Through complex changes, byproducts of the muscle stores of carbohydrates and fats can enter the Krebs cycle, an array of enzymes that modify the structure of the carbohydrate and fat byproducts so they can release energy. Glucose and free fatty acids may enter the cell from the bloodstream. When carbohydrate and fat byproducts eventually combine with oxygen, large amounts of ATP may be produced. The oxygen system is utilized during endurance exercises lasting longer than 4 or 5 minutes.*

The lactic acid energy system. *Muscle glycogen can be broken down without the utilization of oxygen. This process is called* anaerobic glycolysis. *ATP is produced rapidly, but lactic acid is the end product. Lactic acid can be a major cause of fatigue in the muscle. The lactic acid system is utilized during exercise bouts of very high intensity conducted at maximal rates for about 1 to 2 minutes.*

The ATP-PC energy system. *ATP and PC are high-energy phosphates stored in the muscle that can provide energy very rapidly. ATP (adenosine triphosphate) is stored in the muscle in limited amounts and can be used for many body processes, including muscular contraction. The ATP stores are used for fast, all-out bursts of power that last about 1 second. ATP must be replenished from other sources in order for muscle contraction to continue. PC (phosphocreatine) is stored in the muscle in limited amounts and can be used to rapidly synthesize ATP. ATP and PC are called phosphagens and together represent the ATP-PC energy system. This system is utilized for quick, maximal exercises, such as sprinting, lasting about 1 to 6 seconds.*

Through a series of complex metabolic processes in the body, oxygen is eventually utilized in order to release the chemical energy of carbohydrate and fat stored in the body. During rest, most of this chemical energy is utilized to provide energy for our basic metabolic functions. In the process, heat is liberated (thermal energy), which helps to keep our body temperature at about 98.6° F. When we exercise, about 25 percent of the energy we produce by oxidation of carbohydrate and fat is converted into mechanical energy (muscle contraction to actually move the body). However, about 75 percent of the energy produced during exercise is still released as heat (thermal energy).

Thus, in the human body, chemical energy can be converted to either thermal or mechanical energy. Since oxygen is the key to the energy release, the amount of oxygen used can be equated to measures of chemical, thermal, and mechanical energy. There are numerous units of measurement used to express energy in the different forms in which it exists. An international system of units has been developed in order to standardize measurements. However, in the United States, the Calorie still appears to be the most popular means of expressing energy, both for exercise and for food. For practical purposes, we shall use it as the basic unit of measurement for human energy. The Calorie is especially relevant when exercise is used as a means to control body weight.

A calorie, or gram calorie, is the amount of heat necessary to raise the temperature of 1 gram of water one degree Celsius. A kilocalorie, or **Calorie** (with a capital C), is 1,000 gram calories. We shall refer only to the Calorie in this text. Oxygen in itself does not contain any Calories, but carbohydrate and fat do. Oxygen releases the Calories from the carbohydrate and fat. For a given amount of oxygen, carbohydrate provides a slightly greater amount of Calories than fat. For example, 1 liter (1,000 milliliters) of oxygen will release 5.05 Calories from carbohydrate and 4.70 Calories from fat. However, without losing a great deal of accuracy, we can state that 1 liter of oxygen equals approximately 5.0 Calories. The average person consumes about .25 of a liter (250 milliliters) of oxygen per minute at rest and about 3 to 3.5 liters per minute during maximal exercise. Highly trained athletes may consume as much as 6.0 liters

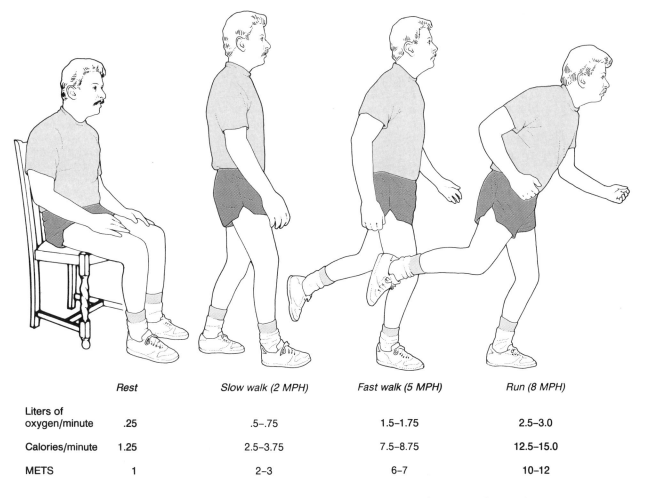

	Rest	Slow walk (2 MPH)	Fast walk (5 MPH)	Run (8 MPH)
Liters of oxygen/minute	.25	.5–.75	1.5–1.75	2.5–3.0
Calories/minute	1.25	2.5–3.75	7.5–8.75	12.5–15.0
METS	1	2–3	6–7	10–12

1 liter oxygen/minute = 5 Calories/minute

Figure 3.3 *Energy equivalents in oxygen consumption, Calories, and METS. This figure depicts three means of expressing energy expenditure during four levels of activity. These values are for an average male of 154 pounds (70 kg). If you weigh more or less, the values will increase or decrease accordingly for oxygen consumption and Calories, but not for the MET because it is based on body weight.*

per minute during exercise. Thus, in the average individual, the caloric expenditure may vary from 1.25 per minute during rest (.25 L × 5 = 1.25 Calories) to about 15 per minute during maximal exercise (3 L × 5 = 15 Calories).

The **MET** is another related energy concept. One MET represents energy consumption during rest. By technical definition, 1 MET equals 3.5 milliliters (ml) of oxygen consumption per kilogram of body weight per minute (the resting metabolic rate). For the average individual, 10 to 12 METS would represent hard exercise.

Finally, an energy term you might find in nutritional scientific literature is the **megajoule (MJ).** A joule is a very small amount of work, defined as the energy needed to move one newton (about 0.22 pounds) through a distance of one meter (about 3.28 feet). A kilojoule (kJ) is 1,000 joules, while a megajoule (MJ) is 1,000,000 joules. In case you see the energy values of foods expressed in kJ, it may be important for you to know that one Calorie equals about 4.2 kJ. One MJ equals about 240 Calories.

Figure 3.3 represents some of the interrelationships between oxygen uptake, Calories, and METS during rest and at different levels of exercise.

Aerobic Fitness

Although the basic principles for training the oxygen energy system have been established for a long time, it was not until 1968 that the term *aerobics* came into popular usage with the publication of a book of the same name by Dr. Kenneth Cooper. This classic fitness book served a major role in America's fitness revolution.

Aerobic fitness is probably the single most important health component of physical fitness. **Aerobic fitness** represents the ability of the cardiovascular and respiratory systems to accommodate the oxygen needs of the muscular system over a sustained period of time, as in endurance events such as distance running, swimming, and bicycling. A number of other terms are associated with aerobic fitness—cardiovascular

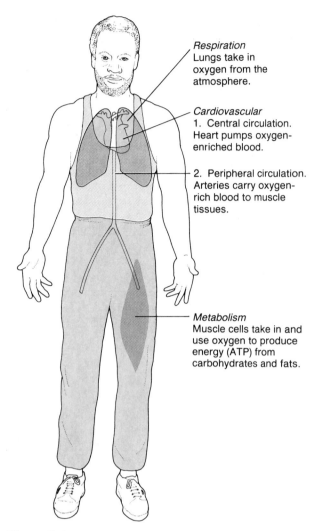

Respiration
Lungs take in oxygen from the atmosphere.

Cardiovascular
1. Central circulation. Heart pumps oxygen-enriched blood.

2. Peripheral circulation. Arteries carry oxygen-rich blood to muscle tissues.

Metabolism
Muscle cells take in and use oxygen to produce energy (ATP) from carbohydrates and fats.

Figure 3.4 *Physiological processes involved in oxygen uptake.*

Table 3.2 Human Physiological Functions Related to Aerobic Fitness

Respiration
1. Lung ventilation. Ability to take in sufficient air
2. Lung perfusion. Ability to distribute blood to key parts of the lungs
3. Diffusion capacity. Ability of oxygen to go from lungs to blood rapidly

Central Circulation
1. Heart rate. Ability to sustain high heart rate
2. Stroke volume. Ability of heart to pump sufficient amounts of blood in each beat
3. Hemoglobin level. Ability to transport adequate amounts of oxygen by binding with hemoglobin
4. Blood volume. Ability to maintain optimal amount of blood in vascular system

Peripheral Circulation
1. Blood flow. Ability of blood to deliver oxygen and nutrients to exercising muscles
2. Capillary density. Ability to develop adequate number of capillaries in muscle tissue
3. Diffusion capacity. Ability of oxygen to go from blood capillaries into muscle cells

Metabolism
1. Energy stores. Ability to store adequate energy in muscle cells
2. Muscle fiber types. Ability to possess a greater proportion of aerobic muscle fibers to anaerobic fibers
3. Muscle myoglobin. Ability to bind oxygen within the muscle cell
4. Mitochondria and oxidative enzymes. Ability to use oxygen to produce ATP in muscle cell

endurance, cardiovascular fitness, cardiorespiratory fitness, aerobic endurance, and physical working capacity—and have the same essential meaning. Other associated terms are aerobic capacity and maximal oxygen uptake.

Aerobic fitness is a complex component of physical fitness. It involves the interaction of numerous physiological processes in the cardiovascular, respiratory, and muscular systems, including the capacity of the lungs to take up oxygen, the capacity of the blood in the lungs to pick up oxygen, the capacity of the heart to pump this oxygenated blood to the muscle tissues, and the capacity of the tissues to extract the oxygen from the blood and use it to generate energy in the form of ATP via the oxygen system. Thus, the combined cardiovascular and respiratory systems are the oxygen supply mechanism for the muscles. As the energy demands of the muscles increase, so do the demands on the cardiovascular and respiratory systems in order to supply increased levels of oxygen. Refer to figure 3.4 for an overall schematic of these systems as they relate to oxygen consumption.

A number of physiological processes are critical components of aerobic fitness. These physiological processes may be grouped under four general areas of physiological functioning during exercise: respiration, central circulation, peripheral circulation, and metabolism. The important aerobic fitness aspects of each of these general areas are listed in table 3.2. Respiration is responsible for taking adequate amounts of oxygen into the lungs and blood; central circulation generates the force to pump the blood; peripheral circulation transports the oxygenated blood throughout the body; metabolism uses the oxygen in the muscle cells to produce ATP.

The interaction of these four physiological functions determines the level of aerobic fitness. The most common measure of aerobic fitness that evaluates the effectiveness of these physiological functions is **maximal oxygen consumption,** or $\dot{V}O_{2MAX}$ (pronounced vee-oh-two-max). It represents the interaction of the cardiovascular and respiratory systems to deliver oxygen to the muscles, and the ability of muscles to use the oxygen to generate energy. $\dot{V}O_{2MAX}$ is usually expressed in two ways: first, as liters of O_2 per minute (L O_2/min); second, as milliliters of O_2 per kilogram of body weight per minute (ml O_2/kg/min). $\dot{V}O_{2MAX}$ is partially dependent upon body weight. The larger the individual, the greater the potential $\dot{V}O_{2MAX}$. All other things equal, a 200-pound man has twice the $\dot{V}O_{2MAX}$ of a 100-pound man (perhaps 4 liters versus

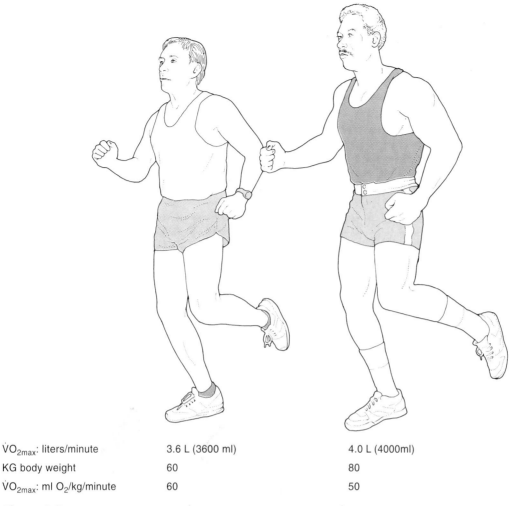

$\dot{V}O_{2max}$: liters/minute	3.6 L (3600 ml)	4.0 L (4000ml)
KG body weight	60	80
$\dot{V}O_{2max}$: ml O_2/kg/minute	60	50

Figure 3.5 *Maximal oxygen uptake ($\dot{V}O_{2MAX}$). The best way to express $\dot{V}O_{2MAX}$ is in milliliters of oxygen per kilogram (kg) of body weight per minute (ml O_2/kg/minute). As noted in the figure, the smaller individual has a lower $\dot{V}O_{2MAX}$ in liters, but a higher $\dot{V}O_{2MAX}$ when expressed relative to weight. In this case, the smaller individual has a higher degree of aerobic fitness.*

2 liters). For this reason, it is best to express $\dot{V}O_{2MAX}$ relative to body weight. Expressed in this way, a 132-pound person (Subject A) with a $\dot{V}O_{2MAX}$ of 3.0 liters is considered aerobically equivalent to a 176-pound person (Subject B) with a $\dot{V}O_{2MAX}$ of 4.0 liters. To illustrate:

Subject A

 132 lbs ÷ 2.2 = 60 kg
 3.0 liters = 3000 ml
 3000 ml O_2 ÷ 60 kg = 50 ml O_2/kg/min

Subject B

 176 lbs ÷ 2.2 = 80 kg
 4.0 liters = 4000 ml
 4000 ml O_2 ÷ 80 kg = 50 ml O_2/kg/min

In this example, both subjects A and B have an identical $\dot{V}O_{2MAX}$ when expressed per unit of body weight. On the other hand, figure 3.5 illustrates how an individual may have a lower $\dot{V}O_{2MAX}$ in liters, but a higher value when expressed in milliliters/kilogram body weight.

Although $\dot{V}O_{2MAX}$ is a very important measure of aerobic fitness, it does not represent the total concept of aerobic fitness. Of equal or greater importance is the ability to exercise at a higher percentage of your $\dot{V}O_{2MAX}$ without experiencing fatigue. Figure 3.6 illustrates this concept. The figure represents the possible effects of an aerobic exercise training program over a six-month period. Note that the $\dot{V}O_{2MAX}$ does increase somewhat; a 10 to 20 percent increase is about all that can be expected in most inactive individuals. However, the ability to perform at a greater percentage of $\dot{V}O_{2MAX}$ increases much more. In essence, you have improved your steady-state threshold.

In exercise, the **steady-state threshold** is that point where you are able to supply enough oxygen to meet the oxygen demands of the exercise; the contribution of anaerobic energy sources is minimal. If you exercise at an intensity above the steady-state threshold, the contribution of energy from the lactic acid energy system, an anaerobic system, will increase rapidly since you are now not able to provide enough oxygen to meet your energy demands. Other terms associated with the steady-state threshold include **anaerobic threshold,** lactic acid threshold, or onset of blood lactic acid (OBLA). Exercising above your steady-state threshold increases your

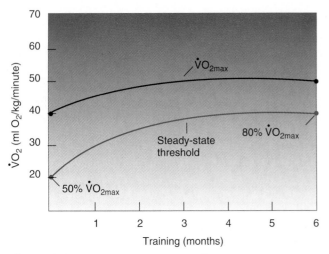

Figure 3.6 *The effect of training upon $\dot{V}O_{2MAX}$ and the steady-state threshold. Training increases both your $\dot{V}O_{2MAX}$ and your steady-state threshold, which is the ability to work at a greater percentage of your $\dot{V}O_{2MAX}$ without producing excessive lactic acid—a causative factor in fatigue. For example, before training, the $\dot{V}O_{2MAX}$ may be 40 ml, while the steady-state threshold is only 20 ml (50% of $\dot{V}O_{2MAX}$). After training, $\dot{V}O_{2MAX}$ may rise to 50 ml, but the steady-state threshold may rise to 40 ml (80% of the $\dot{V}O_{2MAX}$).*

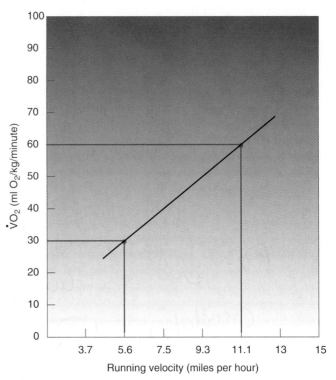

Figure 3.7 *Oxygen uptake necessary to prevent fatigue at different running speeds. The greater your running speed, the more oxygen you need. In order to prevent fatigue, the amount of oxygen needed should be under your steady-state threshold.*

oxygen debt, a term often used to label the extra amount of oxygen you consume immediately after the completion of intense exercise; it is the amount of oxygen above your normal resting level. A number of physiological factors contribute to the magnitude of the oxygen debt, but excess production of lactic acid is also important; it stimulates respiration to help you return the blood pH, or acidity, back to normal.

As you may recall, this increased production of lactic acid speeds up the onset of fatigue. By raising your steady-state threshold through training, you may be able to perform at 80 percent of your $\dot{V}O_{2MAX}$, as compared to only 50 percent before training. You will be able to perform at a greater percentage of your maximal ability without accumulating excessive amounts of lactic acid that could cause you to fatigue or slow down.

What are the implications of this concept? Figure 3.7 illustrates the effect of oxygen uptake on the ability to run long distances at a particular speed without the early onset of fatigue. In general, although individuals may vary, at an oxygen delivery rate of 30 ml/kg, running speed is only about 5.6 miles per hour (MPH); at 60 ml/kg, speed almost doubles to about 11.1 MPH. For an individual who could only do about an 11-minute mile before training, the training effect in this case reduces the time to approximately 5.5 minutes.

In summary, we can see that aerobic fitness may be expressed in terms of $\dot{V}O_{2MAX}$ and the percentage of $\dot{V}O_{2MAX}$ at which an individual is able to sustain exercise. Both of these factors may be improved by a proper training program. More importantly, the major determinants of $\dot{V}O_{2MAX}$ are the physiological functions of the cardiovascular, respiratory, and muscular systems, which will improve and bring significant benefits to the health of the individual.

Measurement of Aerobic Fitness

Now that we know what aerobic fitness is, how do we measure it in a given individual? As mentioned previously, $\dot{V}O_{2MAX}$ is probably the best single indicator of aerobic fitness and should be expressed in relation to the body weight of the individual (ml O_2/kg/min). The two general means to measure aerobic fitness include direct tests of $\dot{V}O_{2MAX}$ and indirect tests utilized to predict aerobic fitness or $\dot{V}O_{2MAX}$.

A variety of test protocols measure $\dot{V}O_{2MAX}$ directly, but the general procedure is to monitor oxygen consumption while an individual exercises to exhaustion. This test is usually done on a motor-driven treadmill or on a bicycle ergometer, although other exercise modes may also be used. The work load is gradually increased and, through the use of sophisticated monitoring devices and gas analyzers, the maximal level of oxygen uptake is recorded at or near exhaustion. An illustration is provided in figure 3.8. This type of test requires considerable time and expense, making it impractical for use with large numbers of individuals. However, if the facilities are available, this test does provide the most valid measure. With the increasing popularity and decreased cost of computers that are combined with electronic means to analyze respiratory gases, it is anticipated that direct tests will become increasingly more available for aerobic fitness assessment.

At the present time, however, a number of indirect tests are often used to assess aerobic fitness. The two most common are distance runs and step tests.

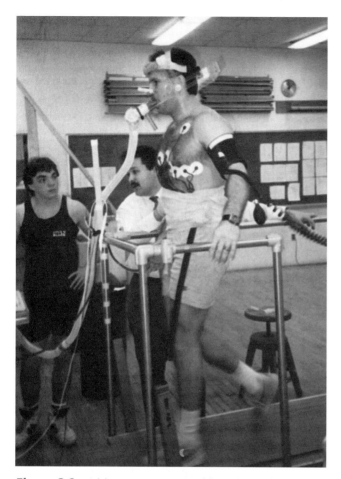

Figure 3.8 *A laboratory stress test. A laboratory stress test with a 12-lead EKG and measurement of maximal oxygen uptake ($\dot{V}O_{2MAX}$) can provide some highly technical data related to cardiovascular-respiratory function.*

Over the years, Dr. Kenneth Cooper has collected and analyzed data on thousands of individuals relative to $\dot{V}O_{2MAX}$ and performance in distance running, distance swimming, and distance cycling. Based upon his analysis, Cooper suggests that a given performance on his running, swimming, or bicycling test is indicative of a certain level of $\dot{V}O_{2MAX}$. His research, and resultant fitness programs, are presented in a series of books. The most recent of these is *The Aerobics Program for Total Well-Being.*

Cooper's tests are designed for men and women between the ages of thirteen and sixty. An individual may take any of the following tests:

1. 3-mile walking test (no running)
2. 1½-mile running test
3. 12-minute walking/running test
4. 12-minute swimming test
5. 12-minute cycling test

For the 12-minute tests, the goal is to cover as great a distance as possible during the allotted time; finishing in the shortest time possible is the criterion in the 1½- and 3-mile tests. To conduct these tests, you will need accurately

measured distances and a stopwatch. An indoor and outdoor track are excellent for the running, walking, and cycling tests; a 25-yard (or longer) pool is appropriate for the swimming test. Scoring tables for the 3-mile walking test and the 1½-mile running test are presented in Appendix B.

Although there is general agreement that these types of indirect tests do measure the ability to produce aerobic energy over a prolonged period of time, they may not be highly accurate predictors of $\dot{V}O_{2MAX}$. The factors that contribute to running, swimming, and bicycling performance are complex; they include $\dot{V}O_{2MAX}$ and other factors such as steady-state threshold, body fatness, and mechanical efficiency. Nevertheless, they appear to be some of the best practical means available to assess aerobic fitness. Moreover, since the steady-state threshold is a component of aerobic fitness, and body fat is a health-related component of fitness, these indirect tests do appear to be useful as fitness measuring techniques. Improved performance would most likely be due to increased fitness levels.

Laboratory Inventory 3.3 (at the end of the book) may be used to predict $\dot{V}O_{2MAX}$ and assess aerobic fitness. Be sure to read the instructions prior to taking any of the distance tests. Sedentary individuals should exercise regularly for several weeks before taking any of the tests. A recommended sequence is

1. Train 2 weeks; take 3-mile walking test.
2. Train 4 more weeks; take 3-mile walking test or 1½-mile running test.
3. Train 6 more weeks; take 1½-mile running test.
4. Repeat 1½-mile running test about once a month to check on progress.

Another indirect technique commonly used to measure aerobic fitness involves the heart rate response during the recovery period after an exercise step test. Since the heart rate is the most rapidly obtainable measure of the cardiovascular response to exercise, it has commonly been used to predict $\dot{V}O_{2MAX}$ or to assess aerobic fitness. Unfortunately, research has shown that the heart rate response to various step tests is not a good predictor of $\dot{V}O_{2MAX}$ or even of performance on the other indirect tests such as distance runs. However, the heart rate response may be useful in evaluating the effect of a conditioning regimen on a given individual. One of the beneficial effects of aerobic exercise training is a lower resting heart rate and a lower heart rate response to a submaximal exercise task. Hence, the results of a step test administered prior to the initiation of a conditioning program could be compared with the results of a test administered toward the conclusion of the program. A lowered heart rate response would be indicative that the heart has become more efficient. This should serve to motivate the individual to continue the training program. This may be the most valuable use of the step test. Laboratory Inventory 3.4 describes the protocol for a step test, but you could actually design your own to help measure your progress during training.

Both the Cooper test and step tests are useful in measuring certain aspects of cardiovascular-respiratory fitness;

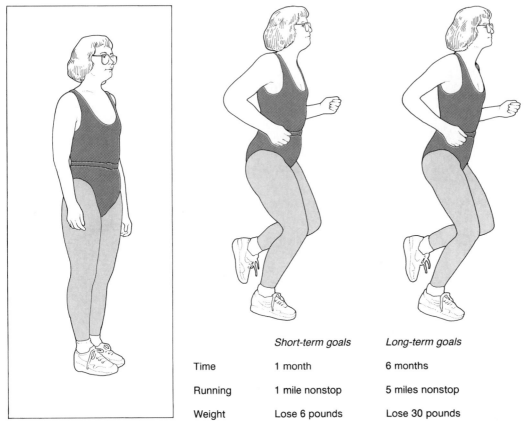

	Short-term goals	Long-term goals
Time	1 month	6 months
Running	1 mile nonstop	5 miles nonstop
Weight	Lose 6 pounds	Lose 30 pounds

Figure 3.9 *Goal setting is an important factor in an exercise program.*

however, the Cooper test does not monitor heart rate, and the step test, except for those who participate primarily in step aerobics, is not normally selected as an aerobic exercise in a training program to improve fitness. However, the Rockport Walking Institute, in cooperation with medical researchers at the University of Massachusetts, developed a fitness evaluation test that combines walking with measurement of heart rate. Laboratory Inventory 3.5 provides you with information relative to the conduct and interpretation of the Rockport Fitness Walking Test. For those who use walking as an aerobic exercise mode, this test would be excellent to monitor progress.

In order to achieve valid and reliable results for these tests, as well as for any fitness test, identical protocol must be used each time the test is taken. If walking or running, the same course should be used, if possible, and the step height and stepping cadence should remain the same for step tests. Extraneous factors such as the environmental temperature and wind conditions may influence test results. Try to minimize these extraneous influences whenever possible.

Exercise tests can be used to establish short-term and long-term goals. The results of these tests may also provide excellent data for evaluating progress during an exercise program.

Prescription for Aerobic Exercise

A general outline for an exercise prescription for aerobic fitness should include goals, mode of exercise, a warm-up period, a stimulus period, and a warm-down period. Although research does provide sufficient information to enable us to offer exercise recommendations to the general population, it is important to note that the exercise dosage, as with many medications, may need to be prescribed carefully for individuals with certain preexisting risks. Although such risks are relatively rare in the average young college student, and most healthy middle-aged adults can initiate an exercise program without risk, you should be aware of your personal medical background. You should check the guidelines in chapter 2 on pages 18–19 and the Revised Physical Activity Readiness Questionnaire in Laboratory Inventory 2.2 to see whether you should seek medical clearance before you undertake your own exercise program.

Goals

As illustrated in figure 3.9, the goals you set for yourself should be of two types—short-term and long-term. They should be personal goals and should reflect why you are initiating an aerobic fitness program. For example, a short-term goal may be to lose 5 pounds of body fat in 1 month, while a long-term goal may be to lose 30 pounds in 6 months. Another example is a short-term goal of nonstop jogging for 1 mile and a long-term goal of entering and completing a 10-kilometer road race. When you achieve your short-term goal, a new short-term goal should be established as you progress toward your long-term goal. It is important to remember that no initial short-term goal is too small, nor is any new short-term goal

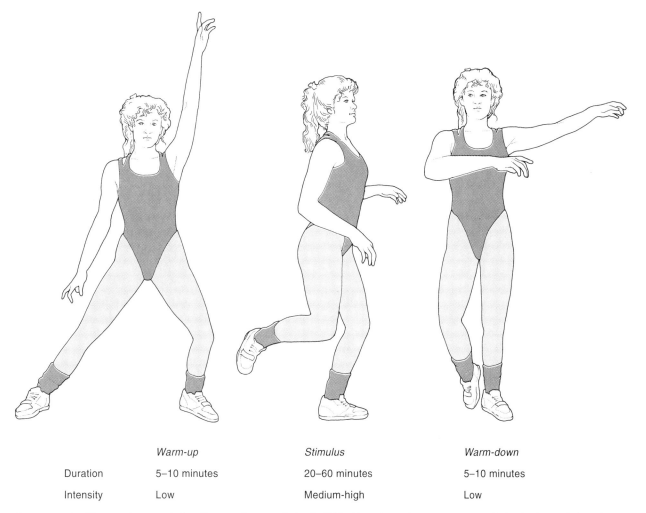

	Warm-up	Stimulus	Warm-down
Duration	5–10 minutes	20–60 minutes	5–10 minutes
Intensity	Low	Medium-high	Low

Figure 3.10 *The exercise prescription. The exercise prescription is divided into three phases: warm-up period, stimulus period, and warm-down period. The stimulus period is the key.*

too small in the progress towards your long-term goal. The initial goals you establish will be dependent upon your initial level of physical fitness. If you have been completely sedentary, your initial goal may be simply to walk more each day, such as 10 minutes at a time. On the other hand, if you are somewhat fit, you may establish somewhat higher initial goals.

Mode of Exercise

The mode of exercise represents the aerobic activity choice you participate in to achieve aerobic fitness. You may use a wide variety of physical activities for this purpose. This topic is discussed in a later section of this chapter.

Warm-Up and Warm-Down

A proper warm-up and warm-down are important components of the aerobic exercise prescription (see fig. 3.10). Both may help to prevent excessive strain on the heart and may also be helpful in the prevention of muscular soreness or injuries.

The warm-up precedes the stimulus period and may be done in several ways. It may be general in nature, such as calisthenics, or be specific to the type of exercise you plan to do, such as initially exercising at a lower level of intensity of the actual mode of exercise. Some stretching exercises, such as those illustrated in chapter 5, are also helpful in the warm-up period. Five to 10 minutes should provide an adequate warm-up time.

For most aerobic-type exercise, it is probably better to warm up the specific muscles to be used. For example, if you plan to use jogging as your mode of aerobic exercise, you should stretch your leg muscles gently at first and then jog at a slower than normal pace for several minutes. Breaking a sweat is a good external sign that you have sufficiently elevated your body temperature; by using a specific type of warm-up, the temperature of your exercising muscles will also be increased.

At the end of your stimulus period, a gradual tapering of exercise intensity will provide an appropriate warm-down (cool-down). If you are jogging, simply slow your pace and gradually begin to walk. A warm-down may take about 5 to 10 minutes to get your heart rate near normal. Complete your warm-down by gently stretching the muscles you have used. Since your muscles are now warm from the exercise, they are easier to stretch; such stretching may help to improve your flexibility and prevent muscle stiffness.

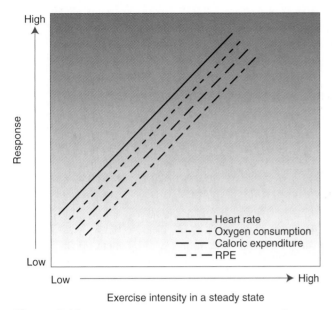

Figure 3.11 *The relationship among various measures of energy expenditure. Heart rate, oxygen consumption, caloric expenditure, and RPE are, in general, directly related to the intensity of the exercise under steady-state conditions, i.e., when the oxygen supply is adequate for the energy cost of the exercise.*

Stimulus Period

The **stimulus period** is based upon the overload principle and is the most important part of any exercise program. It is the heart of the exercise prescription for aerobic fitness. As illustrated in figure 3.11, several important physiological and psychological measures increase in proportion to an increase in exercise intensity, two of which may serve as practical guides for you to monitor your exercise intensity.

The two major components of the stimulus period are intensity and duration of exercise. In any exercise session, these two components are usually inversely related. In other words, if intensity is high, duration is short, and if intensity is low, duration is long. Frequency (the number of exercise sessions per week) is also an important part of the exercise prescription. A number of medical groups, including the American Heart Association (AHA), the Federation Internationale de Sports Medicine (FISM), and the American College of Sports Medicine (ACSM), have made specific recommendations concerning the quality and quantity of exercise for developing and maintaining cardiorespiratory fitness in adults. The recommendations from these groups are slightly different, but the differences are very minor.

The recommendations of the ACSM, which follow, are based on an exhaustive review of the pertinent research. They will be used as the basis for developing an aerobic fitness program here, although they may be modified somewhat under certain circumstances. Such modifications will be noted where appropriate.

1. Intensity of training. 60 to 90 percent of maximum heart rate (HR_{MAX}) or 50 to 85 percent of maximum oxygen uptake ($\dot{V}O_{2MAX}$) or HR_{MAX} reserve (see definition).

2. Duration of training. 20 to 60 minutes of continuous aerobic activity.

3. Frequency of training. 3 to 5 days per week.

The Threshold Stimulus

The intensity of exercise is the most important component of the stimulus period; in order to receive the optimal benefits from the exercise program, you must attain a certain **threshold stimulus,** the minimal stimulus intensity that will produce a training effect. The intensity of exercise can be expressed in a number of different ways, such as percentage of $\dot{V}O_{2MAX}$, Calories/minute, or heart rate. In general, there is a high degree of relationship among these variables during exercise at a steady state. For example, the heart rate may reflect a certain level of oxygen consumption or caloric expenditure. Since the heart rate is easily obtained, it is usually used to determine the threshold level of exercise intensity. Another means to judge exercise intensity is the **RPE,** or **rating of perceived exertion,** your psychological perception of how strenuous the exercise is that you are doing.

The Target Heart Rate

How do you determine your threshold level? Let's look at two ways—the heart rate and RPE. To obtain the heart rate, press lightly with the index and middle fingers on the carotid artery, located just under the jawbone and beside the Adam's apple. Do not use your thumb as it also has a pulse, and do not press hard on the carotid artery, for it may cause a reflex slowing of the beat in some persons. The radial artery pulse is obtained by placing your fingers on the inside of the wrist on the thumb side. These are the two most common locations for monitoring pulse rate, but other locations (the temple, inside the upper arm, and directly over the heart) may be used (see fig. 3.12).

To obtain the heart rate per minute, simply count the pulse rate for 6 seconds and add a zero. Resting and recovery heart rates are easily obtainable, since they may be taken while you are motionless, but it is difficult to manually monitor the heart rate while exercising. Wireless devices, usually consisting of a chest strap and a special wrist watch, are commercially available to accurately monitor your heart rate during exercise. Research has shown that the exercise heart rate correlates very highly with the heart rate during the early stages of recovery. Hence, to monitor exercise heart rate, secure the pulse *immediately* upon cessation of exercise and count the beats for 6 seconds. This provides a reliable measure of exercise heart rate, although it may be slightly lower due to the beginning of the recovery effect. If it is difficult for you to monitor your heart rate for 6 seconds, then use a 10-second period and multiply the count by six to obtain your heart rate per minute. Laboratory Inventory 3.1 gives you some practical experience in palpating your heart rate. You probably should use 30 seconds to determine your resting heart rate; multiply your results by two. It may also be better to measure your resting pulse early in the morning, just after rising. Additionally, for the calculations, you should take your

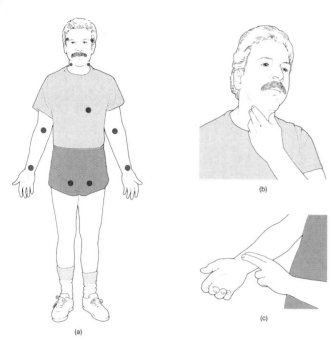

Figure 3.12 *Palpation of the heart rate. The pulse rate may be taken at a variety of body locations (a), but the two most common locations are (b) the neck (carotid artery) and (c) the wrist (radial artery).*

resting heart rate in the position in which you will exercise, for example lying down if you swim, seated if you cycle, or standing if you walk or run.

One of the most prevalent techniques to determine the threshold stimulus for exercise is based upon the **maximal heart rate reserve (HR$_{MAX}$ reserve),** the reserve difference between the resting heart rate and the maximum heart rate. Your resting heart rate corresponds to your resting oxygen consumption, or resting metabolic rate, while your maximal heart rate is achieved at your maximal oxygen consumption. As your heart rate increases from resting to maximal, so too does your oxygen consumption, so exercising at a percentage of your HR$_{MAX}$ reserve may be roughly comparable to the percentage of your $\dot{V}O_{2MAX}$. Research has indicated that the percentage of the HR$_{MAX}$ reserve during exercise is generally higher than the percentage of $\dot{V}O_{2MAX}$, particularly at lower levels of submaximal exercise. For example, exercising at 65 percent of the HR$_{MAX}$ reserve may only be comparable to 50 percent of the $\dot{V}O_{2MAX}$, but the relationship becomes closer as the exercise task approaches HR$_{MAX}$ levels. Also, the relationship may vary with the type of physical activity. In particular, arm exercises may increase the heart rate disproportionately to the oxygen consumption, and the percent of the HR$_{MAX}$ reserve may be much greater than the percent of $\dot{V}O_{2MAX}$. Nevertheless, monitoring the heart rate during exercise provides useful information relative to increases in energy expenditure for most aerobic activities.

If you have not been physically active in some time, it may not be advisable for you to engage in strenuous physical activity in order to determine your actual maximal heart rate (HR$_{MAX}$), but there are ways to predict it based upon your age. Although there are individual variations, a general guide for the prediction of HR$_{MAX}$ in women and untrained men is 220 minus the person's age. For physically trained men, the formula 205 minus one-half the person's age may be more appropriate. Based upon the first formula, a forty-year-old untrained individual would have a predicted HR$_{MAX}$ of 180. Using the second formula, a trained forty-year-old male would have a predicted HR$_{MAX}$ of 185. Keep in mind, however, that there is considerable individual variation relative to predicted HR$_{MAX}$. For example, a forty-year-old man may predict a HR$_{MAX}$ of 180, yet it may be 200, 160, or even much lower if he was a victim of coronary heart disease.

There is rather widespread general agreement that, in order to obtain a training effect, the heart rate response should be increased above the resting level by about 50–85 percent of the HR$_{MAX}$ reserve. Recent research has revealed that lower levels, 45 percent, may also be effective, particularly in individuals with poor levels of physical fitness.

Continuing with our example of the forty-year-old man, we can calculate the heart rate range needed to elicit a training effect. This is called the **target heart rate range,** or **target HR.** In order to complete the calculations, we need to know the age-predicted HR$_{MAX}$ and the resting heart rate (RHR); the latter should be determined under relaxed circumstances. If we assume a RHR of 70 and a HR$_{MAX}$ of 180, the following formula would give us the target range:

$$\text{Target HR} = X\% \ (\text{HR}_{MAX} - \text{RHR}) + \text{RHR}$$

For the 50 percent threshold level, the target heart rate for our example would be calculated as follows:

$$.5 \ (180 - 70) + 70 =$$
$$.5 \ (110) + 70 = 55 + 70 = 125$$

For the 85 percent level, the target heart rate would be:

$$.85 \ (180 - 70) + 70 =$$
$$.85 \ (110) + 70 = 93 + 70 = 163$$

Thus, in order to achieve a training effect, our forty-year-old man needs to train within a target HR range of 125–163.

If you wish to bypass the calculations, table 3.3 presents the target HR ranges for various age groups with RHR between 45 and 90 beats/minute. Simply find your age group and RHR in the headings and locate your target HR range. The table is based on a predicted HR$_{MAX}$ of 220 – age.

In general, this table is a useful guide to the threshold heart rate and target HR range. However, there is considerable variability in HR$_{MAX}$ among individuals, particularly in the older age groups. If your true HR$_{MAX}$ is below the predicted value (220 – age), the target HR range in the table would be higher than the recommended level. If your true HR$_{MAX}$ is higher than the predicted value, the target HR range in the table is lower than the recommended level. Although the target HR range might vary by a few beats, if your actual HR$_{MAX}$ is slightly higher or lower than the predicted value, you will still receive a good training effect—assuming you are in the middle of the range.

Table 3.3 Target Heart Rate Zones Using the HR$_{MAX}$ Reserve Method

RHR	Age											
	15–19	20–24	25–29	30–34	35–39	40–44	45–49	50–54	55–59	60–64	65–69	70–74
45–49	125	123	120	118	115	113	110	108	105	103	100	98
	180	175	171	167	163	158	154	150	146	141	137	133
50–54	127	125	122	120	117	115	112	110	107	105	102	100
	181	176	172	168	164	159	155	151	147	142	138	134
55–59	130	128	125	123	120	118	115	113	110	108	105	103
	181	176	172	168	164	159	155	151	147	142	138	134
60–64	132	130	127	125	122	120	117	115	112	110	107	105
	182	177	173	169	165	160	156	152	148	143	139	135
65–69	135	133	130	128	125	123	120	118	115	113	110	108
	183	178	174	170	166	161	157	153	149	144	140	136
70–74	139	135	132	130	127	125	122	120	117	115	112	110
	184	179	175	171	167	162	158	154	150	145	141	137
75–79	140	138	135	133	130	128	125	123	120	118	115	113
	184	180	176	172	168	163	159	155	151	146	142	138
80–84	142	140	137	135	132	130	127	125	122	120	117	115
	185	181	177	173	169	164	160	156	152	147	143	139
85–89	145	143	140	138	135	133	130	128	125	123	120	118
	186	181	177	173	169	164	160	156	152	147	143	139

The target zone (50–85 percent threshold) is based upon the median figure for each age range and resting heart rate range.

Once you have been training for a month or so, you may desire to determine your HR$_{MAX}$ in the specific activity you do. You may use the procedures described in Laboratory Inventory 3.2, modifying it dependent upon your aerobic exercise. For example, recent research has revealed that HR$_{MAX}$ is lower in swimming, possibly as much as 10 to 15 beats per minute, so the target heart rate may be slightly lower if this mode of exercise is used. William McArdle of Queens College recommends use of the formula 205 minus age to predict maximal heart rate while swimming.

The Target RPE

Although the target heart rate approach is a sound means for monitoring exercise intensity and may add enjoyment to your workouts (an important factor in exercise adherence), it is not the only technique available. You may also wish to use the RPE scale developed by Gunnar Borg. This scale was originally designed to reflect heart rate responses by adding a zero to the rating. You simply rate the perceived difficulty or strenuousness of the exercise task according to the scale in table 3.4. For example, at an RPE of 9 (very light) your heart rate should be about 90. If you are running, how do your legs feel? Do they feel light and easy to move, or are they heavy, or possibly beginning to ache or burn? How is your breathing? Are you breathing easily and able to carry on a conversation, or are your sentences shortened to a few words. In general, how does your total body feel? Is the exercise too easy, or are you working too hard? A new ten-point rating scale has been developed by Borg, but the American College of Sports Medicine notes that the original one is still useful since it is based on the heart rate response to exercise.

Table 3.4 The RPE Scale

6	14
7 very, very light	15 hard
8	16
9 very light	17 very hard
10	18
11 fairly light	19 very, very hard
12	20
13 somewhat hard	

When you determine your exercise heart rate, it is a good idea to associate an appropriate RPE value with it. For example, at an exercise heart rate of 150 you might make a mental note of the exercise difficulty and assign a value of 15, or hard, to that level of exercise intensity. With practice, you can learn to use the RPE to gauge the intensity for different modes of exercise. Research has shown that the RPE can be an effective means to measure exercise intensity in healthy individuals, particularly at heart rates above 150 beats/minute. You may adjust the RPE to reflect heart rate during certain conditions, such as pregnancy. A general rule of thumb is the so-called talk test: If you cannot maintain a conversation with a friend while exercising, you are probably exercising too hard. Rod Dishman, an expert in exercise psychology, suggests that you select a *preferred* level of exertion, i.e., an exercise intensity that you favor but which is also safe and health-promoting, in order to enhance your ability to adhere to your exercise program.

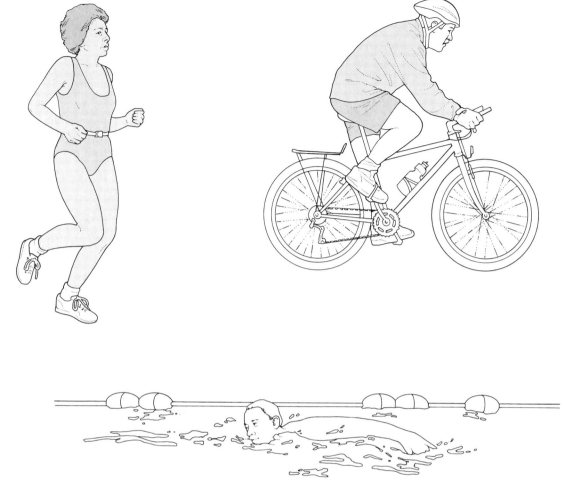

Figure 3.13 *Aerobic-mode exercises such as running, bicycling, or swimming must involve large muscle groups.*

Modes of Aerobic Exercise

Aerobic exercises involve large muscle groups in a rhythmical manner (fig. 3.13). The muscles of the legs compose a good portion of the total body musculature, so exercises such as rapid walking, running, and bicycling have a high potential for developing aerobic fitness. The major muscles in the chest and back, which are actively involved in most arm movements, are also relatively large and may be used to obtain an aerobic training effect. Most types of swimming strokes depend primarily upon the arms for movement. Some forms of exercise, such as cross-country skiing and rowing, use both the arms and the legs rather vigorously. Although many different types of activities may be used to develop the cardiovascular system, you should recall the principal of specificity, whereby the muscles that develop are specific to the type of exercise that is used.

Needless to say, there are many good large muscle rhythmical activities that may be used to improve aerobic fitness. Table 3.5 presents a variety of physical activities grouped according to their potential for development of aerobic fitness. Keep in mind, however, that in order for these activities to be effective, they must adhere to the overload principle. The exercise intensity must pass the threshold level, that level must be maintained for a set duration, and the exercise must be done frequently. For example, bicycling possesses high potential for improving your aerobic fitness, but if the intensity level is low, such as in leisurely cycling around your neighborhood, then the potential for aerobic fitness is also low. In chapter 7, some additional guidelines will be presented when we discuss the role of aerobic exercise in a weight control program.

One of the most important factors regarding your chosen mode of exercise is enjoyment. To be effective in the long run (no pun intended), you should select an activity that you enjoy, that has a recommended intensity level, and that can be performed over a long period of time. If you do not enjoy jogging or running, other activities may be substituted. Fast walking (with vigorous arm action) has been shown to be a very effective aerobic exercise for all age groups, while swimming, bicycling, aerobic dancing, step aerobics, slide aerobics, in-line skating (rollerblading), tennis, handball, racquetball, or a variety of other activities, including the use of exercise machines for rowing, stair climbing, or cross-country

Table 3.5 The Potential of Various Physical Activities for the Development of Aerobic Fitness

High Potential	Moderate Potential	Low Potential
Aerobic dancing	Basketball	Archery
Aerobic walking	Calisthenics	Baseball
Bicycling	Downhill skiing	Bowling
Cross-country skiing	Field hockey	Football
Hiking uphill	Handball	Golf
In-line skating	Racquetball	Softball
Jogging	Soccer	Volleyball
Rope jumping	Squash	
Rowing	Tennis (singles)	
Running		
Running in place		
Skating		
Slide aerobics		
Stair climbing		
Stationary bicycling		
Step aerobics		
Swimming		
Water aerobics		

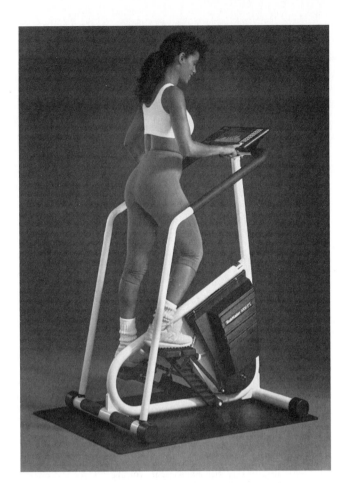

Figure 3.15 *Stair climbing machines can provide an effective aerobic workout.*

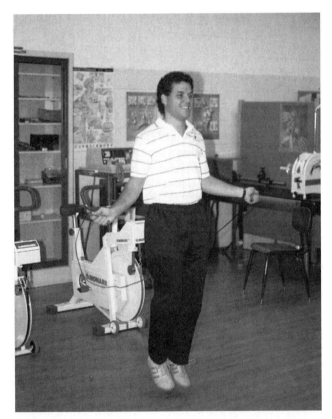

Figure 3.14 *Rope jumping may be an excellent indoor aerobic exercise.*

skiing, may produce a greater feeling of enjoyment and may elicit an aerobic fitness training effect. Enjoy your exercise. Try to make it a lifelong habit.

Practicality is a key point. You may enjoy swimming, tennis, racquetball, and a variety of other sports, but lack of facilities, poor weather conditions, no partner, or high costs may limit your ability to participate. For the person who travels frequently, this may be a major concern. Practicality is the major reason that a walking-jogging-running program is stressed in this book. This mode of aerobic training is not superior to other modes of equal intensity, duration, and frequency, but it can be done almost anytime and anywhere—which is not the case for many other types of aerobic activities. All you need are a good pair of shoes and proper clothing to suit the weather. Nothing short of an injury should deter you from your planned daily exercise routine, be it fast walking, jogging, or running. You may not learn to enjoy jogging, but it can be a very practical substitute on those days when you cannot participate in your regular physical activity. Other practical modes of aerobic exercise include aerobic dancing, rope jumping, and stair climbing (figs. 3.14, 3.15).

Implementing an Aerobic Fitness Program

Now that you have all this information about aerobic exercise, how do you begin your own personal program? In this section, we discuss some general guidelines for selecting your aerobic exercise program, show you a technique to determine the exercise intensity necessary to elicit your target heart rate or target RPE, discuss the concept of progression, and provide you with some sample exercise programs that satisfy the principles set forth in the preceding section.

After finishing this section, you should be able to complete Laboratory Inventory 3.6, an aerobic exercise prescription and contract.

General Guidelines

One of the most important factors to consider before beginning your aerobic fitness program is your current level of physical fitness. If you are sedentary or have been inactive for some time, you should begin with a less vigorous activity such as aerobic walking. As you improve your physical fitness, the intensity of the exercise program may be increased. Review the practical suggestions on pages 18–19 concerning health status and the initiation of an aerobic fitness program. In general, if you are young and healthy (twenties or early thirties) and have no coronary risk factors, it is probably safe to begin an aerobic exercise program without a medical examination. Otherwise, check with your physician.

The time of day you exercise is immaterial, for the effects will be the same if you train in the morning, afternoon, or evening. The key point is to schedule your exercise as a part of your regular daily activities. Allot yourself that 40 to 60 minutes for a total workout at least three days each week. If you regularly exercise in the evening but have something else scheduled on the evening of your exercise day, then try to work the exercise into your schedule earlier in the day, maybe getting up an hour earlier than usual. Commitment is a key to developing a lifetime fitness program. Make exercise a part of your life-style.

Versatility is an important consideration. Learn a variety of modes of aerobic exercise. You may prefer handball as your exercise mode, but lack of a partner or playing facilities may eliminate this means of exercise. Jogging is a good substitute. You may enjoy running outdoors because of the variety of scenery and the fresh air, but inclement weather may force you to exercise indoors. Aerobic dancing, rope jumping, stationary running or a wide variety of exercise machines are good indoor substitutes.

Associated with versatility is the concept of **cross-training,** or doing a variety of aerobic exercises during the course of your weekly training schedule. Cross-training may help keep motivation high, may help to prevent overuse injuries, and may help you maintain training if an injury prevents you from doing your favorite exercise. For example, if you experience a running injury to the foot, you may be able to cycle, run in deep water using various support devices (aqua-running), or other nonimpact activities in order to maintain aerobic fitness. Have a backup exercise plan.

Determination of Your Target Heart Rate and Target RPE

As you may recall from our previous discussion, exercise intensity is a key factor in developing aerobic fitness. Duration and frequency are basically self-evident; that is, you exercise for 20 to 60 minutes on three or four days per week. However, you must determine the intensity of exercise necessary to elicit your target heart rate. Laboratory Inventory 3.1 introduces you to heart rate palpation techniques; Laboratory Inventory 3.2 enables you to determine the level of exercise intensity for your target zone.

Since the concept of the target HR or RPE is so important, let us illustrate with an example of Laboratory Inventory 3.2 for someone who is twenty years old and has a RHR of 70. From table 3.3, the target HR range is 135 (50 percent) to 179 (85 percent).

This person takes the test outlined in Laboratory Inventory 3.2 with the following results:

Test	Time	RPE	HR	Minutes/Mile
1	7:30	12	125	15:00
2	6:00	15	150	12:00
3	4:00	17	174	8:00
4	3:15	19	193	6:30

Obviously, as the speed increases for each test, so do the heart rate and RPE. In this case, the RPE correlates fairly well with the heart rate, i.e., adding a zero to the RPE approximates the heart rate response. In this example, the first test at a pace of $7\frac{1}{2}$ minutes for a $\frac{1}{2}$ mile does not reach the target zone because the heart rate of 125 is below the 50 percent threshold of 135. Test two does reach the threshold value with a heart rate of 150. Tests three and four lead to higher heart rates, with test four exceeding the 85 percent level of the target HR range. The data are plotted in figure 3.16. The RPE offers a means of judging the intensity of the exercise when you do not have a known distance or a watch to determine your pace or heart rate.

To determine the speed for these tests, simply double the time for the $\frac{1}{2}$ mile and you have the time per mile. In our example, the first test was a 15-minute mile, and subsequent tests were 12-, 8-, and $6\frac{1}{2}$-minute miles.

The exercise intensity necessary to achieve the target heart rate should be developed specific to the type of exercise program you are going to do. For example, if you plan to swim for your aerobic exercise, then you should use the swim test protocol at different speeds to determine your heart rate response. It should be noted that the HR_{MAX} is generally lower (about 10 to 15 beats) when swimming than running, so the target HR range for swimming might be 8 to 10 beats lower. This is due to the different body position for exercise in swimming. The heart can pump more blood per beat while the body is in a horizontal position rather than in a vertical position as in running. Other aqua-exercises, like running in deep water, may decrease the heart rate response. A lower HR_{MAX} has also been noted during bicycling. Thus, it may be advisable to determine your HR_{MAX} specific to your mode of exercise once you become conditioned. Using your RHR

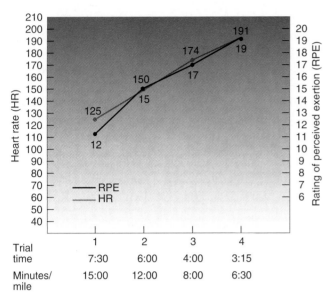

Trial
time   7:30   6:00   4:00   3:15

Minutes/
mile   15:00   12:00   8:00   6:30

Figure 3.16   *Plot of heart rate and RPE in determination of threshold heart rate for a $^1/_2$ mile run/walk.*

and your HR_{MAX} for a specific type of exercise, you can calculate your target HR range from the table on page 38.

Progression

Progression of exercise intensity is an important concept. The intensity of exercise necessary to elicit the target heart rate at the higher levels of the target HR range may be too severe for some beginners; hence, the initial stages of the training program, especially for the habitually sedentary individual, should be mild to moderate. For a forty-year-old individual with a RHR of 72, the target HR might be in the range of 126 to 164. Obviously, the intensity of exercise needed to produce an HR of 126 is much less than that needed for an HR of 164. During the early stages of training, the 126 HR may be tolerated easily, while a 164 HR may produce a rapid onset of fatigue or intolerance. Hence, the intensity of the exercise may be regulated toward the lower end of the target range during the early weeks of training, increasing gradually so that the HR begins to approach the upper limits of the target range.

It is important to reiterate that individuals who have been sedentary should begin their exercise programs no higher than the 50 percent level of the heart rate reserve, possibly only 40 to 45 percent. Many individuals start out at too high a work load and experience problems. It will take time to get back in shape and improve your fitness level. Start slowly, following the progressive programs offered later in this chapter. Training at a lower intensity level at first will still improve your fitness.

A modified training program, such as the walk-jog-walk program described below, to produce a varying HR response during the exercise period may be advisable. For example, the individual may walk at a pace sufficient to achieve an HR of 126 for several minutes; increase the intensity by jogging to achieve an HR of 164 for several minutes; then walk again to reduce the heart rate to the lower levels of the target range. By alternating intensity levels, the HR can be made to

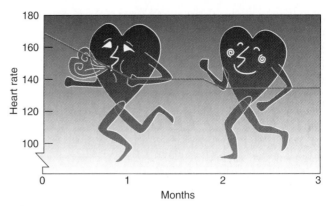

Figure 3.17   *As you become trained over several months, your heart-rate response to a standard exercise, such as running a 10-minute mile, decreases significantly. Thus, to hit your target HR, you may have to increase your exercise intensity.*

vary from the lower to upper levels of the target HR range. Let your RPE also serve as a guide to exercise intensity.

As the body begins to adapt to the exercise routine over the weeks, the intensity, duration, and/or frequency may be increased. For example, one of the effects of training is a decrease in both the resting HR and the HR and RPE responses to a given work load. For example, initially, you may be able to reach a target heart rate of 160 by running a mile in 10 minutes. However, as you become conditioned, that same speed may elicit a heart rate of only 140 (see fig. 3.17). Hence, you must increase your intensity, or speed, in order to continue to elicit the target heart rate of 160. Eventually, you progress to a training level that helps maintain the desired target heart rate. The resting HR also decreases as you become better conditioned, and this decrease then modifies the heart rate reserve. Check your RHR periodically in order to calculate the changes in your threshold HR. Mathematically, the minimal threshold decreases, because your resting heart rate is lower. But, a lower resting heart rate also means you have an increase in the number of heart beats in order to get to this minimal threshold. Also, you become able to work at higher threshold levels (70 to 80 percent), so a good training effect still occurs.

It is important to keep in mind that using your heart rate as a guide to exercise intensity is not an exact science, so getting your heart rate somewhere in the target range will still give you a good training effect, as will the use of your target RPE.

Aerobic Exercise Programs

Although diverse modes of aerobic exercise may be used to elicit a training effect for the cardiovascular system, only three of the more practical ones are described here. They can be done alone and with a minimum of equipment. However, these examples may be modified and applied to many other forms of structured physical activity, such as cycling, swimming, or a variety of aerobic exercise machines.

Aerobic Walk-Jog-Run Programs

There is a wide variety of methods to initiate an aerobic exercise program of walking, jogging, or running. The key is to

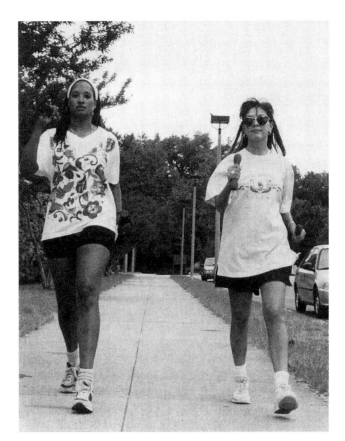

Figure 3.18 *Brisk aerobic exercise is an excellent mode of exercise to develop cardiovascular fitness.*

begin slowly, gradually increasing the exercise intensity as you become better conditioned. Leisurely walking is not usually an adequate stimulus to reach the target heart rate range, although it may still confer some health benefits, as noted later in this chapter. To reach the recommended level of 50 to 85 percent of HR_{MAX} reserve, the walking pace must be brisk. Walking at a faster-than-normal pace is often called **aerobic walking,** and many recent research studies have shown that it may be an adequate stimulus to improve aerobic fitness in individuals of varying fitness levels, particularly so with vigorous arm action and/or carrying of hand weights. The energy expenditure of vigorous aerobic walking can parallel that of jogging.

One style of aerobic walking is to bend your elbows at a 90° angle, clench your fists loosely, and move your arms naturally, making as wide an arc as possible, with your elbows coming up to chest level in the front and to the shoulder blade level in the back. Your stomach should be tightened in order to tuck your pelvis bone back to help avoid arching the lower back. The path of your feet should be as wide as your shoulders. You should land on your heel with the foot at about a 45° angle to the ground, rolling your foot naturally on the outside to your toes, and then pushing off vigorously (fig. 3.18). Research indicates that most individuals self-select a pace fast enough to achieve an appropriate target heart rate and RPE.

Table 3.6 details a walking program for individuals who may be at a low level of physical fitness, so jogging may be too strenuous for them. Individuals with excess body fat should also start with such a walking program. The target heart rate method should be used here and may be adjusted downward during the initial week, maybe to a level of 40 to 50 percent. As you improve your fitness, you may wish to include skipping in your walking program; it is more strenuous and will help to increase your heart rate, but it is also more likely to cause injuries due to the increased force of foot impact.

Jogging and running are strenuous activities and will usually be effective means for reaching your target heart rate. Table 3.7 provides for a rapid progression to jogging, using an interval training approach. **Interval training** was developed primarily for athletes, but its principles of alternating rest and exercise periods may also be applied to aerobic training for the nonathlete. Again, the heart rate and RPE should be monitored during this program to check whether you are within the target range.

Aerobic Dancing

By now, you should know the meaning of the word *aerobic* as it relates to exercise. And, for most of us, dancing is fun. Combining the two, we have a fun way to exercise. Exercise to music has been around for years, but it was not until the 1970s that aerobic dancing was developed. In essence, **aerobic dancing** is simply exercising to music. In a stricter sense, such as the method pioneered by Jackie Sorensen, aerobic dancing has been choreographed to contain certain percentages of (1) simple vigorous dance steps to improve aerobic capacity, (2) stretching movements to improve flexibility, and (3) muscle-toning movements (fig. 3.19).

Aerobic dancing has become increasingly popular in the past ten years, particularly among women. As a result, a number of organizations have been developed to capitalize on this trend—some reputable, others not. If you are interested in joining a commercial aerobic dance program, you should ask questions to see if it meets the guidelines set forth in this chapter and in chapter 12.

What are the qualifications of the instructor and is she/he certified by a recognized national association, such as the American College of Sports Medicine?
Does the program screen for medical problems?
Does the program use the ACSM exercise prescription guidelines in relation to intensity, duration, and frequency?
Is the program progressive in nature?
Does the program allow for a warm-up and a warm-down period?

Research has shown that both high-impact and low-impact (soft) aerobic dancing are effective means to reach the target HR range. High-impact aerobic dancing is more vigorous as the legs are lifted higher and the foot may land with greater impact; in soft aerobics, one foot usually remains in contact with the exercise surface. Step aerobics, use of hand weights, and water aerobics can help to modify exercise intensity. Well-designed aerobic dance programs can improve aerobic fitness comparable to walk-jog programs.

Table 3.6 Sample Aerobic Walking Program*

	Warm-Up	Target Zone Exercising	Warm-Down	Total Time
Week 1	Walk slowly 5 minutes	Walk briskly 5 minutes	Walk slowly 5 minutes	15 minutes
Week 2	Walk slowly 5 minutes	Walk briskly 7 minutes	Walk slowly 5 minutes	17 minutes
Week 3	Walk slowly 5 minutes	Walk briskly 9 minutes	Walk slowly 5 minutes	19 minutes
Week 4	Walk slowly 5 minutes	Walk briskly 11 minutes	Walk slowly 5 minutes	21 minutes
Week 5	Walk slowly 5 minutes	Walk briskly 13 minutes	Walk slowly 5 minutes	23 minutes
Week 6	Walk slowly 5 minutes	Walk briskly 15 minutes	Walk slowly 5 minutes	25 minutes
Week 7	Walk slowly 5 minutes	Walk briskly 18 minutes	Walk slowly 5 minutes	28 minutes
Week 8	Walk slowly 5 minutes	Walk briskly 20 minutes	Walk slowly 5 minutes	30 minutes
Week 9	Walk slowly 5 minutes	Walk briskly 23 minutes	Walk slowly 5 minutes	33 minutes
Week 10	Walk slowly 5 minutes	Walk briskly 26 minutes	Walk slowly 5 minutes	36 minutes
Week 11	Walk slowly 5 minutes	Walk briskly 28 minutes	Walk slowly 5 minutes	38 minutes
Week 12	Walk slowly 5 minutes	Walk briskly 30 minutes	Walk slowly 5 minutes	40 minutes

From week 13 on, check your pulse periodically to see if you are exercising within your target heart rate range. As you become more fit, walk faster to increase your heart rate toward the upper levels of your target range. Follow the principle of progression.

Note: If you find a particular week's pattern tiring, repeat it before going on to the next pattern. You do not have to complete the walking program in 12 weeks. Remember that your goals are to continue getting the benefits you are seeking and to enjoy your activity. Listen to your body and progress less rapidly, if necessary.

*Program should include *at least* three exercise sessions per week.

Source: U.S. Department of Health and Human Services.

Table 3.7 Sample Aerobic Jogging Program (Interval Training)*

	Warm-Up	Target Zone Exercising	Warm-Down	Total Time
Week 1	Stretch and limber up 5 minutes	Walk (nonstop) 10 minutes	Walk slowly 3 minutes; stretch 2 minutes	20 minutes
Week 2	Stretch and limber up 5 minutes	Walk 5 minutes; jog 1 minute; walk 5 minutes; jog 1 minute	Walk slowly 3 minutes; stretch 2 minutes	22 minutes
Week 3	Stretch and limber up 5 minutes	Walk 5 minutes; jog 3 minutes; walk 5 minutes; jog 3 minutes	Walk slowly 3 minutes; stretch 2 minutes	26 minutes
Week 4	Stretch and limber up 5 minutes	Walk 5 minutes; jog 4 minutes; walk 5 minutes; jog 4 minutes	Walk slowly 3 minutes; stretch 2 minutes	28 minutes
Week 5	Stretch and limber up 5 minutes	Walk 4 minutes; jog 5 minutes; walk 4 minutes; jog 5 minutes	Walk slowly 3 minutes; stretch 2 minutes	28 minutes
Week 6	Stretch and limber up 5 minutes	Walk 4 minutes; jog 6 minutes; walk 4 minutes; jog 6 minutes	Walk slowly 3 minutes; stretch 2 minutes	30 minutes
Week 7	Stretch and limber up 5 minutes	Walk 4 minutes; jog 7 minutes; walk 4 minutes; jog 7 minutes	Walk slowly 3 minutes; stretch 2 minutes	32 minutes
Week 8	Stretch and limber up 5 minutes	Walk 4 minutes; jog 8 minutes; walk 4 minutes; jog 8 minutes	Walk slowly 3 minutes; stretch 2 minutes	34 minutes
Week 9	Stretch and limber up 5 minutes	Walk 4 minutes; jog 9 minutes; walk 4 minutes; jog 9 minutes	Walk slowly 3 minutes; stretch 2 minutes	36 minutes
Week 10	Stretch and limber up 5 minutes	Walk 4 minutes; jog 13 minutes	Walk slowly 3 minutes; stretch 2 minutes	27 minutes
Week 11	Stretch and limber up 5 minutes	Walk 4 minutes; jog 15 minutes	Walk slowly 3 minutes; stretch 2 minutes	29 minutes
Week 12	Stretch and limber up 5 minutes	Walk 4 minutes; jog 17 minutes	Walk slowly 3 minutes; stretch 2 minutes	31 minutes
Week 13	Stretch and limber up 5 minutes	Walk 2 minutes, jog slowly 2 minutes; jog 17 minutes	Walk slowly 3 minutes; stretch 2 minutes	31 minutes
Week 14	Stretch and limber up 5 minutes	Walk 1 minutes; jog slowly 3 minutes; jog 17 minutes	Walk slowly 3 minutes; stretch 2 minutes	31 minutes
Week 15	Stretch and limber up 5 minutes	Jog slowly 3 minutes; jog 17 minutes	Walk slowly 3 minutes; stretch 2 minutes	30 minutes

From week 16 on, check your pulse periodically to see if you are exercising with your target zone. As you become more fit, try exercising within the upper range of your target zone.

Note: If you find a particular week's pattern tiring, repeat it before going on to the next pattern. You do not have to complete the jogging program in 15 weeks. Remember that your goals are to continue getting the benefits you are seeking and to enjoy your activity.

*Program should include *at least* three exercise sessions per week.

Source: U.S. Department of Health and Human Services.

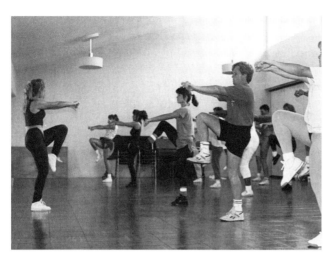

Figure 3.19 *Aerobic dancing can be an effective means of improving cardiovascular fitness for both males and females.*

It may be quite expensive to enroll in a commercial aerobic dance class, but most colleges and universities offer physical education classes for credit or free workouts through recreation or student activities programs. Another option is to design your own aerobic exercise program to music. Although it may take some time and effort, you will be able to exercise to music you really enjoy. Simply follow these steps.

1. Compile a number of your favorite records that have good 4-count beats to them. Use your stopwatch to count the total number of 4-count beats per minute (4-count BPM); 1–2–3–4 would be one 4-count beat. If a record had thirty 4-count BPM and if you exercised with the beat, you would do thirty repetitions of a 4-count exercise each minute.

2. Select records with different 4-count BPM. Use the following as a guide to developing your aerobic dance workout.

Exercise Phase	4-Count BPM	Time (Minutes)
Warm-up	20–30	5–10
Stretching	15–20	3–5
Stimulus	35–45	15–45
Warm-down	20–30	5–10

3. Select the exercises you will do for each phase; arrange them in a logical sequence. Determine how many exercises you want to do for each song; if a song has forty 4-count BPM and is 5 minutes long, you could do 5 different exercises for one minute each, or forty repetitions for each.

4. Use a high-quality tape to record your songs in the sequence of warm-up, stretching, stimulus, and warm-down. Design a program to fit your needs, about 30 to 60 minutes total time.

5. Check your heart rate responses before, during, and after your dance or exercise routine. Determine your target HR from table 3.3.

Still another option is to purchase one of the many videotapes on aerobic dancing exercise for home use. There are a number of good programs on the market that are relatively inexpensive. Some package deals are available, e.g., videotape, step-bench, and hand weights.

You may also apply the concept of interval training to aerobic dancing. Simply intersperse your more active stimulus periods with periods of less intense exercise, such as stretching or walking in place.

Another recent innovative approach is **circuit aerobics,** a form of exercise in which aerobic dancing and resistance exercises, such as weight lifting, are combined. Such programs provide an adequate aerobic stimulus and also facilitate the development of muscle tone. Some additional information will be presented in the next chapter.

In the beginning, if you want to start with a less intense aerobic dancing program, try the low-impact or soft aerobics versions in which there is less jarring motion of the legs to the floor. Done properly, they may be vigorous and provide an excellent aerobic workout, and they are less likely than the high-impact version to lead to injury. Both high- and low-impact aerobic dance styles can be high intensity, requiring 10–11 Calories per minute. Step benches and hand weights can also be used to increase exercise intensity.

Rope Jumping

A number of recent research studies have shown that rope jumping may be a very effective means to achieve the target HR range and thus is an effective mode for an aerobic fitness program. In fact, it may be too strenuous for the sedentary individual who is just beginning an exercise program. For such a person, a walking-jogging program might precede a rope-jumping program. In these studies, the turn rates for the rope varied from 66 to 160 per minute (RPM).

Rope jumping at a high RPM requires skill, but you can learn the skill through practice. You are more prone to foot and knee injuries due to the repeated force of foot impact. Using a padded landing surface may help to prevent injuries.

In order to individualize a rope-jumping program in relation to your target HR range, simply follow the protocol of Laboratory Inventory 3.2 and vary the RPM of the rope for each test. Heavier, weighted ropes are available that will increase the exercise intensity; however, they may be more likely to contribute to injuries.

Other Aerobic Activities

Although the emphasis here has been on a walk-jog-run mode of training, a wide variety of activities may be utilized to elicit an aerobic training effect. For those who desire to exercise indoors, particularly during inclement weather, rope jumping, aerobic sliding, stationary jogging, or stair climbing may be effective. Moreover, a host of exercise machines are available. Treadmills may be used for a walk-jog-run program, but stationary bicycles, rowing apparatus, and cross-country skiing machines may also be used to provide adequate aerobic exercise stimulus. Many of these exercise

Table 3.8 Motivation for Running at Different Levels of Consciousness

	Consciousness I	Consciousness II	Consciousness III
Activity	Jogging	Running	Racing
Weekly Mileage	5–15	30–50	50 and up
Type of Training	Jog/walk	Long slow distance	Hard day/easy day
Short-Term Goal	Aerobic points	Finish a marathon	Qualify for Boston Marathon
Long-Term Goal	Avoid heart disease	Improve best times	Age-group awards
Primary Motivation	Health and appearance	Accomplishment	Success

Source: From Hal Higdon, in The Runner, *4:52–53. Copyright © 1983 Hal Higdon. Reprinted by permission of the author.*

devices use modern computer technology to motivate you to exercise, such as a video display of you racing a rival in a 2,500-meter rowing race. Some interactive video games monitor your heart rate so that you must increase it in order to escape from some type of danger, adding fun and excitement to home exercise programs. One advantage of some home exercises is that you may be able to do two things at one time. You may not only exercise, but study, read, or watch television at the same time. Become a super spud instead of a couch potato.

The interested student should consult Dr. Kenneth Cooper's most recent book on aerobics, *The Aerobics Program for Total Well-Being,* for aerobic data on such activities as basketball, bicycling, swimming, stationary running, and many others. An alternative method is to select exercises presented in chapter 7 as means to control body weight. These exercises are based upon approximate caloric expenditure per minute. Appendix C has been developed to facilitate the implementation of this approach.

In essence, however, the application of the overload principle, using the target HR as the method to determine exercise intensity, may be used with almost any mode of exercise to develop your personal aerobic exercise program. Exercise in your target zone for 20 to 60 minutes at least three to four days per week.

Aerobic Competitive Sports

Although improvement of your personal health or appearance may be the primary motivation for initiating a fitness program, your motivational stimulus may change as you become more fit. Hal Higdon, an accomplished runner and a popular writer on the running scene, described three levels of consciousness through which many runners progress after initiating their personal fitness program (see table 3.8). Although accomplishment and success may replace health and appearance as the primary motivational factors for exercising, the health-related benefits will be the same, and possibly of a greater magnitude

If you get into training for athletic competition, you may ask yourself, how good can I be? What are my physical limitations and how may these guide me in determining my fitness objectives above and beyond those necessary for health? The two key determinants responsible for your success in athletics are genetics and training.

Genetics, the traits and characteristics we inherit from our parents, endow some of us with the physical ability to be very strong or very fast, while others may have inherited the capability for endurance activities. Somatotype, or body build, is also inherited. Some individuals are predisposed toward a muscular body, while others may have a tendency toward leanness or heaviness. The upper limits of such factors as maximal oxygen uptake and muscle fiber type, important determinants of endurance capacity, are estimated to be over 90 percent determined by your genetic endowment.

What do these genetic limitations mean to you? Let us explore the role of genetic endowment relative to maximal oxygen uptake, a very important determinant of endurance capacity. Individuals such as Belayneh Dinsamo from Ethiopia and Ingrid Christensen from Norway, male and female world record holders for the marathon, inherited a high maximal oxygen uptake capacity and, hence, the potential for world-class performance. However, they would not have become world record holders if they had not undergone an intensive program of physical training to not only develop their maximal oxygen uptake to its greatest capacity, but to exercise at a high percentage of their maximum without inducing early fatigue. The rest of us, even if we trained as intensively as Belayneh and Ingrid, would not be able to reach their performance levels because we do not have their genetic potential. However, with a proper training program, almost all of us could complete a 26.2-mile marathon. A proper training program will increase your maximal oxygen uptake toward its genetic potential and will increase your ability to perform at a higher percentage of that maximum without fatigue. Thus, although genetics may set the upper limits, an optimal performance within your own genetic limitations can still be attained with proper training.

Although there are sophisticated laboratory techniques to determine physiological and biomechanical characteristics essential for success in various sports, for most of us the proof is in our performances. For example, a friend of mine has been trying for a number of years to break the 3-hour barrier in the marathon; he even has a personalized license plate on his car, 2:59:59. He has established a specific measure of how good he believes he can be, and his achievement of that objective will be the proof he needs to substantiate that belief.

There are a number of opportunities to become involved in competitive sports that are aerobic in nature, but the most common involve running, cycling, swimming, and the combination

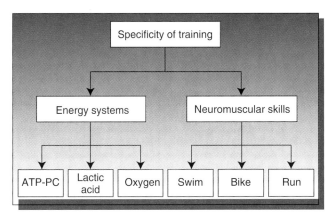

Figure 3.20 *Specificity of training. There are two general aspects of training specificity. First, if you want to improve a particular energy system, exercise at an intensity level that stresses that particular system. Second, the training effect is better if you use the actual activity for which you are training. For example, if you want to improve in swimming, you should swim to train the specific neural patterns and muscle groups involved.*

of the three, triathloning. If you enjoy running, you may get involved in competition such as a 10K road race (10 kilometers or 6.2 miles), and often the first goal is simply to finish the race. In subsequent races, your goal may be to run faster than the last race, to establish a personal record (PR), or to eventually place in the top five in your age group. In order to become more competitive, you will need to train harder. You will still use the same general training principles of overload, progression, and specificity. However, one or two workouts per week should be devoted to higher levels of intensity, training at race pace or faster for shorter distances, often referred to as interval, tempo, or repetition training. These workouts should stress specific energy systems and muscle groups (see fig. 3.20). It is beyond the scope of this book to discuss such training methods in detail. Most communities, and some colleges and universities, have clubs that focus on training and competition in aerobic sports, including aerobic dancing. Local contacts may be stores that market running or cycling equipment or the recreational sports department on campus, for such organizations can often provide resources to help guide you in your training.

Although training for sports competition may enhance your motivation to adhere to an aerobic exercise program, it may not confer any additional health benefits beyond a threshold maximal level of aerobic exercise, as discussed below. Moreover, such training programs often increase markedly in intensity and duration, two factors that may increase risks, particularly injuries, associated with overtraining.

Aerobic Leisure and Unstructured Physical Activity

One of the major reasons for the decline in the fitness of Americans is an increasingly sedentary life-style; one of the major villains is excessive television viewing. Because so many Americans are completely sedentary, and because even a certain minimal level of aerobic exercise may confer some health benefits, there may be considerable value in simply getting people to increase the amount of exercise they do during their daily activities and leisure time. This is the major thrust of recent exercise initiatives advanced by governmental agencies such as the Centers for Disease Control and Prevention and professional organizations such as the American College of Sports Medicine. As mentioned in chapter 2, the ACSM has introduced a program entitled *Exercise Lite,* and the address to receive information on this program is on page 16. Two excellent books, *Fitness Without Exercise* by Bryant Stamford and Porter Shimer and *Living with Exercise* by Steven Blair, have focused on this approach to health-related fitness. The major thesis in both books is "just get moving."

As mentioned in chapter 2, unstructured physical activity includes many of the usual activities of daily living, such as climbing stairs, gardening, and housework. In order to increase the amount of aerobic energy we expend in these activities, we may have to make them somewhat structured, mostly by increasing two components of the exercise prescription, frequency and duration. Blair suggests giving yourself occasional reminders, perhaps taping the words *Move* or *Exercise* on your refrigerator at home, the dashboard of your car, or your telephone at work. This strategy may help remind you to climb the stairs more at home or at work (frequency) or to park your car some distance from your office so you need to walk farther (duration). You can probably think of dozens of ways to incorporate more unstructured physical activity into your daily schedule, depending upon your particular life-style, but one idea is to simply take three to six mini-walks during the course of the day. Three 10-minute walks will provide you with 30 minutes of exercise, a recommended daily goal. Don't just sit, but stand, walk, move!

What you do during your leisure time may also help improve your health, for a number of sports or recreational activities of low intensity may confer some health benefits. For example, research has shown that playing golf three times a week, walking eighteen holes, would improve serum cholesterol levels. Other activities, such as softball, badminton, soccer, racquet sports, and dancing, will also help increase energy expenditure. Appendix C lists a wide variety of recreational activities and related levels of caloric expenditure. Such activities may also enhance opportunities for social interaction, and, for those with families, may provide for some quality family time.

As noted in chapter 2, involvement in leisure activities and increased frequency and duration of unstructured physical activity may confer some health benefits, but possibly not to the level associated with a structured aerobic exercise program. Nevertheless, these types of activities are highly recommended, not only because of possible health benefits, but because they may stimulate interest and participation in more structured aerobic exercise programs.

Benefit-Risk Ratio

Medicines are developed because they provide some benefits to us. However, the dosage has to be appropriate. In the same way, the "dosage" of exercise must be considered. There is some debate about exactly how much exercise is needed to reap certain health benefits, but some general recommendations are available. Based primarily upon epidemiological research that involves the relationship between physical activity and all causes of mortality, it appears that a minimal threshold level of physical activity, structured or unstructured, that may confer some health benefits is the equivalent of approximately 500 Calories per week. We shall deal with exercise and caloric expenditure in chapter 7 and learn how to use Appendix C, but you can peruse Appendix C at this time to determine approximately how many Calories per minute you use for a wide variety of physical activities. As an example, however, 500 Calories would be the equivalent of about 8 miles of leisurely walking per week for an average-sized adult male, or just over a mile per day.

There also appears to be a dose-response relationship between physical activity and reduced mortality rates. Research conducted with Americans by Blair and Paffenbarger suggests that increased benefits will occur with a weekly energy expenditure of 2,000 Calories or more, which may be achieved through unstructured or structured physical activity or a combination of the two. A recent study by Morris, who pioneered the relationship between exercise and mortality in his landmark 1953 report, supports these findings of Blair and Paffenbarger. However, in order to be effective, Morris contends that the intensity of the physical activity in the British subjects he studied needed to be moderately intense, also referred to as being vigorous or causing the individual to be "out of breath" at times. Such activity included swimming, badminton, tennis, football (soccer), rowing, jogging, and brisk walking. Lee and others recently reported similar findings with American men. For a structured exercise program, 2,000 Calories per week would be the equivalent of jogging 15–20 miles or walking about 32 miles. For jogging, an appropriate plan would be 4–5 miles four days per week.

Based on the available data, a recommended short-range goal would be to increase physical activity to 500 Calories per week, with a long-range goal of 2,000 Calories or more per week. Although some research suggests that vigorous aerobic activity or structured aerobic exercise programs, such as those adhering to the ACSM guidelines, might be more beneficial, simply increasing the frequency and duration of unstructured and leisure-time physical activity will confer significant health benefits, particularly for those who have been completely sedentary.

Risks

Medicines may also be associated with a certain degree of risk to the patient. For example, penicillin and other antibiotics help cure infections. However, some individuals are allergic to penicillin. For them, the allergic reaction may be more serious than the infection it was designed to cure. In a related manner, although exercise will elicit health benefits in most individuals, it may not be advisable for others, such as those with certain cardiac complications. Moreover, exercise may pose some risk even to the apparently healthy individual.

The risks of exercise can be categorized under five general headings: hidden heart problems, muscular soreness and injuries, heat illnesses, cold-weather running risks, and safety concerns.

Hidden Heart Problems

One of the most popular forms of exercise to sweep the United States in the past quarter-century is an aerobic program of jogging and running. Periodically, however, the communications media question the safety of such an exercise program by publishing such articles as "Running is dangerous to your health" or "Jogging can kill you." Occasionally, you will also read in the newspaper that a jogger died while exercising. Such incidents are likely to raise a question in your mind about the actual safety of an exercise program. Several startling incidents were the cardiac deaths of Jim Fixx, the middle-aged author of a best-selling book on running, while running on a country road, and Hank Gathers, a young collegiate basketball standout who collapsed and died during an intercollegiate contest.

This issue has been studied by several groups of researchers, and they suggest that a small (though not negligible) risk exists of acute cardiovascular problems (such as heart attack) for adults participating in a vigorous exercise program. The prevalence of such problems is most common in individuals who are susceptible to cardiovascular disorders. These deaths occur mostly in susceptible individuals who may be participating in competitive events that overexcite the heart, who are heavy smokers, or who do not exercise on a regular basis. The death rate during jogging is about seven times greater than the estimated death rate during more sedentary activities, but only in susceptible individuals. There have been no deaths reported for those whose hearts were tested and found to be healthy. Most reported deaths during jogging are in middle-aged individuals who already had a diseased heart, such as Jim Fixx.

However, one often reads of sudden deaths in young, highly-trained athletes who do not appear to have diseased hearts. In recent reviews of such deaths, atherosclerotic heart disease was not a very common occurrence, although it was noted in several cases. The most common cause in cardiac deaths for those under thirty years of age was a structural cardiovascular abnormality that appeared to interfere with normal heart function. Again, although different in nature, a cardiovascular problem existed in these victims prior to exercise, such as Hank Gathers.

Although the heart-health benefits far outweigh the risks for most individuals, exercise may aggravate existing hidden heart problems. Individuals who may be prone to coronary heart disease should consult a physician before initiating an exercise program. This topic was covered previously; you may want to consult pages 18–19 for a review, particularly if you are over thirty-five years of age.

Whether or not you have had a medical examination, you should be aware of symptoms occurring during or after exercise that may be indicative of cardiovascular problems. Stop exercising and consult a physician if you experience any of the following (fig. 3.21):

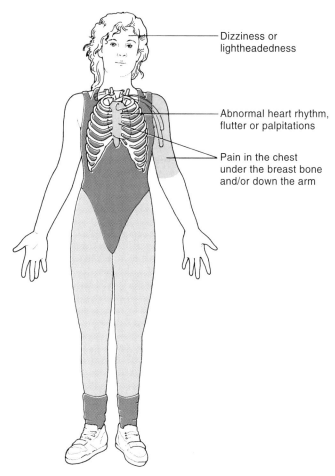

Dizziness or
lightheadedness

Abnormal heart rhythm,
flutter or palpitations

Pain in the chest
under the breast bone
and/or down the arm

Figure 3.21 *Body signals to stop exercising. If you experience
any of these symptoms during exercise, stop immediately and rest.
Consult a physician if they persist.*

1. Dizziness, light-headedness, confusion, or fainting.
2. Irregular pulse rate or palpitations of the heart (flutters, or changes rate very rapidly—either too fast or too slow), known as arrhythmias.
3. Pain or sensation of pressure in the chest or under the breastbone; such pain may radiate to the left arm, left shoulder, or the jaw.
4. Unaccustomed shortness of breath during exercise.

Muscular Soreness and Injuries

If you develop and implement an exercise program properly, you should experience little problem as you continue to train. The key to avoiding problems is to start easily and to progress slowly. However, most individuals overdo it at one time or another and eventually end up with either sore muscles or an injury.

Basically there are two types of muscle soreness. *Acute soreness* occurs during exercise and appears to be due to inadequate circulation to the exercising muscle. The lack of blood flow leads to an accumulation of metabolic by-products of exercise in the muscle. These by-products can stimulate pain receptors and cause pain or soreness, which usually disappears when you stop exercising. A second type, called *delayed soreness,* usually occurs 24 to 48 hours after an exercise period and may persist for several days. This type of muscle soreness is usually caused by exercise bouts that involve repetitive, strenuous muscle contractions. For example, as you run downhill, you put a tremendous stress on the leg muscles as they try to control your body from moving too fast (due to gravity's pull). In aerobic dance, you may land repeatedly on your toes, which will overwork the muscles in your lower leg. This stress appears to tear the connective tissue and/or muscle fibers, causing inflammation that, according to the most current theory, may be the cause of the delayed soreness. A stretching program may be helpful for relief, but generally rest and/or reduced activity levels for several days are necessary to let the soreness run its course and gradually fade away.

Muscle soreness will usually limit exercise for a few days at the most. However, an injury may incapacitate you for weeks or months—depending upon its type and severity. All individuals who become physically active can, at one time or another, expect to be injured. Certain types of activities predispose to a specific injury (bruised palms in handball, heel bruises in running). In many cases, injuries can be prevented by the use of proper equipment, technique, and conditioning, but even these factors are not able to prevent some acute injuries that happen very suddenly (a sprained ankle due to uneven terrain, a sprained wrist incurred during a fall).

A common cause of several types of injuries is overuse, particularly during the early stages of an exercise program. The exercise may be too intense, too long, or too frequent, not allowing sufficient time for recovery. As you begin an exercise program, you make rapid gains in fitness; this often encourages you to overexert yourself. For example, your normal progression on a jogging program may call for a 2-mile jog, but you may feel good and decide to do 5 miles that day. The next day you feel some tenderness in your shin bone, Achilles tendon, or knee. It may not be sore enough to prevent you from running, so you continue to overdo it. Eventually, the pain gets so severe that you must stop training due to a case of shinsplints, Achilles tendinitis, or chondromalacia of the knee. You are a victim of the overuse syndrome. Hence, one of the keys to injury prevention is to follow a proper progression in your training program and to avoid sudden increases in the intensity and duration of exercise.

Since walking, jogging, running, aerobic dance, and rope jumping are recommended aerobic exercises, several of the main injuries that occur are highlighted in table 3.9. Most of these injuries are due to overuse and the force of impact when you land, so walking may be less likely to lead to such injuries. Poor foot mechanics may also be a contributing factor to injury.

Table 3.9   Common Injuries in Running, Aerobic Dance, and Rope Jumping

Injury	Symptoms	Cause	Prevention/Treatment
Plantar fasciitis; an inflammation of the plantar fascia, a tough band of tissue on the bottom of your foot	Tenderness or pain on the bottom of the foot near the heel	Landing on hard surfaces Inadequate cushioning in shoes Landing on toes Running uphill	Exercise on soft surfaces Use well-cushioned shoes or customized orthotics Ice after exercise Rest if pain is severe; switch to other exercises like cycling
Achilles tendinitis; an inflammation in the Achilles tendon on the lower back portion of your calf	Tenderness, swelling, or pain where the Achilles attaches to the back of your heel or where the tendon emerges from your muscle	Overuse causes tears in the tendon Landing on toes Running uphill, excessively stretching the tendon Inadequate cushioning in heel Poor foot biomechanics	Stretching and warm-up Proper shoes or orthotics inserts Use of a heel lift, such as a sponge insert Ice and anti-inflammatory drugs Rest if pain is severe
Shinsplints; a general term for pain around the tibia (shin); most common form is inflammation of tendons	Tenderness, swelling, or pain just behind and above the bony protrusion (malleolus) on the inside of the lower leg	Poor foot biomechanics leading to overpronation; the foot rolls to the inside excessively Running consistently on a road with an inclination (camber) Excessive running mileage; rapid increase in number of miles/week Excessive aerobic dancing; high impact on toes	Proper shoes or orthotics to prevent poor biomechanics Exercise on soft surfaces Ice and anti-inflammatory drugs Rest if pain is severe; switch to other aerobic exercises
Chondromalacia; a softening of the cartilage around the kneecap (patella)	Tenderness or pain near the top of the kneecap; movement, such as climbing stairs, will elicit pain; may hear a crunching sound while moving the kneecap around with your fingers	Excessive movement of the kneecap while exercising irritates the cartilage under the kneecap Poor foot biomechanics	Proper shoes or orthotics to correct faulty foot biomechanics Strengthen your quadriceps (thigh) muscles Ice and anti-inflammatory drugs Rest if pain is severe; switch to other aerobic exercises
Iliotibial band injury; inflammation of the iliotibial band, a strong layer of connective tissue near the outside area of the knee	Tenderness or severe pain on the lateral outside part of your knee; bending of the knee, such as squatting, will elicit pain	Overuse injury caused by excessive exercise Poor foot biomechanics	Decrease intensity and duration of exercise Ice and anti-inflammatory drugs Proper shoes or orthotics to correct poor foot biomechanics Complete rest may be required; switch to other aerobic exercises
Stress fracture; a small crack in a bone, usually in the foot or shin bone	Tenderness, pain, and possible swelling in the area of the fracture	Excessive exercise placing too much stress on the foot or shin Exercising on hard surfaces Poor foot biomechanics	Exercise on soft surfaces Proper cushioning in shoes Adequate stretching before and after exercise Complete rest if stress fracture is diagnosed
Stitch in the side	Pain, mild to severe, during exercise occurring just under the lower part of the rib cage	Unknown, but believed due to inadequate blood supply or oxygen to the diaphragm or other respiratory muscles	Stop exercising, stretch arm by raising arm overhead. Massage area. If onset is mild, try shallow breathing

Space does not permit a full coverage of all the means to prevent injuries in all types of activities, but the following may be helpful.

1. Warm up thoroughly before your activity. Stretching exercises for the Achilles tendon and groin area are helpful before and after jogging or running. See chapter 5 for appropriate stretching exercises.

2. Do not progress too rapidly in the early stages of training. Take it easy and follow a gradual progression.

3. Listen to your body. Minor aches and pains are early warning signals. If they persist when you are resting, lay off for a day or so to help avoid developing a more serious condition. Minor aches and pains may be relieved by rest, anti-inflammatory agents such as ibuprofen or aspirin, or the application of ice to the injured area.

4. Try to avoid situations that may change your running biomechanics and lead to ankle, knee, or hip problems. Avoid running too much in one direction on a slanted road. Keep the soles of your shoes in good repair so that one side is not worn down excessively. Avoid a lot of either uphill or downhill running. Check your shoes for proper fit so your foot does not roll in toward the inside excessively.

5. Avoid hard surfaces (concrete surfaces for jogging and hard floors for aerobic dancing and rope jumping), as persistent impact may contribute to shinsplints.

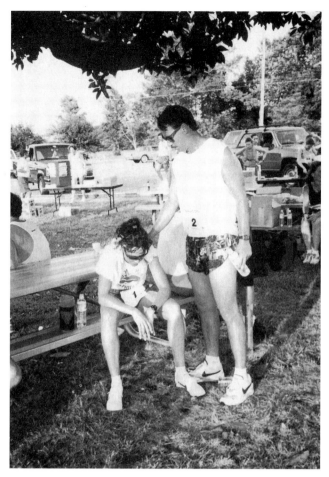

Figure 3.22 *If proper precautions are not taken, exercise in the heat may lead to weakness or severe heat injury.*

6. If you are injured, substitute other aerobic activities that do not aggravate the injury. Cycling, rowing, cross-country skiing, or exercise machines may help preserve cardiorespiratory fitness. If you have access to a pool, you may be able to maintain your aerobic fitness through water exercises. For example, you may run in the low end of the pool if the water is about chest level. The buoyancy will reduce the force of your foot impact. Flotation vests are also available to keep your head out of the water in the deep end. Wearing a pair of running shoes will help to increase the resistance and give you a better training effect. Special inflatable cuffs for your ankles provide both buoyancy and resistance.

Heat Illnesses

Be aware of the signs of heat illnesses when exercising in hot weather. Excessive fatigue, weakness, nausea, and cramps may be indicative of heat exhaustion (fig. 3.22). Headache, disorientation, and a high body temperature may signal the onset of heat stroke. If you experience these symptoms, stop exercising, seek a cool place to rest, and drink cool fluids.

The following suggestions may be helpful in the prevention of heat illnesses.

1. Check the temperature and humidity conditions before exercising. Adjust your intensity as needed. Hot, humid conditions cause fatigue sooner, so slow your pace or decrease the duration of your activity. A heat index for heat disorders is presented in figure 3.23.

2. Exercise in the cool of the morning or evening in order to avoid the heat of the day.

3. Exercise in the shade, if possible, in order to avoid radiation from the sun.

4. Wear as little clothing as possible. That which is worn should be loose to allow air circulation, white to reflect radiant heat, and porous to permit evaporation to occur. Some of the new sportswear available satisfy these criteria. In particular, avoid the use of plastic or rubberized sweatsuits; such suits may increase your sweat rate, but since evaporation is prevented, your body temperature may increase rapidly.

5. Drink fluids periodically. If on a long training run, have your route planned so you know where some watering holes may be (gas stations or other public sources of water). Take frequent water breaks, consuming about 6 to 8 ounces of water every 15 minutes or so. During exercise, thirst is not an adequate stimulus to replace water losses, so you should drink before you get thirsty. To help cool down after exercising, pour water over your head and chest.

6. Replenish your water daily. Keep a record of your body weight. For each pound you lose, drink 1 pint of fluid. Your body weight should be back to normal before your next exercise workout.

7. Hyperhydrate if you plan to perform prolonged strenuous exercise in the heat. This means drinking about 16 to 32 ounces of fluid 30 to 60 minutes prior to exercising.

8. Replenish lost electrolytes (salt) if you have sweat excessively. Put a little extra salt on your meals unless you have a problem with high blood pressure that is aggravated by excess sodium. Eat foods high in potassium, such as bananas and citrus fruits. Additional information on nutrition is presented in chapter 6.

9. If you are sedentary, overweight, or older, you are less likely to tolerate exercise in the heat and should, therefore, use extra caution.

10. If you are going to compete in a sport that is held under hot environmental conditions, you must become acclimatized to exercise in the heat. You can do this by exercising in the heat for seven to fourteen days before the event, but exercise at a much reduced intensity. Your body will gradually adjust to exercise in the heat, but you still will not be able to perform as well as you do in cooler weather.

If you are monitoring your heart rate as a guide to your training intensity, you will probably note that you have a higher exercise heart rate at a lower exercise intensity while performing in the heat. The need to channel extra blood to

Relative humidity (%)

Air temp (°F)	0	5	10	15	20	25	30	35	40	45	50	55	60	65	70	75	80	85	90	95	100
140	125																				
135	120	128																			
130	117	122	131																		
125	111	116	123	131	141																
120	107	111	116	123	130	139	148														
115	103	107	111	115	120	127	135	143	151												
110	99	102	105	108	112	117	123	130	137	143	150										
105	95	97	100	102	105	109	113	118	123	129	135	142	149								
100	91	93	95	97	99	101	104	107	110	115	120	126	132	138	144						
95	87	88	90	91	93	94	96	98	101	104	107	110	114	119	124	130	136				
90	83	84	85	86	87	88	90	91	93	95	96	98	100	102	106	109	113	117	122		
85	78	79	80	81	82	83	84	85	86	87	88	89	90	91	93	95	97	99	102	105	108
80	73	74	75	76	77	77	78	79	79	80	81	81	82	83	85	86	86	87	88	89	91
75	69	69	70	71	72	72	73	73	74	74	75	75	76	76	77	77	78	78	79	79	80
70	64	64	65	65	66	66	67	67	68	68	69	69	70	70	70	70	71	71	71	71	72

Heat index (or apparent temperature)

Heat index/heat disorders

Heat index	Possible heat disorders for people in higher risk groups
130° or higher	Heatstroke/sunstroke highly likely with continued exposure.
105° – 130°	Sunstroke, heat cramps, or heat exhaustion likely, and heatstroke possible with prolonged exposure and/or physical activity.
90° – 105°	Sunstroke, heat cramps and heat exhaustion possible with prolonged exposure and/or physical activity.
80° – 90°	Fatigue possible with prolonged exposure and/or physical activity.

Figure 3.23 *The heat index, or apparent temperature, is based on the combination of air temperature and relative humidity. For any given air temperature, the heat index increases with increased levels of relative humidity. A guide to heat disorders based on the heat index is provided.*

both your muscles and skin (for cooling purposes) imposes an additional work load on the heart. Consequently, exercise intensity must be reduced somewhat in order not to exceed the recommended target HR range. Research has shown the RPE to be an effective means to evaluate appropriate exercise intensity under warm environmental conditions.

Cold-Weather Running

Cold weather does not usually pose a problem if you dress properly for it. Some general suggestions are

1. Cover your head, hands, and wrists. Your head and neck can lose up to 40 percent of your body heat, and you feel warmer if your hands and wrists are warm.

2. Wear several layers of light clothing with a windbreaker on the outside. Some of the newer cold-weather running gear is designed to be lightweight yet very warm and allows sweat to dissipate without getting your clothing too wet. Rainproof running gear is also available.

3. Check the prevailing wind conditions. It is usually best to go out against the wind and return with the wind at your back. Since the wind chill is less when the wind is with you, you are less likely to chill down if your clothes are wet with sweat produced while exercising in several layers of clothing. Cover your ears, nose, and face to prevent frostbite in very cold, windy conditions.

4. Do not remain outside after finishing your workout. You are likely to cool down rapidly. Change to dry clothing and seek a warmer environment.

Properly dressed, you can exercise outside in almost any weather. However, if you would prefer to stay inside and avoid the cold, home aerobic exercise programs such as stationary bicycling, treadmill running, jogging in place, stair climbing, rope skipping, and aerobic dancing can be beneficial alternatives. Some shopping malls open early in the morning for mall walking.

Safety Concerns

As with injuries, space will not permit a full coverage of the safety concerns associated with all aerobic activities, but the following suggestions may be helpful.

1. Use proper equipment, such as eye goggles for handball and racquetball sports or wrist, elbow, and knee protectors for in-line skating.
2. Joggers and runners should be on the lookout for cars. Be cautious at all intersections. If you must run on the road, run facing traffic.
3. Do not use headphones; if you do, keep the volume at a level so you can still hear traffic.
4. Wear light-colored clothing or reflective material at night. Do not assume that drivers see you.
5. Avoid heavy traffic areas. Research has shown that running in polluted air exposes you to potentially harmful effects of carbon monoxide. If you must run in such areas, try to run on the side of the road where the wind is blowing the automobile pollutants away from you.
6. Avoid exercising in areas with severe smog; pollutants such as ozone and nitrogen oxides may be damaging to your lungs.
7. Bicyclists should use all safety devices available, including reflectors, flags, and a safety helmet. Ride in the direction of traffic. Obey traffic lights and signs. Seek out bike trails, not busy roads.
8. Never swim alone.
9. Females should be cautious running alone at night. Other guidelines for female runners are presented in chapter 10.

Other Risks

There are other risks associated with exercise, usually with overtraining. As you get involved in an exercise program and begin to experience success, you may feel that if a little bit is good, then a lot is better. Such may not be the case, and, actually, too much exercise may be counterproductive. As mentioned above, it may predispose you to overuse injuries, but overtraining may also lead to more serious conditions, which will be discussed in later chapters. For example, in chapter 8, we shall note that although exercise may be used to reduce stress, it may actually increase stress in those who become overzealous in pursuit of exercise goals. Overtraining may also predispose females to menstrual dysfunctions, possibly contributing to premature osteoporosis, a topic that will be discussed in chapter 10. Additionally, overtraining may interfere with optimal functioning of the immune system, possibly predisposing one to upper respiratory tract infections.

As with all life-style behavior changes recommended in this book, moderation is the key.

Benefits

Epidemiological research supports a significant relationship between aerobic physical activity and reduced rates of mortality or increased longevity, while experimental research has provided us with data relative to the underlying mechanisms of this relationship. A more detailed discussion of this relationship is presented in chapter 11, while other health-related benefits of exercise are presented in chapters 7–10. As an overview, the following are some of the major potential benefits of aerobic exercise as they relate to health enhancement. According to Morris, however, it is important to note that these benefits may be transient; aerobic exercise needs to be continuing and current. Fitness cannot be stored.

Potential Benefits of Aerobic Exercise

1. Reduces risk of heart attack by
   a. increasing blood serum HDL cholesterol levels, the "good" cholesterol
   b. decreasing blood serum triglyceride levels
   c. reducing high blood pressure
   d. reducing the desire to smoke
   e. improving the efficiency of the heart
2. Reduces risk of developing certain forms of cancer
3. Reduces risk of developing noninsulin-dependent diabetes
4. Reduces excess body weight and helps to maintain optimal weight
5. Reduces risk of developing osteoporosis
6. Increases resistance to stress, anxiety, and fatigue; enhances mood and lowers depression
7. Increases stamina, strength, and working ability
8. Improves self-esteem

A proper aerobic exercise program, in conjunction with a proper diet and other Positive Health Life-style practices, can produce lifelong health benefits.

References

Books

American College of Sports Medicine. 1995. *Guidelines for graded exercise testing and exercise prescription.* 5th edition. Philadelphia: Lea & Febiger.

Blair, S. 1991. *Living with exercise.* Dallas: American Health Publishing Company.

Bouchard, C., et al., eds. 1994. *Physical activity, fitness, and health.* Champaign, Ill.: Human Kinetics.

Cooper, K. 1982. *The aerobics program for total well-being.* New York: M. Evans.

Daniels, J., R. Fitts, and G. Sheehan. 1978. *Conditioning for distance running.* New York: John Wiley & Sons.

Editors of *Runner's World.* 1994. *Running injury free.* Emmaus, Pa.: Rodale Press.

Feinstein, A. 1992. *Training the body to cure itself: How to use exercise to heal.* Emmaus, Pa.: Rodale Press.

Heyward, V. 1991. *Advanced fitness assessment and exercise prescription.* Champaign, Ill.: Human Kinetics.

LaFavore, M. 1992. *Men's health advisor.* Emmaus, Pa.: Rodale Press.

McArdle, W., et al. 1991. *Exercise physiology.* Philadelphia: Lea & Febiger.

National Heart, Lung and Blood Institute. 1981. *Exercise and your heart.* Washington, D.C.: U.S. Government Printing Office.

The Rockport Company. 1987. *Walking.* Marlboro, Mass.: The Rockport Company.

Stamford, B., and P. Shimer. 1990. *Fitness without exercise.* New York: Warner Books.

Williams, M. 1995. *Nutrition for fitness and sport.* Dubuque, Iowa: Brown & Benchmark Publishers.

Reviews

Ainsworth, B., et al. 1993. Compendium of physical activities: Classification of energy costs of physical activities. *Medicine and Science in Sports and Exercise* 25:71–80.

American College of Sports Medicine. 1990. ACSM position stand: The recommended quantity and quality of exercise for developing and maintaining cardiorespiratory and muscular fitness in healthy adults. *Medicine and Science in Sports and Exercise* 22:265–74.

American Heart Association. 1990. Special report: Exercise standards. *Circulation* 82:2286–2322.

Bernhardt, D., and G. Landry. 1994. Chest pain in active young people. Is it cardiac? *Physician and Sportsmedicine* 22 (June): 70–85.

Birk, T., and C. Birk. 1987. Use of ratings of perceived exertion for exercise prescription. *Sports Medicine* 4:1–8.

Blair, S. 1993. 1993 C. H. McCloy research lecture: Physical activity, physical fitness, and health. *Research Quarterly for Exercise and Sport* 64:365–76.

Blair, S., et al. 1985. Relationships between exercise or physical activity and other health behaviors. *Public Health Reports* 100:172–80.

Borg, G. 1973. Perceived exertion: A note on "History" and methods. *Medicine and Science in Sports* 5:90–93.

Case, W. 1994. Relieving the pain of shinsplints. *Physician and Sportsmedicine* 22 (April): 31–32.

Davison, R., and S. Grant. 1993. Is walking sufficient exercise for health? *Sports Medicine* 16:369–73.

DeBenedette, V. 1990. Are your patients exercising too much? *Physician and Sportsmedicine* 18 (August): 119–22.

DeBenedette, V. 1991. Exercise that'll bowl you over. *Physician and Sportsmedicine* 19 (March): 180–84.

Dishman, R. 1994. Prescribing exercise intensity for healthy adults using perceived exertion. *Medicine and Science in Sports and Exercise* 26:1087–94.

Draper, D., and G. Jones. 1990. The 1.5 mile run revisited—An update in women's times. *Journal of Physical Education, Recreation, and Dance* 61 (September): 78–80.

Durstine, J., and W. Haskell. 1994. Effects of exercise training on plasma lipids and lipoproteins. *Exercise and Sport Sciences Reviews* 22:477–521.

Franklin, B. 1993. Heed your heart's warnings. *Physician and Sportsmedicine* 21 (April): 16.

Franklin, B., et al. 1994. Exercise and cardiac complications. Do the benefits outweigh the risks? *Physician and Sportsmedicine* 22 (February): 56–68.

Friedewald, V., and D. Spence. 1990. Sudden cardiac death associated with exercise: The risk-benefit issue. *American Journal of Cardiology* 66:183–88.

Goldfine, H., et al. 1991. Exercising to health. *Physician and Sportsmedicine* 19 (June): 81–93.

Gudat, U., et al. 1994. Physical activity, fitness and non-insulin-dependent (Type II) diabetes mellitus. In *Physical activity, fitness, and health,* eds. C. Bouchard, et al. Champaign, Ill.: Human Kinetics.

Hagerman, F. 1992. Energy metabolism and fuel utilization. *Medicine and Science in Sports and Exercise* 24 (Supplement): S309–S314.

Haskell, W. 1994. Dose-response issues from a biological perspective. In *Physical activity, fitness, and health,* eds. C. Bouchard, et al. Champaign, Ill.: Human Kinetics.

Haskell, W. 1994. Health consequences of physical activity: Understanding and challenges regarding dose-response. *Medicine and Science in Sports and Exercise* 26:649–60.

Higdon, H. 1988. Base fitness. *The Walking Magazine.* February/March: 38–43.

Kibler, W., et al. 1992. Musculoskeletal adaptations and injuries due to overtraining. *Exercise and Sport Sciences Reviews* 20:99–126.

Kohl, H., and K. Powell. 1994. What is exertion-related sudden cardiac death? *Sports Medicine* 17:209–12.

Kuehls, D. 1995. First aid: A complete guide to preventing and treating the five most common running injuries. *Runner's World* (February): 36–44.

Lee, I-M. 1994. Physical activity, fitness, and cancer. In *Physical activity, fitness, and health,* eds. C. Bouchard, et al. Champaign, Ill.: Human Kinetics.

Lee, I-M., et al. 1995. Exercise intensity and longevity in men. *Journal of the American Medical Association* 273:1179–84.

Levin, S. 1991. Overtraining causes Olympic-sized problems. *Physician and Sportsmedicine* 19 (May): 112–18.

Martinsen, E. 1990. Benefits of exercise for the treatment of depression. *Sports Medicine* 9:380–89.

McAuley, E. 1994. Physical activity and pyschosocial outcomes. In *Physical activity, fitness, and health,* eds. C. Bouchard, et al. Champaign, Ill.: Human Kinetics.

McKeag, D., and C. Dolan. 1989. Overuse syndromes of the lower extremity. *Physician and Sportsmedicine* 17 (July): 108–23.

Mersy, D. 1991. Health benefits of aerobic exercise. *Postgraduate Medicine* 90:103–12.

Millard-Stafford, M. 1992. Fluid replacement during exercise in the heat. *Sports Medicine* 13:223–33.

Morris, J. 1994. Exercise in the prevention of coronary heart disease: Today's best buy in public health. *Medicine and Science in Sports and Exercise* 26:807–14.

Munnings, F. 1991. Exercise: Is any time the prime time? *Physician and Sportsmedicine* 19 (May): 101–4.

Newsholme, E., et al. 1991. A biochemical mechanism to explain some characteristics of overtraining. *Medicine and Sports Science* 32:79–93.

Noakes, T. 1993. Fluid replacement during exercise. *Exercise and Sport Sciences Reviews* 21:297–330.

O'Toole, M. 1992. Prevention and treatment of injuries to runners. *Medicine and Science in Sports and Exercise* 24 (Supplement): S360–S363.

Paffenbarger, R., et al. 1994. Some interrelationships of physical activity, physiological fitness, health, and longevity. In *Physical activity, fitness, and health,* eds. C. Bouchard, et al. Champaign, Ill.: Human Kinetics.

Pate, R., and C. Macera. 1994. Risks of exercising: Musculoskeletal injuries. In *Physical activity, fitness, and health,* eds. C. Bouchard, et al. Champaign, Ill.: Human Kinetics.

Polivy, J. 1994. Physical activity, fitness and compulsive behaviors. In *Physical activity, fitness, and health,* eds. C. Bouchard, et al. Champaign, Ill.: Human Kinetics.

Powell, K., and S. Blair. 1994. The public health burdens of sedentary living habits: Theoretical but realistic estimates. *Medicine and Science in Sports and Exercise* 26:851–56.

Renstrom, A. 1993. Mechanism, diagnosis, and treatment of running injuries. *Instructional Course Lectures* 42:225–34.

Roberts, W. 1992. Managing heatstroke. On-site cooling. *Physician and Sportsmedicine* 20 (May): 17–28.

Rosenson, R. 1993. Low levels of high-density lipoprotein cholesterol (hypoalphalipoproteinemia). An approach to management. *Archives of Internal Medicine* 153:1528–38.

Sallis, J., and P. Nader. 1990. Family exercise: Designing a program to fit everyone. *Physician and Sportsmedicine* 18 (September): 130–36.

Sonstroem, R., and W. Morgan. 1989. Exercise and self-esteem: Rationale and model. *Medicine and Science in Sports and Exercise* 21:329–37.

Stamford, B. 1990. Exercise and air pollution. *Physician and Sportsmedicine* 18 (September): 153–54.

Stamford, B. 1992. Exerting yourself: Listening to your body's signals. *Physician and Sportsmedicine* 20 (February): 187–88.

Stamford, B. 1993. Tracking your heart rate for fitness. *Physician and Sportsmedicine* 21 (March): 227–28.

Stamford, B. 1994. Making a splash. Let water workouts soothe your body. *Physician and Sportsmedicine* 22 (June): 105–6.

Suominen, H. 1993. Bone mineral density and long term exercise. An overview of cross-sectional athlete studies. *Sports Medicine* 16:316–30.

Thompson, P. 1993. Athletes, athletics, and sudden cardiac death. *Medicine and Science in Sports and Exercise* 24:270–80.

Thompson, P., and M. Fahrenbach. 1994. Risks of exercising: Cardiovascular including sudden cardiac death. In *Physical activity, fitness, and health,* eds. C. Bouchard, et al. Champaign, Ill.: Human Kinetics.

van Mechelen, W. 1992. Running injuries. A review of the epidemiological literature. *Sports Medicine* 14:320–35.

Williams, J., and R. Eston, 1989. Determination of the intensity dimension in vigorous exercise programs with particular reference to the use of the rating of perceived exertion. *Sports Medicine* 8:177–89.

Williford, H., et al. 1989. The physical effects of aerobic dance. A review. *Sports Medicine* 8:335–45.

Wood, P., and M. Stefanick. 1994. Physical activity, lipid and lipid protein metabolism and lipid transport. In *Physical activity, fitness, and health,* eds. C. Bouchard, et al. Champaign, Ill.: Human Kinetics.

Specific Studies

Angelopoulos, T., et al. 1993. Effect of repeated exercise bouts on high density lipoprotein-cholesterol and its subfractions HDL2-C and HDL3-C. *International Journal of Sports Medicine* 14:196–201.

Auble, T., et al. 1987. Aerobic requirements for moving handweights through various ranges of motion while walking. *Physician and Sportsmedicine* 15 (June): 133–40.

Ballor, D., et al. 1990. Exercise training attenuates diet-induced reduction in metabolic rate. *Journal of Applied Physiology* 68:2612–17.

Berry, M., et al. 1992. A comparison between two forms of aerobic dance and treadmill running. *Medicine and Science in Sports and Exercise* 24:946–51.

Boone, J., et al. 1993. Postexercise hypotension reduces cardiovascular responses to stress. *Journal of Hypertension* 11:449–53.

Clement, D., et al. 1993. Exercise-induced stress injuries to the femur. *International Journal of Sports Medicine* 14:347–52.

Debusk, R., et al. 1990. Training effects of long versus short bouts of exercise in healthy subjects. *American Journal of Cardiology* 65:1010–13.

DeMeersman, R. 1993. Heart rate variability and aerobic fitness. *American Heart Journal* 125:726–31.

Dimsdale, J., et al. 1984. Postexercise peril: Plasma catecholamines and exercise. *Journal of the American Medical Association* 251:630–32.

Dolgener, F., et al. 1994. Validation of the Rockport Fitness Walking Test in college males and females. *Research Quarterly for Exercise and Sport* 65:152–58.

Dunbar, C., et al. 1992. The validity of regulating exercise intensity by ratings of perceived exertion. *Medicine and Science in Sports and Exercise* 24:94–99.

Duncan, J., et al. 1991. Women walking for health and fitness. How much is enough? *Journal of the American Medical Association.* 266:3295–99.

Eckerson, J., and T. Anderson. 1992. Physiological response to water aerobics. *Journal of Sports Medicine and Physical Fitness* 32:255–61.

Garber, C., et al. 1992. Is aerobic dance an effective alternative to walk-jog exercise training? *Journal of Sports Medicine and Physical Fitness* 32:136–41.

Glass, S., et al. 1992. Accuracy of RPE from graded exercise to establish exercise training intensity. *Medicine and Science in Sports and Exercise* 24:1303–7.

Greer, N., and F. Katch. 1982. Validity of palpation recovery pulse rate to estimate exercise heart rate following four intensities of bench step exercise. *Research Quarterly for Exercise and Sport* 53:340–43.

Kingwell, B., and G. Jennings. 1993. Effects of walking and other exercise programs upon blood pressure in normal subjects. *Medical Journal of Australia* 158:234–38.

Kurokawa, T., and T. Ueda. 1992. Validity of ratings of perceived exertion as an index of exercise intensity in swimming training. *Annals of Physiology and Anthropology* 11 (May): 277–88.

Maw, G., et al. 1993. Ratings of perceived exertion and affect in hot and cool environments. *European Journal of Applied Physiology* 67:174–79.

Morris, J., et al. 1990. Exercise in leisure time: Coronary attack and death rates. *British Heart Journal* 63:325–34.

Murase, Y., et al. 1989. Heart rate and metabolic responses to participation in golf. *Journal of Sports Medicine and Physical Fitness* 29:269–72.

O'Neill, M., et al. 1992. Accuracy of Borg's ratings of perceived exertion in the prediction of heart rates during pregnancy. *British Journal of Sports Medicine* 26:121–24.

Scharff-Olson, M., et al. 1992. The heart rate $\dot{V}O_{2MAX}$ relationship of aerobic dance: A comparison of target heart rate methods. *Journal of Sports Medicine and Physical Fitness* 32:372–77.

Smith, J., et al. 1982. Failure of the Karvonen formula to accurately estimate training heart rate in coronary artery disease patients. *Medicine and Science in Sports and Exercise* 14:149.

Snyder, A., et al. 1993. Exercise responses to in-line skating: Comparisons to running and cycling. *International Journal of Sports Medicine* 14:38–42.

Solis, K., et al. 1988. Aerobic requirements for and heart rate responses to variations in rope jumping techniques. *Physician and Sportsmedicine* 16 (March): 121–28.

Spelman, C., et al. 1993. Self-selected exercise intensity of habitual walkers. *Medicine and Science in Sports and Exercise* 25:1174–79.

Stanforth, D., et al. 1993. Aerobic requirement of bench stepping. *International Journal of Sports Medicine* 14:129–33.

Sun, M., and J. Hill. 1993. A method for measuring mechanical work and work efficiency during human activities. *Journal of Biomechanics* 26:229–41.

Swain, D., et al. 1994. Target heart rates for the development of cardiorespiratory fitness. *Medicine and Science in Sports and Exercise* 26:112–16.

Town, G., and S. Bradley. 1991. Maximal metabolic responses of deep and shallow water running in trained runners. *Medicine and Science in Sports and Exercise* 23:238–41.

Tucker, L., and G. Friedman. 1990. Walking and serum cholesterol in adults. *American Journal of Public Health* 80:1111–13.

Weltman, A., et al. 1990. Percentages of maximal heart rate, heart rate reserve and $\dot{V}O_{2MAX}$ for determining endurance training intensity in male runners. *International Journal of Sports Medicine* 11:218–22.

Wichmann, S., and D. Martin. 1992. Exercise excess: Treating patients addicted to fitness. *Physician and Sportsmedicine* 20 (May): 193–200.

4

MUSCULAR STRENGTH AND ENDURANCE

Key Terms

accommodating resistance
backward pelvic tilt
circuit weight training
curl-up
fast twitch, glycolytic fiber
fast twitch, oxidative,
    glycolytic fiber
hernia

hip flexion
isokinetic muscle contraction
isometric contraction
isotonic concentric contraction
isotonic eccentric contraction
muscle endurance
muscle fibers

muscle strength
myofibrils
psoas major
rectus abdominis
rectus femoris
repetition maximum (RM)
resistance training

sacroiliac
slow twitch, oxidative fiber
spinal flexion
strength-endurance continuum
tendon
Valsalva phenomenon
variable resistance

Key Concepts

- Your muscles contain a mixture of different muscle fiber types, some designed for speed and power, others for endurance.

- Resistance training increases muscle size by various mechanisms. The most important appears to be an increase in the size of the individual muscle fibers.

- The two major principles underlying all resistance-training programs are the overload principle and the progressive resistance exercise principle; however, others (such as specificity, exercise sequence, and recuperation) are important.

- Although resistance training generally has not been recognized as an acceptable means for training the cardiovascular system, current research suggests resistance training may confer some moderate cardiovascular health benefits.

- Intense resistance training may be contraindicated for individuals with certain health problems, such as hernia, high blood pressure, coronary heart disease, and low back pain.

- Although resistance training is regarded as a relatively safe exercise program, exercisers should be aware of proper breathing techniques, the use of spotters, safe use of equipment, and proper lifting techniques for each exercise.

- Resistance-training programs may be designed to exercise each of the three human energy systems.

- As long as the major principles underlying a resistance-training program are followed, the various methods of training, such as free weights or machines, appear to be equally effective in producing gains in strength, endurance, and muscle mass.

- A resistance-training program that exercises all of the major muscle groups in the body is the best technique to gain lean body mass.

- To strengthen the abdominal muscles, you need to do exercises that either flex the spine or rotate the pelvic bone backwards.

- Improper abdominal exercises may actually contribute to the development of low back problems.

- Circuit aerobics combines aerobic and resistance-training exercises, leading to gains in cardiovascular fitness and muscular strength and endurance.

INTRODUCTION

The fitness movement that began in the late 1960s and early 1970s centered around aerobic exercise. Millions of individuals became engaged in a variety of aerobic activities, and literally thousands of health spas developed around the country to capitalize on this emerging interest in fitness, particularly aerobic dancing for females. A number of fitness spas existed prior to this aerobic fitness movement, even a national chain with spas in most major cities. However, their focus was not on aerobics, but rather on weight training for their primarily male clientele. **Resistance training,** or weight training, exercise programs are designed to develop muscle mass, strength, and endurance. These fitness spas did not seem to benefit financially from the aerobic fitness movement to better health, since medical opinion at that time suggested that weight-training programs conferred few, if any, health benefits. In recent years, however, weight training has again become increasingly popular for males and for females. Many current programs focus not only on developing muscular strength and endurance but on aerobic fitness as well.

Historically, most physical-fitness tests have usually included measures of muscular strength and endurance, not for health-related reasons, but primarily because such fitness components have been related to performance in athletics. However, in recent years, evidence has shown that training programs designed primarily to improve muscular strength and endurance might also confer some health benefits as well. The American College of Sports Medicine (ACSM) now recommends that resistance training be part of a total fitness program for healthy Americans. Increased participation in such training is one of the specific physical activity and fitness objectives promoted by the United States Department of Health and Human Services in *Healthy People 2000: National Health Promotion and Disease Prevention Objectives.*

Resistance training may contribute to health-related fitness in several ways. First, it is generally accepted that resistance-training programs do not improve the efficiency or health of the cardiovascular system comparable to the benefits from an aerobic-training program. However, increased muscular strength and endurance levels will reduce the stress of many work tasks, such as lifting heavy objects, and thus may result in less stress on the heart. Other cardiac risk factors, such as high blood pressure and poor serum lipid profiles, may be favorably modified by properly prescribed resistance training. In this regard, muscular strength and endurance training is even incorporated in many cardiac rehabilitation programs.

Second, resistance-training programs have been shown to alter body composition, primarily by increasing muscle mass and decreasing total body fat and percent body fat—changes that are believed to be healthful. In chapter 7, we will explore the role of resistance training in programs to either gain or lose weight.

Third, appropriate resistance training may help prevent the development of osteoporosis by helping to maximize increases in bone density.

Fourth, resistance training may help prevent the development of adult-onset diabetes by preventing the loss of muscle mass during the aging process. An increased muscle mass may help prevent impairment to insulin sensitivity and glucose tolerance, two factors associated with the development of diabetes.

Fifth, resistance training may confer significant benefits relative to psychological, or mental, health. Most young adults use resistance training as a means to improve their physical appearance; such improvement may help them to psychologically feel better about themselves.

Finally, improvement in muscular strength and endurance may help to prevent some common injuries, particularly the syndrome of low back pain. In combination with appropriate flexibility programs to be discussed in the following chapter, the development of strength and endurance in the abdominal muscles may be one of the best means to prevent injury and resultant pain to the low back region.

In this chapter, we shall present a brief overview of the muscular system, the basic principles of exercise as related to resistance training, the benefit/risk ratio of resistance training, general guidelines to program design, a basic resistance-training program, exercises specifically for the abdominal muscles, and programs focusing upon development of muscular strength and endurance as well as aerobic fitness .

The Muscular System

The primary purpose of most weight-training programs is to improve the size, shape, and function of the muscular system. Athletes involved in the sport of bodybuilding want to maximize their muscle size, but they also want to highlight muscle shape in order to receive higher ratings from the judges. In the sports of weight lifting and power lifting, athletes are primarily interested in developing the strength necessary to lift several hundred pounds. Other athletes, such as swimmers, may be interested in developing both strength and endurance in the specific muscles used in their stroke. Most of us, however, do not lift weights for athletic competition; we lift weights to look better physically. But as we train with weights to improve our appearance, we also improve our muscular strength and endurance.

In this section we shall look briefly at the structure and function of the muscular system, the determinants of muscle strength and endurance, and muscular hypertrophy.

Muscle Structure

Figure 4.1 represents a cross section of various parts of a muscle. The entire muscle, such as the biceps, is composed of bundles of muscle tissue. The bundles are composed of a number of **muscle fibers,** the actual muscle cells. The muscle fiber is composed of **myofibrils,** the contractile units within the muscle fiber. Finally, the myofibrils are composed of thin protein filaments that interact and slide by one another during contraction. Figure 4.2 is a schematic of the sliding filaments.

The whole muscle—the bundles and the muscle fibers—is covered by layers of connective tissue that bind the tissue and the fibers together. The connective tissue blends together and forms the **tendon,** such as the biceps tendon that can be felt in the front bend of the elbow, which attaches to the bones. When your muscle contracts and shortens, the force is transmitted through the tendon to bones in the forearm, and thus the elbow bends.

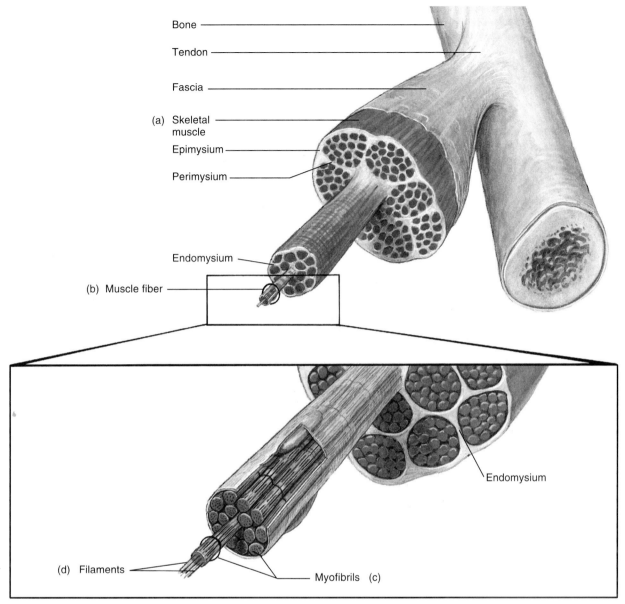

Bone

Tendon

Fascia

(a) Skeletal muscle

Epimysium

Perimysium

Endomysium

(b) Muscle fiber

Endomysium

(d) Filaments

Myofibrils (c)

Figure 4.1 *Muscle structure. The whole muscle (a) is composed of separate bundles of individual muscle fibers (b). Each fiber is composed of numerous myofibrils (c), each of which contains thin protein filaments (d) arranged so they can slide by one another to cause muscle shortening or lengthening. Various layers of connective tissue surround the muscle fibers, bundles, and whole muscles, which eventually bind together to form the tendon.*

Muscle Function

In chapter 3, you were introduced to the three different human energy systems. You may recall that ATP is the immediate source of energy for muscle contraction, and that the three energy systems are designed to replenish ATP stores at varying rates. In terms of the speed at which each of the three systems restores ATP, the ATP-PC system is the fastest, the lactic acid system is fast, while the oxygen system is the slowest. You may wish to review the characteristics of the three human energy systems in table 3.1 and in figure 3.2 on pages 27–28.

The use of muscle biopsy techniques has revealed that humans possess several different types of muscle cells, or muscle fibers. A needle is inserted into a muscle, a piece of muscle is extracted, and it is stained for its physiological, or functional, characteristics. These physiological characteristics relate to the human energy systems.

In general, we have three different muscle fiber types in each muscle, and these fiber types have been classified by the speed at which they contract and also by their predominant energy system. Figure 4.3 presents a schematic of these three fiber types.

The **slow twitch, oxidative fiber** type is characterized by a slower rate of muscle contraction; it primarily uses the oxygen energy system, which replenishes ATP slowly. We use the slow twitch fiber mainly in aerobic endurance activities. In the scientific literature, this fiber type is often referred to as Type I, or slow oxidative (SO).

The **fast twitch, oxidative, glycolytic fiber** type is characterized by a faster speed of contraction; it may use both the oxygen and lactic acid (rapid glycolytic) energy systems to replenish ATP. This fiber type is used in both aerobic and anaerobic type activities. It is referred to as the Type IIa fiber, or fast, oxidative, glycolytic fiber (FOG).

The **fast twitch, glycolytic fiber** type is characterized by a very fast speed of contraction; it primarily uses the lactic acid energy system and has the ability to use ATP rapidly. This fiber type is used primarily in fast, anaerobic type activities. It is also the largest of the three fiber types. It is referred to as the Type IIb fiber, or fast glycolytic (FG).

Most skeletal muscles in the body contain all three fiber types, but in different proportions. Muscle contraction is complex, as is the etiology of fatigue, and a detailed discussion of both is beyond the scope of this text. However, in general, since the slow, oxidative muscle fiber uses the oxygen energy system, it is very resistant to the development of fatigue. Since both of the fast twitch muscle fibers use the lactic acid energy system, they are more prone to develop fatigue early, particularly the fast twitch, glycolytic fiber.

Although a muscle biopsy provides the most accurate means to evaluate your muscle fiber type, several noninvasive predictive methods are available, although the predictive accuracy may not be very high. The interested reader is referred to the articles by Waldron and by Suter and her colleagues.

Muscular Strength and Endurance

In the preceding chapter we discussed the development of aerobic endurance, which uses the oxygen energy system. When doing an activity such as aerobic walking or jogging, you use a large muscle mass, your legs, to help lift your body weight on each step. By exercising at a speed within the capacity of your oxygen energy system, the steady state, you are able to exercise continuously for a long period of time. Aerobic endurance is primarily dependent upon the oxidative, or aerobic, muscle fibers to produce ATP to meet your energy needs. Aerobic training improves the oxidative capacity of all muscle fibers, even the fast glycolytic fibers. On the other hand, muscular strength and muscular endurance, particularly powerful short-term exercise tasks, are primarily dependent upon energy production via the two anaerobic energy systems, the ATP-PC and the lactic acid systems, particularly as they function in the fast twitch muscle fibers. Resistance training primarily improves the ATP-PC and lactic acid energy systems.

Muscle strength, the ability of a muscle or muscle group to develop force in one maximal effort, is dependent upon a large number of factors. For our purposes, the main factors are the size, type, and number of muscle fibers in the muscle and the ability of the nervous system to fully activate these fibers. The greater the number and size of fast-twitch muscle fibers you

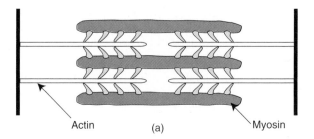

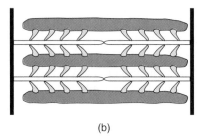

Figure 4.2 (a) Sliding protein filaments. (b) The muscle shortens when thin protein filaments (actin) are pulled inward by projections from thick protein filaments (myosin).

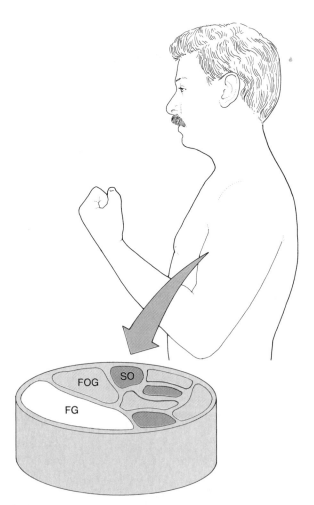

Figure 4.3 The three muscle fiber types. This schematic of a muscle shows three different muscle fiber types. SO is the slow, oxidative fiber type; FOG is the fast, oxidative, glycolytic fiber type; and FG is the fast glycolytic fiber type.

possess and the greater your ability to use them, the greater will be your muscle strength. Although the total strength you can develop is determined by your genetic background, you can maximize your potential through a proper training program.

Muscle endurance, often known as local muscle endurance or anaerobic endurance, is defined as the ability of a muscle or muscle group to repeatedly exert force by use of the anaerobic energy systems. It is distinguished from aerobic endurance in that fatigue usually occurs in a relatively short period of time. For example, lifting your body weight in a pull-up may lead to fatigue rapidly because the muscle groups involved in the pull-up are not able to produce ATP at a rate to meet your needs. Local muscular endurance, like muscular strength, is dependent upon a number of different factors, but probably the most important factor is the capacity of the lactic acid energy system to generate ATP.

As you might suspect, there are a wide variety of muscular strength and endurance tests available. If you have ever attempted to do as many pull-ups or push-ups as you could, you have tested the muscular endurance of several different muscle groups. Laboratory Inventories 4.1 and 4.2 provide an opportunity to test yourself for muscular strength and/or endurance in several basic exercises. By using a similar protocol, you may be able to develop your own tests of strength and endurance for any weight-training exercise you choose.

In a later section, we will discuss various resistance-training programs to improve muscular strength and endurance, but for now let's look at the major result of such programs and at why most of us engage in resistance training to increase muscle mass, or muscle size.

Muscle Hypertrophy

Muscle hypertrophy means increased muscle size. Resistance-training exercises place a heavy overload on the muscle cell, and one hypothesis suggests that this overload may slightly damage the muscle tissue. The muscle cells then respond to this stress by rebuilding and over time increase in size. It may do so in several possible ways. First, the individual muscle cells and myofibrils may simply increase their size by incorporating more protein. Second, the myofibrils in each cell may increase in number, which will increase the size of each muscle fiber. Third, the amount of connective tissue around each muscle fiber and around each bundle of muscle may increase and thicken, leading to an overall increase in the size of the total muscle. Finally, the muscle fibers themselves may increase in number, an effect known as muscle hyperplasia.

Although all of these are proposed mechanisms to explain muscle hypertrophy, the first three are fairly well established and are the most likely causes for the hypertrophy experienced by most of us when we train with weights. Research using muscle biopsies has revealed a significant increase in the size of individual muscle fibers, primarily the fast-twitch fibers, following a 10-week resistance-training program. Such increases help improve muscular strength and endurance and may be important components in body weight-control programs. Although females do not normally experience the same amount of hypertrophy that males do, they do experience proportional gains in strength and endurance. Moreover, recent research with young women has revealed a significant increase in muscle-cell size when they engaged in an intense, concentrated resistance-training program. Research has also shown significant muscular hypertrophy in older men and women as well, even those in their sixties and seventies.

Although muscle hypertrophy may take some time to develop, strength gains may occur more rapidly, even in 2 weeks. Strength may actually double or even triple in 3 months time in some individuals. In the early phases of training, strength gains may be due to adaptations in the nervous system, such as becoming more skilled at lifting, but eventually muscular hypertrophy becomes the predominant factor.

Principles of Resistance Training

In chapter 2 we discussed a variety of principles important in the design of any exercise program. Those principles relative to resistance training include overload, progressive resistance, specificity, exercise sequence, and recuperation. In the last chapter we discussed interval training and introduced terms such as *exercise intensity* and *recovery*. Before we discuss each principle, let's look at some important terms as they apply to resistance training. Although resistance may be applied in a variety of ways, this chapter will emphasize the use of weights.

Repetition simply means the number of consecutive times you do a specific exercise. Intensity is determined by the weight, or resistance, that is lifted. A term used to describe the interrelationship between repetitions and intensity in weight training is **repetition maximum (RM).** If you perform an exercise such as a bench press and lift 150 pounds once, but you cannot do a second repetition, you have done one repetition maximum, or 1RM. If you bench press a lighter weight, say 120 pounds for five repetitions, but cannot do a sixth, you have done five repetition maximum, or 5RM. A set is any particular number of repetitions, such as five or ten. The total volume of work you do in a single workout is the product of sets, repetitions, and resistance. For example, if you bench press three sets with five repetitions and a resistance of 100 pounds, your total volume of work is 1,500 pounds ($3 \times 5 \times 100$). The recovery period may represent the rest intervals between sets in a single workout or the rest interval between each workout during the week.

The Overload Principle

The overload principle is the most important principle in all resistance-training programs. The use of weights places a greater than normal stress on the muscle cell. This overload stress stimulates the muscle to grow—to become stronger—in order to effectively overcome the increased resistance imposed by the weights.

To overload the muscle you must increase the volume of work it must do. There are basically two ways to do this. One is to increase the amount of resistance or weight that you use; the other way is to increase the number of repetitions and sets you do. Although there is no single best combination of sets and repetitions, usually one to three sets with 5–12RM provide an

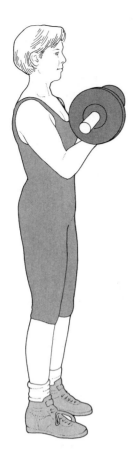

Week:	1	4	7	10	13	16
Weight:	50	50	60	60	70	70
Repetitions:	8	12	8	12	8	12
Sets:	3	3	3	3	3	3

Figure 4.4 *The principle of progressive resistance exercise (PRE) states that as you get stronger, you need to progressively increase the resistance in order to continue to gain strength and muscle.*

adequate stimulus for muscle growth. The ACSM recommendation is one set of 8–12 repetitions for minimum strength gains. If you know your 1RM, you should be able to do 5 to 10 RM if you use 70 to 80 percent of your 1RM value. For example, if your bench press 1RM is 150 pounds, you should be able to do at least 5RM with 80 percent of that value, or 120 pounds ($.80 \times 150$).

The Principle of Progressive Resistance Exercise (PRE)

As the muscle continues to get stronger during your training program, you must increase the amount of resistance, the overload, in order to continue to get the proper stimulus for sustained muscle growth. As noted in chapter 2, this is known as progressive resistance exercise and is another basic principle of resistance training.

Following a learning period, a recommended program for beginners is one to three sets with 8RM in each set. The first step is to determine the maximum amount of weight that you can lift for eight repetitions. If you can do more than eight repetitions, the weight is too light and you need to add more

poundage. As you get stronger during the succeeding weeks, you will be able to lift the original weight more easily. When you can perform twelve repetitions, add more weight to force you back down to eight repetitions; this is the progressive resistance principle. Over several months time, the weight will probably need to be increased several times as you continue to get stronger. Such a transition is illustrated in figure 4.4.

The Principle of Specificity

Specificity of training is a broad principle with many implications for resistance training, including specificity for various sports movements, strength gains, endurance gains, and bodyweight gains. For example, a swimmer who wanted to gain strength and endurance for a stroke should attempt to find a resistance-training program that exercises the specific muscles in a way as close as possible to the form used in that stroke. If you want to gain muscle mass in a certain part of the body, those muscles must be exercised.

The Principle of Exercise Sequence

Your exercise routine should be based upon the principle of exercise sequence. This means that if you have ten exercises in your routine, they should be arranged in a logical order so that fatigue does not limit your lifting ability. Another general recommendation is to exercise the larger muscles first and the smaller muscle groups later in the sequence of exercises. For example, the first exercise in a sequence of ten might stress the quadriceps muscle, the second the abdominals, the third the pectorals, and so forth. After you perform one full set of each of the ten exercises, you then do a complete second set, followed by a third set. This approach may be best for beginners.

Another popular option is to do three sets of the same exercise, with a rest between each set; then do three sets of the second exercise, and so on. This approach may be a little more fatiguing since you are using the same muscle group in three successive sets, but it appears to be very effective.

The Principle of Recuperation

Resistance training, if done properly to achieve the greatest gains, imposes a rather severe stress on the muscles, requiring a period of recovery both during the workout and between workouts. Research has shown that exercises of 5 to 10RM can lead to rapid depletion of ATP and PC in the muscles; however, most of these high-energy compounds may be restored in about 2 to 3 minutes' recovery. Thus, several minutes should intervene between sets if you are using the same exercise. Additionally, for beginners, resistance training should generally be done about three days per week, with a rest or recuperation day in between. This day of rest allows sufficient time for your muscle to repair itself and to synthesize new protein as it continues to grow.

These general principles should serve as guidelines during the beginning phase of your resistance-training program and should be used to guide your progress during the first three months of the basic resistance-training program described later in this chapter.

Benefits and Risks of Resistance Training

In the past, most of the benefits derived from resistance training were thought to be of importance only to athletes, but increasing evidence suggests that resistance training may also confer some health benefits for others. On the other hand, although resistance training is generally considered safe, there are some potential risks if proper precautions are not taken.

Benefits

As might be expected, for those athletes involved in sports in which high levels of muscular mass, strength, power, and endurance are important, resistance-training programs may confer some very significant benefits. Such findings are supported by numerous research studies. Furthermore, some recent research has even found that resistance training may increase maximal oxygen uptake, although the gains do not appear to be comparable to those that may be derived from aerobic training. Thus, many athletes may benefit from a properly designed resistance-training program specific to their individual needs.

But what health benefits might accrue from resistance training? Although it is not clear exactly how much muscular strength and endurance is necessary for good health, research generally supports a positive association between resistance training and a variety of health benefits.

The increase in strength and muscular endurance through resistance training may help prevent injuries. In particular, injury resulting in low back pain may be prevented by developing a balance of strength and flexibility of the abdominals and back extensors. Strength training, another way to prevent injuries, may also help to maintain balance and prevent falls, particularly in the elderly.

Another benefit may involve improved mental health. Although a number of factors determine our state of mental health, an important one is our self-concept, or how we view ourselves. Our self-concept may be influenced markedly by our body image, or how we feel about our bodies. Do we look the way we want to look? Such feelings may be revealed by tests of body image, which have been used in studies to investigate the effect of resistance training. In this regard, several studies with college-aged males revealed a significant improvement in body image and self-concept following a 16-week resistance-training program. The students who improved the most were those who perceived their body image to be less than ideal at the beginning of the program. Resistance-training programs have also improved strength in the elderly, even those in their nineties, with accompanying feelings of increased independence and sense of well-being.

Still another benefit may occur in body weight-control programs. One of the problems associated with low-Calorie diets to lose body fat is that muscle protein is also lost at the same time. The reason for this is complex, but, in general, if there is insufficient carbohydrate in the diet to provide glucose, which is essential for brain functions, the liver converts muscle protein into glucose. This loss of muscle tissue may lead to a decrease in resting metabolism, which may be counterproductive on a weight-loss program since energy expenditure would be decreased. Some research has shown that resistance training may help to prevent this loss of muscle tissue by stimulating muscle hypertrophy. As shall be noted in chapter 7, aerobic exercise may also be effective in this regard.

Recent evidence also suggests that resistance training may stimulate increases in bone mineral content, and could complement weight-bearing exercise, such as running, as a means to enhance optimal bone development. Such training may help to increase bone mineral content during the growth years to age twenty-five and possibly help retard bone loss in later years.

Some data are also available suggesting that resistance training, particularly programs such as circuit aerobics (described later in this chapter), may help to reduce risk factors associated with coronary heart disease, although the benefits are not as great as those derived from an aerobic exercise program. In reviews of the available literature, Fleck and Kraemer, as well as Stone and Wilson, noted that resistive weight training may help lower the resting heart rate, reduce the strain on the heart during exercise, decrease blood pressure, and elicit beneficial changes in serum lipid levels. Although Kokkinos and Hurley, in a major review, noted that most resistance-training studies report favorable changes in blood lipids, they recommend additional research to control some possible methodological problems in previous studies. Obesity and diabetes are also risk factors for coronary heart disease. As noted previously, resistance training may be an effective adjunct to a weight loss program, while Soukup and Kovaleski indicate resistance training may help prevent adult-onset diabetes by preventing the loss of muscle mass, an effect that may improve insulin sensitivity, glucose tolerance, and blood sugar control. Some of these beneficial effects may be related to the total volume of work done; a greater total volume of work may be done with less resistance and more repetitions. This might introduce a significant aerobic component during the workout, as suggested by Wallace and others in a recent study.

Risks

The risks associated with resistance training fall into two general categories—those associated with preexisting health problems that may be aggravated by resistance training and those associated with unsafe weight-lifting practices that may lead to injury.

Preexisting Health Problems

Several health problems may be aggravated during resistance training due to the increased pressures that occur within the body, such as when you strain to lift heavy weights and hold your breath at the same time. Such straining will increase the resistance to blood flow so the blood pressure in your arteries rises dramatically, possibly to levels of 300 to 400 mmHg or more. Fortunately, since the pressure surrounding your arteries also increases, there is little danger for most healthy individuals. However, for individuals with high blood pressure or weak points in their arterial walls, resistance training may lead to excessive pressures and possible rupture of the artery.

Individuals with resting blood pressures over 90 mmHg diastolic or 140 mmHg systolic should consult with their physician before engaging in heavy resistance training.

Lifting with the arms and straining exercises also increase the stress on the heart. Individuals with heart disease should consult their cardiologist about safe resistance-training programs. Although such programs may be used in a cardiac rehabilitation program, they should be individually prescribed.

Individuals with a **hernia,** a weakness in the abdominal wall, should refrain from strenuous weight lifting; the increased pressure in the abdominal area may cause a rupture. Low back problems may also be aggravated by lifting improperly.

Individuals who have any of these problems should seek medical advice prior to initiating a resistance-training program.

Safety Concerns

Resistance training is generally regarded as a relatively safe sport, particularly if these guidelines are followed.

1. Learn to breathe properly. During the most strenuous part of the exercise you are likely to hold your breath. This is a natural response; it helps stabilize your chest cavity in order to provide a more stable base for your muscles to function. Usually the breath hold is short, and no problems occur. However, if prolonged, it may increase the chances of suffering some of the problems noted previously, such as a hernia.

   Also associated with prolonged breath holding is a response known as the **Valsalva phenomenon,** which may lead to a possible blackout. Here is what happens. As you reach a sticking point in your lift and strain to overcome it, you normally hold your breath; this causes your glottis to close over your windpipe and the pressure in your chest and abdominal area to rise rapidly. This pressure provides resistance to blood flow, reducing the return of blood to the heart, and eventually leads to decreased blood flow to the brain and a possible blackout. Additionally, the Valsalva maneuver exaggerates the increase in blood pressure during resistance exercises, and although a brief Valsalva maneuver is unavoidable when doing near maximal exercises, its effect may be minimized by proper breathing.

   A recommended breathing system that will help to minimize these adverse effects is to breathe out while lifting the weight and breathe in while lowering it. You should breathe through both your mouth and nose while exercising. Practice proper breathing when you learn new resistance-training exercises.

2. When using free weights, use spotters when doing exercises that may be potentially dangerous, such as the bench press. If you are doing a bench press alone and reach a sticking point in your lift, the Valsalva phenomenon may lead to serious consequences if you lose control of the weight directly above your head. The use of various machines, such as Nautilus® and Universal Gym®, helps eliminate the need for spotters.

3. If using free weights, place lock collars on the bar ends so the plates do not fall off and cause injury to the feet. Again, the use of machines eliminates this safety hazard. However, do not attempt to change weight plates on machines while they are being used. Your fingers may get caught between the weights.

4. Warm up with proper stretching exercises. The next chapter on flexibility provides you with some guidelines.

5. Use light weights to learn the proper technique of a given exercise so you do not strain yourself if an improper technique is used. When the proper technique is mastered, the weights may be increased.

6. Avoid exercises that may cause or aggravate low back problems. A properly fitted weight belt may help prevent low back injury when lifting heavy weights and many resistance-training machines provide support for the back. Try to prevent an excessive forward motion or stress in the lower back region. Figure 4.5 illustrates some positions to be avoided. Additional information is provided in chapter 5.

7. Lower weights slowly. If you lower them rapidly, your muscles have to contract rapidly in order to slow the weights down as you reach the starting position. This necessitates the development of a large amount of force that may tear some muscle and connective tissue and cause muscle soreness.

Program Design Considerations

There are numerous types of resistance-training programs available to you; all of them will help you gain strength and endurance if they adhere to the basic principles discussed earlier in this chapter. The type of training program you develop for yourself will be dependent not only upon your specific goals, but also upon the equipment available to you.

Goals and the Strength-Endurance Continuum

As is probably obvious to you, there is an inverse relationship between the amount of weight you can lift and the number of repetitions you can do. If your 1RM in the bench press is 150 pounds, you can do more repetitions with 100 pounds than you can with 140 pounds. The **strength-endurance continuum** is a training concept that focuses upon the interrelationship between resistance and repetitions. As depicted in figure 4.6, to train for strength you must combine high resistance with a low number of repetitions. Conversely, to train for endurance, you must combine a low resistance with a high number of repetitions.

Since the ATP-PC energy system predominates in strength and power activities and the oxygen system is involved in aerobic endurance activities, resistance-training programs may be designed to train all three of the human energy systems.

To train the anaerobic ATP-PC system for strength and power, select a resistance of about 85 to 90 percent of your 1RM. With this resistance, you will be able to do only several

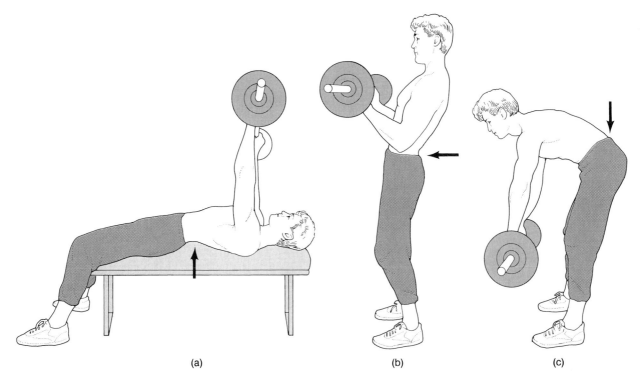

(a)   (b)   (c)

Figure 4.5 *Avoid exercises or body positions that place excessive stress on the low back region. Poor form in exercises like (a) the bench press and (b) the curl exaggerates the lumbar curve. Be sure to keep the lower back as flat as possible. Exercises similar to (c) the bentover row place tremendous forces on the lower back because the weight or resistance is so far in front of the body.*

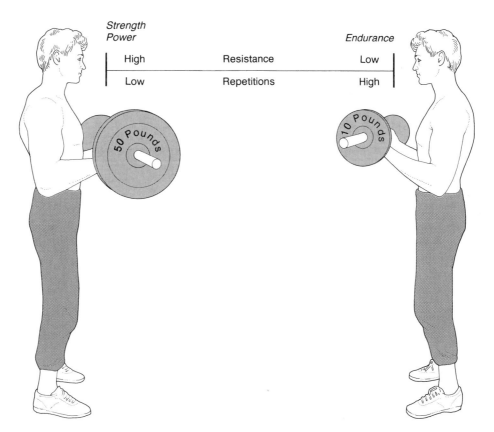

Strength Power		Endurance
High	Resistance	Low
Low	Repetitions	High

Figure 4.6 *The strength-endurance continuum. To gain strength, you need to train on the strength end of the continuum; to gain endurance, you need to train on the endurance end of the continuum.*

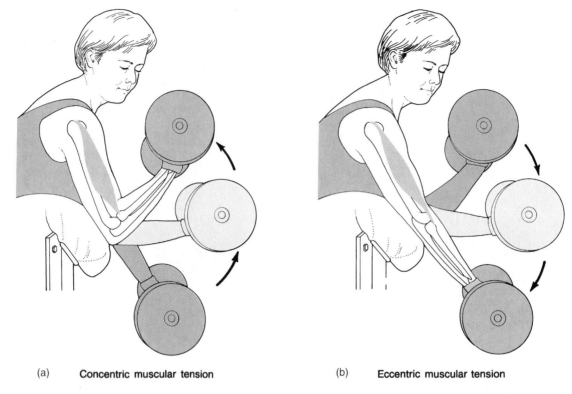

(a) Concentric muscular tension	(b) Eccentric muscular tension

Figure 4.7   *Isotonic concentric and eccentric muscle contractions in the biceps curl. (a) Lifting the weight upwards is caused by shortening of the muscle fibers, or a concentric contraction. (b) Lowering the weight to the starting point is caused by the force of gravity; the biceps muscle helps to lower the weight slowly through an isotonic eccentric contraction. The muscle is developing force to shorten, but the force is less than that exerted by gravity. Thus, the muscle is being lengthened.*

repetitions; you are on the strength end of the continuum. Since this type of lifting will rapidly deplete your ATP and PC stores, you will need to rest 2 to 3 minutes between sets. Do the same exercise in several consecutive sets.

To train the anaerobic lactic acid energy system, or the ability to do high-intensity exercise for 1 to 2 minutes, select a resistance of about 65 to 80 percent of your 1RM. You will be able to do more repetitions with this lower resistance, and you should produce significant amounts of lactic acid. By resting only about 1 minute between sets, you will put more stress on the lactic acid system, because recovery will not be complete. Do the same exercise in several consecutive sets.

To train the aerobic oxygen system, select a resistance of about 30 to 60 percent of your 1RM. This low resistance should enable you to do a high number of repetitions; you are near the endurance end of the continuum. Rest periods between sets should be relatively brief, about 20 to 30 seconds, since you should not be accumulating significant amounts of lactic acid. This type of resistance training is usually incorporated into programs known as circuit training. Although you may do the same exercise in consecutive sets, many circuit-training programs alternate exercises from one part of the body to another. The last section in this chapter focuses upon circuit aerobics. It should be noted that although this type of resistance training is designed to stress the oxygen system, the gains are only moderate in comparison to those achieved with the aerobics-training program described in the preceding chapter.

You may desire to modify your body appearance through weight training. If you wish to improve your muscle tone and reduce body fat, the circuit aerobics program described later in this chapter may be appropriate. It will help you burn Calories as a means to reduce body fat, but the resistance-training exercises will also help to improve muscle tone throughout your body.

Types of Muscle Contraction

Relative to resistance training, there are basically four different types of muscle contraction—isometric, isotonic concentric, isotonic eccentric, and isokinetic. Let's look at a simple resistance-training exercise, the biceps curl, to explain these terms. The biceps curl is done by holding a weight in your hands with your arms straight down in front of your body, palms facing away from your body. Using your biceps muscle (and several others), you curl the weight towards your shoulder by bending your elbows and then lower it back to the starting position (fig. 4.7).

An **isometric contraction** involves no shortening of the muscle. It occurs when the muscular force you generate is inadequate to overcome the resistance. For example, if your 1RM for the biceps curl is 80 pounds and you attempted to lift 100 pounds, no movement would occur. Your muscle is attempting to shorten, but it cannot because the resistance is too great.

There are two types of isotonic contractions. An **isotonic concentric contraction** represents muscle shortening

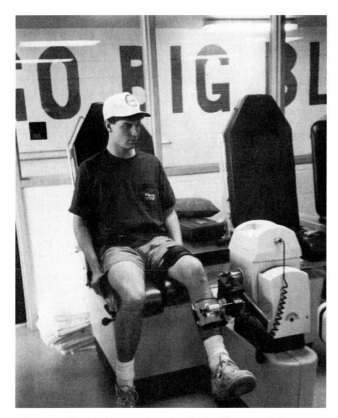

Figure 4.8 Machines such as the Kin-Com® are needed to control the speed of muscle shortening. Muscle shortening at a set speed is known as an isokinetic contraction.

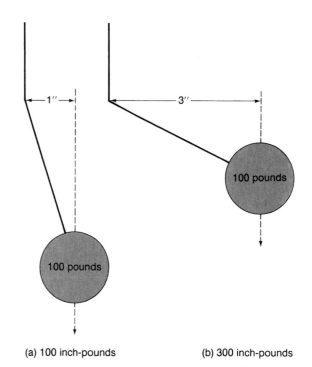

(a) 100 inch-pounds   (b) 300 inch-pounds

Figure 4.9 The total amount of resistance created by a weight is the product of the weight times the perpendicular distance to the fulcrum, the elbow joint in this example. In position (a), the total resistance is 100 inch-pounds, or 100 pounds times one inch. In position (b), the total resistance is now 300 inch-pounds, or 100 pounds times three inches.

(fig. 4.7a), sometimes referred to as a positive contraction. It occurs when you are able to curl the weight, a weight lower than your 1RM. The biceps muscle shortens and provides the force for you to move the weight against the pull of gravity, which of course is attempting to pull the weight back to earth. When you lower the weight, your biceps muscle is still contracting, but now it is classified as an **isotonic eccentric contraction,** and the muscle is actually lengthening (fig. 4.7b), sometimes referred to as a negative contraction. Gravity is the force that is attempting to pull the weight down, and your biceps muscle is opposing this gravitational pull so the weight is lowered slowly. For example, if gravity is pulling the 100-pound weight to earth, and your biceps is providing 90 pounds of force to counteract this gravitational pull, then the net gravitational force is only 10 pounds.

If your biceps did not provide some resistance to gravity, the weight would drop rapidly due to gravitational forces. If you then tried to stop the rapid fall of the weight by contracting your biceps, the force might be so great that some of your muscles and connective tissue might tear. A slow, controlled eccentric contraction, involved in all isotonic exercises when you lower the weight, poses no problem, but if the movement is rapid, muscle soreness or tissue damage may occur.

An **isokinetic muscle contraction** is one in which the muscle can shorten only at a set speed. In order to control the speed of your biceps curl, a machine or device of some type is necessary to provide a resistance that changes depending upon how much force you exert (fig. 4.8). If you exert a strong force in an attempt to do a fast curl, the resistance will increase so that you can move only as fast as the machine will allow. If you exert a lesser force, the resistance will decrease, again permitting you to move at the speed set by the machine. The term **accommodating resistance** is used to describe the machines or devices used for isokinetic contractions, such as the Kin-Com® and Hydra-Gym®, that use either electrical forces or hydraulic fluid to provide the accommodating resistance. If you exert your maximal force throughout the entire range of motion in the curl, theoretically you will receive maximal resistance at each point throughout that range.

Some machines used for isotonic concentric and eccentric exercises provide a **variable resistance,** which is slightly different from accommodating resistance. As you move the weight in an isotonic contraction, the resistance actually changes. For example, in the biceps curl illustrated in figure 4.9, the resistance provided by the weight is the product of the weight times the perpendicular distance to the elbow joint. To simplify, we might say that in the starting position of the curl, the resistance is 100 inch-pounds; as you move the weight upward, the resistance may increase to 300 inch-pounds. Also, as your muscle shortens, its ability

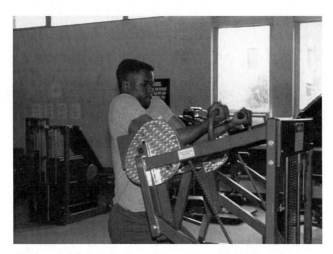

Figure 4.10 *Nautilus® machines use devices known as cams to automatically adjust the resistance as you move through the range of motion in an exercise.*

to exert force changes due to a number of factors. Thus, your biceps are stronger in some positions than in others. For example, in the starting position for the curl, your biceps might have the ability to generate 100 pounds of force, but as you curl through the range of motion, your ability changes, so that in another position it may be able to generate 150 pounds of force. In essence, then, the theory is that by lifting only 100 pounds, the force you can generate in the starting position, you are not adequately stressing your muscle when it reaches the position where it can generate 150 pounds. Unfortunately, the increases in the resistance and the increases in your strength potential do not match perfectly as you lift the weight. Thus, machines such as Nautilus® have devices called cams designed to automatically change the resistance arm as you curl the weight so that you will have the optimal resistance through the full range of motion (fig. 4.10). Although the idea is basically sound, the construction of the cams is based upon the average values of strength data obtained from large groups of people. If your strength curve varies from that average, the cam will not provide you with the optimal resistance throughout the range of motion.

Methods of Training

There are numerous methods to train with resistance, but each method is based upon one or more of the four basic types of muscle contraction. You can train isometrically with almost any immovable object. You may train isotonically with free weights such as barbells and dumbbells, but many machines like Nautilus® and Universal Gym® provide variable resistance for isotonic contractions. In order to train isokinetically, you will need some machine or device that will provide accommodating resistance to control your speed of contraction. Which method should you choose?

A number of research studies have been conducted to determine which of these methods is best, but most of this research focused upon strength and power gains. The results of many of these studies are contradictory, particularly when isotonic and isokinetic programs are compared. However, at the present time it is probably safe to say that isotonic and isokinetic programs are comparable in their ability to produce gains in strength as well as gains in muscle mass.

Although you may train isometrically, it does not appear to be a popular technique because you do not see any actual work being accomplished. Maximal isometric exercises also tend to invoke a powerful Valsalva response, which may increase the blood pressure excessively. Since isokinetic exercises necessitate the use of complex machines, usually expensive ones, most individuals train isotonically either with free weights or with apparatus such as Nautilus®. Again, research has shown very little difference between free weights or machines as a means to increase strength or muscle mass, so the choice is up to you. In comparison to machines, free weights are less expensive and allow the performance of a wider variety of exercises. However, they may also require a greater degree of skill, the presence of spotters, greater attention to safety precautions, and more time, due to the need to change weights often.

All methods may be effective provided the basic principles of resistance training, particularly the overload principle and the progressive resistance principle, are followed.

A Basic Resistance-Training Program for Muscular Strength, Muscular Endurance, and Increased Muscle Mass

In this section, you find one exercise for each of the major body areas. Since barbells and dumbbells appear to be the most common means of doing resistance training, this is the method utilized. However, as mentioned previously, other apparatus such as the Nautilus®, Universal Gym®, and others can also be used effectively to gain weight and strength. Most of the exercises described here using barbells or dumbbells have similar counterparts on other apparatus, and a schematic of such machines is illustrated with each exercise.

Note that muscles seldom operate alone, and that most resistance-training exercises stress more than one muscle group. Thus, keep in mind that although an exercise may be listed specifically for the chest muscle, it may also stress the arm and shoulder muscles. The exercises described in this section generally stress more than one body area, although their main effect is on the area noted.

These eight exercises stress most of the major muscle groups in the body, and thus provide an adequate stimulus for gaining body weight and strength through an increase in muscle mass. Literally hundreds of different resistance-training exercises and techniques to train are available; if you become interested in diversifying your program (such

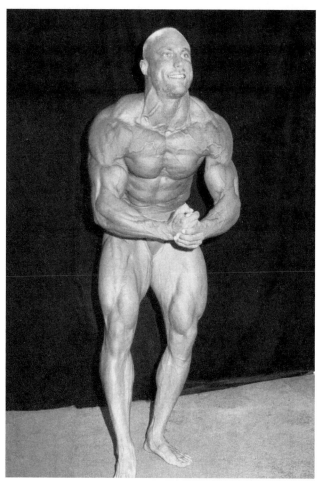

Figure 4.11 *Bodybuilders use a variety of techniques to maximize individual muscle development.*

6. Exercise two to three days per week; in each succeeding day try to do as many repetitions as possible for each exercise in each set. When you can do twelve repetitions each after a month or so, add more weight to the bars so you can do only eight repetitions.

7. Repeat Step 6 as you progressively increase your strength.

Abdominal Strength and Endurance

As shall be noted in the next chapter, stretching exercises to improve the flexibility of the lumbar region are very important in the prevention of low back pain, but so too are exercises to strengthen the abdominal musculature. A wide variety of exercises help improve abdominal strength, but some may actually predispose an individual to low back problems rather than help prevent them. In order to understand why, let us look at the movements that occur in some of these exercises and at the primary muscles involved.

For our discussion, it is important to understand the difference between flexion of the spine and flexion of the hip. **Spinal flexion** occurs only between the vertebrae in the spinal column. If you lie flat on the floor on your back and then begin to curl your head, neck, and shoulders forward while keeping your lower back flat against the floor, you are doing spinal flexion. This movement is often called the **curl-up** or trunk curl; we shall refer to it later. It is important to realize that no movement occurs where the spine joins the pelvis. This is an immovable joint called the **sacroiliac** joint where the sacrum (part of the spine) fuses with the iliac bones of the pelvis.

The muscles we are primarily interested in are the abdominals, particularly the **rectus abdominis.** The rectus abdominis is illustrated in figure 4.20a. As the rectus abdominis contracts, it causes one of two movements. First, it pulls on the ribs. Because the ribs are attached to the spine, this causes spinal flexion. Second, it pulls up on the lower part of the pelvic bone, thus tilting it backward and helping to flatten out the lower back. Thus, exercises that highlight spinal flexion or tilting the pelvis backward help to strengthen the abdominal muscles. These movements are presented in figures 4.20b and 4.20c.

Hip flexion occurs only at the hip joint, the joint between the pelvic bone and the thigh bone. As illustrated in figure 4.21, if you stand and lift one leg forward, you are doing hip flexion; if you keep your back straight and bend over to touch your toes, you are also doing hip flexion. In some exercises, you may do both spinal flexion and hip flexion. For example, spinal flexion occurs in the early phase of a full sit-up, but after about 30 degrees, hip flexion takes over. It is also important to realize that, although the pelvic bone usually moves in order to facilitate spine and thigh movements, it may also be moved independently. For example, if you stand with your back against a wall and simply pull in your stomach to flatten your back against the wall, you are primarily moving the pelvic bone.

Several muscles that cause hip flexion may also act on the spine or pelvis. A deep muscle, the **psoas major,** is primarily

as getting involved in bodybuilding as depicted in fig. 4.11), consult a book specific to resistance training. Several may be found in the reference list at the end of this chapter.

The beginner should adhere to the following procedure using the basic resistance-training program.

1. Learn the proper technique for each exercise with a light weight, possibly only the bar itself or the lowest weight on the machine, for 2 weeks. Do ten to twelve repetitions of each exercise to develop form. Do not strain during this initial learning phase.

2. For each exercise, determine the maximum weight that you can lift for eight repetitions after the 2-week learning phase.

3. Do one set of the eight exercises in the sequence as listed on figures 4.12 through 4.19.

4. Since the exercise sequence is designed to stress different muscle groups in order, not much recuperation is necessary between exercises—possibly only 30 seconds or so.

5. Do one to three complete sets. You may wish to rest 2 to 3 minutes between sets.

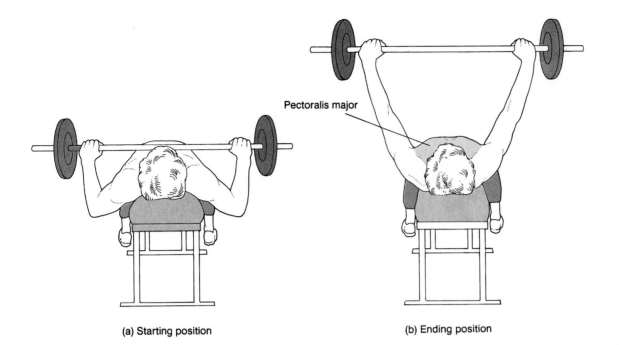

(a) Starting position

(b) Ending position

Pectoralis major

Figure 4.12 *The bench press. The bench press primarily develops the pectoralis major muscle group in the chest; it also develops the deltoid in the shoulder and the triceps at the back of the arm. The weight machine (c) exercises the same muscles.*

Chest
Figure 4.12

Exercise	Bench press
Chest Muscles	Pectoralis major
Other Muscles	Deltoid, triceps
Sets	1–3
Repetitions	8–12, PRE concept
Safety	Have spotter stand between bar to assist as fatigue sets in.
Equipment	Bench with support for weight, or two spotters to hand weight to you.
Description	Lie supine on bench. Use wide grip for chest development. Secure bar and lower *slowly* to chest. Press bar straight up to full extension. Do not arch back.

(c) Weight machine for pectoralis major

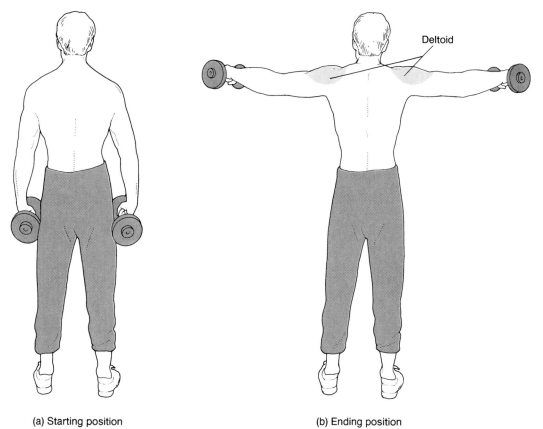

(a) Starting position

(b) Ending position

Deltoid

Figure 4.13 *Standing lateral raise. The standing lateral raise primarily develops the deltoid muscle in the shoulder; the trapezius in the upper back and neck area is also trained. The weight machine (c) exercises the same muscles.*

Shoulders
Figure 4.13

Exercise	Standing lateral raise
Shoulder Muscles	Deltoid
Other Muscles	Trapezius
Sets	1–3
Repetitions	8–12, PRE concept
Safety	Do not arch back.
Equipment	Dumbbells
Description	Stand with dumbbells in hands at sides. With palms down, bend arms slightly at the elbows and raise straight arms sideways to shoulder level. Return slowly to starting position.

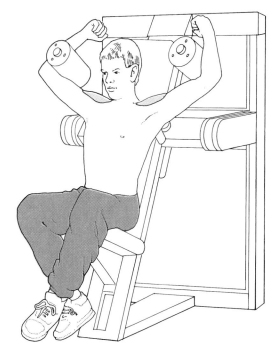

(c) Weight machine for the deltoids

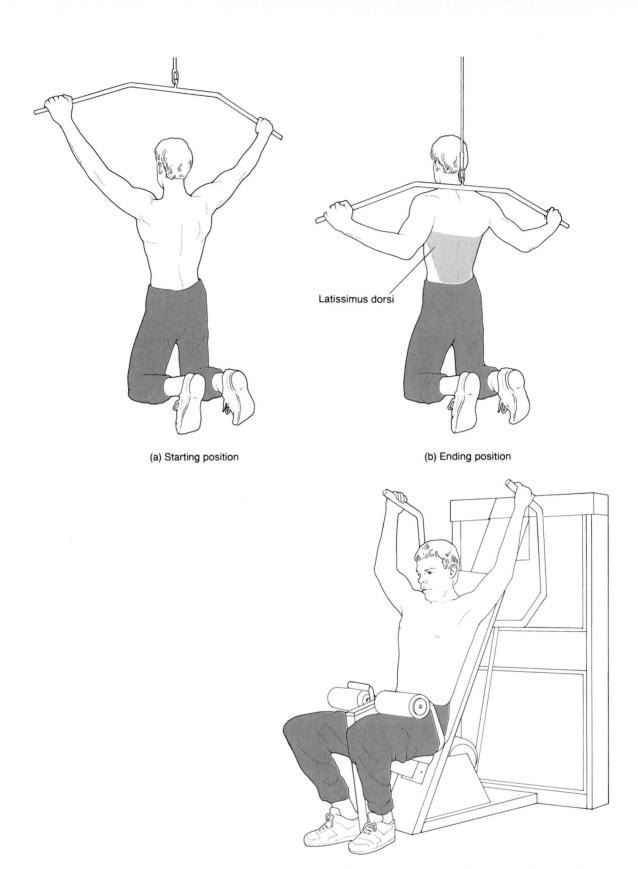

(a) Starting position

(b) Ending position

Latissimus dorsi

(c) Another type of machine for the latissimus dorsi

Figure 4.14A *The lat machine pull down. The lat machine pull down trains the latissimus dorsi in the back and side of the upper body, but it also develops the biceps on the front of the upper arm and the pectoralis major in the chest. Another type of weight machine (c) exercises the same muscles.*

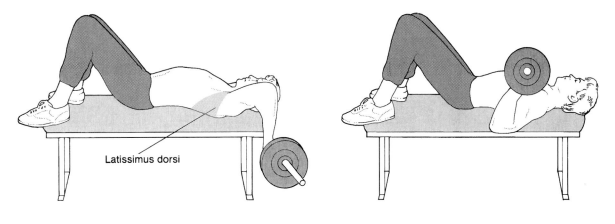

(a) Starting position   (b) Ending position

Latissimus dorsi

Figure 4.14B *The bent-arm pullover. The bent-arm pullover trains the latissimus dorsi and develops the pectoralis major. The weight machine in figure 4.14A trains the same muscles.*

Back
Figure 4.14A

Exercise	Lat machine pull down
Back Muscles	Latissimus dorsi
Other Muscles	Biceps, pectoralis major
Sets	1–3
Repetitions	8–12, PRE concept
Safety	A very safe exercise
Equipment	Lat machine
Description	From seated or kneeling position, take a wide grip at arm's length on the bar overhead. Pull bar down until it reaches back of the neck. Return slowly to starting position.

Note: If a lat machine is not available, the bent arm pullover may be substituted.

Figure 4.14B

Alternate Exercise	Bent-arm pullover
Back Muscles	Latissimus dorsi
Other Muscles	Pectoralis major
Sets	1–3
Repetitions	8–12, PRE concept
Safety	Do not arch back. Start with light weights when learning the technique.
Equipment	Bench
Description	Lie supine on bench, entire back in contact with the bench, feet on the bench, knees bent. Hold weight on chest with elbows bent. Swing weight over head, just brushing hair, and lower as far as possible without taking back off the bench. Keeping elbows in, return the weight to the chest.

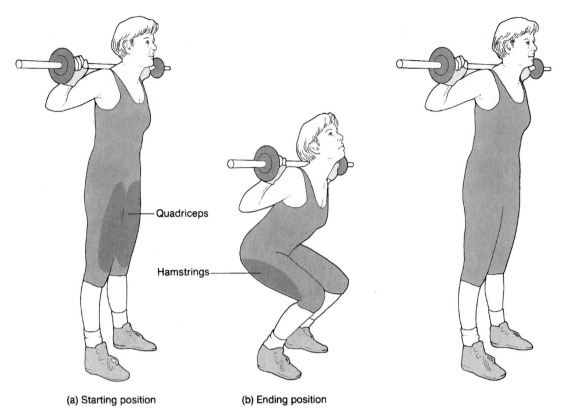

(a) Starting position   (b) Ending position

Figure 4.15 *The half-squat or parallel squat. The half-squat develops the quadriceps muscle group on the front of the thigh and the hamstrings on the back of the thigh. The weight machines (c) develop the same muscles.*

Thigh
Figure 4.15

Exercise	Half-squat or parallel squat
Thigh Muscles	Quadriceps (front), hamstrings (back)
Other Muscles	Gluteus maximus
Sets	1–3
Repetitions	8–12, PRE concept
Safety	Have two spotters to assist if using free weights. Keep back straight. Drop weight behind you if you lose balance. Do not squat more than halfway down.
Equipment	Squat rack if available. Pad the bar with towels if necessary.
Description	In standing position, take bar from squat rack or spotters and rest on the shoulders behind the head. Squat until thighs are parallel to ground or until buttocks touch a chair at this parallel position. Do not squat beyond halfway. Keep back as straight as possible. Return to standing position.

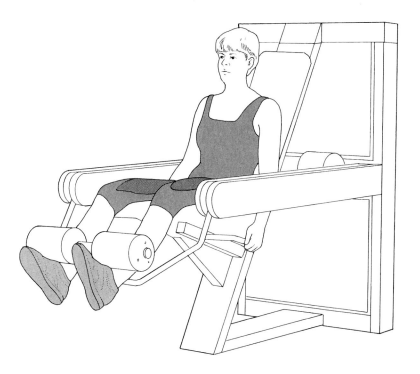

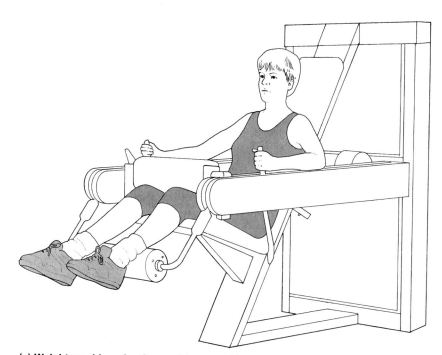

(c) Weight machines for the quadriceps and hamstrings muscle group

Figure 4.15— *Continued*

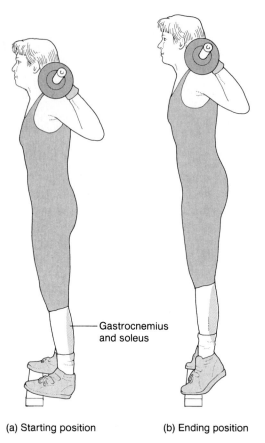

(a) Starting position   (b) Ending position

Figure 4.16 *Heel raise. The heel raise develops the two major calf muscles—the gastrocnemius and the soleus. Machines are also available to exercise these muscles.*

Gastrocnemius and soleus

Calf
Figure 4.16

Exercise	Heel raises
Calf Muscles	Gastrocnemius, soleus
Other Muscles	Deep calf muscles
Sets	1–3
Repetitions	8–12, PRE concept
Safety	Have two spotters if you use free weights.
Equipment	Squat rack, if available. Pad the bar with a towel if necessary.
Description	Place bar on back of shoulders as in squat exercise. Rise up on your toes as high as possible, and then return to standing position. Place the toes on a board so heels can drop down lower than normal. Point toes in, out, and straight ahead during different sets in order to work the muscles from different angles.

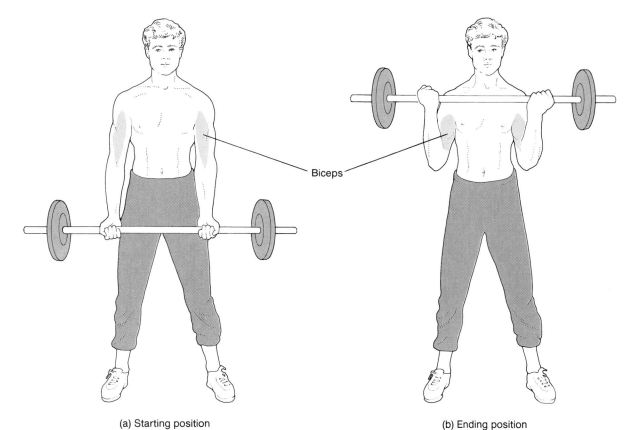

(a) Starting position

(b) Ending position

Figure 4.17 *The standing curl. The standing curl strengthens the biceps muscle in the front of the upper arm as well as several other muscles in the region that bend the elbow. The weight machine (c) trains the same muscles.*

Front of arm
Figure 4.17

Exercise	Standing curl
Arm Muscle	Biceps
Other Muscles	Several elbow flexors
Sets	1–3
Repetitions	8–12, PRE concept
Safety	Do not arch back. Place back against wall to control arching motion.
Equipment	Curl bar if available
Description	Stand with weight held in front of body, palms forward. Place back against wall. Bend the elbows and bring the weight to the chest. Lower it slowly.

(c) Weight machine for the biceps

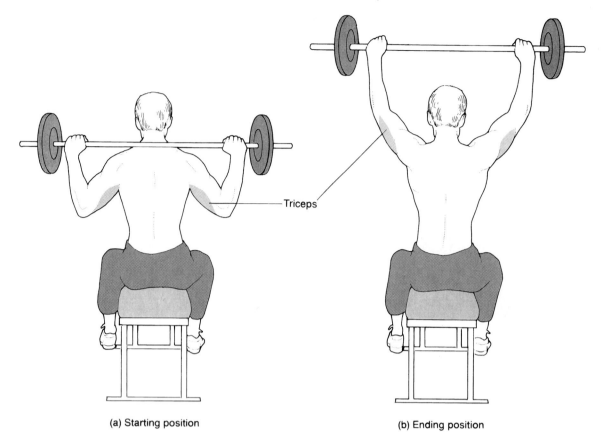

(a) Starting position   (b) Ending position

Figure 4.18 *The seated overhead press. The seated overhead press primarily develops the triceps muscle on the back of the upper arm; the exercise also trains the trapezius in the upper back and neck. The weight machine (c) develops the same muscles.*

Back of arm
Figure 4.18

Exercise	Seated overhead press
Arm Muscle	Triceps
Other Muscles	Trapezius, deltoid
Sets	1–3
Repetitions	8–12, PRE concept
Safety	Do not arch back excessively. Have spotter available as fatigue sets in.
Equipment	Bench or chair
Description	Sit on bench with weight held behind the head near the neck. Hands should be close together, elbows bent. Straighten elbows and press weight over head to arm's length. Lower weight slowly to starting position.

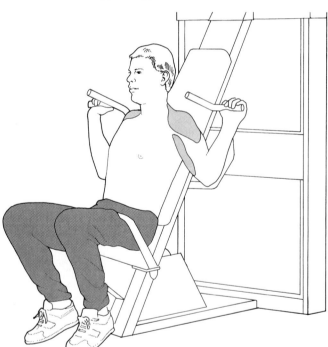

(c) Weight machine for the triceps

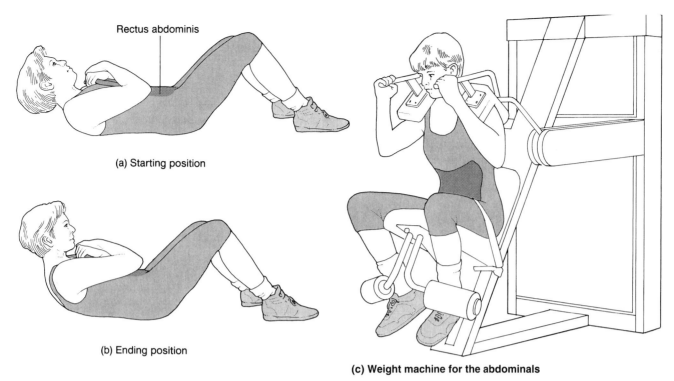

Rectus abdominis

(a) Starting position

(b) Ending position

(c) Weight machine for the abdominals

Figure 4.19 *The curl-up. The curl-up trains the rectus abdominis and the oblique abdominis muscles. The weight machine (c) strengthens the same muscles.*

Abdominal area
Figure 4.19

Exercise	Curl-ups
Abdominal Muscles	Rectus abdominis
Other Muscles	Oblique abdominis muscles
Sets	1–3
Repetitions	8–12, PRE concept
Safety	Develop sufficient abdominal strength before using weights with this exercise. Do not arch back when exercising.
Equipment	Free weight plates; incline sit-up bench if available.
Description	Lie on back, knees bent with heels close to buttocks, hands should hold weights on chest. Curl up about a third to half way. Return to starting position slowly.

Note: This exercise may be done without weights, but with an increased number of repetitions. See the next section for more information on the sit-up exercise.

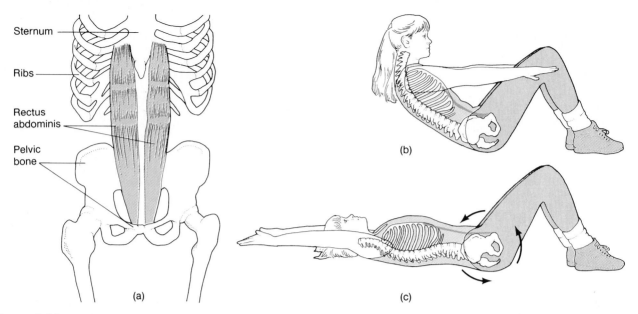

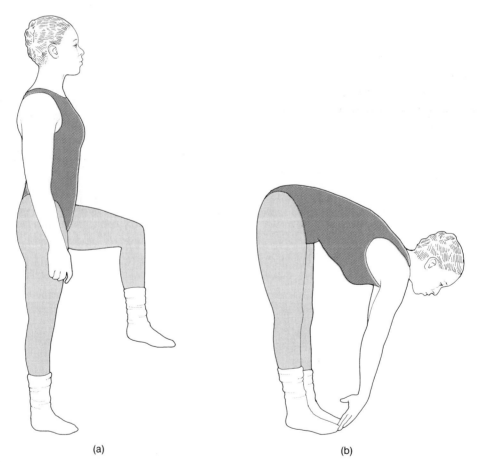

Figure 4.20 (a) The rectus abdominis muscle connects to the ribs and to the lower part of the pelvic bone. Contraction of the rectus abdominis can cause (b) spinal flexion or (c) backward pelvic tilt.

Figure 4.21 Hip flexion occurs at the joint between the pelvic bone and the thigh bone. Both (a) and (b) are examples of hip flexion. (B is not a highly recommended exercise.)

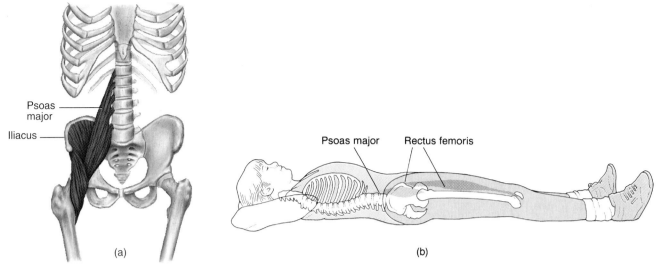

Figure 4.22 *The effect of the psoas major on the spine. The psoas major is shown in (a). In the straight leg position, (b), the psoas major may pull forward on the lower spine area, thus increasing the lumbar lordosis. This is particularly true if the abdominal muscles are weak. The rectus femoris can also pull forward on the pelvis and increase the lumbar lordosis.*

a hip flexor, but as you can see in figure 4.22, it may also pull forward on the lumbar spine area. The **rectus femoris** (see fig. 4.22), the main muscle in the front of the thigh, is also a hip flexor, but it can also pull forward on the pelvic bone. The actions of both of these muscles may cause an increased curve in the lumbar area, which is exactly the opposite of the purpose of abdominal exercises. Thus, exercises that increase this forward curve should be avoided as much as possible.

One good way to help avoid the adverse effects of the psoas major and rectus femoris muscles is simply to flex the hips in the starting position for abdominal exercises. Figure 4.23 illustrates one possible method. In this position the psoas major and rectus femoris are shortened somewhat so they are not in a position to increase the lumbar curve. Do not anchor your feet, for holding them down will increase the role of these muscles and decrease the effect on the abdominals.

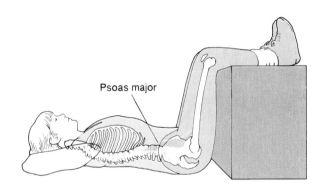

Figure 4.23 *The bent-knee position. By bending the knees while on the back, thus flexing the hips, the psoas major and rectus femoris are somewhat shortened and have a lesser tendency to accentuate the curve in the low back area. Putting the feet flat on the floor with the knees bent achieves the same effect.*

Recommended and Nonrecommended Abdominal Exercises

Individuals with lower levels of abdominal strength may need to progress gradually from the less strenuous to the more difficult abdominal exercises. For those with very low levels of abdominal strength, the pelvic tilt should be used as the primary exercise, with eventual progression through the various levels of the modified curl-up.

A. Backward pelvic tilt (fig. 4.20c). Do ten repetitions of 15 seconds each. The **backward pelvic tilt** is an excellent abdominal exercise that can be done almost any time of the day. You can do it sitting, standing, or lying down. Simply contract your abdominal muscles to tuck in your stomach and flatten out your lower back. For example, you may stand with your back against a wall and attempt to flatten your lower back so that it touches the wall. These tummy tucks help to stretch tight muscles in your lower back region while strengthening your abdominal muscles.

B. Curl-up with modifications (fig. 4.24a–e). Research has shown that the curl-up exercise is very effective for increasing abdominal strength and is least likely to create increased pressure in the lumbar area. The curl-up should be performed to the point where only the shoulder blades are lifted off the floor. For each level, work up to fifty repetitions before progressing to the next level.

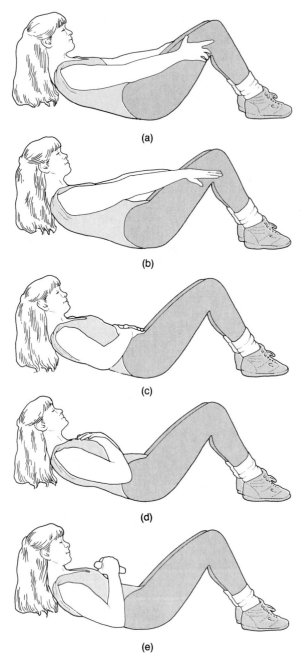

(a)

(b)

(c)

(d)

(e)

Figure 4.24 *The curl-up. The curl-up involves only spinal flexion. Sit up part way (about 30°), and return slowly to the starting position. Do not anchor the feet. Figures (a) through (e) show progressive increases in difficulty. (a) If the abdominal muscles are very weak, pull yourself up by holding on to your thighs. (b) Hold arms straight down in front. (c) Fold your arms across your stomach. (d) Cross your arms over your chest with fingertips on opposite shoulders. (e) Hold weights on your chest.*

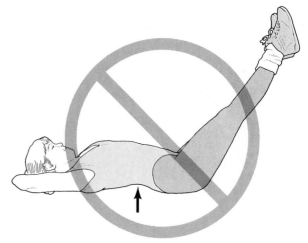

Figure 4.25 *Slow leg lowering. Exercises such as this help to strengthen the abdominal muscles, but they may place a tremendous stress on the low back area. If you do exercises like this, keep the lower back flat against the floor throughout.*

Level 1—Grasp back of both thighs with your hands and assist the curl-up by pulling yourself up. Go back slowly (fig. 4.24a).

Level 2—Place hands at sides of legs, arms straight as in figure 4.24b. Curl up with no pulling assistance. Go back down slowly.

Level 3—Cross arms on stomach. Do curl-up. Go back down slowly (fig. 4.24c).

Level 4—Fold arms across chest. Do curl-up. Go back down slowly (fig. 4.24d).

Level 5—Place weights on chest. Do curl-up. Be sure lower back maintains contact with the floor. Go back down slowly. Only do this exercise after you are able to complete Level 4 comfortably. Start with light weights (e.g., 5 pounds) and follow the progression noted earlier in this chapter (fig. 4.24e).

A number of other exercises may be used to develop abdominal strength, but you should avoid those that cause an increased lumbar curve as shown in figure 4.25. It is important to incorporate the backward pelvic tilt in all exercises. Always try to keep the lower part of the back flat against the supporting surface, an action that will ensure that the abdominal muscles are being exercised.

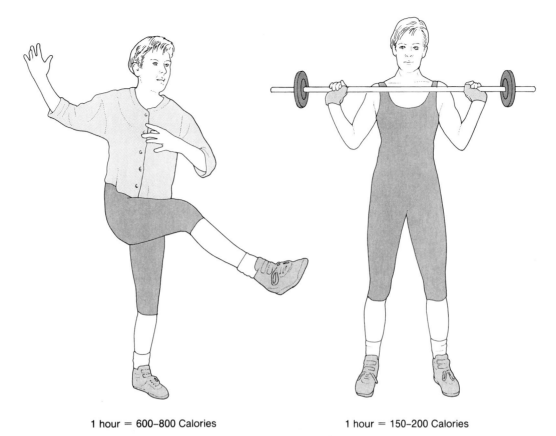

1 hour = 600–800 Calories   1 hour = 150–200 Calories

Figure 4.26 *All modes of exercise increase caloric expenditure. However, an hour of regular weight training expends only about one-third to one-fourth as many Calories as vigorous aerobic activity. Combining aerobic exercises with weight training (circuit aerobics) helps burn more Calories than weight training alone; it also provides cardiovascular health benefits while increasing muscular strength and endurance.*

Circuit Aerobics

Although the principles underlying the development of an aerobic-training program and a resistance-training program are similar, the purposes of each are rather different. An aerobic exercise program is designed to improve the efficiency of the cardiovascular system; the basic purpose of a resistance-training program is to increase muscle size, strength, and endurance.

One form of resistance training that has been used to provide some moderate benefits to the cardiovascular system is **circuit weight training,** a method in which the individual moves rapidly from one exercise to the next. Generally, this type of program has used lighter weights with greater numbers of repetitions, thus increasing the aerobic component of training.

A newer version of this method is circuit aerobics. Circuit aerobics may be done in a variety of ways, but basically it involves an integration of aerobic and resistance-training exercises. It is actually a form of interval aerobic training, but instead of resting or doing a lower level of aerobic activity during the recovery interval, you do resistance-training exercises. Circuit aerobics may offer you benefits such as improved cardiovascular fitness, increased caloric expenditure for loss of body fat, improved muscular strength and endurance, and increased muscle tone in body areas not normally stressed by aerobic exercise alone (fig. 4.26).

If interested, you may develop your own program. How you design it depends upon the facilities and equipment available. One technique would be to integrate the self-constructed aerobic dance exercise program presented in the last chapter with the resistance-training program presented in this chapter. Simply do the aerobic exercise bout for 2 to 4 minutes and follow it with one of the resistance-training exercises during a 1- to 2-minute recovery period. If you integrate eight aerobic dance exercises with eight resistance-training exercises, you may have a complete workout in 30 to 60 minutes, including warm-up and warm-down.

Try it. It can be a great indoor workout that will provide you with the combined benefits of both aerobic and resistance-training exercise programs.

References
Books

Bouchard, C., et al., eds. 1994. *Physical activity, fitness, and health.* Champaign, Ill.: Human Kinetics.

Feinstein, A. 1992. *Training the body to cure itself: How to use exercise to heal.* Emmaus, Penn.: Rodale Press.

Fleck, S., and W. Kraemer 1988. *Designing resistance training programs.* Champaign, Ill.: Life Enhancement Publications.

Heyward, V. 1991. *Advanced fitness assessment and exercise prescription.* Champaign, Ill.: Human Kinetics.

United States Department of Health and Human Services. 1991. *Healthy people 2000: National health promotion and disease prevention objectives.* Washington, D.C.: U.S. Government Printing Office.

Westcott, W. 1982. *Strength fitness.* Boston: Allyn and Bacon.

Reviews

American College of Sports Medicine. 1990. ACSM position stand: The recommended quantity and quality of exercise for developing and maintaining cardiorespiratory and muscular fitness in healthy adults. *Medicine and Science in Sports and Exercise* 22:265–74.

Aoyagi, Y., and R. Shephard. 1992. Aging and muscle function. *Sports Medicine* 14:376–96.

Biering-Sorensen, F., et al. 1994. Physical activity, fitness, and back pain. In *Physical activity, fitness, and health,* eds. C. Bouchard, et al. Champaign, Ill.: Human Kinetics.

Blimkie, C. 1993. Resistance training during preadolescence. Issues and controversies. *Sports Medicine* 15:389–407.

Dudley, G. 1988. Metabolic consequences of resistive-type exercise. *Medicine and Science in Sports and Exercise* 20:S158–S161.

Effron, M. 1989. Effects of resistive training on left ventricular function. *Medicine and Science in Sports and Exercise* 21:694–97.

Evans, W. 1992. Exercise, nutrition, and aging. *Journal of Nutrition* 122:796–801.

Evans, W., and W. Campbell. 1993. Sarcopenia and age-related changes in body composition and functional capacity. *Journal of Nutrition* 123:465–68.

Ewart, C. 1989. Psychological effects of resistive weight training: Implications for cardiac patients. *Medicine and Science in Sports and Exercise* 21:683–88.

Fleck, S. 1988. Cardiovascular adaptations to resistance training. *Medicine and Science in Sports and Exercise* 20:S146–S151.

Fleck, S., and J. Falkel. 1986. Value of resistance training for the reduction of sports injuries. *Sports Medicine* 3:61–68.

Fleck, S., and W. Kraemer. 1988. Resistance training: Basic principles. *Physician and Sportsmedicine* 16 (March): 160–71.

Fleck, S., and W. Kraemer. 1988. Resistance training: Exercise prescription. *Physician and Sportsmedicine* 16 (June): 69–81.

Fleck, S., and W. Kraemer. 1988. Resistance training: Physiological responses and adaptations. *Physician and Sportsmedicine* 16 (April): 108–23.

Fleck, S., and W. Kraemer. 1988. Resistance training: Physiological responses and adaptations. *Physician and Sportsmedicine* 16 (May): 63–76.

Foran, B. 1985. Advantages and disadvantages of isokinetics, variable resistance, and free weights. *National Strength Coaches Association Journal* 7:24–25.

Franklin, B. 1989. Aerobic exercise training programs for the upper body. *Medicine and Science in Sports and Exercise* 21:S141–S148.

Goldberg, A. 1989. Aerobic and resistive exercise modify risk factors for coronary heart disease. *Medicine and Science in Sports and Exercise* 21:669–74.

Hopp, J. 1993. Effects of age and resistance training on skeletal muscle: A review. *Physical Therapy* 73:361–73.

Humphrey, D. 1988. Abdominal muscle strength and endurance. *Physician and Sportsmedicine* 16 (February): 201–2.

Kokkinos, P., and B. Hurley. 1990. Strength training and lipoprotein-lipid profiles: A critical analysis and recommendations for further study. *Sports Medicine* 9:266–72.

Kraemer, W., et al. 1988. A review: Factors in exercise prescription of resistance training. *National Strength and Conditioning Association Journal* 10:36–41.

Munnings, F. 1993. Strength training. Not only for the young. *Physician and Sportsmedicine* 21 (April): 133–40.

National Strength Coaches Association. 1985. Strength training and conditioning for the female athlete. *National Strength Coaches Association Journal* 7:10–29.

National Strength Coaches Association. 1987. Breathing during weight training. *National Strength Coaches Association Journal* 9:17–24.

Pauletto, B. 1986. Choice and order of exercises. *National Strength Coaches Association Journal* 8:71–73.

Plowman, S. 1992. Physical activity, physical fitness, and low back pain. *Exercise and Sport Sciences Review* 20:221–42.

Risser, W. 1990. Musculoskeletal injuries caused by weight training. Guidelines for prevention. *Clinics in Pediatrics* 29:305–10.

Schafer, J. 1991. Prepubescent and adolescent weight training: Is it safe? Is it beneficial? *National Strength and Conditioning Association Journal* 13:39–46.

Schatz, M. 1993. Boosting abdominal strength without back pain. *Physician and Sportsmedicine* 21 (April): 153–54.

Skinner, J., and P. Oja. 1994. Laboratory and field test for assessing health-related fitness. In *Physical activity, fitness, and health,* eds. C. Bouchard, et al. Champaign, Ill.: Human Kinetics.

Snyder-Mackler, L. 1989. Rehabilitation of the athlete with low back dysfunction. *Clinics in Sports Medicine* 8:717–29.

Soukup, J., and J. Kovaleski. 1993. A review of the effects of resistance training for individuals with diabetes mellitus. *Diabetes Education* 19:307–12.

Stamford, B. 1987. Isometric exercise. *Physician and Sportsmedicine* 15 (October): 191.

Stone, M., and G. Wilson. 1985. Resistive training and selected effects. *Medical Clinics in North America* 69:109–22.

Waldron, M. 1994. Determining muscle fiber type. *Runner's World* 29 (February): 34.

Weltman, A., and B. Stamford. 1982. Strength training: Free weights vs. machines. *Physician and Sportsmedicine* 10 (November): 197.

Specific Studies

Ballor, D., et al. 1988. Resistance weight training during caloric restriction enhances lean body weight maintenance. *American Journal of Clinical Nutrition* 47:19–25.

Boyden, T., et al. 1993. Resistance exercise training is associated with decreases in serum low-density lipoprotein cholesterol levels in premenopausal women. *Archives of Internal Medicine* 153:97–100.

Donnelly, J., et al. 1993. Muscle hypertrophy with large-scale weight loss and resistance training. *American Journal of Clinical Nutrition* 58:561–65.

Fiatarone, M., et al. 1990. High-intensity strength training in nonagenarians. Effects on skeletal muscle. *Journal of the American Medical Association* 263:3029–34.

Gettman, L., et al. 1982. A comparison of combined running and weight training with circuit weight training. *Medicine and Science in Sports and Exercise* 14:229–34.

Gleeson, P., et al. 1990. Effects of weight lifting on bone mineral density in premenopausal women. *Journal of Bone Mineral Research* 5:153–58.

Gundewall, B., et al. 1993. Primary prevention of back symptoms and absence from work. A prospective randomized study among hospital employees. *Spine* 18:587–94.

Heinrich, C., et al. 1990. Bone mineral content of cyclically menstruating female resistance and endurance trained athletes. *Medicine and Science in Sports and Exercise* 22:558–63.

Hortobagyi, T., and F. Katch. 1990. Role of concentric force in limiting improvement in muscular strength. *Journal of Applied Physiology* 68:650–58.

Knowlton, R., et al. 1987. Plasma volume changes and cardiovascular responses associated with weight lifting. *Medicine and Science in Sports and Exercise* 19:464–68.

Konig, M., and K. Biener. 1990. Sport-specific injuries in weight lifting. *Schweizerische Zeitschrift fur Sportmedizine* 38:25–30.

Kraemer, W., et al. 1987. Physiological responses to heavy resistance exercise with very short rest periods. *International Journal of Sports Medicine* 8:247–52.

Lacerte, M., et al. 1992. Concentric versus combined concentric-eccentric isokinetic training programs: Effect on peak torque of human quadriceps femoris muscle. *Archives of Physical Medical Rehabilitation* 73:1059–62.

Lander, J., et al. 1990. The effectiveness of weight belts during the squat exercise. *Medicine and Science in Sports and Exercise* 22:117–26.

MacDougall, J., et al. 1985. Arterial blood pressure response to heavy resistance exercise. *Journal of Applied Physiology* 58:785–90.

Petersen, S., et al. 1989. The influence of high-velocity circuit resistance training on VO$_{2MAX}$ and cardiac output. *Canadian Journal of Sport Sciences* 14:158–63.

Pollock, M., et al. 1989. Effect of resistance training on lumbar extension strength. *American Journal of Sports Medicine* 17:624–29.

Pyka, G., et al. 1994. Muscle strength and fiber adaptations to a year-long resistance training program in elderly men and women. *Journal of Gerontology* 49:M22–M27.

Ricci, B., et al. 1981. Biomechanics of the sit-up. *Medicine and Science in Sports and Exercise* 13:54–59.

Sale, D., et al. 1994. Effect of training of the blood pressure response to weight lifting. *Canadian Journal of Applied Physiology* 19:60–74.

Snow-Harter, C., et al. 1990. Muscle strength as a predictor of bone mineral density in young women. *Journal of Bone Mineral Research* 5:589–95.

Staron, R., et al. 1990. Muscle hypertrophy and fast fiber type conversions in heavy resistance-trained women. *European Journal of Applied Physiology* 60:71–78.

Suter, E., et al. 1993. Muscle fiber type distribution as estimated by cybex testing and by muscle biopsy. *Medicine and Science in Sports and Exercise* 25:363–70.

Tesch, P., et al. 1986. Muscle metabolism during intense, heavy-resistance exercise. *European Journal of Applied Physiology* 55:362–66.

Tucker, L. 1987. Effect of weight training on body attitudes: Who benefits most. *Journal of Sports Medicine and Physical Fitness* 27:70–78.

Virvidakis, K., et al. 1990. Bone mineral content of junior competitive weightlifters. *International Journal of Sports Medicine* 11:244–46.

Wallace, M., et al. 1991. Acute effects of resistance exercise on parameters of lipoprotein metabolism. *Medicine and Science in Sports and Exercise* 23:199–204.

Wilson, G., et al. 1993. The optimal training load for the development of dynamic athletic performance. *Medicine and Science in Sports and Exercise* 25:1279–86.

5

FLEXIBILITY

Key Terms

ballistic stretching exercises
dynamic flexibility
elastic fibers

flexibility
hamstrings
kyphosis

lordosis
proprioceptive neuromuscular
   facilitation (PNF)

soft tissues
static flexibility

Key Concepts

■ Flexibility may be an important health-related fitness component. Proper flexibility may be helpful in the prevention of low back pain, the improvement of posture and physical appearance, and the prevention of minor injuries associated with everyday life and planned aerobic exercise programs.

■ The soft tissues of the body, such as muscles, tendons, ligaments, and connective tissue, contain elastic fibers that can be stretched in order to improve flexibility.

■ Although both static stretching and ballistic stretching techniques may improve flexibility, the static stretching technique is recommended because the slow movement is less likely to cause an injury. One popular static stretching technique is proprioceptive neuromuscular facilitation (PNF).

■ In order to improve flexibility, the muscle must be overloaded (stretched beyond its normal range of motion) and held in position for about 15 to 60 seconds three times a day.

■ The key to flexibility exercises for the low back area is to flatten out the forward curve in the lumbar area—as it would appear if you curled yourself up into a ball.

■ Joggers and runners may benefit from flexibility exercises for several body areas—the low back region, the hamstrings, the calf muscles or Achilles tendon, and the groin muscles.

■ You can develop a flexibility program for almost any joint or muscle group in the body simply by stretching that muscle group and using the basic guidelines relative to overload and progression.

INTRODUCTION

Although flexibility has not received the attention that other health-related fitness factors such as aerobic fitness have, it is usually included in fitness tests associated with a Positive Health Life-style. In general, improved flexibility is believed to be important in the prevention of certain injuries and in the correction of poor posture.

Flexibility is simply the range of motion that the bones may go through at the various joints in your body. Flexibility is specific to each joint and is primarily limited by the nature or structure of the joint. For example, the elbow joint is constructed like a hinge. You may bend the forearm forward fairly freely, but it becomes locked when you extend it to its limit. Thus, the hinge structure of the elbow joint limits the range of motion to about 160 degrees (see fig. 5.1a). Moreover, the hinged joint allows movement only forward and backward. On the other hand, joints such as the shoulder, constructed like a ball and socket, allow movement in all directions and permit a greater range of motion (see fig. 5.1b, c, d).

If flexibility were limited only by the structure of the joint, we would not be able to improve it through a flexibility program because we could not change the basic joint structure. However, other body tissues, called **soft tissues,** also limit flexibility. These tissues include the muscles and the sheaths of tissue that surround them, the connective tissue (tendons and ligaments), and the skin. These tissues possess varying amounts of **elastic fibers,** that permit them to change their lengths (see fig. 5.2). Thus, as we move our bodies, the elasticity, or flexibility, of these soft tissues usually allows for a normal range of motion. However, if the body assumes a certain position for a prolonged period of time, then the soft tissues will adjust to that position. An example is illustrated in figure 5.3, which depicts a condition of round shoulders caused by habitual slouching of the shoulders. The soft tissues in the chest area have become rather shortened and tight, whereas those in the upper back region have become lengthened. Fortunately, a proper exercise program can help increase flexibility by lengthening those soft tissues, primarily the muscle tissue, that have become shortened and by strengthening those that have lengthened.

The major thrust of the flexibility exercise programs presented in this chapter is to help prevent or relieve low back pain, a common health problem discussed in detail in chapter 11. Combined with exercises presented in the previous chapter to strengthen the abdominal muscles, improved flexibility in various muscle groups appears to be an important component of preventive medicine.

Improved flexibility may be helpful for other reasons related to improved health. Postural problems caused by shortened soft tissues may be ameliorated. Such changes in body posture may improve physical appearance and body image, important components related to mental health. Furthermore, the current thinking among many medical advisors is that flexibility exercises are important in preventing some of the common injuries associated with aerobic exercise programs such as jogging, running, and aerobic dance. Since aerobic exercise is advocated in this book as a major component of the Positive Health Life-style, proper flexibility exercises for muscles involved in these activities may help you continue to exercise without injury. In their position stand on exercise programs for healthy adults, the American College of Sports Medicine recommends that flexibility exercises be incorporated in the warm-up or warm-down for aerobic or resistance exercises. Finally, improved flexibility will help you to move more easily, such as when turning your head to back out a car.

In addition, flexibility is an important factor for success in many sports. Athletes who participate in sports that require a great deal of flexibility may need to increase flexibility to the maximum possible. A good example of maximum flexibility is the cheerleader or gymnast doing a split. It is important to note that if you are training for a particular sport, the exercise program you develop to improve your flexibility must be specific to that sport. For example, a swimmer might be particularly interested in improved flexibility in the shoulder area, whereas a hurdler in track may want improved hip and leg flexibility. The principles underlying the development of a basic flexibility program may be applied to training the appropriate muscle groups for sports as well.

The flexibility exercises presented in this chapter are designed for three different purposes: to help prevent or relieve low back pain, to improve posture (such as the correction of **kyphosis** [round shoulders]), and to stretch soft tissues that are commonly injured in aerobic exercise programs, particularly jogging and running. But first, let's look at some of the basic principles underlying the development of a flexibility exercise program ∎

Principles of Flexibility Exercises
Types of Flexibility and Methods of Training

Flexibility may be subdivided into two different types: static and dynamic. **Static flexibility** represents the range of motion that you may achieve through a slow steady stretch to the limits of the joint movement. **Dynamic flexibility** is characterized by the range of motion obtained when moving a body part rapidly to its limits. A variety of different programs using either static or dynamic stretching techniques have been developed to improve flexibility.

Static techniques simply use slow stretching exercises. You may do these exercises by yourself, using the force of gravity to gradually stretch your muscles. For example, if you hang from a pull-up bar by your hands, the muscles of your chest are stretched as gravity exerts its force to pull you down. You may also have another individual apply a gradual stretching force, such as the technique illustrated in figure 5.4a, to stretch the chest muscles. This technique is often known as passive stretching.

A static stretching technique popular with athletic trainers is **proprioceptive neuromuscular facilitation,** or **PNF.** A full discussion of the neurological basis of PNF is beyond the scope of this text, but basically the movements involved help you relax the muscle so that stretching may be facilitated. There are a number of different PNF techniques, but one that is effective involves a five-step protocol involving a prestretch, isometric contraction, relaxation,

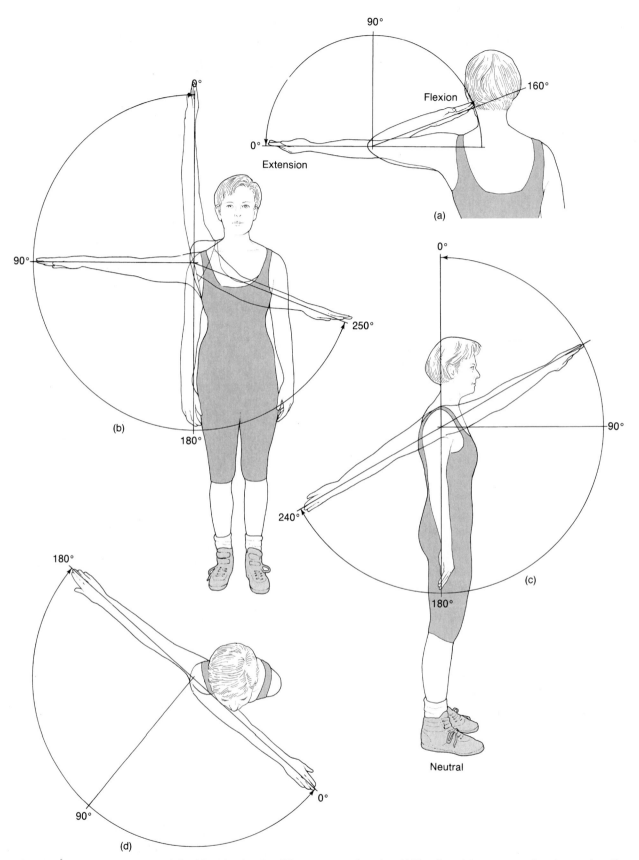

Figure 5.1 *The elbow joint and shoulder joint showing different ranges of motion. (a) The elbow joint may move in only one plane through a range of about 160°. (b–d) The shoulder joint permits 180° of motion or more in three planes.*

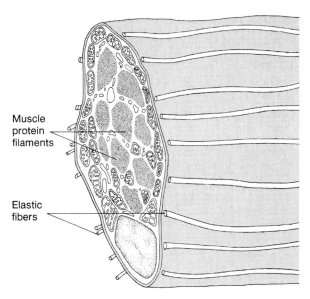

Figure 5.2 *Elastic fibers are found throughout the body, including the muscle tissues as illustrated here. These elastic fibers may be shortened under such circumstances as habitual poor posture, or they may be lengthened through a flexibility exercise program.*

Muscle protein filaments

Elastic fibers

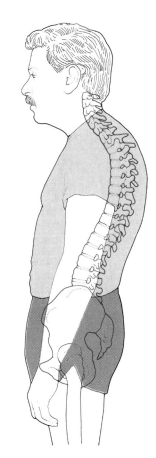

Figure 5.3 *Round shoulders. Round shoulders are accompanied by a stretching of the muscles in the upper back region and a tightening, or shortening, of muscles in the chest area.*

concentric contraction, and a poststretch; this technique is often referred to as the slow-reversal-hold-relax (SRHR) maneuver. For example, to stretch your chest muscles as in figure 5.4a, you follow this procedure:

1. Prestretch—Your partner prestretches your chest muscles gently by pulling back on your elbows for about 6 seconds.

2. Isometric contraction—Your partner provides increased resistance to you by holding your elbows back as you contract your chest muscles isometrically for about 6 seconds in an attempt to bring your elbows forward.

3. Relaxation—You and your partner relax for about 2 seconds.

4. Concentric contraction—You actively contract your back muscles, not your chest muscles, concentrically to pull your elbows back; when you pull your elbows as far back as you can, you hold for 6 seconds, continuing to contract the back muscles.

5. Poststretch—Your partner again pulls back gradually on your elbows to stretch your chest muscles, holding for about 10 seconds.

Similar techniques may be applied to other muscle groups, such as the hamstrings, illustrated in figure 5.4b.

You may also use the PNF technique without a partner, as illustrated in figure 5.4c to stretch the calf muscles and Achilles tendon. Using the same five-step protocol, apply force with a towel or thick rope to prestretch the calf (Step 1), and to provide resistance by pulling back on your foot as you isometrically contract your calf muscles in an attempt to push your foot forward (Step 2). Relax (Step 3), then contract the muscles on the front of your leg in an attempt to move your toes toward your leg (Step 4), then stretch the calf in the post-stretch by pulling back with the towel (Step 5).

Although PNF has been shown to be one of the most effective means to improve flexibility, research has shown that the basic static technique is also very effective.

Some machines are available to provide the force for static stretching. For example, some Nautilus® machines are designed to put your muscles on stretch prior to lifting, as illustrated for the chest muscles in figure 5.5. Recently, some health spas have used machines to exercise you passively; basically, you just lie there and let the machine do the work for you. Although these latter machines may help improve flexibility, they do nothing for aerobic fitness (fig. 5.6).

Ballistic stretching exercises, or bouncing type exercises, are usually used in a dynamic flexibility program. For example, to improve dynamic flexibility of the chest muscles, you might do a number of elbow-flinging exercises. Your starting position is similar to that depicted in figure 5.4a or figure 5.15. You vigorously and repeatedly move your elbows backwards to the limits of their flexibility.

Most flexibility exercises may be done using both static and ballistic techniques. For example, from a standing position, you could bend over slowly, touch your fingers to the

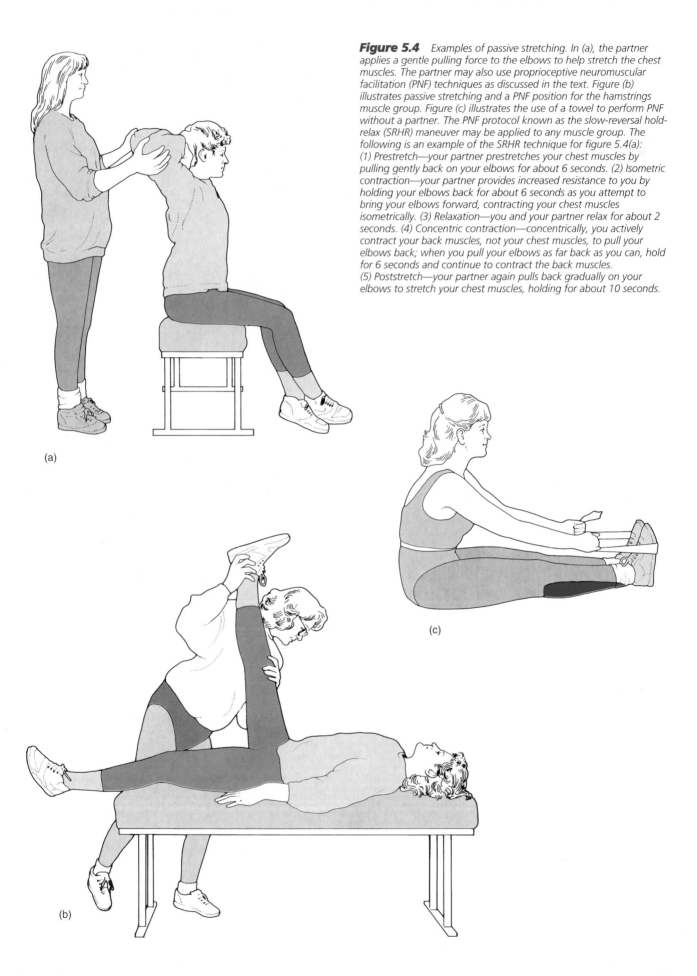

Figure 5.4 *Examples of passive stretching. In (a), the partner applies a gentle pulling force to the elbows to help stretch the chest muscles. The partner may also use proprioceptive neuromuscular facilitation (PNF) techniques as discussed in the text. Figure (b) illustrates passive stretching and a PNF position for the hamstrings muscle group. Figure (c) illustrates the use of a towel to perform PNF without a partner. The PNF protocol known as the slow-reversal hold-relax (SRHR) maneuver may be applied to any muscle group. The following is an example of the SRHR technique for figure 5.4(a): (1) Prestretch—your partner prestretches your chest muscles by pulling gently back on your elbows for about 6 seconds. (2) Isometric contraction—your partner provides increased resistance to you by holding your elbows back for about 6 seconds as you attempt to bring your elbows forward, contracting your chest muscles isometrically. (3) Relaxation—you and your partner relax for about 2 seconds. (4) Concentric contraction—concentrically, you actively contract your back muscles, not your chest muscles, to pull your elbows back; when you pull your elbows as far back as you can, hold for 6 seconds and continue to contract the back muscles. (5) Poststretch—your partner again pulls back gradually on your elbows to stretch your chest muscles, holding for about 10 seconds.*

(a)

(b)

(c)

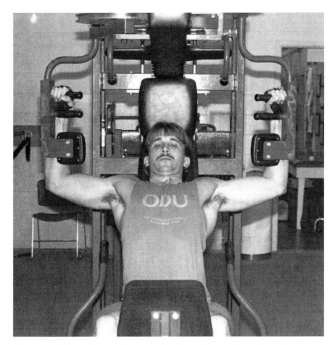

Figure 5.5 *The Nautilus Double Chest® may force the chest muscles into a stretched position prior to the start of strength training exercises.*

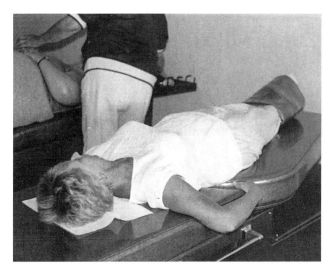

Figure 5.6 *Some fitness spas contain passive exercise machines designed to improve flexibility and muscle tone.*

floor and hold this position (remain static) for a period of time. On the other hand, you could move rapidly to touch the floor, straighten up rapidly, and repeat this ballistic exercise several times. Although research has shown that both types of exercise programs will equally improve flexibility, there appears to be a trend away from the ballistic exercises and toward the static type. The major reason for this is that ballistic exercises may exceed the normal range of motion and tear the muscle tissue or connective tissue. For example, as you bounce down to touch your toes as described, the soft tissues in the lower back are stretched rapidly, which may actually initiate a reflex muscle contraction; at the end of the movement, the muscles contract to stop your back from flexing too far forward. The stress created may exceed the elasticity of the soft tissues in the lower back and may damage the discs in the spinal column as well. The result may be a disabling back injury or muscle soreness. This does not mean that all individuals should refrain from all ballistic flexibility exercises. Many athletes, for example, may include ballistic exercises in their training regimen, since such movements may be an inherent part of their sport. However, for the vast majority of us, a static stretching program is an effective and safer approach.

Measurement of Flexibility

The techniques used to measure flexibility are specific to each joint in the body and usually involve devices such as goniometers and protractors to measure range of motion in degrees (fig. 5.7). Unless we have had an injury, most of us have normal ranges of motion in most joints throughout our body, so measurement of specific joints is of minor concern to us. If you do have some concern about specific joint flexibility, medical specialists or allied health personnel such as physical therapists

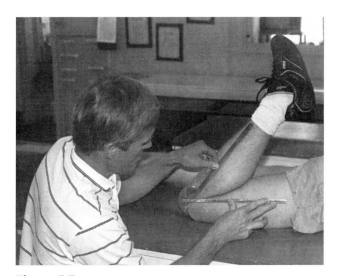

Figure 5.7 *Devices such as goniometers and protractors are used to measure the range of motion or flexibility of a joint.*

or athletic trainers may be able to provide an evaluation for you.

In health-related fitness tests, the most commonly used measure of flexibility involves the sit-and-reach test, which basically measures flexibility in several major muscle groups involved in the etiology of low back pain—the lower back muscles in the lumbar region of the spine and the hamstring muscles at the back of the thigh. Such tests are often known as low back-hamstring muscle flexibility tests.

There are several caveats to consider in using the sit-and-reach test as a measure of low back health. First, Jackson and Langford indicate that no hard research data are available demonstrating that low back flexibility is important in preventing low back pain. Other research actually indicates that the sit-and-reach test, as well as a modified sit-and-reach test that adjusts the test score for arm length, are not very good measures of lower back muscle flexibility, although they may be good indicators of hamstring flexibility. Thus, the use of these tests is based on the concept of logical validity, i.e., it may be logical to assume that muscle groups that lose flexibility, such as the hamstrings and lower back muscles, may contribute to the development of low back pain or injury by changing the normal relationship between the pelvic bone and the lower spine, or by being more prone to injury if overstretched.

Although it is not known for certain how much flexibility you need for good health, including prevention of low back pain, Laboratory Inventory 5.1 may provide you with some guidelines for the sit-and-reach test. Other tests of flexibility are found in Laboratory Inventories 5.2 and 5.3.

Basic Guidelines for a Flexibility Program

Static stretching exercise programs appear to be the safest way to improve flexibility for most individuals. In order to improve flexibility, however, you must adhere to the same basic principles of training that underlie the development of other fitness components. In essence, the principles of overload (intensity, duration, and frequency), progressive resistance, and specificity are the bases for your flexibility program. Some flexibility exercises may be done in conjunction with progressive relaxation training techniques, which you will learn in chapter 8.

The following specific guidelines should be followed for a beginning static stretching program:

1. For intensity, the muscle must be stretched, or overloaded, beyond its normal range of motion. Stretch until you feel mild to moderate tension, tightness, or discomfort. You should not stretch to a point of excessive pain; this may cause an injury in itself. Be very cautious when stretching the muscles in the low back area. Pain indicates trouble.

2. For duration, hold this static position for about 15 to 60 seconds. Repeat three or four times. In the beginning, stretch 15 seconds and use the principle of progression to increase it to 60 seconds. When you can hold a set position for 60 seconds, stretch a little further and hold the new position for 15 seconds. Continue with this progression principle.

3. For frequency, you may do flexibility exercises on a daily basis if you desire, but at least three to four days per week appear to be necessary for flexibility improvement to occur. Many of the exercises in the following sections can be done any time of the day. You are only limited by your imagination as to how these exercises may be worked into your daily schedule.

4. For specificity, select those exercises designed to improve flexibility in a specific body area. Try to do several exercises for each area that interests you.

5. Stretching before doing aerobic exercise should be a gentle, slow, steady stretch, particularly if the muscles are relatively cold.

6. Since a warm muscle has a decreased resistance to stretching, a good time to stretch is after your aerobic exercise bout and warm-down.

7. Use Laboratory Inventory 5.1 to evaluate your progress for improving flexibility in the low back-hamstring area and Laboratory Inventories 5.2 and 5.3 for other body areas.

8. Avoid ballistic stretching of injured muscles.

9. Avoid exercises involving an increased forward curvature in the lower back area, creating the hollow back look. See figures 4.25 on page 82 or 5.12 on page 95.

10. You may use the PNF techniques with a partner or by yourself by following the instructions on pages 87–89.

Flexibility Exercises for the Low Back Area

An increased hyperextension of the inward curve of the lower back area is known as **lordosis,** also called swayback, and it is believed to contribute to the development of low back pain.

The key to flexibility exercises for the low back area is to flatten out the forward curve in the lumbar region of the spine, which is lumbar spinal flexion. This movement is depicted in figure 5.8. Another way to flatten the lumbar spine is to rotate the hips backward. This movement, illustrated in figure 5.9, was introduced in the previous chapter and should be a part of all flexibility and abdominal exercises for the low back area. These movements help to stretch the tight muscles in the lower back region and those muscles, such as the psoas major, which tend to pull the hips forward.

When doing flexibility exercises for the low back area you should be especially cautious. Although a mild degree of discomfort is normally needed to improve flexibility of the muscle groups in this area, it should be the type of discomfort associated with muscle stretching. If you experience any pain, particularly a sharp pain, discontinue the exercise immediately. For those who do suffer from low back pain, select those exercises that will flatten your lower back and also those that help relieve the pain when you are in the stretched position. Figures 5.8, 5.9, 5.10, and 5.11 illustrate some useful exercises to improve flexibility in the low back area; these exercises may also relieve low back pain and be helpful in the prevention and treatment of pain associated with dysmenorrhea, or painful menstruation.

Research by Fairweather and Sidaway has shown that visualization techniques may enhance the effectiveness of lower back stretching exercises. For example, when doing an exercise such as depicted in Figure 5.9, they had subjects imagine themselves lying on their backs on a toboggan with their legs over the curved-up end which pressed back against their thighs. From this position the subjects visualized their seats slinging downward to fit the curve of the toboggan, thus helping to flatten out the lumbar curve.

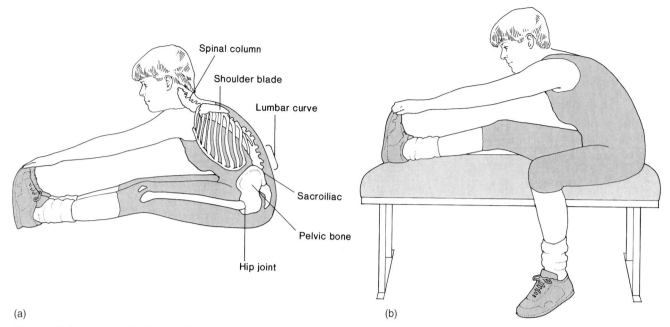

(a)

Spinal column

Shoulder blade

Lumbar curve

Sacroiliac

Pelvic bone

Hip joint

(b)

Figure 5.8 Lumbar spinal flexion, forward curvature in the spine, occurs primarily in the spine itself, with little or no movement at the hip joint. The lumbar curve tends to flatten out or reverse its direction, as illustrated in the forward bend. A good exercise to improve flexibility in the low back area is shown in (a). Bend forward slowly while sitting, reaching as far as you can until you experience mild discomfort. Hold a static position for 15–60 seconds. Repeat three times. An alternative approach is to do unilateral stretching of each leg as illustrated in (b). Alternate each leg for 15–60 seconds. Repeat three times for each leg.

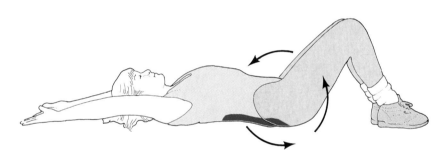

Figure 5.9 Backward pelvic tilt exercise. Lie on back with knees bent and feet flat on floor. Tighten the abdominal muscles and other muscles necessary to flatten the lower back against the floor. This exercise may also be done standing against a wall or sitting in a chair. Hold static position for 15–60 seconds. Repeat three times.

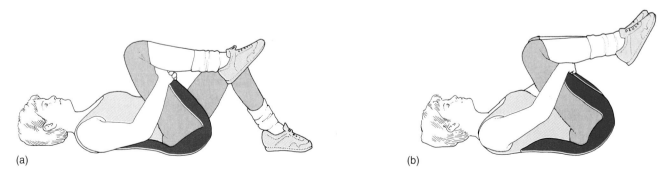

(a)

(b)

Figure 5.10 Single or double knee to chest. Lie with back on the floor, knees bent, and feet flat on the floor. In single knee exercise (a), draw one knee to the chest and pull it in tightly with the arms until you feel tension. In double knee exercise (b), draw both knees in. Pull tightly for 15–60 seconds. Repeat three times each for single knee or total of three times for double knee exercise.

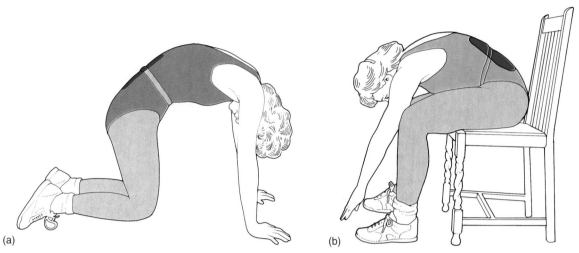

Figure 5.11 *(a) The cat stretch position. Take a deep breath, drop your head, and arch your lower back upwards by pulling in with your abdominal muscles. Hold for 15–60 seconds. Repeat three times. (b) You can also mimic the cat position while seated, something you can do throughout the day.*

It is important to reiterate that certain exercises may contribute to low back injury, such as those that cause an excessive increase in the lumbar curve as noted in figure 5.12. If you desire to do such exercises to improve the strength or flexibility of the lumbar region by actually accentuating the lumbar curve, figure 5.13 demonstrates an exercise that may be recommended. The bent-arm cobra should be done very gently, avoiding any sensation of pain in the low back area. Additionally, some exercises that flatten the lumbar curve may not be advisable. For example, both exercises in figure 5.14 have been advocated to increase flexibility in the low back region, but position (a) may place an excessive stress on the muscles in the lower back as the individual begins to straighten up, while this yoga position (b) may overload the spine in the neck region.

Flexibility Exercises for Round Shoulders

In the condition of round shoulders, the muscular forces in the chest and upper back are out of balance. The chest muscles are shortened and stronger while those in the back are lengthened and weaker, thus allowing the shoulders to be pulled forward. Exercises to help correct this condition should be designed to increase the length or flexibility of the chest muscles and to strengthen the back muscles. Several exercises for round shoulders are depicted in figures 5.15, 5.16, and 5.27b.

Flexibility Exercises for Tight Upper Back and Neck

Excess tension often contributes to tightness in the upper back and neck, which may be relieved by a variety of flexibility exercises. Figure 5.17 illustrates a simple exercise for stretching tight muscles in the upper back region. Flexibility exercises for the neck should not use a full circle rotation, for some impingement may occur in the neck vertebrae. Instead, gently lower your chin to your chest and gently roll your head from side to side. See figure 5.18 for proper and improper neck flexibility exercise.

Flexibility Exercises for Joggers, Runners, and Other Aerobic Exercisers

Joggers, runners, swimmers, bicyclists, aerobic dancers, and other aerobic exercisers often may develop minor aches, pains, or minor injuries in various parts of their bodies, particularly during the beginning stages of an exercise program. Those who are strong advocates of flexibility exercises for joggers, runners, and other exercisers suggest that these minor injuries may be prevented by a proper flexibility exercise program. The theory that a more flexible muscle may be less susceptible to injury appears to be sound. At the least, since improved flexibility should not be

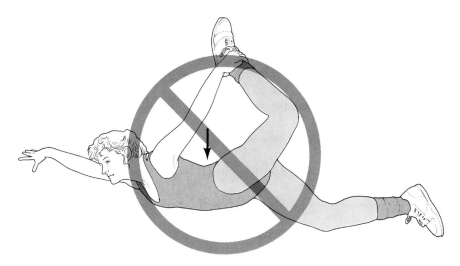

Figure 5.12 *Avoid exercises that increase the lumbar curve by placing excessive stress on the lower back region. This hyperextension of the lumbar spine is called lordosis.*

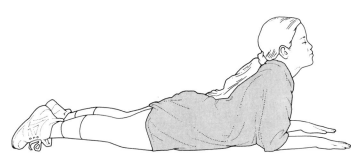

Figure 5.13 *Bent-arm cobra. Lie flat on your stomach, toes pointed, with arms bent at the elbow and hands flat on the floor. From this position, while keeping your pelvis on the floor slowly raise your head and upper body until you feel mild tension in the lower back area. Do not overstretch; avoid the sensation of pain. Hold static position for 15–60 seconds. Repeat three times. It is extremely important to keep the pelvis on the floor so as to avoid an excessive increase in the lumbar curve.*

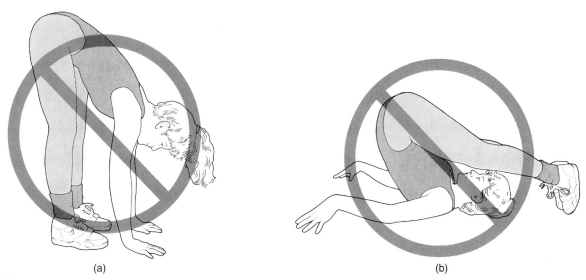

(a)   (b)

Figure 5.14 *Some exercises that flatten the lumbar curve should be avoided. In (a), excessive stress may be placed upon the muscles and ligaments of the lower back region when straightening up, particularly with knees locked. This exercise may be safer when done with the knees slightly bent. The yoga position in (b) may subject the neck region to injury.*

harmful, joggers, runners, and other aerobic exercisers may want to do flexibility exercises for five body areas that are commonly subject to minor injuries.

First, the low back area may be prone to injury through improper running form or overuse injuries in a variety of aerobic activities. The exercises suggested for relief or prevention of low back pain presented earlier in this chapter are highly recommended.

Second, the **hamstrings,** a muscle group at the back of the thigh, should be stretched. Some of the exercises for low back pain, such as those in figures 5.8 and 5.10, help improve hamstring flexibility. Other more strenuous exercises for hamstring flexibility are depicted in figures 5.19 and 5.20.

Third, the calf muscles in the back of the lower leg should be stretched to prevent possible problems with the Achilles tendon, a common injury among joggers, runners, and aerobic dancers. Two examples of appropriate flexibility exercises are presented in figure 5.21.

The fourth general area to stretch includes the hip and thigh, including the groin, muscle areas that often tighten up or become aggravated in runners. Figures 5.22, 5.23, 5.24, and 5.25 are common flexibility exercises for these muscle groups. These exercises may also contribute to the relief of low back pain.

Fifth, stretching the lateral trunk muscles and the underlying respiratory muscles, as illustrated in figure 5.26, may help relieve, and possibly help prevent, the stitch-in-the-side phenomenon in runners. Although this finding is based on anecdotal evidence, it may possibly help by relieving a muscle spasm or other underlying cause of the pain.

You can develop a flexibility exercise program for any joint in your body simply by finding a safe position that puts the muscles around that joint on stretch and by following the guidelines provided earlier. A towel or thick rope may be a very simple yet effective means to help you stretch almost any joint in your body. Figure 5.27 illustrates two stretches that may be done with a towel.

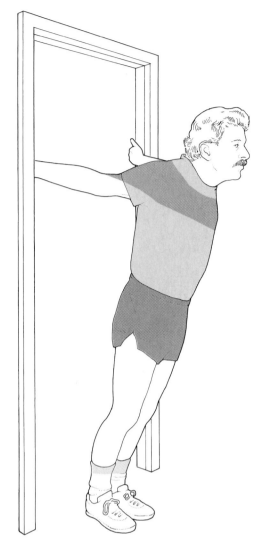

Figure 5.15 *Doorway stretch. Stand in a doorway with arms outstretched and placed against wall on one side of the doorway. Lean forward gradually until tension and mild discomfort is experienced in muscles of the chest. Hold static position for 15–60 seconds. Repeat three times.*

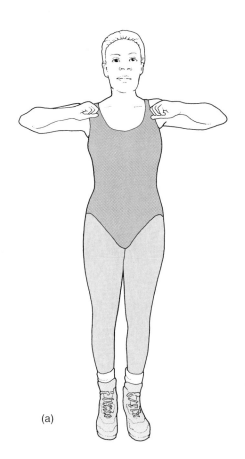

Figure 5.16 Isometric chest stretcher. (a) In standing or sitting position, raise arms sideways to shoulder level with elbows bent and hands near the chest. (b) Try to move your elbows back sideways as far as possible by pulling your shoulder blades together. Hold static position for 15–60 seconds. Repeat three times. Alternatively, (c) lock your hands or hold a towel behind you as shown, raising arms back and up as far as possible. Hold for 15–60 seconds.

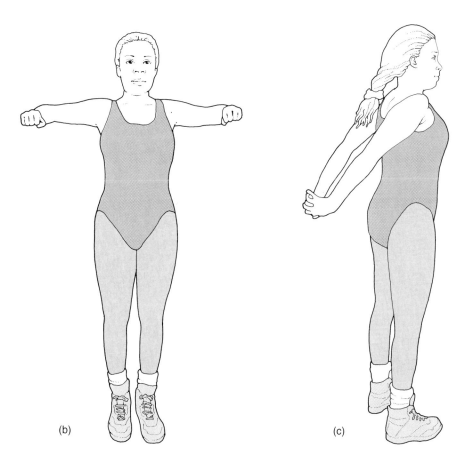

(a)

(b)

(c)

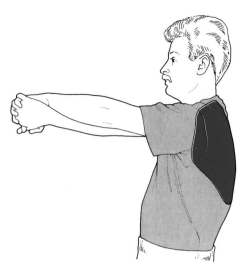

Figure 5.17 Isometric upper back stretcher. Cross your arms out in front of you as shown, putting your hands together with your thumbs pointed towards the floor. Stretch as far forward as possible to a point of tightness. Hold static position for 15–60 seconds. Repeat three times.

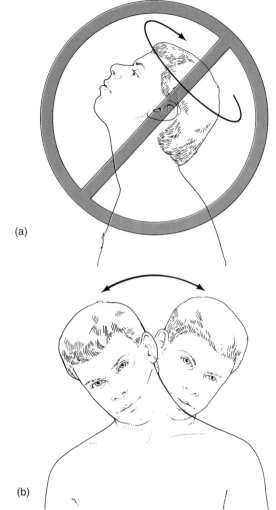

(a)

(b)

Figure 5.18 Neck flexibility exercise. (a) Do not rotate your head in a full circle. (b) Instead, lower your chin gently to your chest and roll carefully side to side. Stretch to a point near your shoulder and hold for 15–60 seconds. Repeat three times for each side.

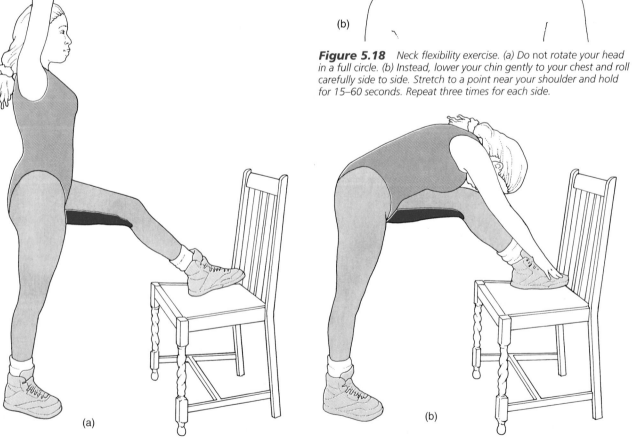

(a)   (b)

Figure 5.19 Hurdle stretch for hamstrings. (a) Place one leg out on some type of support. (b) Bend forward at the waist, keep back straight, and try to place your head as close to your leg as possible as you develop tightness, not pain, in your hamstrings. Keep knee bent slightly. Flatten back upward to also help stretch low back area. Hold forward position for 15–60 seconds. Repeat three times for each leg.

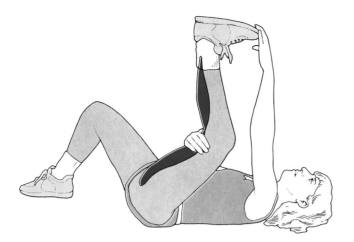

Figure 5.20 *Hamstring stretcher. Lie on your back with your knees bent and feet flat on the floor. Raise one leg and grasp toes with hand on same side. Grasp back of thigh with opposite hand. Pull down on toes, push heel towards the ceiling, and pull down on thigh until you feel tightness in the hamstrings. Hold 15–60 seconds. Repeat three times for each leg.*

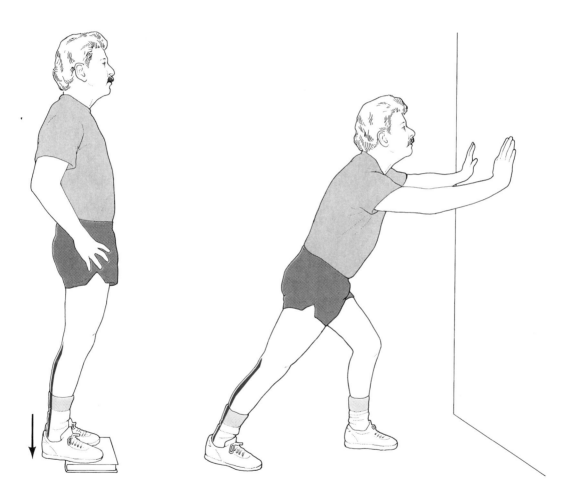

Figure 5.21 *Achilles stretcher. In (a), place the balls of feet on a solid object like a book, stair step, or street curb, and then lower the heel about two inches below the top surface. Hold static position for 15–60 seconds. Repeat three times. An alternate approach is illustrated in (b). Place your hands against a wall or tree for balance. Bend the knee of the front leg and keep the rear leg straight with the heel flat on the floor. Move your hip forward slowly until you feel stretch and tension in the calf of the rear leg. Hold for 15–60 seconds. Repeat three times for each leg. There are two major muscles in the calf, the gastrocnemius and the soleus. Keep your back leg straight to stretch the gastrocnemius, and then bend your back leg knee slightly to focus on the soleus.*

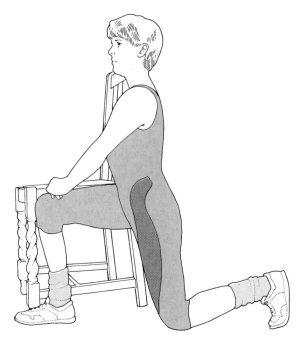

Figure 5.22 *Hip and thigh stretcher. Hold onto a chair or other object for balance. To stretch hip and thigh, place one leg out in front with the knee directly over the foot. Place knee and foot of trailing leg on the floor. Press hips forward to stretch upper thigh and deep hip muscles until you feel tightness. Keep back straight. Hold forward position 15–60 seconds. Repeat three times for each leg.*

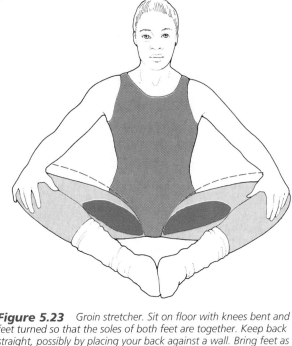

Figure 5.23 *Groin stretcher. Sit on floor with knees bent and feet turned so that the soles of both feet are together. Keep back straight, possibly by placing your back against a wall. Bring feet as close to crotch as possible. While in this position, push down on knees until mild tension or tightness is experienced in the groin muscle. Hold this position for 15–60 seconds. Repeat three times. Caution: Avoid this exercise if undue pain is experienced in the knees.*

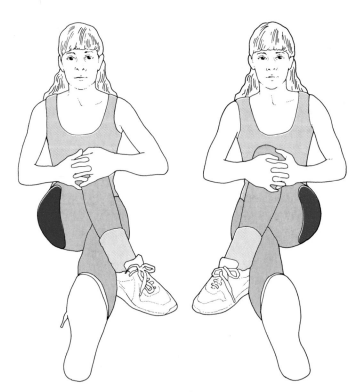

Figure 5.24 *Lateral hip stretcher. In seated position, cross one leg over the other straight leg. Grasp knee on the outside and pull towards opposite side of chest until you feel tightness, but not pain. Do both sides. Hold position 15–60 seconds. Repeat three times.*

Benefits/Risks

The benefits of improved flexibility are more difficult to study than those associated with aerobic and resistance training. Flexibility-training programs will increase the range of motion in the joints that are stretched, and this may help prevent low back pain and may benefit performance in certain athletic endeavors, as noted previously. However, the benefit most often associated with enhanced flexibility is the prevention of injury during exercise. The results of epidemiological studies are inconsistent, probably because so many variables other than a flexibility-exercise program can contribute to sports injuries. Experimental studies of flexibility training and prevention of injuries are difficult to conduct with humans, but laboratory studies with animals have suggested that stretching programs will improve the viscoelastic properties of tendons so that an increased load is tolerated before the tendon tears. If we can generalize these findings to humans, improved flexibility may help prevent overstretching-type injuries.

Improved flexibility may also enhance relaxation by decreasing tension in the muscle. Relaxation techniques for stress management incorporating a form of flexibility exercise are discussed in chapter 8.

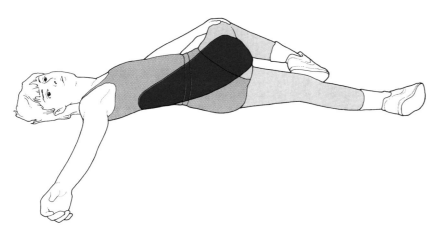

Figure 5.25 *The chiropractic stretch. To stretch hips, buttocks, and lower back, lie on back and cross one leg over the other as shown, pulling the knee gently to the floor with your opposite hand. Hold for 15–60 seconds. Repeat three times for both sides.*

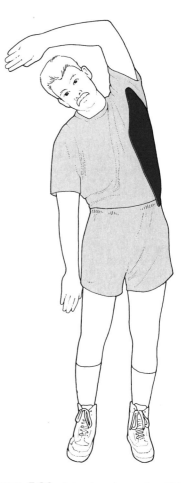

Figure 5.26 *Lateral trunk stretcher. This stretch may be used to relieve or prevent the stitch-in-the-side occurrence. Stretch arm overhead as shown, reaching opposite arm down the leg. Do both sides, but focus on the side that gets the stitch. Hold 15–60 seconds. Repeat three times.*

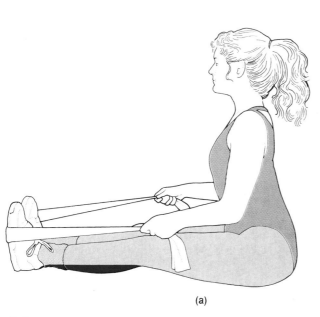

(a)

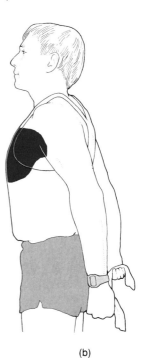

(b)

Figure 5.27 *A towel may be a simple yet effective means to stretch the muscles around most joints in the body. In (a) the towel is used to stretch the Achilles tendon and calf muscles, while in (b) the towel is used to stretch the chest muscles.*

References

Books

Anderson, B. 1980. *Stretching*. California: Shelter Publications.

Corbin, C., and R. Lindsey. 1993. *Concepts of physical fitness*. Dubuque, Iowa: Wm. C. Brown.

Feinstein, A. 1992. *Training the body to cure itself: How to use exercise to heal*. Emmaus, Penn.: Rodale Press.

Heyward, V. 1991. *Advanced fitness assessment and exercise prescription*. Champaign, Ill.: Human Kinetics.

Johnson, B., and J. Nelson. 1986. *Practical measurements for evaluation in physical education*. New York: Macmillan.

Schatz, M. 1992. *Back care basics: A doctor's gentle yoga program for back and neck pain relief*. Berkeley, Calif.: Rodmell Press.

Reviews

American College of Sports Medicine. 1990. ACSM position stand: The recommended quantity and quality of exercise for developing and maintaining cardiorespiratory and muscular fitness in healthy adults. *Medicine and Science in Sports and Exercise* 22:265–74.

Consumers Union. 1993. Safe alternatives to risky exercises. *Consumer Reports on Health* 5:100–101.

Corbin, C., and L. Noble. 1980. Flexibility. *Journal of Physical Education and Recreation* 51 (June): 23–24, 57–60.

Cornelius, W. 1985. Flexibility: The effective way. *National Strength Coaches Association Journal* 7:62–64.

Cornelius, W. 1990. Modified PNF stretching: Improvement in hip flexion. *National Strength and Conditioning Association Journal* 12:44–46.

Findelstein, H., and R. Roos. 1990. Ontario study raises doubt about stretching. *Physician and Sportsmedicine* 18 (January): 48–49.

Gauthier, M. 1987. Continuous passive motion: The no-exercise exercise. *Physician and Sportsmedicine* 15 (August): 142–48.

Liemohn, W. 1988. Flexibility and muscular strength. *Journal of Health, Physical Education, Recreation, and Dance* 59 (September): 37–40.

Lindsey, R., and C. Corbin. 1989. Questionable exercises—Some safer alternatives. *Journal of Physical Education, Recreation, and Dance* 60:26–32.

Lubell, A. 1989. Potentially dangerous exercises: Are they harmful to all? *Physician and Sportsmedicine* 17 (January): 187–92.

Olson, E. 1993. Beating back pain. *Running Times* 199 (August): 32–37.

Parniapour, M., et al. 1990. Environmentally induced disorders of the musculoskeletal system. *Medical Clinics of North America* 74:347–55.

Rimmer, J. 1990. Flexibility and strength exercises for persons with arthritis. *Clinical Kinesiology* 44:90–96.

Sady, S., et al. 1982. Flexibility training: Ballistic, static, or proprioceptive neuromuscular facilitation. *Archives of Physical Medicine and Rehabilitation* 63:261–63.

Schatz, M. 1994. Easy hamstring stretches. *Physician and Sportsmedicine* 22 (January): 115–16.

Schatz, M. 1994. Safe stretches for your inner thighs. *Physician and Sportsmedicine* 22 (May): 101–2.

Sharpe, G., et al. 1988. Exercise prescription and the low back: Kinesiological factors. *Journal of Physical Education, Recreation, and Dance* 59:74–78.

Skinner, J., and P. Oja. 1994. Laboratory and field tests for assessing health-related fitness. In *Physical activity, fitness, and health*, eds. C. Bouchard, et al. Champaign, Ill.: Human Kinetics.

Waldron, M. 1994. Stretching: The next generation. *Runner's World* 29 (February): 76–81.

Wathen, D. 1987. Flexibility: Its place in warm-up activities. *National Strength Coaches Association Journal* 9:26–27.

Specific Studies

Blackburn, S., and L. Portney. 1981. Electromyographic activity of basic musculature during Williams' flexion exercises. *Physical Therapy* 61:878–85.

Carlson, C., et al. 1990. Muscle stretching as an alternative relaxation training procedure. *Journal of Behavior Therapy and Experimental Psychiatry* 21:28–38.

Cornelius, W., and K. Craft-Hamm. (1988). Proprioceptive neuromuscular facilitation flexibility techniques: Acute effects on arterial blood pressure. *Physician and Sportsmedicine* 16 (April): 152–61.

Etnyre, B., and E. Lee. 1988. Chronic and acute flexibility of men and women using three different stretching techniques. *Research Quarterly for Exercise and Sport* 59:222–28.

Fairweather, M., and B. Sidaway. 1993. Ideokinetic imagery as a postural development technique. *Research Quarterly for Exercise and Sport* 64:385–92.

Jackson, A., and N. Langford. 1989. The criterion-related validity of the sit and reach test: Replication and extension of previous findings. *Research Quarterly for Exercise and Sport* 60:384–87.

Kujala, U., et al. 1992. Subject characteristics and low back pain in young athletes and nonathletes. *Medicine and Science in Sports and Exercise* 24:627–32.

Minkler, S., and P. Patterson. 1994. The validity of the modified sit-and-reach test in college-age students. *Research Quarterly for Exercise and Sport* 65:189–92.

Shephard, R., et al. 1990. On the generality of the "sit and reach" test: An analysis of flexibility data for an aging population. *Research Quarterly for Exercise and Sport* 61:326–30.

Sullivan, M., et al. 1992. Effect of pelvic position and stretching method on hamstring flexibility. *Medicine and Science in Sports and Exercise* 24:1383–89.

Taylor, D., et al. 1990. Viscoelastic properties of muscle-tendon units. The biomechanical effects of stretching. *American Journal of Sports Medicine* 18:300–309.

Williford, H., and J. Smith. 1985. A comparison of proprioceptive neuromuscular facilitation and static stretching techniques. *American Corrective Therapy Journal* 39:30–33.

6

▼▼▼

BASIC NUTRITION FOR HEALTHFUL EATING

Key Terms

amino acids
antioxidant
antipromoters
apoprotein
beta-carotene
carcinogens
cholesterol
coenzymes
complex carbohydrates
cruciferous vegetables
Daily Reference Value (DRV)
Daily Value (DV)
dietary fiber
eicosanoids
essential amino acids

fatty acids
Food Exchange System
Food Guide Pyramid
free radicals
glucose
glycerol
glycogen
HDL (high-density lipoproteins)
hidden fat
hydrogenated fats
iron-deficiency anemia
key nutrient concept
lactovegetarian
LDL (low-density lipoproteins)
legumes

lipids
lipoprotein
megadose
monounsaturated fatty acids
nutraceuticals
nutrient density
nutrients
omega-3 fatty acids
osteoporosis
ovolactovegetarian
ovovegetarian
phytochemicals
polyunsaturated fatty acids
promoters
protein complementarity

Recommended Dietary
   Allowances (RDA)
Reference Daily Intake (RDI)
saturated fatty acids
semivegetarian
simple carbohydrates
trans fatty acids
triglycerides
vegetarian
VLDL (very low-density
   lipoproteins)
water-insoluble fibers
water-soluble fibers

Key Concepts

■ Poor nutrition is one of the major health problems in the United States today.

■ The human body has a need for over fifty different nutrients found in six general classes—carbohydrates, fats, proteins, vitamins, minerals, and water.

■ Carbohydrates, particularly complex carbohydrates, are regarded as one of the most important components of a healthful diet.

■ Although a certain amount of dietary fat is necessary to obtain several essential nutrients, excessive intake of total fat, saturated fat, and cholesterol is associated with an increased risk of several chronic diseases.

■ The protein in foods from animal sources contains a proper blend of the nine essential amino acids needed in a diet; proper combinations of different plant foods also provide a comparable blend of these essential amino acids.

■ Vitamin and mineral supplements are not necessary for an individual on a well-balanced diet; however, women should pay particular attention to foods rich in calcium and iron.

■ For the physically active person who exercises in the heat, water prevents an excessive rise in body temperature.

■ If your diet is composed of natural, wholesome foods and is adequate in the eight key nutrients—protein, vitamin A, vitamin C, thiamin, riboflavin, niacin, iron, and calcium—you should be receiving an ample supply of all the nutrients essential to humans.

■ Some foods contain a greater proportion of key nutrients than other foods and thus have a greater nutrient density or nutritional value.

■ Nutritional labeling can be a valuable asset in selecting healthful foods with high nutrient density.

■ The Food Guide Pyramid and the six Food Exchange Lists are practical means to enable you to obtain a well-balanced diet.

■ Foods rich in antioxidant nutrients, such as vitamin E, vitamin C, and beta-carotene, may help prevent the development of certain chronic diseases, such as coronary heart disease and some forms of cancer.

■ A dozen general recommendations for healthier nutrition include (1) maintaining a healthful body weight, (2) consuming a wide variety of natural foods, particularly fruits, vegetables, and whole-grain products, (3) eating foods rich in calcium and iron, (4) eating adequate amounts of protein from both animal and plant sources, (5) increasing the dietary proportion of complex carbohydrates and natural sugars, increasing the intake of dietary fiber, (6) moderating consumption of refined sugar, (7) choosing a diet low in total fat, saturated fat, and cholesterol, (8) moderating sodium and salt intake, (9) maintaining an adequate intake of fluoride, (10) avoiding dietary supplements in excess of the Recommended Dietary Allowances (RDA), (11) eating fewer foods containing questionable additives, and (12) moderating alcohol consumption.

■ Although a vegetarian diet may be a healthful way to obtain needed nutrients, so too is a well-balanced diet containing wisely selected animal products.

INTRODUCTION

When the current fitness boom materialized nearly thirty years ago, some enthusiasts claimed that exercise was a panacea for a variety of chronic diseases. One physician even reported that anyone who completed a marathon, a 26.2-mile run, was immune to coronary heart disease, a claim repeatedly shown to be false. As noted in the previous chapters, a properly developed exercise program is a very important component of a Positive Health Life-style, but unfortunately, extravagant claims that exercise is a cure-all are not valid. Proper nutrition is of equal or even greater importance in the prevention of certain chronic diseases.

Nutrition is usually defined as the sum total of the processes involved in the intake and utilization of food substances by living organisms. From a health standpoint, the most important factors relative to the prevention of disease are the biochemical and physiological functions of the various nutrients in foods as they are processed in our bodies. It is theorized that some nutrients cause health problems, while other nutrients prevent them. Indeed, Hippocrates, the Greek physician known as the father of medicine, recognized the value of nutrition in the prevention of disease, declaring "Let food be your medicine, and medicine be your food." Today, we know that foods contain compounds known as **phytochemicals** (plant chemicals) that may affect various body functions. The term **nutraceuticals** has been applied to such chemicals in foods that may act as drugs or medicine to promote medical or health benefits.

A deficiency or excess of any nutrient may lead to acute health problems. Experimentation with the effects of nutrient deficiencies or excesses on both animals and humans may be conducted under well-controlled conditions in a nutrition research laboratory. For example, such research has shown that an iron deficiency will lead to anemia, while excessive iron consumption will lead to liver damage and possible death. Unfortunately, it is much more difficult to design an experimental study to investigate the effect of a particular nutrient upon the development of chronic diseases in humans.

Most chronic diseases have a genetic basis; if one of your parents has had coronary heart disease or cancer, you have an increased probability of contracting that disease. Such diseases may go through three stages: initiation, promotion, and progression. Your genetic predisposition may lead to the initiation stage of the disease, but factors in your environment promote its development and eventual progression. In this regard, some nutrients are believed to be **promoters** that lead to the progression of the disease, while other nutrients are believed to be **antipromoters** that deter the initiation process from progressing to a serious health problem. What you eat plays an important role in the development or progress of a variety of chronic diseases, such as coronary heart disease, diabetes, high blood pressure, osteoporosis, obesity, and a variety of different cancers. In this regard, the National Cancer Institute estimates that one-third of all cancers are linked in some way to diet (see fig. 6.1).

A number of research techniques have been used in attempts to determine what nutrients are possible promoters or antipromoters in the development of chronic diseases. This is a difficult area of study. These diseases take considerable time, many years, to develop. Furthermore, it is nearly

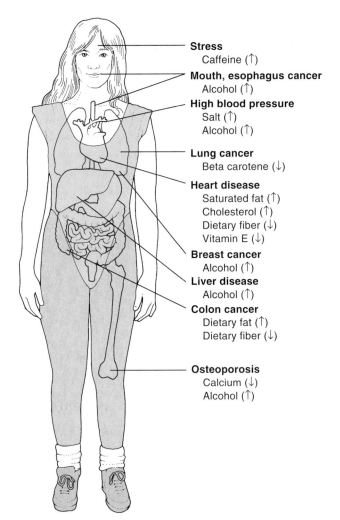

Figure 6.1 *Some possible health problems associated with poor dietary habits. An upward arrow (↑) indicates excessive intake while a downward arrow (↓) indicates low intake or deficiency.*

impossible to precisely control the intake of nutrients in the diets of large groups of people. Thus, most of the currently available evidence has been derived from epidemiological studies that compare characteristics of different populations. For example, population groups that consume diets high in fat generally have a greater incidence rate of heart disease when compared to populations that consume a low-fat diet. It is important to reiterate that although epidemiological research may show a statistical relationship between two variables, such as a high-fat diet and coronary heart disease, there is not necessarily a cause-and-effect relationship. Although causality may be inferred from epidemiological research, this relationship must be determined by properly designed experiments. Although some quality experimental research has been conducted under well-controlled laboratory conditions, most studies have used animals, not humans; however, data from long-term human studies are becoming increasingly available.

Because the prevention of chronic diseases is of critical importance, thousands of studies have been and are being conducted in order to discover the intricacies of how various nutrients may affect our health. Particular interest is focused on nutrient function in body cells at the molecular level, the interaction effect of various nutrients, and the identification of other protective factors in certain foods. All of the answers are not in, but sufficient evidence is available to provide us with some useful, prudent guidelines for healthful eating practices, as suggested in several major reports, *Rationale of the Diet-Heart Statement of the American Heart Association, Diet and Health: Implications for Reducing Chronic Disease Risk* and *Healthy People 2000: National Health Promotion and Disease Prevention Objectives.*

The Public Health Service, a branch of the U.S. Department of Health and Human Services, in their report entitled *Healthy People 2000: National Health Promotion and Disease Prevention Objectives,* noted that poor nutrition is one of the major health problems in our country. In this regard, a variety of nutritional risk-reduction objectives have been developed for the year 2000. Among the most relevant for this chapter are the following:

1. Reduce dietary fat intake to an average of 30 percent of Calories or less and average saturated-fat intake to less than 10 percent of Calories

2. Increase complex-carbohydrates and fiber-containing foods in the diets to five or more daily servings for vegetables (including legumes) and fruits, and to six or more daily servings for grain products

3. Increase to at least 50 percent the proportion of overweight people aged twelve and older who have adopted sound dietary practices combined with regular physical activity to attain an appropriate body weight

4. Increase calcium intake so that at least 50 percent of youth aged twelve through twenty-four and 50 percent of pregnant and lactating women consume three or more servings daily of foods rich in calcium, and at least 50 percent of people aged twenty-five and older consume two or more servings daily

5. Decrease salt and sodium intake so that at least 65 percent of home-meal preparers prepare foods without adding salt, at least 80 percent of people avoid using salt at the table, and at least 40 percent of adults regularly purchase foods modified or lower in sodium

6. Reduce iron deficiency to less than 3 percent among children and among women of childbearing age

7. Increase to at least 85 percent the proportion of people aged eighteen and older who use food labels to make nutritious food selections

These objectives represent an updating of an earlier version proposed in 1980 when health objectives were established for the 1990s. To help implement these earlier objectives, various governmental agencies, professional health associations, community health organizations, and consumer health groups promoted legislation and applied political pressure to the food industry to increase the provision of foods believed to be more healthful. Because of their efforts, we have more choices of healthier foods today. Relative to fat, for example, the meat industry has used genetic techniques to provide leaner beef, national bakeries produce fat-free Danish rolls, and many national fast-food chains provide a variety of low-fat menu items. However, we still have an abundance of high-fat products available. In order to achieve the health-related benefits of these products, you have to know which foods are lower in fat, and you have to choose them rather than the high-fat varieties.

Over the past decade, these same health organizations have promoted educational programs to help Americans adopt more healthful diets, and although recent research suggests that the diet of some health-conscious Americans appears to be changing for the better, there is still considerable room for improvement for the majority of the population. As suggested by the risk-reduction objectives above, many Americans still have unhealthy eating habits, which may be related to poor nutritional knowledge. For example, in a recent study of over 2,300 individuals, even those who should be knowledgeable concerning healthy eating habits, such as university graduate students, health-care workers, and health-club attendees, Schapira and others reported that 80 percent were unaware of the major health recommendations regarding fat intake and could not calculate the fat content of a food product. As mentioned in chapter 1, awareness through proper knowledge may be the initial step in a behavior modification program.

To relate nutrition to health in simplistic terms, most Americans eat more food than they need and eat less of the food they need more. The purpose of this chapter is to provide you with current nutritional knowledge and recommendations believed to promote health and prevent disease so you can plan and eat a healthier diet, the Healthy American Diet. The three major sections in this chapter deal with the major nutrients and implications for health, the basis of diet planning, and general guides to healthier eating. The following chapter will discuss the role of diet in weight control.

The Major Nutrients

The food we eat provides us with a variety of **nutrients,** specific substances found in food that perform one or more biochemical or physiological functions in the body. Six general classes of nutrients are considered necessary in human nutrition. They are carbohydrates, fats, proteins, vitamins, minerals, and water. Within several of these general classes (notably proteins, vitamins, and minerals), there are a number of specific nutrients necessary for life. For example, over a dozen vitamins are needed for optimal physiological functioning. Although several of these nutrients may be manufactured in our bodies, such as vitamin D through the action of sunlight on the skin, the vast majority need to be obtained through the diet.

Table 6.1 represents the specific nutrients known to be essential or probably essential to humans at this time. Some of the nutrients listed have been shown to be essential for various animals and are theorized to be essential for humans. It is possible that this list may be expanded in the future as more accurate analytical methods are developed to study the effects of certain nutrients or phytochemicals in human nutrition. Although carbohydrates are not an essential nutrient in the strictest sense, many nutritionists consider dietary fiber, which is primarily carbohydrate, a specific necessity in the diet for prevention of certain health problems.

These nutrients perform three major functions. First, they provide energy for human metabolism. Carbohydrates

Table 6.1 Essential Nutrients

1. Proteins (Essential Amino Acids)

Histidine	Phenylalanine
Isoleucine	Threonine
Leucine	Tryptophan
Lysine	Valine
Methionine	

2. Fats (Essential Fatty Acids)

Linoleic	Alpha-Linolenic

3. Carbohydrates

Fiber

4. Vitamins

Water-soluble	**Fat-soluble**
B Complex	A (Retinol)
B_1 (Thiamin)	D (Calciferol)
B_2 (Riboflavin)	E (Tocopherol)
Niacin	K (Phylloquinone)
B_6 (Pyridoxine)	
Pantothenic acid	
Folacin	
B_{12} (Cyanocobalamin)	
Biotin	
C (Ascorbic acid)	

5. Minerals

Calcium	Iron	Selenium
Chloride	Magnesium	Silicon
Chromium	Manganese	Sodium
Cobalt	Molybdenum	Sulfur
Copper	Nickel	Tin
Fluoride	Phosphorus	Vanadium
Iodine	Potassium	Zinc

6. Water

Essential nutrients are necessary for human life. An inadequate intake may result in disturbed body metabolism, certain disease states, or death.

Some of the nutrients listed have been shown to be essential for various animals and are probably essential for humans. Essential nutrients, or nutrients from which they may be formed, must be obtained from the foods we eat.

and fats are the prime sources of energy. Second, nutrients are used to build and repair body tissues. Protein is the major building material for muscles, other soft tissues, and enzymes, while certain minerals such as calcium and phosphorus make up the skeletal framework. Third, nutrients are used to help regulate body processes. Vitamins, minerals, and proteins work closely together to maintain the diverse physiological processes of human metabolism. For example, hemoglobin in the red blood cell (RBC) is essential for the transportation of oxygen to the muscle tissue via the blood. Hemoglobin is a complex combination of protein and iron; however, other minerals and vitamins are needed for its synthesis and for full development of the RBC.

As mentioned previously, a deficiency or excess of any nutrient may lead to disease or to some health problem. Since space does not permit a detailed discussion of each specific nutrient, we will cover briefly the general role of each major nutrient in human metabolism and focus upon some of the major health implications as supported by current epidemiological or experimental research.

Carbohydrates

Carbohydrates are the basic foodstuffs formed when energy from the sun is harnessed in plants. They are organic compounds that contain carbon, hydrogen, and oxygen in various combinations. Their major function in human nutrition is to provide a source of energy. Carbohydrates contain four Calories per gram. They are one of the least expensive forms of Calories to produce, and, hence, represent one of the major food supplies for the vast majority of the world's population.

In general terms, carbohydrates may be categorized as either simple or complex. **Simple carbohydrates,** usually known as sugars, occur naturally in some foods, particularly fruits. Although there are many different types of sugars, the most common one in the typical American diet is sucrose, or plain table sugar. The **complex carbohydrates** are commonly known as starches; the vast majority of carbohydrates in the plant world are in this form, including grain products such as wheat, rice, and corn, **legumes** such as beans and peas, and all vegetables. Some food exchanges high in carbohydrate content are found in table 6.2. A more detailed discussion of the food exchange system is presented later in this chapter.

For the most part, all dietary carbohydrates are digested and eventually converted to **glucose,** a simple carbohydrate absorbed into the blood from the intestines. Blood glucose may have several metabolic fates. It may be utilized directly by some tissues, such as the brain, for energy, or it may be stored in the liver or muscles as **glycogen** (a complex carbohydrate). Excess blood glucose may be excreted in the urine or converted into fat and stored in the body's adipose tissue. Figure 6.2 illustrates the general fates of blood glucose.

Health Implications of Dietary Carbohydrates

In the past, dietary carbohydrates have had a poor reputation in the mind of the general public, particularly in those attempting to lose body weight. Now, carbohydrates, particularly complex carbohydrates, are considered to be one of the most important components of a healthy diet. They are rich in many nutrients (vitamins and minerals), are the major source of fiber in the diet, and may also serve as the basis for a low-Calorie diet.

Dietary fiber is the carbohydrate in plants that is resistant to digestive enzymes; hence, it leaves some residue in the digestive tract. Although the nature of dietary fiber is complex, in simplistic terms dietary fiber exists in two basic forms: water-soluble fibers and water-insoluble fibers. **Water-soluble fibers** include gums and pectins, while the

Table 6.2 Foods High in Carbohydrate Content

Starch/bread exchange	Fruit Exchange	Vegetable Exchange	Milk Exchange	Meat Exchange
Whole grain	Apples	Corn	Ice milk	Chestnuts
Brown rice	Applesauce	Green peas	Skim milk	Kidney beans
Buckwheat groats	Apricots	Hominy	Yogurt, fruit	Lentils
Bulgur	Bananas	Lima beans		Navy beans
Corn tortillas	Blackberries	Potatoes		Split peas
Granola	Blueberries	Rutabaga		
Oatmeal	Cantaloupe	Squash		
Ready-to-eat cereal*	Cherries	Sweet potatoes		
Rye crackers	Dried fruits	Taro		
Whole-wheat bread	Figs	Tomatoes		
Whole-wheat cereals	Oranges			
Whole-wheat crackers	Peaches			
Whole-wheat pasta	Pears			
Whole-wheat rolls	Pineapple			
Enriched	Plums			
Bagels	Raspberries			
Biscuits	Tangerines			
Cornbread				
Crackers				
English muffins				
Grits				
Macaroni				
Noodles				
Pasta				
Ready-to-eat cereal*				
White bread				
White rice				

May be whole-wheat or enriched depending on the brand.

major **water-insoluble fibers** are cellulose, hemicellulose, and lignin (a non-carbohydrate). Increasing the intake of complex carbohydrates will lead to an increase in dietary fiber. There is considerable epidemiological evidence and some experimental evidence that increased fiber intake may help reduce the incidence rates of colon cancer and other intestinal disorders. For example, a recent meta-analysis of thirteen studies revealed an inverse relationship between intakes of dietary fiber and risk of colon cancer. In addition, some studies have also reported reduced cholesterol levels in the blood following a diet high in soluble fibers.

Exactly how dietary fiber may be protective is not known, but several mechanisms have been proposed. First, fiber may add bulk to the contents of the large intestine and hence dilute any possible cancer-causing agents (**carcinogens**) that might attack cell walls. Second, the additional bulk stimulates peristalsis and speeds up the transit time of food through the intestines. Thus, any carcinogenic agent present will have less time to function. Third, fiber may bind with carcinogens so that they are excreted by the bowel. Fiber also may bind with and lead to the excretion of bile salts, which contain cholesterol; normally the bile salts are reabsorbed into the body, but excretion of bile salts, along with their cholesterol content, may help reduce serum cholesterol levels. Fourth, fiber slows down gastric (stomach) emptying and thereby slows glucose

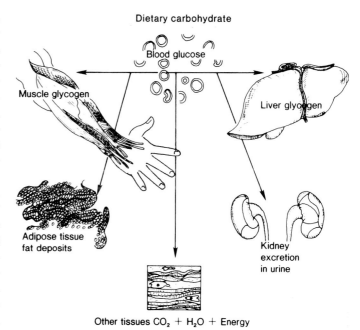

Figure 6.2 *Fates of blood glucose. After assimilation into the blood, glucose may be stored in the liver or muscles as glycogen or may be utilized as a source of energy by these and other tissues, particularly the nervous system. Excess glucose may be partially excreted by the kidneys, but major excesses are converted to fat and stored in the adipose tissues.*

absorption in the small intestine. This effect may lead to better control of blood sugar and may also lengthen the sensation of fullness or satiety, which may be important to individuals on weight loss diets. Fifth, soluble fibers may be fermented in the large intestine to short chain fatty acids (SCFA). SCFA may confer several benefits; they may be absorbed and transported to the liver where they may suppress cholesterol synthesis, possibly helping to decrease serum cholesterol levels, and they also may interfere with the promotion phase of carcinogenesis in the colon, preventing colon cancer. Sixth, diets high in fiber are usually low in fat and cholesterol, which may support these overall healthful effects. Other independent mechanisms also may be functioning. For example, nutraceuticals such as glucarate and sulforaphane, which have recently been isolated from vegetables such as broccoli, may interfere with cancer development, at least as shown in laboratory animals. It should be noted that some of these health benefits, such as decreased serum cholesterol levels associated with dietary fiber intake, occur even when the diet is already low in dietary constituents that may raise serum cholesterol, such as fat.

Although this area is still under investigation, several hypotheses link potential health benefits to the specific type of fiber consumed. Foods that are rich in the water-insoluble type of fiber, such as whole-wheat products, wheat-bran cereals, brown rice, and lentils, are more likely to increase the fecal bulk, maximizing the dilutant effect and speed of transit through the colon, and hence helping prevent diseases of the large intestine and rectum. Foods richer in water-soluble fiber, such as apples, bananas, citrus fruits, and oats, have more of a binding effect and are theorized to be more likely to reduce serum cholesterol. However, it should be noted that research has now shown that oat bran or wheat products added to the diet are equally effective in lowering serum cholesterol. Foods rich in both soluble and insoluble fiber, such as kidney beans, navy beans, and green peas, may provide both benefits.

The National Research Council has cautioned that data relative to a protective effect of fiber per se against the development of certain chronic diseases are inconclusive at present. Nevertheless, the council recognizes the value of the epidemiological data supportive of a protective effect of a diet high in whole-grain products, legumes, fruits, and vegetables. Its current recommendation is to obtain approximately 25–40 grams of dietary fiber through the consumption of natural wholesome foods, not fiber supplements. It is important to recognize that the health benefits attributed to fiber may be associated with the form in which the fiber is consumed, as part of a whole, natural food containing other potential health-promoting nutrients such as vitamins, rather than by consumption of a purified supplement form.

Table 6.3 presents the average fiber content in some common foods. High-fiber foods in the six food exchanges are also highlighted in Appendix A.

If you consume the typical American diet, approximately 20–25 percent of your daily caloric intake is derived from refined sugars, such as ordinary table sugar and the high-fructose corn syrup added to numerous processed foods. Over the years,

Table 6.3 Fiber Content in Some Common Foods

Beans	7–9 grams per ½ cup, cooked
Vegetables	3–5 grams per ½ cup, cooked
Fruits	1–3 grams per piece
Breads and cereals	1–3 grams per serving
Bran cereal	5–13 grams per ounce
Nuts and seeds*	2–5 grams per ounce

Nuts and seeds are also high in fat.

refined sugar has been alleged to contribute to a wide variety of health disorders, such as dental caries, diabetes, cardiovascular disease, obesity, the premenstrual syndrome (PMS), hyperactivity in children, mental illness, and even accelerated aging. Although the role carbohydrates, including refined sugars, may play in the development of several of these health problems is still under investigation, the National Research Council, in its major treatise on *Diet and Health,* stated that with the exception of dental caries, there is minimal evidence linking refined sugar intake per se to specific health problems. Nevertheless, many health organizations around the world have recommended a reduced intake of refined sugars, generally to amounts less than 10 percent of the daily caloric intake. Because refined sugar contains no nutrients, but only Calories, its intake should be limited in any well-balanced diet. Moreover, sugary foods are also usually high in fat.

Fat

The fats in our diet are technically known as **lipids,** a general term for a number of different water-insoluble compounds found in the body. The two major lipids of dietary importance to humans are triglycerides and cholesterol.

Triglycerides are the true fats, the type we normally consume in our diet. They are composed of two different compounds—glycerol and fatty acids. **Glycerol,** an alcohol, is a clear, colorless syrupy liquid that is similar to carbohydrate.

Fatty acids, one of the components of fat, are chains of carbon and hydrogen atoms that vary in the degree of hydrogen saturation. A **saturated fatty acid** contains a full quota of hydrogen; unsaturated fatty acids may absorb more hydrogen. These latter fatty acids may be classified as **monounsaturated** (capable of absorbing two or more hydrogen ions), and **polyunsaturated fatty acids** (capable of absorbing four or more hydrogen ions). Saturated fats are usually solid; unsaturated fats are usually liquid at room temperature. **Hydrogenated fats** or oils have been treated by a process that adds hydrogen to some of the unfilled bonds, thus hardening the fat or oil. In essence, the fat becomes more saturated with a possible realignment of hydrogen atoms, creating a form of hydrogenated or partially hydrogenated fatty acids known as **trans fatty acids. Omega-3 fatty acids** are a special class of polyunsaturated fatty acids found primarily in fish. Some derivatives of specific fatty acids formed by oxidation in the body have some potent biologic functions. These derivatives are collectively known as **eicosanoids,** an example being the prostaglandins. Eicosanoids possess hormone-like properties

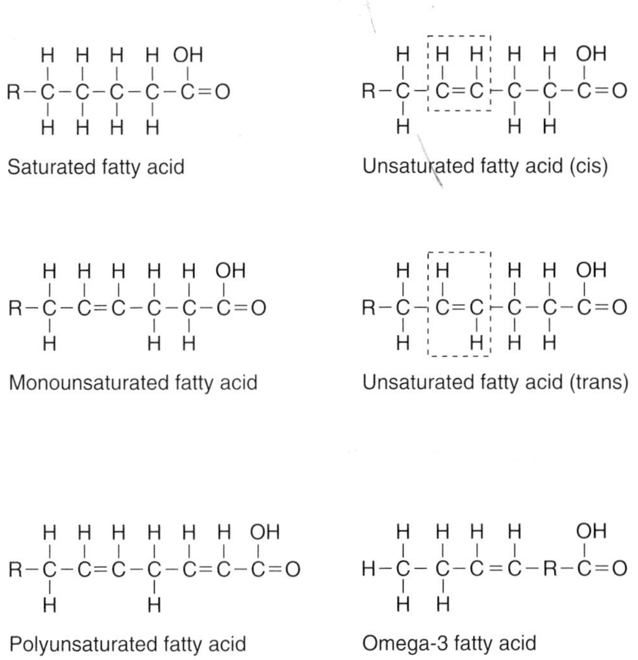

Figure 6.3 *Structural differences between saturated and unsaturated fatty acids. Note the double bonds between carbon atoms in the unsaturated fatty acid. These indicate that more hydrogen atoms may be added. One double bond is present in a monounsaturated fatty acid, while two or more are found in polyunsaturated fatty acids. In the omega-3 fatty acids, the double bond is located three carbons from the last, or omega, carbon. The R represents the radical, or the presence of many more C—H bonds. In the hydrogenation process, the cis configuration (both hydrogen ions at the double bond on the same side) may be changed to the trans configuration.*

that influence a number of physiological functions that may affect health, particularly those derived from omega-3 fatty acids, whose theorized health benefits will be discussed later in this chapter. Figure 6.3 represents the structural differences among fatty acids.

Cholesterol is not a fat; it is a fatlike, pearly substance that is an essential component in the formation of the cell membrane and several hormones. Some cholesterol is obtained in the diet; however, the liver manufactures most of the cholesterol needed by your body from fatty acids and other products derived from carbohydrate and protein.

The fat content in foods can vary from 100 percent, as found in most cooking oils, to less than 1 percent, as found in most fruits and vegetables. Some foods obviously have a high fat content: butter, oils, shortening, margarine, and visible fat on meat. In other foods, the fat content may be high but not as obvious. This is known as **hidden fat.** For example, whole milk, cheese, nuts, desserts, crackers, potato chips, and a wide variety of commercially prepared foods may contain considerable amounts of fat. Each gram of fat contains nine Calories. Table 6.4 presents the percentage of Calories in the fat contained in some common foods. Some examples of hidden fat are illustrated in figure 6.4.

Cholesterol is found only in animal food products; it is not found in fruits, vegetables, nuts, grains, or other plant sources. Table 6.5 represents some foods from the

Table 6.4 Fat and Saturated Fat Content in Some Common Foods

Food Exchange	Total Fat (% Calories)	Saturated Fat (% Calories)
Meat List		
Bacon	80	30
Beef, lean only	32	13
Ham	70	23
Hamburger, regular	62	29
Chicken, breast	23	8
Sausage, pork	79	29
Haddock	32	6
Eggs, whole	67	22
Beans, dry navy	4	—
Peanut butter	76	19
Milk List		
Milk, whole	48	28
Milk, skim	trace	trace
Cheese, cheddar	62	39
Vegetable List		
Beans, green	trace	trace
Carrots	trace	trace
Potatoes	trace	trace
Fruit List		
Bananas	trace	trace
Oranges	trace	trace
Starch/Bread List		
Bread	12	—
Cake, plain sheet	31	8
Crackers*	40	—
Doughnuts	43	7
Macaroni	5	—
Macaroni and cheese	46	20
Oatmeal	13	—
Pancakes, wheat	30	—
Rolls, dinner	22	7
Fat List		
Butter	99	54
Margarine*	99	19
Oil, corn	100	10
Salad dressing, French	68	14

Dashes indicate no value was found, although it is believed some is present.

*May be high in trans fatty acids

Source: *U.S. Department of Agriculture.*

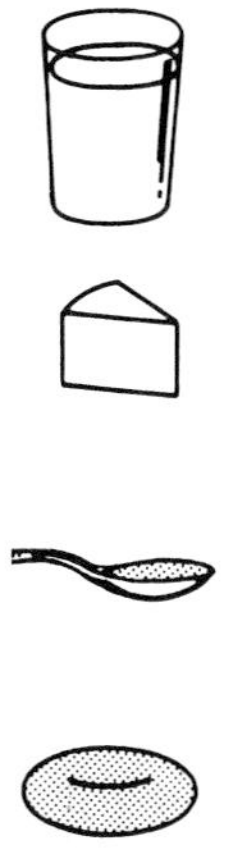

	Calories	Grams of Fat	Percentage Fat Calories
8 ounces whole milk	150	8	48%
1 ounce cheddar cheese	115	9	70%
1 tablespoon peanut butter	95	8	76%
1 doughnut	100	5	45%

Figure 6.4 *Hidden fat. Many of the foods we consume may contain significant numbers of Calories in the form of hidden fat.*

Table 6.5 Cholesterol Content in Some Common Foods

Food	Amount	Cholesterol (Milligrams)
Meat List		
Beef	1 oz	25
Pork, ham	1 oz	25
Poultry	1 oz	23
Fish	1 oz	21
Shrimp	1 oz	45
Lobster	1 oz	25
Sausage	2 links	45
Tuna, salmon	1 oz	20
Frankfurter	1	50
Bacon	1 strip	5
Eggs	1	220
Liver	1 oz	120
Milk List		
Milk, whole	1 c	27
Milk, 2%	1 c	15
Milk, skim	1 c	7
Butter	1 tsp	12
Margarine	1 tsp	0
Cream cheese	1 tbsp	18
Ice milk	1 c	10
Ice cream	1 c	85
Starch/Bread List		
Whole grains and nuts contain no cholesterol but cholesterol may be added in the preparation of some foods (such as eggs in French toast or other baked foods).		
Bread	1 slice	0
Biscuit	1	17
Pancake	1	40
Sweet roll	1	25
French toast	1	130
Doughnut	1	28
Cereal, cooked	1 c	0
Fruit List		
Fruits contain no cholesterol		
Vegetable List		
Vegetables contain no cholesterol		

Source: U.S. Department of Agriculture.

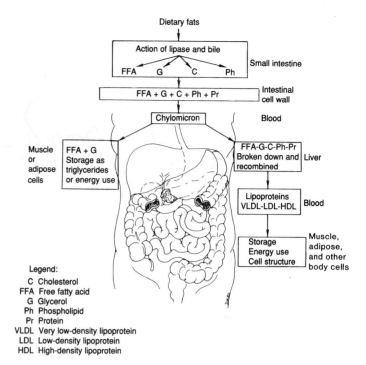

Figure 6.5 *Simplified diagram of fat metabolism. After digestion, fats are carried in the blood as chylomicrons. Through the metabolic processes in the body, fat may be utilized as a major source of energy, used to help develop cell structure, or stored as a future energy source.*

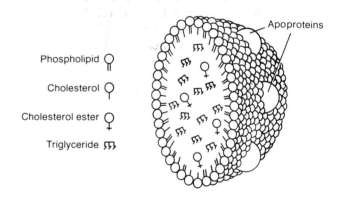

F**Figure 6.6** *Schematic of a lipoprotein. Lipoproteins contain a core of triglycerides and cholesterol esters surrounded by a coat of apoproteins, cholesterol, and phospholipids. The proportion of the protein, cholesterol, triglycerides, and phospholipids varies between the different types of lipoproteins. The apoprotein component regulates the function of the lipoprotein.*

meat and milk exchanges with the cholesterol content in milligrams per serving. Several foods from the starch/bread exchange are also included, indicating that the preparation of some starch/bread products may add cholesterol by including some animal product with cholesterol, mainly egg yolk.

Figure 6.5 presents a diagram of the metabolic breakdown and use of dietary fat. Dietary fat is digested into its constituents (fatty acids, glycerol, and cholesterol) and eventually used for energy, incorporated in the formation of certain cell structures, or stored as fat. Since lipids are insoluble in water, the liver constantly makes compounds called **lipoproteins,** combinations of lipids covered by a protein coat. The protein component, known as an **apoprotein,** allows the lipid to be transported in the blood. Figure 6.6 presents a schematic of a lipoprotein.

Different types of apoproteins, such as A and B, determine the functions of the lipoproteins in the blood. This may have significant health implications, particularly in the development of atherosclerosis, a condition associated with coronary heart disease. For our purposes, the major classifications of lipoproteins, along with their suggested composition and function, are listed below; a graphic illustration is presented in figure 6.7.

VLDL (very low-density lipoproteins). VLDL consist primarily of triglycerides, which are transported to the tissues to deliver fatty acids and glycerol.

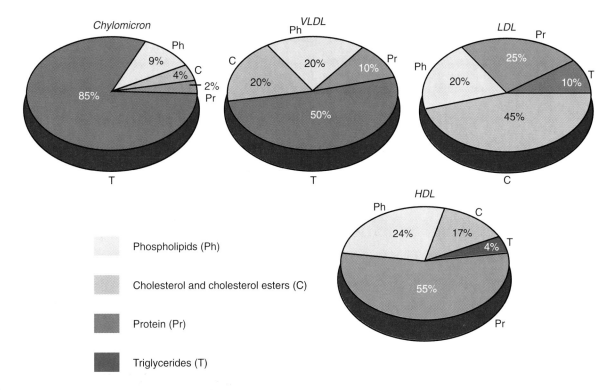

Figure 6.7 *The approximate content of four types of lipoproteins.*

LDL (low-density lipoproteins). LDL contain a high proportion of cholesterol and are associated primarily with B apoproteins. Increased levels of LDL, particularly if oxidized or modified, are associated with increased risk for coronary heart disease. LDL are often referred to as the bad cholesterol, for high levels are believed to contribute to the development of heart disease.

HDL (high-density lipoproteins). HDL contain 50 to 55 percent protein and moderate amounts of cholesterol. Several subclasses of HDL have been identified, such as HDL_2 and HDL_3. HDL are associated primarily with A apoproteins. Higher levels of HDL, particularly the HDL_2 component, have been associated with a lessened risk of coronary heart disease. HDL are often referred to as the good cholesterol, for it is believed that they reduce the risk of heart disease.

Health Implications of Dietary Fat and Cholesterol

Although fat is one of the most criticized nutrients, it does play a significant role in human nutrition and physiological functioning. Dietary fat is a source of energy and helps provide essential fatty acids (linoleic and alpha-linolenic fatty acids) and several fat-soluble vitamins (A, D, E, and K) for the regulation of human metabolism. A diet containing about 5 to 10 percent of Calories from fat could satisfy these needs and provide sufficient cholesterol.

Unfortunately, the average American consumes about 36 percent of the dietary Calories from fat (13 percent from saturated fat) and more cholesterol than is needed (between 400–600 milligrams per day). These facts have the National Cancer Institute, the American Heart Association, and the National Academy of Sciences concerned, for excessive consumption of fat and cholesterol has been linked to the development of a number of diseases, most notably coronary heart disease and cancer. Theorized mechanisms are discussed in chapter 11, but the risk factor of main concern is high blood cholesterol. High levels of LDL and low levels of HDL increase the risk of coronary heart disease. Other mechanisms may operate regarding the relationship of dietary fat to the development of certain forms of cancer.

You should know your blood cholesterol level. Due to the impetus of the National Cholesterol Education Program sponsored by the National Heart, Lung, and Blood Institute (NHLBI), many free or low-cost screenings are offered periodically in community hospitals or by other health care providers. Many colleges and universities also offer cholesterol screening examinations. The screen normally gives you only your total cholesterol level. If it is high, other tests may be used to determine the breakdown of LDL and HDL cholesterol. Table 6.6 presents the cholesterol level guidelines recommended by the NHLBI.

It is not only the amount of fat in the diet, but the type of fat that may have health implications. The general guidelines advanced by the Public Health Service, the American Heart Association, and the National Cancer Institute aim to reduce the total amount of fat in the diet to less than 30 percent of caloric intake, to strike a balance in the ratio of saturated, monounsaturated, and polyunsaturated fats to approximately 10 percent of the Calories from each (preferably less than 10 percent from saturated fat, 10–15 percent from monounsaturated fat, and the remainder from polyunsaturated fat), and to reduce cholesterol intake to less than 300 milligrams per day, or possibly less than 100 milligrams per 1,000 Calories consumed.

Table 6.6 Recommended Cholesterol Levels of the National Cholesterol Education Program Sponsored by the National Heart, Lung, and Blood Institute

	Total Cholesterol Classification	LDL Cholesterol Classification	Serum Triglycerides	HDL Cholesterol Classification
Desirable	< 200	< 130	< 200	> 60
Borderline/High Risk	200–239	130–159	200–400	—
High Risk	> 240	> 160	> 400	< 35

Current research suggests that a decrease in the consumption of saturated fats, trans fatty acids, and cholesterol, coupled with a moderate intake of natural dietary sources of polyunsaturated, monounsaturated, and omega-3 fatty acids, may be prudent nutritional health behaviors. Polyunsaturated fats may help decrease total cholesterol, but they also appear to decrease the HDL component. Monounsaturated fats help lower total cholesterol, but, unlike polyunsaturated fats, they have little effect on HDL levels. However, for healthy individuals on a low fat diet, there appears to be little difference between polyunsaturated and monounsaturated fats relative to HDL cholesterol. Eicosanoid derivatives of omega-3 fatty acids may help prevent atherosclerosis by several means, such as lowering blood cholesterol, inhibiting clot formation in the arterial walls, and reducing blood pressure in hypertensives. Practical suggestions to accomplish these dietary changes are presented later in this chapter. The etiology of atherosclerosis and high blood pressure is covered in chapter 11.

Protein

Protein is a complex chemical structure containing carbon, hydrogen, and oxygen—just as carbohydrates and fat do. However, protein has one other essential element, nitrogen. These four elements are combined into a number of different structures called **amino acids.** There are twenty amino acids, all of which can be combined in a variety of ways to form the different proteins necessary for the structure and functions of the human body. Protein is one of our most essential nutrients, for it is the main structural component of all tissues in the body. Since all enzymes are derived from protein, all physiological processes are dependent upon this nutrient.

Protein is contained in foods from both animal and plant sources. Hence, humans obtain their supply of amino acids from these two sources. The human body can synthesize some but not all amino acids. The amino acids that cannot be manufactured in the body are called **essential amino acids;** they must be supplied in the diet. It should be noted that all twenty amino acids are necessary and must be present simultaneously for optimal maintenance of body growth and function. Thus, the utilization of the term *essential* in relation to amino acids is to distinguish those that must be obtained in the diet. The nonessential amino acids are formed in the body.

In general, the proteins we ingest from animal products are superior to those found in plants. This is not to say that an amino acid found in a plant is inferior to the same amino acid found in an animal. They are the same. Let's look at the distribution of all the amino acids in the two food sources to see why animal protein is called a high-quality protein, whereas plant protein is generally called a low-quality protein.

The reasons for the superiority of animal protein are twofold. First, since it contains all the essential amino acids, it is a complete protein. Second, it contains the essential amino acids in the proper proportion. As noted previously, all amino acids must be present simultaneously in order for the body to synthesize them into necessary body proteins. If one essential amino acid is in short supply, protein construction may be blocked. Hence, having the proper amount of animal protein in the diet is a good way to ensure receiving a balanced supply of amino acids. Excellent low-fat sources include skim milk, turkey, and fish.

Proteins usually exist in smaller concentrations in plants and may be lower in several of the essential amino acids. Consequently, individually, most plant foods are unable to meet our total nutritional needs. However, if plant foods are eaten in proper combinations, they can provide a balanced supply of amino acids. An example of a good combination of plant foods that represents a complete protein is that of grain products and beans, such as rice and navy beans. This balanced intake is of extreme importance to strict vegetarians, discussed later in this chapter.

Table 6.7 presents the protein content of some common foods. The average male needs about 56 grams of protein per day, while the average female needs about 44 grams. (To determine your individual need, simply multiply your body weight, in pounds, by 0.36 grams.)

After protein is digested, the amino acids are generally utilized to form body tissues and other protein substances, such as enzymes and hormones. Excess protein may be converted to glucose or fatty acids, and protein waste products may be excreted as urea. Figure 6.8 represents a simplified description of protein metabolism in the human body.

Health Implications of Dietary Protein

Because protein is the source of the essential amino acids so important to human metabolism, a deficiency could be expected to cause serious health problems. Such is the case in some parts of the world where individuals suffer from protein-Calorie malnutrition, but protein intake in the United States appears to be more than adequate to meet the needs of the average American. However, individuals who are on an extremely low-Calorie diet may not obtain sufficient protein and may experience loss of protein tissue, such as muscle. The body cannot store excess protein for use in times of a deficiency; therefore, daily protein intake is important.

Table 6.7 Protein Content in Some Common Foods

Food	Amount	Protein (Grams)
Milk List		
Milk, whole	1 c	8
Milk, skim	1 c	8
Cheese, cheddar	1 oz	7
Yogurt	1 c	8
Meat List		
Beef, lean	1 oz	8
Chicken, breast	1 oz	8
Luncheon meat	1 oz	5
Fish	1 oz	7
Eggs	1	6
Navy beans, cooked	1/2 c	7
Peanuts, roasted	1/4 c	9
Peanut butter	1 tbsp	4
Vegetable List		
Broccoli	1/2 c	2
Carrots	1	1
Peas, green	1/2 c	4
Potato, baked	1	3
Fruit List		
Banana	1	1
Orange	1	1
Pear	1	1
Starch/Bread List		
Bread, wheat	1 slice	3
Bran flakes	1 c	4
Doughnuts	1	1
Spaghetti	1 c	5

Protein (grams) may vary slightly from the food exchange lists since these data were derived from food analyses reported by the United States Department of Agriculture.

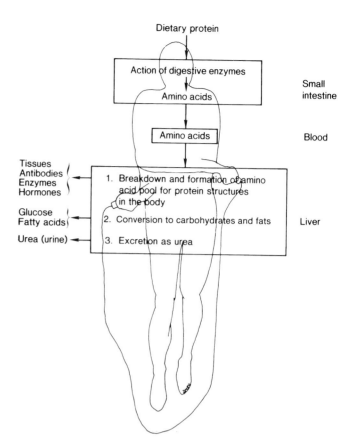

Figure 6.8 *Simplified diagram of protein metabolism. After digestion amino acids are (1) metabolized in the liver forming amino acids needed for new protein synthesis, (2) converted to glucose or fatty acids, or (3) converted to urea. These by-products are then transported by the blood for body use or, in the case of urea, excreted.*

Excessive dietary intake of protein should be avoided by individuals who have a personal or family history of liver or kidney disease. The liver is the major body organ that processes amino acids while the kidney is responsible for excreting protein waste products, such as urea. Excessive protein intake may disturb normal function of these two organs, possibly causing health problems such as acidosis in the blood.

In general, the amount of protein found in the typical American diet is not harmful to the healthy individual. However, animal protein may be accompanied by substantial amounts of saturated fat and cholesterol, both of which are associated with several health problems. Thus, to reduce the intake of fat while maintaining adequate protein intake, you need to be selective in your choice of foods. For example, a glass of whole milk and a glass of skim milk both have about 8 grams of protein, but whole milk has 8 grams of fat compared to only 1 gram or less of fat in the skim milk. Drinking a glass of skim milk instead of whole milk reduces your fat intake by 7 grams and saves you about 60 Calories. Eating more plant proteins may also be a healthful choice.

Vitamins

Vitamins, found in small amounts in most foods, represent a class of complex organic compounds that are essential for the optimal functioning of a great number of physiological processes. Some vitamins, particularly the B vitamins, function as **coenzymes;** they are needed to activate or control the activity of enzymes, those protein compounds that regulate almost all physiological processes in the body, such as digestion, muscle contraction, and the release of energy from foods. Some vitamins, such as C, E, and **beta-carotene** (a precursor of vitamin A) serve as **antioxidants;** they prevent undesired oxidative processes in the body. Vitamin D functions as a hormone.

At the present time the human body needs an adequate supply of thirteen different vitamins. Four of these vitamins are soluble in fat and are obtained primarily from the fat in our diet, while the other nine water-soluble vitamins are distributed rather widely in a variety of foods. A well-balanced diet will satisfy all of the vitamin requirements of most individuals. Some vitamins are also formed in the body from other nutrients that we eat (such as vitamin A from beta-carotene), from the action of sunlight on the skin (vitamin D), or from the action of intestinal bacteria (vitamin K). Table 6.8 highlights the major vitamins, their synonyms, the recommended dietary allowance, some major food sources, their major functions in the human body, and the primary symptoms of a deficiency or excess.

Health Implications of Vitamins

Vitamins continue to be one of the most used and abused nutrients in the United States today. Vitamin-pill manufacturers

Table 6.8 Essential Vitamins

Vitamin Name (Other Terms)	RDA or ESADDI for Adults and Children over Four	Major Sources
Fat-Soluble Vitamins		
Vitamin A (retinol; provitamin carotenoids)	5,000 IU or 1,000 RE ♂ 4,000 IU or 800 RE ♀	Retinol in animal foods: liver, whole milk, fortified milk, cheese. Carotenoids in plant foods: carrots, green leafy vegetables, sweet potatoes, fortified margarine from vegetable oils.
Vitamin D (calciferol)	400 IU or 10 micrograms	Vitamin D fortified foods like dairy products, margarine, and fish oils. Action of sunlight on the skin.
Vitamin E (tocopherol)	10 mg ♂ 8 mg ♀ alpha-TE	Vegetable oils, margarine, green leafy vegetables, wheat germ, whole grain products, egg yolks.
Vitamin K (antihemorrhagic vitamin)	80 micrograms ♂ 65 micrograms ♀	Pork and beef liver, eggs, spinach, cauliflower. Formation in the human intestines by bacteria.
Water-Soluble Vitamins		
Thiamin (vitamin B₁)	1.5 mg ♂ 1.1 mg ♀	Ham, pork, lean meat, liver, whole grain products, fortified breads and cereals, legumes.
Riboflavin (vitamin B₂)	1.7 mg ♂ 1.3 mg ♀	Milk and dairy products, meat, fortified grain products, green leafy vegetables, beans.
Niacin (nicotinamide, nicotinic acid)	19 mg ♂ 15 mg ♀	Lean meats, fish, poultry, whole grain products, beans. May be formed in the body from tryptophan, an essential amino acid.
Vitamin B₆ (pyridoxal, pyridoxine, pyridoxamine)	2 mg ♂ 1.6 mg ♀	Protein foods, liver, lean meats, fish, poultry, legumes, green leafy vegetables.
Vitamin B₁₂ (cobalamin; cyanocobalamin)	2 micrograms	Animal foods only, meat, fish, poultry, milk, eggs.
Folic acid (folacin)	200 micrograms ♂ 180 micrograms ♀	Liver, green leafy vegetables, legumes, nuts.
Biotin	30–100 micrograms	Meats, legumes, milk, egg yolk, whole grain products, most vegetables.
Pantothenic acid	4–7 mg	Beef and pork liver, lean meats, milk, eggs, legumes, whole grain products, most vegetables.
Vitamin C (ascorbic acid)	60 mg	Citrus fruits, green leafy vegetables, broccoli, peppers, strawberries, potatoes.

From Melvin H. Williams, Nutrition for Fitness and Sport, 4th ed. Copyright © 1995 Brown & Benchmark Publishers, Dubuque, Iowa. All Rights Reserved. Reprinted by permission.

and advertisers have perpetuated the myth that the average American diet contains insufficient amounts of vitamins, a potential cause of many diseases. We now have vitamin supplements on the market that have been designed, or so the manufacturers say, to help us combat the stress of everyday life, to help prevent the common cold, and to provide optimal energy for athletic performance.

Vitamins are necessary nutrients. However, exaggerated claims by those with economic interests in vitamin supplements usually are not supported by factual data. Health problems may occur if you experience a dietary vitamin deficiency or an excessive vitamin intake. Table 6.8 presents some of the possible problems associated with a deficiency or excess of each vitamin.

Major Functions in the Body	Deficiency Symptoms	Symptoms of Excess Consumption
Fat-Soluble Vitamins		
Maintenance of epithelial tissue in skin and mucous membranes, formation of visual purple for night vision, bone development.	Night blindness, intestinal infections, impaired growth, xerophthalmia.	Nausea, headache, fatigue, liver and spleen damage, skin peeling, pain in the joints.
Acts as a hormone to increase intestinal absorption of calcium and promote bone and tooth formation.	Rare. Rickets in children and osteomalacia in adults.	Loss of appetite, nausea, irritability, joint pains, calcium deposits in soft tissues such as the kidney.
Functions as an antioxidant to protect cell membranes from destruction by oxidation.	Extremely rare. Disruption of red blood cell membranes, anemia.	General lack of toxicity with doses up to 600 IU.
Essential for blood coagulation processes.	Increased bleeding and hemorrhaging.	Possible clot formation (thrombus), vomiting.
Water-Soluble Vitamins		
Serves as a coenzyme for energy production from carbohydrate; essential for normal functioning of the central nervous system.	Poor appetite, apathy, mental depression, pain in calf muscles, beriberi.	General lack of toxicity.
Functions as a coenzyme involved in energy production from carbohydrates and fats; maintains healthy skin.	Dermatitis, cracks at the corners of the mouth, sores on the tongue, damage to the cornea.	General lack of toxicity.
Functions as a coenzyme for the aerobic and anaerobic production of energy from carbohydrate; helps synthesize fat and blocks release of FFA; needed for healthy skin.	Loss of appetite, weakness, skin problems, pellagra	Nicotinic acid causes headache, nausea, burning and lesions, gastrointestinal itching skin, flushing of face.
Functions as a coenzyme in protein metabolism; necessary for formation of hemoglobin and red blood cells; needed for glycogenolysis and gluconeogenesis.	Nervous irritability, convulsions, dermatitis, sores on tongue, anemia.	Loss of nerve sensation, impaired gait.
Functions as coenzyme for formation of DNA, development of RBC, and maintenance of nerve tissue.	Pernicious anemia, nerve damage resulting in paralysis.	General lack of toxicity.
Functions as coenzyme for DNA formation and RBC development.	Fatigue, gastrointestinal disorders, diarrhea, anemia, neural tube defects.	May prevent detection of pernicious anemia caused by B_{12} deficiency.
Functions as a coenzyme in the metabolism of carbohydrates, fats, and protein.	Rare. May be caused by excessive intake of raw egg whites. Fatigue, nausea, skin rashes.	General lack of toxicity.
Functions as part of coenzyme A in energy metabolism.	Rare. Only produced clinically. Fatigue, nausea, loss of appetite, mental depression.	General lack of toxicity.
Forms collagen essential for connective tissue development; aids in absorption of iron, helps form epinephrine; serves as antioxidant.	Weakness, rough skin, slow wound healing, bleeding gums, scurvy.	Diarrhea, possible kidney stones, rebound scurvy.

The key to adequate vitamin nutrition is to consume a balanced diet of natural foods high in nutrient density. Buy foods in their natural state and properly store them as soon as possible. Prepare them so as to minimize vitamin losses; cook food by steaming or microwaving it rather than by boiling it in water. Table 6.9 presents a list of ten foods, totalling approximately 1,200 Calories, that will provide at least 100 percent of the RDA for every vitamin, assuming adequate sunlight for vitamin D and intestinal synthesis of several other vitamins.

Kim and others reported no increase in longevity among vitamin and mineral supplement users in the United States. However, for some individuals there may be some health benefits associated with several vitamins, such as

Table 6.9 1,200 Calorie Diet Containing at Least 100% of the RDA for Each Vitamin

Food	Amount
Milk, skim, fortified with vitamins A and D	2 cups
Carrot	1 medium
Orange	1 average
Bread, whole wheat	4 slices
Chicken breast, roasted	3 ounces
Broccoli	1 stalk
Margarine	1 tablespoon
Cereal, Grape-nuts	2 ounces
Tuna fish, in water	3 ounces
Cauliflower	1/2 cup

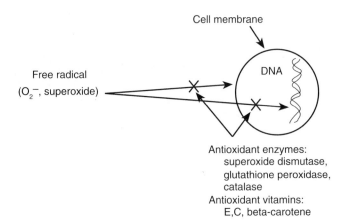

Figure 6.9 *Antioxidant role of vitamins. Some vitamins, serving as antioxidants, may assist naturally occurring antioxidant enzymes in the body to prevent free radicals such as superoxide from attacking cell membranes or the genetic material within the cell. It is theorized that such vitamins protect against cancer and other diseases.*

niacin and folic acid, and some interesting data are emerging in relation to health aspects of the antioxidant vitamins.

Large doses of niacin have been used successfully to lower triglycerides and total and LDL cholesterol and to raise HDL cholesterol. Some health professionals consider niacin the first choice for individuals who may need drugs to lower their serum cholesterol. However, niacin may also cause flushing, burning, and tingling sensations around the face and neck in some individuals, and when taken over long periods, it may contribute to liver problems such as hepatitis and peptic ulcer. Therefore, health professionals recommend that no one take large doses of niacin to reduce serum cholesterol unless under the guidance of a physician.

In 1992, the United States Public Health Service recommended that all women who have the potential to become pregnant should consume 400 micrograms of folic acid daily, which is twice the RDA. Currently, women consume about 200–300 micrograms per day, so they would either have to increase their intake of folate-rich foods or take a supplement of about 200 micrograms. This advice is based on some epidemiological and intervention studies suggesting that increased intake of folic acid may prevent the occurrence of neural tube defects such as spina bifida, or incomplete closure of the bone surrounding the spinal cord; such defects may cause paralysis and affect nearly 2,500 infants per year. Although some investigators suggest more research is needed, 400 milligrams is the RDA for pregnant women, and no adverse effects have been noted in nonpregnant women who have taken such dosages. However, larger doses are not recommended.

Epidemiological evidence has suggested that diets rich in certain vegetables containing beta-carotene, such as carrots, sweet potatoes, and squash, and **cruciferous vegetables** (a plant family with flowers of a crosslike design), such as broccoli, cauliflower, cabbage, and brussel sprouts, may be helpful in the prevention of cancer. Although the mechanism whereby these vegetables may provide this protective effect is not known, one hypothesis was noted previously, i.e., the presence of nutraceuticals, such as sulforaphane, that may act as anticarcinogens. Another hypothesis is that the antioxidant effect exerted by beta-carotene or other antioxidants naturally occurring in plants, such as phytic acid and vitamins C and E, may assist antioxidant enzymes already present in the body to block the possible carcinogenic action of **free radicals** (especially reactive particles, such as superoxide and hydrogen peroxide, produced in the body that are thought to damage cell membranes) in the body on the cell membrane or DNA as illustrated in figure 6.9. It is important to note that these epidemiological studies have supported the health benefits of eating foods rich in beta-carotene and other antioxidants, not vitamin supplements.

However, free radicals are also thought to contribute to the development of atherosclerosis (see chapter 11), and some research suggests vitamin E, an antioxidant, may help to prevent cardiovascular disease by blocking this action. Two recent epidemiological studies associated high intakes of vitamin E with a reduced risk for coronary heart disease. Rimm and others reported a reduced risk in men, while Stampfer and others reported a reduced risk in women. Prevention of the oxidation of LDL cholesterol and the subsequent formation of atherosclerosis is theorized to be the primary underlying mechanism. In these studies, the greatest reduction in risk for coronary heart disease was associated with those groups of subjects who took vitamin E supplements. Although these epidemiologic studies are encouraging, the investigators stress the point that such studies only document an association, not a cause-and-effect relationship, that needs to be supported by intervention studies. Currently, a number of clinical intervention trials are underway to evaluate the health benefits of antioxidant vitamin supplementation, and hopefully data from these clinical trials will be available in the near future to provide us with information as to whether or not antioxidant vitamin supplementation provides us with any significant health benefits above and beyond those associated with the Healthy American Diet.

Some recent national surveys note slight deficiencies in several nutrients, particularly the water-soluble vitamins, in the diets of some Americans. However, these surveys indicate only a deficiency in the diet and do not report any disease symptoms. If an individual is not receiving a balanced diet for some reason, a simple balanced vitamin supplement will not do any harm. There are a number of preparations on the market that contain the daily RDA of most vitamins. If you are on a balanced diet, the only damage sustained by consuming such products is to the pocketbook.

At the present time, megadoses of vitamins are not recommended. A **megadose** is defined as an amount which is ten times the RDA (lower for vitamin A [only five times] and vitamin D [only two times]). Future research may document health benefits of antioxidant supplements, but in general, if the vitamin content of the body is adequate, excess vitamin intake does not serve any useful purpose and may function as a drug and be harmful. There are more than 4,000 cases of vitamin/mineral overdoses in the United States each year, resulting in about thirty fatalities, particularly among young children. Two good reviews of possible adverse effects of excessive vitamin supplementation are one presented by Snodgrass and another by Cook and McDermott.

Minerals

You may recall the periodic table containing all of the known elements on earth hanging on the wall in your high school or college chemistry class. At latest count, there are 110 known elements, 78 of them occurring naturally and the remainder man-made. A number of the natural elements are essential to human body structure and function.

A mineral is an inorganic element found in nature. The term is usually reserved for solid elements. In nutrition, the term *mineral* is used to list those elements that are essential to life processes. Currently, twenty-five minerals are known to be essential in human nutrition, and they perform a wide variety of functions in the body. Seven elements and minerals (carbon, oxygen, hydrogen, nitrogen, sulfur, calcium, and phosphorus) are used as building blocks for such body tissues as bones, teeth, muscles, and other organic structures. Minerals are also important in a number of regulatory functions in the body. Some of the physiological processes regulated or maintained by minerals include muscle contraction, nerve impulse conduction, acid-base balance of the blood, body water supplies, blood clotting, and normal heart rhythm. Table 6.10 lists 16 minerals essential to human nutrition and briefly covers their major food sources, body functions, and health problems associated with deficiency or excess consumption.

Health Implications of Mineral Nutrition

As with each individual vitamin, a deficiency or excess of any mineral may lead to serious health problems. Although an adequate dietary intake of all minerals is important, calcium, iron, and sodium are three minerals that appear to have significant health implications in the typical American diet.

Research suggests that calcium intake among adults, particularly women, is below the recommended level. Because calcium is the primary constituent of bone tissue, calcium deficiency, particularly in older women, may lead to **osteoporosis,** a decrease in bone mass that makes a person more susceptible to fractures in the hip, wrist, and spine (see chapter 11 for more detailed information on osteoporosis). Thus, foods high in calcium, particularly dairy foods, should

be stressed in the diet throughout life, particularly so during the growth years up to age twenty-five in order to maximize bone mass.

Iron is commonly found to be slightly deficient in the diet of many Americans, particularly women and teenagers, groups whose iron requirements are higher than the adult male. National surveys have revealed that over 90 percent of women are receiving less than the RDA for iron. Inadequate dietary intake or excessive losses of iron may lead to **iron-deficiency anemia,** a condition that may lead to constant weakness and fatigue. The inclusion of high iron foods in the daily diet should be an important concern, particularly for all females and for male teenagers.

Sodium has a wide variety of functions in human metabolism, one function being the maintenance of a normal blood pressure. Although most individuals possess effective control systems to maintain a proper balance of sodium in the body, excessive intake of sodium has been associated with the development of high blood pressure in individuals who are labeled salt sensitive or sodium sensitive. Apparently, their bodies do not effectively regulate sodium balance. Since there may be 15 to 20 million Americans who may be sodium sensitive, it is recommended that sodium and salt in the diet be consumed in moderation.

Some guidelines for obtaining adequate amounts of dietary calcium, iron, and sodium are presented later in this chapter.

Excessive intake of one mineral, usually through supplements, may impair the absorption of other essential minerals. For example, excessive intake of calcium will impair the absorption of iron. Moreover, many minerals may be toxic to the body if consumed in excess. It is very difficult to consume excessive amounts of minerals through natural foods, but megadoses provided by excessive intake of mineral supplements may seriously impair normal physiological functions. For example, of every 1,000 Americans approximately two to three have a genetic predisposition to hemochromatosis and store excess iron in their livers. Prolonged consumption of excess iron may cause cirrhosis of and ultimate destruction of the liver. Thus, as with vitamins, individuals should not consume megadoses of mineral supplements, which may be three to five times the RDA, unless under the guidance of a health professional.

Water

Water is a clear, tasteless, odorless fluid. It is a rather simple compound composed of two parts hydrogen and one part oxygen (H_2O). Of all compounds essential in the chemistry and functioning of living forms, water is the most important. Most other nutrients essential to life can be utilized by the human body only in their combination with water. It provides the medium within which other nutrients may function.

Water provides the essential building material for cell protoplasm. It is the main transportation mechanism in the body, conveying oxygen, nutrients, hormones, and other compounds to the cells for their use. Additionally, it helps regulate the acid-base balance in the body and plays a major role in the regulation of body temperature, particularly during exercise in the heat.

Table 6.10 Essential Minerals in Human Nutrition

Major Mineral with RDA and ESADDI	Major Food Sources	Major Body Functions	Deficiency Symptoms	Symptoms of Excessive Consumption
Calcium 1,200 mg age 11–25 800 mg adults	All dairy products: milk, cheese, ice cream, yogurt; egg yolk; dried beans and peas; dark green vegetables; cauliflower	Bone formation; enzyme activation; nerve impulse transmission; muscle contraction; cell membrane potential	Osteoporosis; rickets; impaired muscle contraction; muscle cramps	Constipation; inhibition of trace mineral absorption. In susceptible individuals: heart arrhythmias; kidney stones; calcification of soft tissues
Phosphorus 1,200 mg age 11–25 800 mg adults	All protein products: meat, poultry, fish, eggs, milk, cheese, dried beans and peas; whole grain products; soft drinks	Bone formation; acid-base balance; cell membrane structure; B vitamin activation; organic compound component, e.g., ATP-CP, 2,3-DPG	Rare. Deficiency symptoms parallel calcium deficiency. Muscular weakness.	Rare. Impaired calcium metabolism; gastrointestinal distress from phosphate salts
Magnesium 350 mg ♂ 280 mg ♀	Milk and yogurt; dried beans; nuts; whole grain products; fruits and vegetables, especially green leafy vegetables	Protein synthesis; metalloenzyme; 2,3-DPG formation; glucose metabolism; smooth muscle contraction; bone component	Rare. Muscle weakness; apathy; muscle twitching; muscle cramps; cardiac arrhythmias	Nausea; vomiting; diarrhea
Sodium 500–2400 mg	Most processed foods: canned, packaged, luncheon meats; pretzels; crackers; snacks; soy sauce.	Primary positive ion in extracellular fluid; nerve impulse conduction; muscle contraction; acid-base balance; blood volume homeostasis	Hyponatremia; muscle cramps; nausea; vomiting; loss of appetite; dizziness; seizures; shock; coma	Hypertension (high blood pressure) in susceptible individuals
Chloride 750–3600 mg	Same as sodium.	Primary negative ion in extracellular fluid; nerve impulse conduction; hydrochloric acid formation in stomach	Rare; may be caused by excess vomiting and loss of hydrochloric acid; convulsions	Hypertension, in conjunction with excess sodium
Potassium 2,000–5,800 mg	All fruits and vegetables: bananas, oranges, potatoes; milk; yogurt.	Primary positive ion in intracellular fluid; same functions as sodium, but intracellular; glucose transport into cell	Hypokalemia; loss of appetite; muscle cramps; apathy; irregular heart beat	Hyperkalemia; inhibit heart function
Iron 15 mg ♀ 12 mg ♂ age 11–18 10 mg adult p♂	Organ meats such as liver; meat, fish and poultry; shellfish, especially oysters; dried beans and peas; whole-grain products; green leafy vegetables; broccoli; dried apricots, dates, figs, raisins; iron cookware	Hemoglobin and myoglobin formation; electron transfer; essential in oxidative processes	Fatigue; anemia; impaired temperature regulation; decreased resistance to infection	Hemochromatosis; liver damage

The requirement for body water depends upon the body weight of an individual. Under normal environmental temperatures and activity levels, the average adult female needs about 2,000 milliliters, or 2 liters (slightly more than 2 quarts), of water per day to maintain adequate water balance in the body; adult males need about 2,800 milliliters. Body water balance is maintained when the intake of water matches the output of body fluids. Urinary output is the main avenue for water loss; insensible perspiration, which is not visible, is almost pure water and makes a significant contribution to body water losses. A small amount of water is lost in the feces and through exhaled air in breathing. Fluid intake of beverages is the main source of water to replenish losses. Solid foods also contribute water in two different ways. First, food contains water in varying amounts; certain foods such as lettuce, celery, melons, and most fruits contain about 90 percent water. Many others contain more than 60 percent—even bread, an outwardly dry-appearing food, contains 36 percent water. Second, the metabolism of foods for energy produces water; fat, carbohydrate, and protein all produce water when

Table 6.10   (continued)

Mineral with RDA and ESADDI	Major Food Sources	Major Body Functions	Deficiency Symptoms	Symptoms of Excessive Consumption
Copper 1.5–3.0 mg	Organ meats, liver; meat, fish and poultry; shellfish; nuts; eggs; bran cereals; avocado; broccoli; banana	Proper use of iron and hemoglobin in the body; metalloenzyme involved in connective tissue formation and oxidations	Rare; anemia	Rare; nausea; vomiting
Zinc 15 mg ♂ 12 mg ♀	Organ meats; meat, fish, poultry; shellfish, especially oysters; dairy products; nuts; whole-grain products; vegetables, asparagus, spinach	Cofactor of many enzymes involved in energy metabolism, protein synthesis, immune function, sexual maturation, and sensations of taste and smell	Depressed immune function; impaired wound healing; depressed appetite; failure to grow; skin inflammation	Increased LDL and decreased HDL cholesterol; impaired immune system; nausea; vomiting; impaired copper absorption
Chromium 50–200 micrograms	Organ meats such as liver; meats; oysters; cheese; whole-grain products; asparagus; beer; stainless steel cookware	Enhances insulin function as glucose tolerance factor	Glucose intolerance; impaired lipid metabolism	Rare from dietary sources
Selenium 70 micrograms ♂ 55 micrograms ♀	Meat, fish, poultry; organ meats such as kidney, liver; seafood; whole grains and nuts from selenium-rich soil	Cofactor of glutathione peroxidase, an antioxidant enzyme	Rare; cardiac muscle damage	Nausea; vomiting; abdominal pain; hair loss
Cobalt not established; part of vitamin B_{12}	Meat; liver; milk	Component of vitamin B_{12}; promotes development of red blood cells	Not found in humans	Nausea; vomiting; death
Fluoride 1.5–4.0 mg	Milk; egg yolk; seafood; drinking water in fluoridated communities	Helps form bones and teeth	Higher incidence of dental cavities	Discolored teeth
Iodine 150 micrograms	Iodized salt; seafood; vegetables	Helps in the formation of thyroid hormones	Goiter, an enlarged thyroid gland	Depressed thyroid gland activity
Manganese 2.0–5.0 mg	Whole grain products; dried beans and peas; leafy vegetables; bananas	Part of many enzymes involved in energy metabolism; bone formation; fat synthesis	Poor growth	Weakness; nervous system problems; mental confusion
Molybdenum 75–250 micrograms	Liver; organ meats; whole grain products; dried beans and peas	Works with riboflavin in enzymes involved in carbohydrate and fat metabolism	Not found in humans	Rare

broken down into energy. This water is often called metabolic water. Table 6.11 summarizes daily water loss and intake for the maintenance of water balance.

Health Implications of Water Intake

The body possesses a very effective control system to maintain normal water levels. Several hormones and the sensation of thirst help maintain water balance on a day-to-day basis. The main health problem occurs primarily during exercise in the heat when body water losses greatly exceed fluid intake. In such cases, several different forms of heat illnesses may occur,

such as heat exhaustion and heat stroke. The guidelines presented on page 51, including those dealing with fluid replenishment, should help prevent any serious consequences associated with exercise under warm environmental conditions.

The Basis of Diet Planning

Eating a well-balanced diet is the key to good nutrition. We have all heard this statement at one time or another, but what exactly is a well-balanced diet? A diet needs to be balanced in two aspects. First, it must contain an adequate amount of the

Table 6.11 Daily Water Loss and Intake for Water Balance in an Adult Female

Water Loss

Source	Quantity
Urine output	1100 ml
Water in feces	100 ml
Lungs, exhaled air	200 ml
Skin, insensible perspiration	600 ml
Total	2000 ml

Water Intake

Source	Quantity
Fluids	1000 ml
Water in food	700 ml
Metabolic water	300 ml
Total	2000 ml

fifty or more essential nutrients to sustain growth and/or repair body tissues during the various stages of life. Second, it must be balanced in caloric intake for control of body weight (weight maintenance, gain, or loss, depending upon the individual).

Although everyone needs essential nutrients and a balanced caloric intake in their diet, the proportions differ at varying stages of the life cycle; the infant has different needs than his grandfather, and the pregnant or lactating woman has different needs than her adolescent daughter. Needs also differ between the sexes, particularly the iron content of the diet. Moreover, individual variations in life-style impose different nutrient requirements. A long-distance runner in training for a marathon has some distinct nutritional needs compared to a sedentary colleague. The individual trying to lose weight needs to balance Calorie losses with nutrient adequacy. The diabetic needs strict nutritional counseling for a balanced diet. Thus, there are a number of different conditions that influence nutrient needs and the concept of a balanced diet.

The Recommended Dietary Allowances (RDA)

As is noted in table 6.1, humans need to regularly consume over fifty essential nutrients, but what is an adequate amount of each?

In the United States, the adequate amounts of certain nutrients have been established by the Food and Nutrition Board, National Academy of Sciences—National Research Council. The **Recommended Dietary Allowances (RDA)** represent the levels of intake of essential nutrients considered (in the judgment of the Food and Nutrition Board on the basis of an extensive review of the available scientific knowledge) to be adequate to meet the known nutritional needs of practically all healthy persons in the United States. RDA have been established for energy intake (Calories), protein, eleven vitamins, and seven minerals. Although technically not an RDA, Estimated Safe and Adequate Daily Dietary Intakes (ESADDI) have been developed for two additional vitamins and five minerals.

The RDA should not be construed as the recommended ideal diet. They are not guaranteed to represent total nutritional

needs, for there is insufficient evidence relative to some essential trace elements. Moreover, they are designed for healthy persons, not those needing dietary modifications due to illness.

An individual's diet is not necessarily deficient if it does not include the full RDA daily. A person may be deficient in iron consumption in one day's diet, but can compensate for this during the remainder of the week. A general recommendation to help meet the daily RDA requirements is to select as wide a variety of foods as possible when planning the diet.

Key Nutrient Concept

There are eight essential nutrients that, when found naturally in plant and animal sources, are usually accompanied by the other essential nutrients. These eight nutrients are

protein	vitamin B_2 (riboflavin)
vitamin A	niacin
vitamin C	iron
vitamin B_1 (thiamin)	calcium

Thus, if your diet is adequate in these eight key nutrients, you probably receive an ample supply of all nutrients essential to humans. That is the **key nutrient concept.** Foods that contain these key nutrients should be obtained, as much as possible, from naturally occurring plant and animal food sources.

Table 6.12 presents the eight key nutrients along with the significant plant and animal sources of each.

Nutrient Density

The food supply in the United States is extremely varied; most individuals who consume a wide variety of foods do receive an adequate supply of nutrients. Now many of the foods we eat are processed in some way or another, and some individuals believe that processed foods are not as nutritious as nonprocessed foods. That is not necessarily so. For example, frozen peas may possess greater vitamin content compared to fresh peas because the rapid freezing process minimizes the loss of vitamins that occurs after peas are harvested. Nevertheless, there appears to be some concern that many Americans are not receiving optimal nutrition due to the consumption of excessive amounts of highly processed foods. This may be true, as improper food processing may lead to depletion of key nutrients and the addition of high-Calorie and low-nutrient ingredients. Many of the foods we eat contain too much white flour, refined sugar, and extracted oils, all products of a refinement process. In the bleaching and processing of whole wheat to white flour, at least twenty-two known essential nutrients are removed, including the B vitamins, vitamin E, calcium, phosphorus, potassium, and magnesium. Refined sugar is pure carbohydrate with no nutritional value except Calories. The same can be said for extracted oils, which are pure fat. You may be surprised to learn that about three out of every five Calories in the typical American diet are derived from either sugar or fat, because these are two of the most common additives in processed foods, along with sodium. Most fast foods are also high in fat, sugar, and sodium content, although the fast-food industry is beginning to provide healthier menu choices.

Table 6.12 Eight Key Nutrients and Significant Food Sources from Plants and Animals

Nutrient	RDI	Plant Source	Animal Source	Major Food Exchanges
Protein	56 g	Dried beans and peas, nuts	Meat, poultry, fish, cheese, milk	Meat, milk
Vitamin A	5000 IU	Dark green leafy vegetables, yellow vegetables, margarine	Butter, fortified milk, liver	Fruits, vegetables, fat
Vitamin C	60 mg	Citrus fruits, broccoli, potatoes, strawberries, tomatoes, cabbage, dark green leafy vegetables	Liver	Fruits, vegetables
Vitamin B_1 (thiamin)	1.5 mg	Breads, cereals, pasta, nuts	Pork, ham	Starch/Bread, meat
Vitamin B_2 (riboflavin)	1.7 mg	Breads, cereals, pasta	Milk, cheese, liver	Starch/Bread, milk
Niacin	20 mg	Breads, cereals, pasta, nuts	Meat, fish, poultry	Starch/Bread, meat
Iron	15 mg	Dried peas and beans, spinach, asparagus, prune juice	Meat, liver	Meat, starch/bread
Calcium	1000 mg	Turnip greens, okra, broccoli, spinach, kale	Milk, cheese, mackerel, salmon	Milk, vegetables

When buying food, you should attempt to select foods with significant amounts of the key nutrients and a low to moderate number of Calories. This, in general, is the meaning of **nutrient density.** A food with high nutrient density provides a significant amount of a specific nutrient or nutrients per serving, or for a certain amount of Calories. An example of nutrient density is presented in figure 6.10.

The Food Guide Pyramid and the Food Exchange Lists

The RDA, key nutrients, and nutrient density are important concepts to apply when selecting foods for a balanced diet, but they are not practical approaches in educating the American public about sound nutrition. Hence, some time ago the *food group* approach was developed as a guide to eating that can be easily understood by the average American. The basis of the food group approach is that certain groups of foods contain significant amounts of several of the key nutrients. Different patterns of nutrients are found in various food groups. Table 6.13 represents the key nutrients from across six categories, or groups, of food products. This categorization represents the key nutrient content of each major food group; there is some variation in the proportion of the nutrients found between food groups as well as between different foods within each group. For example, the breads, cereals, rice, and pasta category is a good source of protein, but not as good as the meat, poultry, fish, eggs, dry beans, and nuts category. Within the fruit category, oranges are an excellent source of vitamin C, but peaches are not. Since the American population has a tremendous variety of foods from which to select, it is not difficult to get the necessary amounts of nutrients from among and within the six food categories.

The most recent food guide designed to provide the best nutrition advice for daily food selection is the **Food Guide Pyramid** developed by the United States Department of Agriculture. It is based on some of the guidelines underlying the Healthy American Diet. The Food Guide Pyramid is

Amount	8 ounces	8 ounces	8 ounces	8 ounces
Calories	120	150	90	100
Protein (grams)	0	8*	8*	0
Fat (grams)	0	8	Trace	0
Carbohydrates (grams)	30	12	12	25
Calcium (milligrams)	27	352*	352*	0
Iron (milligrams)	0.5	0.1	0.1	0
Vitamin A (IU)	500*	500*	500*	0
Thiamin (milligrams)	0.2*	0.1	0.1	0
Riboflavin (milligrams)	0.07	0.5*	0.5*	0
Niacin (milligrams)	1.0	0.2	0.2	0
Vitamin C (milligrams)	152*	2	2	0
	Orange juice	Milk, whole	Milk, skim	Cola

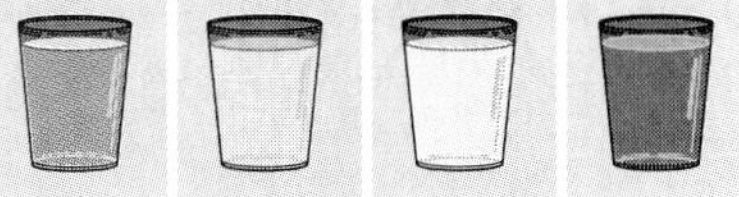

*Significant source of this key nutrient, over 10% of the RDA.

Figure 6.10 *The concept of nutrient density. The key principle is to select foods that are high in nutrients and low in Calories. Compare the nutrient value of the four beverages in this figure. As you can see, orange juice and milk are significant sources of several key nutrients, while cola simply contains Calories in the form of simple carbohydrates. Substituting skim milk for whole milk saves about 60 Calories but does not decrease the key nutrient content, thus increasing the nutrient density.*

designed to provide a visual image of the variety of foods that Americans should eat, the proportion of Calories that should come from each of the food groups, and the use of moderation in consumption of fats, oils, and sweets.

There are five food groups in the Food Guide Pyramid. The base of the pyramid, which should constitute the majority of the daily Calories, is represented by the bread, cereal, rice, and pasta group (6–11 servings), as well as the vegetable group (3–5 servings) and the fruit group (2–4 servings).

Table 6.13 Major Nutrients Found in the Six Food Categories of the Food Guide Pyramid

Milk, Yogurt, Cheese	Meat, Poultry, Fish, Eggs, Dry Beans, Nuts	Breads, Cereals, Rice, Pasta	Vegetable	Fruit	Fats, Oils, Sweets*
Calcium	Protein	Thiamin	Vitamin A	Vitamin A	Vitamin A
Protein	Thiamin	Niacin	Vitamin C	Vitamin C	Vitamin D
Riboflavin	Niacin	Riboflavin			Vitamin E
Vitamin A	Iron	Iron			

Mainly contains Calories. Fat-soluble vitamins found in some foods. Not classified as a food group.

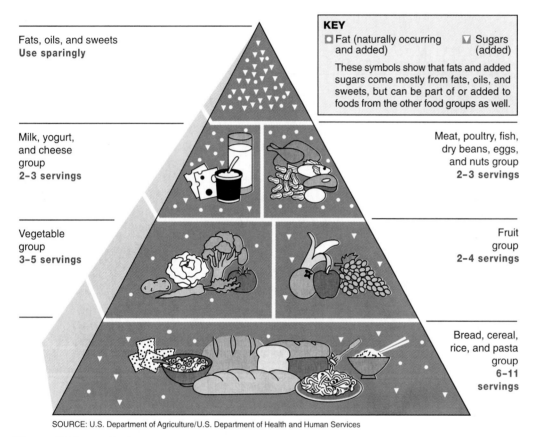

SOURCE: U.S. Department of Agriculture/U.S. Department of Health and Human Services

Figure 6.11 *The food guide pyramid.*

These three food groups are derived from grains and plants. Fewer servings are recommended from the milk, yogurt, and cheese group (2–3 servings) and the meat, poultry, fish, dry beans, eggs, and nuts group (2–3 servings); most of the foods in these two groups are derived from animals. Fats, oils, and sweets (not classified as a group) should be used sparingly. Figure 6.11 depicts the Food Guide Pyramid. Typical serving sizes are presented in table 6.14 while table 6.15 provides general recommendations for various segments of the population. The daily number of servings are based on caloric needs of different individuals.

Although the Food Guide Pyramid represents a significant improvement over previous food guides, it has a few flaws. The Center for Science in the Public Interest, a consumer protection organization concerned primarily with nutrition issues, notes that there is only a hint that meat and dairy products are the largest sources of fat and saturated fat in the average American diet. Also, the pyramid places dry beans and meat in the same category, which may be interpreted as a recommendation to eat less beans. However, dried beans and peas are one of the healthiest food choices for they are low in fat, high in carbohydrate and dietary fiber, and a good source of iron, calcium, and other vitamins and minerals.

A food guide similar to the Food Guide Pyramid is the **Food Exchange System,** a grouping of foods developed by the American Dietetic Association, American Diabetic

Association, and other professional and governmental health organizations (see fig. 6.12). Foods in each of the six exchanges contain approximately the same amount of Calories, carbohydrate, fat, and protein. As with the Food Guide Pyramid, eating a wide variety of foods from the six food exchanges will help guarantee that you receive the RDA for essential nutrients. The basic content of each food exchange is presented in table 6.16. A detailed list of common foods in the various exchange lists and appropriate serving sizes may be found in Appendix A. Laboratory Inventory 6.1 uses the Food Exchange System as a means to evaluate your diet for an appropriate blend of caloric, carbohydrate, fat, and protein intake. Also, because the Food Exchange System has been developed and utilized extensively as a means to balance nutrition and weight control, it is the method utilized in the next chapter as a dietary means to control body weight. More details are presented about the food exchange lists in chapter 7.

Although the use of the Food Guide Pyramid or the Food Exchange System is a valuable means to achieve the RDA for essential nutrients, there may be some problems if foods are not selected wisely. It is easily possible to select the least nutritious foods from each food group or exchange list. In addition, an individual may select foods that might not be considered the most healthful choices on the basis of current nutritional knowledge. A dozen general recommendations are presented later under "Healthier Eating" to serve as guides to food selection whether you use the Food Guide Pyramid or the Food Exchange System.

Food Labels

Although the Food Guide Pyramid and Food Exchange System provide us with a sound means to select a healthy diet, it may not be directly applicable to a large number of food items available to us in the local supermarket. Thus, we may have to rely on food labels to reveal the nutritional quality of a food product. Food manufacturers view labels as a device for persuading you to buy their product instead of a competitor's. Just walk down the cereal aisle next time you visit the supermarket and notice the bewildering number of choices. As manufactured food products multiplied over the years and as competition for your food dollar intensified, food companies began to manipulate their labels to enhance sales. Unfortunately, many of these practices were deceptive, and the consumer had a difficult time determining the nutritional quality of many processed foods. Thus, Congress passed the Nutrition Labeling and Education Act in 1990 designed to establish a set of standards so that when purchasing food most Americans could base their choice of what to eat on sound nutritional information. The latest set of nutritional labeling is based on recommendations for healthier eating, and most of the nutrients which have health implications may be found on food labels.

Table 6.14 Serving Sizes in the Food Guide Pyramid

Pyramid Food Group	Serving Size
Milk, yogurt, cheese	1 cup of milk or yogurt 1½ ounces natural cheese 2 ounces of processed cheese
Meat, poultry, fish, dry beans, eggs, and nuts	2–3 ounces of cooked lean meat, poultry, or fish ½ cup of cooked dry beans 1 egg 2 tablespoons peanut butter
Bread, cereal, rice, and pasta	1 slice of bread 1 ounce of ready-to-eat cereal ½ cup of cooked cereal, rice, or pasta
Vegetable	1 cup of raw leafy vegetables ½ cup of other vegetables, cooked or chopped raw ¾ cup vegetable juice
Fruit	1 medium apple, banana, or orange ½ cup of chopped, cooked, or canned fruit ¾ cup of fruit juice
Fats, oils, sweets (Not an official food group)	No serving size

Table 6.15 Daily Number of Servings with the Food Guide Pyramid

	Many Women, Older Adults	Children, Teen Girls, Active Women, Most Men	Teen Boys, Active Men
*Calorie level**	About 1,600	About 2,200	About 2,800
Bread group servings	6	9	11
Vegetable group servings	3	4	5
Fruit group servings	2	3	4
Milk group servings	2–3+	2–3+	2–3+
Meat group servings	2, for a total of 5 ounces	2, for a total of 6 ounces	3, for a total of 7 ounces
Total fat (grams)	53	73	93

*These are the Calorie levels if you choose low fat, lean foods from the five major food groups and use foods from the fats, oils, and sweets group sparingly. The total fat in grams is based on a diet containing 30 percent of Calories from fat.

+Women who are pregnant or breastfeeding, teenagers, and young adults to age 24 need 3 servings.

Source: United States Department of Agriculture

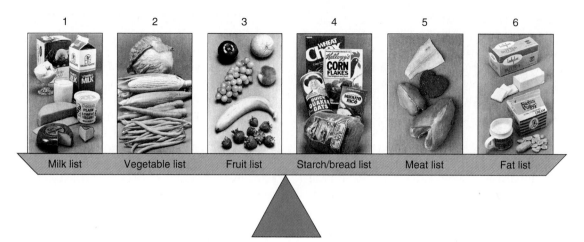

1	2	3	4	5	6
Milk list	Vegetable list	Fruit list	Starch/bread list	Meat list	Fat list

Figure 6.12 *The key to sound nutrition is a balanced diet high in nutrients and low in Calories. For balance, select a wide variety of foods from among and within the Exchange Lists (Appendix A).*

Table 6.16 Carbohydrate, Fat, Protein, and Calories in the Six Food Exchanges

Food Exchange	Carbohydrate	Fat	Protein	Calories
Vegetables	5	0	2	25
Fruits	15	0	0	60
Fat	0	5	0	45
Meat				
Lean	—	3	7	55
Medium fat	—	5	7	75
High fat	—	8	7	100
Starch/Bread	15	trace	3	80
Milk				
Skim	12	trace	8	90
Lowfat	12	5	8	120
Whole	12	8	8	150

Carbohydrate, fat, and protein in grams.

1 g carbohydrate	*= 4 Calories*
1 g fat	*= 9 Calories*
1 g protein	*= 4 Calories*

Source: Exchange Lists for Meal Planning. *American Diabetes Association and American Dietetic Association. Chicago: ADA, 1986.*

The new label is called *Nutrition Facts* and it is designed to provide information on the nutrients which are of major concern for consumers. It must contain the following information:

List of ingredients
    Ingredients will be listed in descending order by weight, even on standardized foods such as mayonnaise and bread.
Serving size
    Serving size has been standardized.
Servings per container
Amount per serving of the following:
    Total Calories
    Calories from fat
    Total fat
    Saturated fat
    Cholesterol
    Sodium
    Total carbohydrate
    Dietary fiber
    Sugars
    Protein
    Vitamin A
    Vitamin C
    Calcium
    Iron
The following may be listed voluntarily:
    Calories from saturated fat
    Polyunsaturated fat
    Monounsaturated fat
    Potassium
    Soluble fiber
    Insoluble fiber
    Sugar alcohols
    Other carbohydrates
    Other essential vitamins and minerals

In order to provide information to help consumers see how foods may be part of a daily diet plan, a new label reference value, the **Daily Value (DV)** has been created. Actually, the DV is based on two other new sets of dietary standards, the **Daily Reference Values (DRVs)** and the **Reference Daily Intakes (RDIs).**

The DRVs cover the macronutrients that are sources of energy, consisting of carbohydrate (including fiber), fat, and protein, as well as cholesterol, sodium, and potassium, which contain no Calories. The DRVs for the energy-producing nutrients are based on the number of Calories consumed daily. On the food label, the percent of the DV that a single serving of a food contains is based on a 2,000 Calorie diet, which has been selected because it is believed to have the greatest public health benefit for the nation. However, the DV may be higher or lower depending on your Calorie needs. Values for some of the macronutrients are also provided for a 2,500 Calorie diet on the food label.

The DRVs for the macronutrients are based on certain minimum and maximum allowances, including the following for a 2,000 Calorie diet:

Total fat: Maximum of 30 percent of Calories, or less than 65 grams.
Saturated fat: Maximum of 10 percent of Calories, or less than 20 grams.
Carbohydrate: Minimum of 60 percent of Calories, or more than 300 grams.
Protein: Based on 10 percent of Calories. Applicable only to adults and children over age 4.
Fiber: Based on 11.5 grams of fiber per 1,000 Calories.
Cholesterol: Less than 300 milligrams.
Sodium: Less than 2,400 milligrams.

The Reference Daily Intakes (RDIs) replaces the old United States Recommended Daily Allowances (U.S. RDAs) which was used prior to 1994 as the label reference value for vitamins, minerals, and protein. Although the name has been changed, the values for the RDIs are the same as the old U.S. RDAs, but they may be modified in the near future. The DVs on the food label for vitamins A and C, calcium, and iron are based on the RDIs. Table 6.12 presents the current RDI for the eight key nutrients.

Labels also must disclose certain ingredients, such as sulfites, certain food dyes, and milk proteins, so food-sensitive consumers may avoid foods which may cause allergic responses.

In the past, many terms used on food labels, such as lean and light, had no definite meaning. However, under the new regulations, most terms used have specific definitions, and a summary of these terms is presented in table 6.17.

The new regulations also permit food manufacturers to make health claims if the food meets certain minimum standards. These health claims are permitted because the FDA believes there may be sufficient scientific data supporting a relationship between consumption of a specific nutrient and possible prevention of certain chronic diseases. However, there are several requirements, such as not stating the degree of risk, using only terms such as *may* or *might* reduce health risks, and indicating that other foods may provide similar benefits. Currently, seven health claims are allowed on the label. Although additional constraints may be required before a food may carry a health claim, the following are the key points.

Calcium and osteoporosis—A food must contain 20 percent or more of the DV for calcium.
Fat and cancer—A food must meet the definition for low fat.
Saturated fat and cholesterol and coronary heart disease—A food must meet the definition for low saturated fat, low cholesterol, and low fat.
Fiber-containing grain products, fruits and vegetables and cancer—A food must meet the definition for low fat and be, without fortification, a good source of fiber.
Fruits, vegetables and grain products that contain fiber and risk of coronary heart disease—Fruits and vegetables

must meet the definition for low saturated fat, low cholesterol, low fat, and contain, without fortification, at least 0.6 grams of soluble fiber.
Sodium and hypertension—A food must meet the description for low sodium.

Table 6.17 Definitions of Terms for Food Labels

Free *(None or trivial amount; if the product is inherently free of the ingredient, it must note so on the label.)*

Fat free—Less than 0.5 grams per serving
Saturated fat free—Less than 0.5 grams per serving
Cholesterol free—Less than 2 milligrams per serving
Sugar free—Less than 0.5 grams per serving
Sodium free—Less than 5 milligrams per serving
Calorie free—Less than 5 per serving

Low *(Very little, or low source of)*

Fat—No more than 3 grams of fat
Sodium—Fewer than 40 milligrams
Calories—Fewer than 40
Saturated fat—No more than 1 gram
Cholesterol—Less than 20 milligrams

High or Good Source

Based on daily reference value (DRV); High is 20% or more of the DRV; good source is 10–19%. For example, to be high in fiber, a cereal must have 5 grams because the DRV is 25 grams.

Reduced, Less, or Fewer

At least 25 percent less of a nutrient per serving compared to the particular nutrient in the reference food.

More or Added

Must be 10 percent or more of the daily value for the particular nutrient in the reference food.

Light or Lite

If a food normally derives 50% or more of its Calories from fat, it can be labeled light or lite if it is reduced in fat by 50%. If it derives less than 50% of its Calories from fat, the food must be reduced in fat by at least 50% or reduced in Calories by at least one-third. These foods must carry the percentage reduction. Light in sodium may be used if the sodium content is reduced by 50%.

Lean *(Meat, Fish, and Game)*

Contains fewer than 10 grams of fat, 4 grams of saturated fat, and 95 milligrams of cholesterol per 100 grams.

Extra Lean

Contains fewer than 5 grams of fat, 2 grams of saturated fat, and 95 milligrams of cholesterol per 100 grams.

Fresh

If the food is unprocessed, it must be in its raw state, having not been frozen or subjected to other forms of processing. Fresh does not apply to processed foods such as fresh milk or fresh bread.

Meals and Main Dishes *(per 100 grams)*

Low Calorie is defined as fewer than 120 Calories. To be called light, the meal must meet the definition for a low Calorie or a low fat meal, and it must signify which, e.g., a low Calorie meal. A low cholesterol meal must contain less than 20 milligrams of cholesterol and no more than 2 grams of saturated fat.

The terms refer to one serving. A reference food is a standard food containing set proportions of nutrients.

The New Food Label at a Glance

The new food label will carry an up-to-date, easier-to-use nutrition information guide and will be required on almost all packaged foods. The guide will help people plan a healthy diet. Here is a sample:

Serving sizes are now more consistent across product lines, are stated in both household and metric measures, and reflect the amounts people actually eat.

The list of nutrients covers those most important to the health of today's consumers, most of whom need to worry about getting too much of certain items, such as fat, rather than too few vitamins or minerals, as in the past.

Calories from fat are now shown on the label to help consumers follow dietary guidelines that recommend people get no more than 30% of their calories from fat.

% Daily Value shows how a food fits into the overall daily diet.

Daily Values are based on a daily diet of 2,000 and 2,500 calories. Some daily values show maximums, such as with fat (65 g or less), and others are minimums, as with carbohydrates (300g or more). Individuals should adjust the values to fit their own calorie intake.

Nutrition Facts

Serving Size 1/2 cup (114 g)
Servings Per Container 4

Amount Per Serving
Calories 90   Calories from Fat 30

	% Daily Value*
Total Fat 3 g	5%
Saturated Fat 0 g	0%
Cholesterol 0 mg	0%
Sodium 300 mg	13%
Total Carbohydrate 13 g	4%
Dietary Fiber 3 g	12%
Sugars 3 g	
Protein 3 g	

Vitamin A 80% • Vitamin C 60%

Calcium   4% • Iron   4%

* Percent Daily Values are based on a 2,000 calorie diet. Your daily values may be higher or lower depending on your calorie needs:

	Calories	2,000	2,500
Total Fat	Less than	65 g	80 g
Sat Fat	Less than	20 g	25 g
Cholesterol	Less than	300 mg	300 mg
Sodium	Less than	2,400 mg	2,400 mg
Total Carbohydrate		300 g	375 g
Fiber		25 g	30 g

Calories per gram:
Fat 9 • Carbohydrates 4 • Protein 4

Figure 6.13 *An example of the new food label, Nutrition Facts, with explanatory comments.*

Fruits and vegetables and cancer—Fruits and vegetables that meet the definition for low fat and that, without fortification, are a good source of at least one of the following: dietary fiber, or vitamins A or C.

An example of a Nutrition Fact food label, with some explanatory material, is presented in figures 6.13 and 6.14.

In general, the nutritional information presented on a label may serve as a practical guide for determining nutrient density and choosing foods wisely. For those trying to lose weight, foods with high concentrations of nutrients and low Calorie content may be chosen. Foods with a high iron or calcium content may be chosen for women and children. Nutritional labeling may serve as a useful guide for those who want or need to restrict saturated fats, cholesterol, or sodium in their diets.

In addition, nutrition labeling can help you get the most nutrition for your money. Reading labels carefully and comparing brands and prices may reveal significant savings and no loss of nutrient value when a store or generic brand is purchased instead of one that is nationally advertised. In general, you should look for food products providing the greatest percentages of the DV for the key nutrients at the lowest price.

Healthier Eating

During the past sixty years or so, there has been a gradual but rather significant shift in the dietary habits of most Americans. Changing social customs, improvement in food processing technology, and the advent of the fast-food industry have been

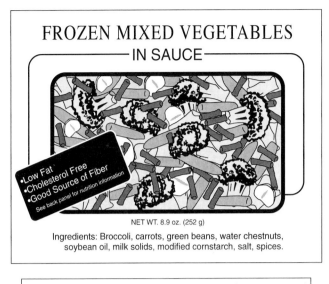

FROZEN MIXED VEGETABLES
— IN SAUCE —

•Low Fat
•Cholesterol Free
•Good Source of Fiber
See back panel for nutrition information

NET WT. 8.9 oz. (252 g)

Ingredients: Broccoli, carrots, green beans, water chestnuts, soybean oil, milk solids, modified cornstarch, salt, spices.

"While many factors affect heart disease, diets low in saturated fat and cholesterol may reduce the risk of this disease."

Figure 6.14 *An example of a food label with an approved health claim.*
Source: Food and Drug Administration 1992

instrumental factors in producing changes in the types of food we eat. At the same time, there has been a rather parallel increase in degenerative types of diseases, such as coronary heart disease and cancer. Thousands of studies have been conducted to investigate the link between nutrition and disease. Although there are some limitations in both the epidemiological and experimental studies conducted, and although there is no absolute proof that dietary changes will enhance the health status of every member of the population, the following dozen recommendations appear to be prudent for most individuals and are based upon the available scientific evidence. These recommendations represent a synthesis of a number of reports from both health and government organizations such as the American Heart Association, the National Cancer Institute, the National Research Council, and the U.S. Department of Health and Human Services, including the comprehensive sources, *Diet and Health: Implications for Reducing Chronic Disease Risk* and *The Surgeon General's Report on Nutrition and Health.* Taken together, these recommendations may be helpful in preventing most chronic diseases, including cardiovascular diseases and cancer. Exercise is also a healthful adjunct to several of these dietary recommendations.

A Dozen Guidelines for Healthier Eating

Contrary to popular belief, healthier eating is not that difficult. Since no single food in and by itself is totally harmful, or for that matter totally healthful, a healthy diet may contain any food you desire. You may have sweets, fats, chocolate, alcohol, or anything you want, but the key is moderation. Eating a half-cup of ice cream after a balanced meal is one thing; sitting down to a quart is another.

To make the general recommendations for healthier nutrition more practical, the following guidelines for the Healthy American Diet have been developed to provide a sound means to achieve them.

1. Maintain a healthy body weight. To avoid becoming overweight, you should consume only as many Calories as you expend daily. Methods of regulating your body weight are presented in detail in the following chapter. An aerobic exercise program and adherence to the concept of nutrient density, which includes a number of the following recommendations, could serve as the basis for a sound weight-control program.

2. Eat a wide variety of natural foods from within and among the Food Guide Pyramid or Food Exchange List food groups. Eating a wide variety of natural foods will assure you of obtaining a balanced and adequate intake of all essential nutrients. Stress foods that are high in the key nutrients (table 6.12).

3. Eat foods rich in calcium and iron. This is particularly true for women and children. Skim or low-fat milk and other low-fat dairy products are excellent sources of calcium. For example, one glass of skim milk provides about one-third the RDI for calcium. Certain vegetables, such as broccoli, are also good sources of calcium. Iron is found in good supply in the meat and starch/bread exchanges. Lean meats should be selected so as to limit fat intake, while whole-grain or enriched products contain more iron than those made with bleached, unenriched white flour. Table 6.10 provides examples of foods rich in calcium and iron.

4. Eat a moderate amount of protein, balancing your intake of plant and animal sources. The recommended dietary goal for protein is about 10–12 percent of the daily Calories. This averages out to about 50 to 60 grams of protein per day; the current American intake is about 100 grams, so we appear to be meeting this dietary goal. However, most of the protein Americans eat is of animal origin. Although animal products are an excellent source of complete protein, they tend to be higher in saturated fats and cholesterol compared to foods high in plant protein. On the other hand, animal protein is usually a better source of dietary iron and other minerals like zinc and copper than plant protein.

   One general health recommendation is to obtain more protein from plant foods. As little as four ounces of meat, fish, or poultry, combined with two glasses of skim milk, will actually provide the average individual with the daily RDA for protein, totalling about 45 grams of high quality protein. Combining this small amount of animal protein with plant foods high in protein, such as whole-grain products, beans and peas, and vegetables, will substantially increase your protein intake and more than meet your needs.

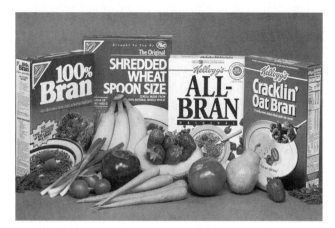

Figure 6.15 *Include in your diet foods high in plant starch and fiber. Eat more fruits, vegetables, and whole-grain products.*

Table 6.18 Daily Allowances for Grams of Fat and Saturated Fat, and Milligrams of Cholesterol*

Total Calories	Fat Calories	Grams of Fat	Grams of Saturated Fat	Milligrams of Cholesterol
1,000	300	33	11	100
1,500	450	50	16	150
2,000	600	66	22	200
2,500	750	83	27	250
3,000	900	100	33	300

*Based on a diet containing 30 percent of Calories as fat with 100 milligrams of cholesterol per 1,000 Calories.

Seafood is another excellent source of protein; it is usually low in fat. In addition, many fish are rich in omega-3 fatty acids.

5. Eat more complex carbohydrates, fiber, and natural sugars. The DRV for a 2,000 Calorie diet is 300 grams of carbohydrate, or 1,200 Calories from carbohydrate. In general, about 60 percent of your daily Calories should come from carbohydrates, about 50 percent from complex carbohydrates and the other 10 percent from simple, natural carbohydrates. To accomplish this, you need to eat more whole-grain products (breads and cereals), legumes (beans and peas), and vegetables and fruits. In particular, eat fruits and vegetables. Stress those high in beta-carotene and vitamin C, such as carrots, peaches, squash, and sweet potatoes. Deep yellow and orange fruits and vegetables, as well as dark green, leafy vegetables are usually good sources of these vitamins. Also, increase your intake of cruciferous vegetables, those from the cabbage family, such as broccoli, cauliflower, brussel sprouts, and all cabbages. These fruits and vegetables appear to protect you against lung, stomach, colon, and rectal cancer. The National Cancer Institute has recently sponsored a campaign called "Five a Day for Better Health," meaning to eat at least five servings of fruits and vegetables daily. The point is stressed that five is the minimum number of servings, and more should be consumed. The following examples may help you increase your daily consumption of fruits and vegetables. Breakfast—Drink fruit juice; add fruit to cereal and pancake batter; make a cholesterol-free omelette with vegetables like onions and green peppers. Lunch—Eat a salad; add broccoli and cauliflower to pasta; add vegetables to soups and sandwiches. Dinner— Eat vegetarian pizzas; make a vegetable-based stew; cook a vegetable stir-fry.

Another benefit of complex carbohydrates is their high fiber content (fig. 6.15). Whole-grain products and numerous vegetables are excellent sources of water-insoluble fiber. Fruits, beans, and products derived from oats, such as oatmeal and oat bran, are rich in the water-soluble type of fiber. The high fiber content of these foods is believed to be important in the prevention of diseases such as cancer of the colon and coronary heart disease as mentioned earlier.

6. Use sugars only in moderation. The recommended dietary goal is to reduce consumption of refined sugar from the current level of 24 percent of the daily Calories to 10 percent or less. Excessive consumption of refined sugar has been associated with high blood triglyceride levels. Sticky sugars are a major contributing factor to dental cavities. Sugars also significantly increase the caloric content of foods without an increase in nutritional value, so they may contribute to body-weight problems.

To meet this goal, you should reduce your intake of common table sugar and products high in refined sugar. Sugar is one of the major additives to processed foods, so check the labels. The amount of sugar must be listed on the food label.

Use natural sugars to satisfy your sweet tooth. Also, artificial sweeteners may be effective in weight-control programs, and their role is discussed in the next chapter.

7. Choose a diet low in total fat, saturated fats, and cholesterol. There is no specific requirement for fat in the diet. However, a need exists for several essential fatty acids and vitamins that are components of fat. Since almost all foods contain some fat, sufficient amounts of the essential fatty acids and fat-soluble vitamins are found in the average diet. Even on a vegetarian diet of fruits, vegetables, and grain products, about 5 to 10 percent of the Calories are derived from fat, thus supplying enough of these essential nutrients. Fat, however, currently comprises about 36 percent of our Calories; the recommended dietary goal is less than 30 percent, which amounts to a DV of 65 grams on a 2,000 Calorie diet. In addition, the amount of saturated fat in the diet should be 10 percent or less, and cholesterol intake should be limited to 300 milligrams or less per day, or about 100 mg per 1,000 Calories. Table 6.18

provides daily allowances for grams of fat and saturated fat and milligrams of cholesterol for diets with varying amounts of Calories.

The basis for the reduction in dietary saturated fats and cholesterol is the assumption that they are associated with high blood levels of triglycerides and cholesterol, a major risk factor associated with atherosclerosis and coronary heart disease. There appears to be enough medical evidence to justify a modification of the diet to lower high blood levels of triglycerides and cholesterol or to prevent their rise in individuals with low to normal levels. The following practical suggestions will help you meet the recommended dietary goal.

a. Eat less meat with high fat content. Avoid hot dogs, luncheon meats, sausage, and bacon. Trim off excess fat before cooking. Eat only lean red meat and more white meat, such as turkey, chicken, and fish, which have less fat. Remove the skin from poultry.

b. Eat only two to three eggs per week. One egg yolk contains about 250 milligrams of cholesterol, close to the limit of 300 milligrams per day. Egg whites have no cholesterol and are an excellent source of high quality protein. You may use commercially prepared egg substitutes; however, some brands are high in fat, so be careful to check the label.

c. Eat fewer dairy products that are high in fat. Switch from whole milk to skim milk. Eat other dairy products made from skim or nonfat milk, such as yogurt and cottage cheese. If you like cheese, switch from hard cheeses to soft cheeses, although most cheeses, except low-fat cottage cheese, are still high in fat and Calories. Some fat-free cheeses are now available with virtually no fat.

d. Eat less butter, which is high in saturated fats, by substituting soft margarine made from liquid oils that are monounsaturated or polyunsaturated, such as corn oil. Avoid margarine made from hydrogenated or partially hydrogenated oils. The hydrogenation process produces the trans form of fatty acids, which is metabolized in the body like saturated fats. Eat butter and margarine sparingly. Some fat-free margarines may be excellent substitutes.

e. Eat fewer commercially prepared baked goods made with eggs and saturated or hydrogenated fats.

f. Limit your consumption of fast foods. Although fast-food chains generally serve grade A foods, most of their products are high in fat. The average fast-food sandwich contains approximately 50 percent of its Calories in fat. Appendix D provides a breakdown of the fat Calories and milligrams of cholesterol in products served by popular fast-food restaurants. Some fast-food restaurants do serve nutrient-dense foods, and the trend is towards lower fat items. Wise choices, such as baked fish, grilled skinless chicken, lean meat, baked potatoes, and salads can provide healthy nutrition. However, much of the fat content is found in sandwich sauces, sour cream, or salad dressings, so order these on the side.

Although diets in China, Italy, and Mexico are generally considered to be more healthful than the typical American diet, many items served in Chinese, Italian, and Mexican fast-food restaurants in the United States, including national chains not typically classified as fast-food outlets, serve high-fat items, for example, fettucini Alfredo, sweet and sour pork, and chile relleno.

g. Check food labels for main ingredients that indicate fat, saturated fat, and cholesterol. You can calculate the percentage of fat Calories per serving of food. Simply divide the total fat Calories by the total Calories and multiply by 100. For example, if one serving of a product contains 300 Calories and there are 180 fat Calories, the product contains 60 percent of the Calories as fat ($180 \div 300 \times 100$). Additionally, if you are on a 2,000 Calorie diet, you have a daily allowance of 65 grams of fat. One serving of this food contains 20 grams of fat, or about 30 percent of your daily fat allowance ($20 \div 65 \times 100$).

h. Broil, bake, or microwave your foods. Limit frying. If you must use oil in your cooking, try to use monounsaturated oils such as olive or canola oil.

i. Eat more fish. Many fish, such as sardines, salmon, tuna, and mackerel, are rich in omega-3 fatty acids. White fish, such as flounder, is very low in fat Calories.

j. Select fat-free products, for example fat-free mayonnaise, if they are available. Artificial fats such as Simplesse® help reduce the total fat content and Calories in the diet and may be an effective means to enjoy the taste of certain foods without the caloric intake. Experts caution, however, that artificial fats are not a panacea but should be used only to complement the Healthy American Diet focusing on whole grains, fruits, vegetables, and meat and milk products low in fat.

Probably the most important single dietary recommendation is to reduce the fat content in your diet. In general, decrease your intake of cholesterol, total fat, and saturated fat, substituting monounsaturated, polyunsaturated, and omega-3 fatty acids for saturated or hydrogenated fats.

8. Use salt and sodium only in moderation. Try to limit sodium intake to less than 2,400 milligrams daily, which is the equivalent of 6,000 milligrams (6 grams) of salt. This lower amount will still provide sufficient sodium for normal physiological functioning. Increased salt intake has been associated with high blood pressure (hypertension), but the National Research Council has indicated that there is little or no direct evidence to suggest that high blood pressure can be produced in an individual with normal blood pressure and normal

dietary intake of salt. On the other hand, hypertensive individuals may be able to reduce their blood pressure by decreasing the amount of salt in the diet.

Sodium is found naturally in a wide variety of foods, so it is not difficult to get an adequate supply. Several key suggestions may help you reduce the salt and sodium content in your diet.

a. Get rid of your salt shaker. One teaspoon of salt is 2,000 mg of sodium; the average well-salted meal contains about 3,000 to 4,000 mg. Put less salt on your food both in your cooking pot and on your table.

b. Reduce the consumption of obviously high-salt foods· such as most pretzels and potato chips, pickles, and other such snacks.

c. Check food labels for sodium content; it must be listed so that you can see the percentage of your DV in one serving. Table 6.19 lists the sodium content in some common foods.

d. Eat more fresh fruits and vegetables, which are very low in sodium. Fruits, both fresh and canned, have less than 8 mg sodium per serving. Fresh and frozen vegetables may have 35 mg or less, but if canned may contain up to 460 mg.

e. Use lite salt, fresh herbs, or nonsodium spices as flavoring alternatives for your food.

9. Maintain an adequate intake of fluoride. This is particularly important during childhood when the primary and secondary teeth are developing, for fluoride helps prevent tooth decay by strengthening the tooth enamel. Your water supply may contain sufficient fluoride naturally or artificially to provide an adequate amount, but if not, fluoride supplements or the use of fluoride toothpaste is recommended.

10. In general, avoid taking dietary supplements in excess of the RDA. As noted previously, dietary supplements of most vitamins and minerals are not necessary for individuals consuming a balanced diet. If you adhere to the recommendations listed here, you are not likely to need any supplementation at all, for the consumption of nutrient-dense foods should guarantee adequate vitamin and mineral nutrition. If you feel a supplement is needed, the ingredients should not exceed 100 percent of the daily RDA for any vitamin or mineral. Many one-a-day vitamin-mineral supplements do adhere to this standard, and the USP (United States Pharmacopeia) designation on the label indicates the product meets superior standards for quality and purity.

Unfortunately, scientific data are not available to provide specific guidelines if you want to purchase supplements that exceed the RDA. However, the Center for Science in the Public Interest (CSPI) used an educated guess approach to offer some prudent guidelines. The following are the highlights of the CSPI recommendations, which may be found in the report by Liebman.

Table 6.19 Sodium Content of Common Foods

Food Exchange Item	Amount	Sodium (mg)
Milk		
Low-fat milk	1 c	120
Cottage cheese		
Creamed	½ c	320
Unsalted	½ c	30
Cheese, American	1 oz	445
Vegetables		
Beans, cooked fresh	1 oz	5
Beans, canned	1 oz	150
Pickles, dill	1 medium	900
Potato, baked	1 medium	6
Fruits		
Banana	1 medium	1
Orange	1 medium	1
Bread-Cereal		
Bread, whole wheat	1 slice	130
Bran flakes	¾ c	340
Oatmeal, cooked	1 c	175
Pretzels	1 oz	890
Meat		
Luncheon meats	1 oz	450
Frankfurter	1 medium	495
Chicken	3 oz	40
Beef, steak	3 oz	70
Pork sausage	1 medium link	170
Tuna, in oil	3 oz	800
Fish (cod, flounder)	1 oz	35
Deviled crab, frozen	1 c	2085
Fats		
Butter, salted	1 tsp	50
Margarine, salted	1 tsp	50
Canned Foods and Prepared Entrees		
Chop suey, canned	1 c	1050
Spaghetti, canned	1 c	1220
Turkey dinner, frozen	1	1735
Chicken noodle soup	5 oz	655
Condiments		
Mustard	1 tbsp	195
Tomato catsup	1 tbsp	155
Soy sauce	1 tbsp	1320

As you can see in this table, the sodium content of foods can vary greatly. In general, canned and processed foods have a much higher sodium content than do fresh foods. Eat fresh meats, fruits, vegetables, and bread products whenever possible, and prepare them with little or no salt. Avoid highly salted foods like pickles, pretzels, soy sauce, and others. Look for low-sodium labels when shopping for canned foods.

Source: U.S. Department of Agriculture.

a. Buy supplements rich in beta-carotene, about 25,000 IU, and low in vitamin A, less than 5,000 IU. Avoid supplements of vitamin A in excess of 5,000 IU.

b. Buy supplements rich in vitamin C, about 250–500 milligrams.

c. Buy supplements rich in vitamin E, about 100–400 IU.

d. Buy a supplement with about 200 micrograms of folic acid to complement the diet in order to get 400 micrograms per day. This is especially important for women who are capable of bearing children.

e. Buy a supplement limited in the minerals iron, copper, and zinc, no more than the RDA for each.

f. Buy a supplement with calcium if you are female and do not consume adequate dietary calcium.

g. Buy the inexpensive house brand of vitamins. Most companies that market vitamins buy their vitamins from the same manufacturers, so the contents in national brands and house brands are similar.

As noted previously, excess supplementation with specific nutrients may elicit some serious adverse health effects. Although the positive health effects of antioxidant vitamins look promising, some investigators note that additional research is needed before specific doses may be recommended. There may be an appropriate balance between free radicals and antioxidants in the body, and upsetting this balance may elicit negative effects. If negative effects do occur, it may take years before they become clinically evident.

Thus, although the CSPI published the recommendations cited above, they, along with most investigators researching the health implications of vitamin supplementation, note there is no guarantee of improved health. Almost all health professionals note we should obtain our vitamin-mineral nutrition through consumption of a wide variety of healthful, natural foods, particularly fruits and vegetables.

11. Eat fewer foods with questionable additives. Although the general consensus appears to be that most additives used in processed foods are relatively safe, several health agencies, such as the CSPI, recommend caution with some. For example, saccharin and nitrates have been linked to the development of cancer in laboratory animals, and other substances such as sulfites and certain food colors may cause allergic reactions in some individuals. Read the labels on processed foods and select those products with the least number of additives. Eating fresh, natural foods is one of the best approaches to avoiding additives.

12. If you drink alcohol, do so in moderation. The current available scientific evidence does not suggest that light to moderate daily alcohol consumption will cause any health problems to the healthy, nonpregnant adult. Light to moderate drinking is based upon a limit of one drink for every 50 pounds of body weight. A drink is defined as one 12-ounce bottle of beer, one 4-ounce glass of wine, or 1.5 ounces of 80-proof distilled spirits. Thus, for an average-sized male of 150 pounds, light to moderate drinking would be three drinks daily. However, excessive alcohol consumption is one of the most serious health problems in our society today, and even small amounts can pose health problems to some individuals. An expanded discussion is presented in chapter 9.

Your health depends on a variety of factors, such as heredity and certain aspects of your environment.

Adherence to these twelve simple dietary guidelines of the Healthy American Diet will not guarantee you good health; however, the available data indicate that dietary changes have the potential to keep you healthy or even to improve upon your current health status. Although it may not appear obvious, the general nature of these dietary recommendations is a shift toward vegetarianism, so it may be important to address the nature of this dietary regimen.

The Vegetarian Diet

The recommendation to eat less meat and more fruits, vegetables, and whole-grain products is suggestive of a vegetarian diet. Vegetarianism is a complex topic and cannot be covered in any depth in this text, but the following information may be helpful to those who are thinking in that direction.

Vegetable, in a broad sense, is a term used for foods that have a plant origin. If we look at our Food Guide Pyramid this excludes most foods normally found in the Milk and Meat Groups (which are primarily animal products) found near the top of the pyramid, but includes those in the Bread, Cereal, Rice, and Pasta Group, as well as the Fruit Group and the Vegetable Group.

There are a variety of types of **vegetarians.** A strict vegetarian, known also as a *vegan,* eats no animal products at all. Most nutrients are obtained from fruits, vegetables, breads, cereals, legumes, nuts, and seeds. **Ovovegetarians** include eggs in their diet, while **lactovegetarians** include foods in the Milk Group, such as cheese and other dairy products. An **ovolactovegetarian** eats both eggs and milk products. These latter classifications are not strict vegetarians, since eggs and milk products are derived from animals. Others may consider themselves vegetarians because they do not eat red meat, such as beef and pork products, although they may eat fish and other sea products. Others even add poultry to their diets. These individuals have been referred to as **semivegetarians.** In practice, then, a vegetarian may range on a continuum from one who eats nothing but plant foods to someone who eats a typical American diet with the exception of red meat. The concern for obtaining a balanced intake of nutrients depends on where a vegetarian is on that continuum.

Although the individual who eats a typical American diet needs to be aware of sound nutritional principles, this knowledge is even more important for the vegetarian, particularly the vegan who eats no animal products whatsoever. If foods are not selected carefully, the vegetarian may suffer nutritional deficiencies of iron, calcium, riboflavin, or protein.

The semivegetarian, ovolactovegetarian, and lactovegetarian may have no difficulty meeting nutrient requirements, with the possible exception of iron, so it is important that all classes of vegetarians include high-quality sources of iron in their diet. Because ovovegetarians do not consume dairy products, which are high in calcium and riboflavin, they need to include foods in their diet that are rich in these two nutrients. The complete vegetarian, the vegan, is most at risk for a

Table 6.20 Combining Foods for Protein Complementarity

Milk and Grains

Pasta with milk or cheese
Rice and milk pudding
Cereal with milk
Macaroni and cheese
Cheese sandwich
*Cheese on nachos

Milk and Legumes

*Creamed bean soups
*Cheese on refried beans

Grains and Legumes

Rice and bean casserole
Wheat bread and baked beans
*Corn tortillas and refried beans
Pea soup and toast
Peanut-butter sandwich

*Low-fat, low-sodium versions should be selected to minimize excessive saturated fat and sodium intake.

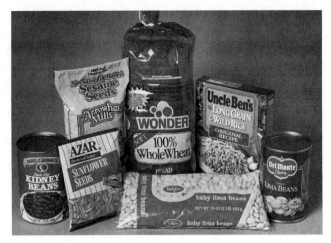

Figure 6.16 *It is important for the vegetarian to eat protein foods that complement each other (e.g., nuts and bread, rice and beans) so that all the essential amino acids are obtained in the diet.*

nutrient deficiency, and therefore must plan her or his diet carefully to obtain adequate amounts of iron, calcium, riboflavin, and protein.

A major concern of the vegan is to obtain adequate amounts of the right type of protein. If you recall our earlier discussion, proteins are classified as either complete or incomplete. A protein is complete if it contains all of the essential amino acids that the human body cannot manufacture. Animal products generally contain complete proteins, while plant proteins are incomplete. However, certain vegetable products may also provide good sources of protein. Grain products such as wheat, rice, and corn, as well as soybeans, peas, beans, and nuts, have a substantial protein content. However, most vegetable products lack one or more essential amino acids in sufficient quantity. They are incomplete proteins and, eaten individually, are not generally adequate for maintaining proper human nutrition. But, if certain plant foods are eaten together, they may supply all of the essential amino acids necessary for human nutrition and may be as good as meat protein.

In order to receive a balanced distribution of essential amino acids, the vegan must eat vegetable foods that possess what is known as **protein complementarity,** in which a vegetable product low in a particular amino acid is eaten together with a food that is high in that same amino acid. Some examples are presented in table 6.20, which also includes ideas to incorporate dairy products. Grains and cereals that are low in lysine need to be complemented by legumes, such as beans, that have adequate amounts of lysine. The low level of methionine in the legumes is offset by its high concentration in the grain products. These types of food combinations are practiced throughout the world. Mexicans eat pinto beans and corn; Chinese eat soybeans and rice. Through the proper selection of complementary foods, the

vegan can get an adequate intake of the essential amino acids (fig. 6.16). Eating complementary foods at one meal helps guarantee that they are properly utilized by the body.

Although the vegetarian diet has not been proven to be healthier than a diet that includes foods in the Meat and Milk Groups, it is based on certain nutritional concepts that may help in the prevention of some degenerative diseases common to industrialized society. First, saturated-fat content in a vegetarian diet is usually low; fats found in plant foods are generally monounsaturated and polyunsaturated. Second, plants do not contain cholesterol, since this compound is found only in animal products. These two factors account for the fact that vegetarians generally have lower blood triglycerides and cholesterol than meat eaters, which may be an important mechanism in the prevention of coronary heart disease. Third, plant foods possess a high fiber content that has been associated with reduced levels of serum cholesterol and the prevention of certain disorders in the intestinal tract. Fourth, plant foods, primarily fruits and vegetables, are rich in antioxidant vitamins and other phytochemicals that may play a role in the prevention of coronary heart disease or cancer. Fifth, if the proper foods are selected, the vegetarian diet supplies more than an adequate amount of nutrients and is rather low in caloric content. Plant foods can be high nutrient density foods, providing bulk in the diet without the added Calories of fat. Hence, the vegetarian diet can be an effective dietary regimen for losing excess body weight.

Choosing to adopt a vegetarian diet is up to the individual and represents a significant change in dietary habits. Anyone desiring to make an abrupt change to a vegetarian diet should do some serious reading on the matter beforehand. Once you have done some reading on vegetarianism, there may be several ways to gradually phase yourself into a vegetarian diet. You may become a partial vegetarian simply by eating less red meat. You may have several meatless days per

Table 6.21 Daily Food Guidelines for a Vegetarian Diet

Starch/Bread Exchange

Servings: 4 or more daily
Note: Use whole wheat or other whole grains. Products made of oats, rice, rye, corn, and whole wheat are good sources of protein, vitamin B, and iron, more so if they are enriched products.

Food examples:

Barley	Macaroni, enriched
Bran flakes	Oatmeal
Bread, whole wheat	Rice, brown
Buckwheat pancakes	Rye wafers
Corn muffins	Spaghetti, enriched
Farina, cooked	Wheat, shredded

Legumes (Meat Exchange)

Servings: 2 or more daily
Note: Good sources of protein, niacin, iron, and Calories.

Food examples:

Great northern beans	Soybeans
Navy beans	Black-eyed peas
Red kidney beans	Split peas
Pinto beans	Chickpeas
Lima beans	Lentils

Nuts and Seeds (Fat Exchange)

Servings: 2 or more daily
Note: Good sources of protein, niacin, and iron. May be excellent snack foods.

Food examples:

Almonds	Pecans
Brazil nuts	Walnuts
Cashew nuts	Sesame seeds
Peanuts	Sunflower seeds
Peanut butter	Pumpkin seeds

Fruit Exchange

Servings: 3 or more daily
Note: Fruits are generally good sources of vitamins and minerals. At least one fruit should come from the citrus group and one from the high-iron group.

Food examples:

Regular	*Citrus*	*High iron*
Apples	Oranges	Dried apricots
Bananas	Orange juice	Dried prunes
Grapes	Grapefruit	Dried dates
Peaches	Grapefruit juice	Dried figs
Pears	Strawberries	Dried peaches
Pineapple	Tomato juice	Raisins
	Lemon juice	Prune juice

Vegetable Exchange

Servings: 2 or more daily
Note: Vegetables are good sources of vitamins and minerals. At least one serving should come from the dark green or deep yellow vegetables.

Food examples:

Regular	*Dark green or deep yellow*
Artichokes	Beans, yellow
Asparagus	Beet greens
Beans, green	Broccoli
Cabbage	Carrots
Cauliflower	Collard greens
Cucumbers	Peas, green
Eggplant	Spinach
Potatoes	Squash
Radishes	Sweet potatoes
Tomatoes	

week, or one or two meatless meals each day (breakfast and lunch). For example, you may skip the ham or sausage at breakfast and have a big salad for lunch. You may wish to substitute white meat, with its generally lower fat content, for red meat. Eat more fish, chicken, and turkey. You may wish to become an ovolactovegetarian, eating eggs and dairy products. These excellent sources of complete protein can be blended with many vegetable products or eaten separately. You may use the above methods as forerunners to a strict vegetarian diet, gradually phasing out animal products altogether as you learn to select and prepare vegetable foods with protein complementarity. Some daily food guidelines for a vegetarian diet are presented in table 6.21.

It should be emphasized, however, that the nonvegetarian who carefully selects foods from the Meat and Milk Group, including lean red meat, may attain the same health benefits as the vegetarian. In fact, a diet with small amounts of lean meat may be healthier than an ovolactovegetarian diet that contains substantial amounts of high-fat cheese and whole milk. The major nutritional difference between a vegetarian and a nonvegetarian diet appears to be the higher content of saturated fats and cholesterol in the latter.

Selection of animal products with low-fat and low-cholesterol content helps to avoid this problem and also assures consumption of a very high-quality protein. The National Research Council, in *Diet and Health,* did not recommend against eating meat, but recommended eating leaner meat in smaller and fewer portions than is customary in the United States.

In summary, the dietary recommendations presented in this chapter, in combination with a properly designed exercise program, represent two of the most essential keys to a Positive Health Life-style. They complement each other nicely relative to the reduction of risk factors associated with the development of such diseases as diabetes, high blood pressure, and coronary heart disease. Moreover, as is noted in the next chapter, a combined exercise-diet program is the most effective type of program for regulating body weight.

As with a sound aerobic exercise program, sound nutritional habits need to be lifelong. The earlier in life you adopt such a sound exercise-nutrition life-style, the greater the possibility of preventing the onset of many of the chronic diseases discussed in chapter 11.

Make time to exercise, but also take time to eat right.

References

Books

Bouchard, C., et al., eds. 1994. *Physical activity, fitness, and health.* Champaign, Ill.: Human Kinetics.

Byrne, K. 1991. *Understanding and managing cholesterol: A guide for wellness professionals.* Champaign, Ill.: Human Kinetics.

Carper, J. 1993. *Food—Your miracle medicine.* New York: HarperCollins.

Gisolfi, C., et al., eds. 1993. *Exercise, heat, and thermoregulation.* Dubuque, Iowa: Brown & Benchmark.

Jacobs, M. 1991. *Vitamins and minerals in the prevention and treatment of cancer.* Boca Raton, Fla.: CRC Press.

Kukreja, R., and M. Hess. 1994. *Free radicals, cardiovascular dysfunction and protection strategies.* Boca Raton, Fla.: CRC Press.

Machlin, L., ed. 1991. *Handbook of vitamins.* New York: Marcel Dekker, Inc.

Moslen, M., and C. Smith, eds. 1992. *Free radical mechanism of tissue injury.* Boca Raton, Fla.: CRC Press.

National Dairy Council. 1992. *Guide to good eating.* 6th ed. Rosemont, Ill.: National Dairy Council.

National Institutes of Health. 1993. *The fifth report of the joint national committee on detection, evaluation, and treatment of high blood pressure.* National Institutes of Health. National Heart, Lung, and Blood Institute. NIH Publication No. 93-1088. January.

National Research Council. Food and Nutrition Board. National Academy of Sciences. 1989. *Recommended dietary allowances.* Washington, D.C.: U.S. Printing Office.

National Research Council. National Academy of Sciences. 1989. *Diet and health: Implications for reducing chronic disease risk.* Washington, D.C.: National Academy Press.

Pal Yu, B. 1993. *Free radicals in aging.* Boca Raton, Fla.: CRC Press.

Sauberlich, H., and L. Machlin, eds. 1992. *Beyond deficiency. New views on the function and health effects of vitamins,* Volume 669. New York: The New York Academy of Sciences.

Shils, M., et al. 1994. *Modern nutrition in health and disease.* Philadelphia: Lea & Febiger.

Smith, L. 1994. *Feed your body right.* New York: M. Evans.

United States Department of Agriculture, Human Nutrition Information Service. 1992. *The Food Guide Pyramid.* Home and Garden Bulletin Number 252. Washington, D.C.: U.S. Government Printing Office.

United States Department of Agriculture and United States Department of Health and Human Services. 1990. *Nutrition and your health: Dietary guidelines for Americans.* Washington, D.C.: U.S. Government Printing Office.

United States Department of Health and Human Services. Public Health Service. 1988. *The Surgeon General's report on nutrition and health.* Washington, D.C.: U.S. Government Printing Office.

United States Department of Health and Human Services. Public Health Service. 1990. *National Cholesterol Education Program Report of the Expert Panel on Population Strategies for Blood Cholesterol Reduction.* Bethesda, Md: National Institutes of Health.

United States Department of Health and Human Services. Public Health Service. 1991. *Healthy people 2000: National health promotion and disease prevention objectives.* Washington, D.C.: U.S. Government Printing Office.

United States Department of Health and Human Services. Public Health Service. 1992. *Eating to Lower Your High Blood Cholesterol.* Bethesda, Md: National Institute of Health.

Williams, M. H. 1995. *Nutrition for Fitness and Sport.* Dubuque, Iowa: Brown Benchmark Publishers.

Reviews

American College of Sports Medicine. 1993. The female athlete triad: Disordered eating, amenorrhea, and osteoporosis—call to action. *ACSM Sports Medicine Bulletin* 28:(1),6.

American Dietetic Association. 1988. Position of the American Dietetic Association: Vegetarian diets. *Journal of the American Dietetic Association* 88:351–55.

American Dietetic Association. 1991. Position of the American Dietetic Association: Fat replacements. *Journal of the American Dietetic Association* 91:1285–88.

American Dietetic Association. 1993. Final food labeling regulations. *Journal of the American Dietetic Association* 93:146–48.

American Dietetic Association. 1993. Position of the American Dietetic Association and the Canadian Dietetic Association: Nutrition for physical fitness and athletic performance for adults. *Journal of the American Dietetic Association* 93:691–96.

American Heart Association, Nutrition Committee. 1993. Rationale of the Diet-Heart Statement of the American Heart Association. *Circulation* 88:3008–29.

Anderson, J., and J. Metz. 1993. Contributions of dietary calcium and physical activity to primary prevention of osteoporosis in females. *Journal of the American College of Nutrition* 12:378–83.

Assmann, G., et al., 1993. High density lipoproteins, reverse transport of cholesterol, and coronary artery disease: Insights from mutations. *Circulation* 87:III-28–III-34.

Ausman, L. 1993. Fiber and colon cancer: Does the current evidence justify a preventive policy? *Nutrition Reviews* 51:57–63.

Badimon, J., et al. 1993. Coronary atherosclerosis: A multifactorial disease. *Circulation* 87:II-3–II-5.

Bang, O. 1990. Dietary fish oils in the prevention and management of cardiovascular and other diseases. *Comprehensive Therapy* 16:31–35.

Beaton, G. 1994. Criteria of an adequate diet. In *Modern nutrition in health and disease,* ed. M. Shils, et al. Philadelphia: Lea & Febiger.

Beilin, L. 1992. Dietary salt and risk factors for cardiovascular disease. *Kidney International Supplement* 37:S90–S96.

Bender, M., et al. 1992. Trends in prevalence and magnitude of vitamin and mineral supplement usage and correlation with health status. *Journal of the American Dietetic Association* 92:1096–1101.

Bendich, A. 1992. Safety issues regarding the use of vitamin supplements. *Annals of the New York Academy of Sciences* 669:300–312.

Block, G. 1992. The data support a role for antioxidants in reducing cancer risk. *Nutrition Reviews* 50:207–13.

Block, G. 1992. Vitamin C status and cancer: Epidemiologic evidence of reduced risk. *Annals of the New York Academy of Sciences* 669:280–92.

Bonkovsky, H. 1991. Iron and the liver. *American Journal of Medical Sciences* 301:32–43.

Bothwell, T., et al. 1989. Nutritional iron requirements and food iron absorption. *Journal of Internal Medicine* 226:357–65.

Breslow, J. 1993. Genetics of lipoprotein disorders. *Circulation* 87:III-16–III-21.

Brown, B., et al. 1993. Lipid lowering and plaque regression: New insights into prevention of plaque disruption and clinical events in coronary disease. *Circulation* 87:1781–89.

Buettner, G. 1993. The pecking order of free radicals and antioxidants: Lipid peroxidation, alpha-tocopherol, and ascorbate. *Archives of Biochemistry and Biophysics* 308:535–43.

Byham, L. 1991. Dietary fat and natural killer cell function. *Nutrition Today* 26:31–36.

Center for Science in the Public Interest. 1991. What's the best diet? *Nutrition Action Newsletter* 18 (December): 7–9.

Center for Science in the Public Interest. 1992. Pyramid scheme foiled. *Nutrition Action Healthletter* 19 (July/August): 3.

Charnock, J., et al. 1992. Dietary modulation of lipid metabolism and mechanical performance of the heart. *Molecular and Cellular Biochemistry* 116:19–25.

Cheah, P., and H. Bernstein. 1990. Colon cancer and dietary fiber: Cellulose inhibits the DNA-damaging ability of bile acids. *Nutrition and Cancer* 13:51–57.

Clark, N. 1993. How safe are artificial sweeteners? *Physician and Sportsmedicine* 21 (February): 45–46.

Colditz, G. 1993. Epidemiology of breast cancer. Findings from the nurses' health study. *Cancer* 71:1480–89.

Connor, W., and S. Connor. 1990. Diet, atherosclerosis, and fish oil. *Advances in Internal Medicine* 35:139–71.

Consumers Union. 1993. What can E do for you? *Consumer Reports on Health* 5:33–36.

Consumers Union. 1994. Can fast food be good food? *Consumer Reports* 59:493–99.

Consumers Union. 1994. Cutting your risk of colon cancer. *Consumer Reports on Health* 6:55–58.

Consumers Union. 1994. Iron: Too much of a good thing? *Consumer Reports on Health* 6:76–77.

Consumers Union. 1995. Cutting cholesterol. More vital than ever. *Consumer Reports on Health* 7:13–14.

Consumers Union. 1995. Fiber bounces back. *Consumer Reports on Health* 7:25–28.

Cook, M., and R. McDermott. 1991. Vitamin supplementation: Changing the view that more is better. *Journal of Health Education* 22:217–23.

Cowley, G., et al. 1993. Vitamin Revolution. *Newsweek* 7 (June):46–51.

Cronin, F., et al. 1993. Translating nutrition facts into action: Helping consumers use the new food label. *Nutrition Today* 28 (September/October): 30–36.

Dattilo, A. 1992. Dietary fat and its relationship to body weight. *Nutrition Today* 27 (January/February): 13–19.

Davidson, M. 1993. Antioxidants and lipid metabolism. Implications for the present and direction for the future. *American Journal of Cardiology* 71(6):32B–36B.

Dinneen, S., et al. 1992. Carbohydrate metabolism in non-insulin-dependent diabetes mellitus. *New England Journal of Medicine* 327:707–12.

Drewnowski, A. 1990. The new fat replacements. A strategy for reducing fat consumption. *Postgraduate Medicine* 87:111–14.

Dwyer, J. 1988. Health aspects of vegetarian diets. *American Journal of Clinical Nutrition* 48:712–38.

Dwyer, J. 1993. Dietary fiber and colorectal cancer risk. *Nutrition Reviews* 51:147–48.

Dwyer, J. 1995. Overview: Dietary approaches for reducing cardiovascular disease risks. *Journal of Nutrition* 125:656S–665S.

Finn, R. 1992. Food allergy—fact or fiction: A review. *Journal of the Royal Society of Medicine* 85:560–64.

Fruchart, J., et al. 1993. Heterogeneity of high density lipoprotein particles. *Circulation* 87:III-22–III-27.

Gaziano, J., et al. 1992. Dietary antioxidants and cardiovascular disease. *Annals of the New York Academy of Sciences* 669:249–59.

Gershoff, S. 1992. Fifty ways to improve your diet. *Tufts University Diet and Nutrition Newsletter* 10 (June):3–6.

Gershoff, S. 1993. Vitamin C (ascorbic acid): New roles, new requirements? *Nutrition Reviews* 51:313–26.

Gotto, A. Jr., 1992. Hypertriglyceridemia: Risks and perspectives. *American Journal of Cardiology* 70:19H–25H.

Graf, E., and J. Eaton. 1990. Antioxidant functions of phytic acid. *Free Radicals in Biology and Medicine* 8:61–69.

Heaney, R. 1990. Calcium intake and bone health throughout life. *Journal of the American Medical Women's Association* 45:80–86.

Herbert, V. 1992. L-Tryptophan. A medicolegal case against over-the-counter marketing of supplements of amino acids. *Nutrition Today* 27 (March/April): 27–30.

Howe, G., et al. 1992. Dietary intake of fiber and decreased risk of cancers of the colon and rectum: Evidence from the combined analysis of 13 case-control studies. *Journal of the National Cancer Institute* 84:1887–96.

Klatsky, A., et al. 1992. Alcohol and mortality. *American College of Physicians Annals of Internal Medicine* 117:646–53.

Kleiner, S. 1993. Sidestepping food sensitivities. *Physician and Sportsmedicine* 21 (March): 59–60.

Kleiner, S. 1994. Antioxidants: Vitamins that do battle. *Physician and Sportsmedicine* 22 (February): 23–24.

Kromhout, D. 1992. Dietary fats: Long-term implications for health. *Nutrition Reviews* 50:49–53.

Kune, G., and L. Vitetta. 1992. Alcohol consumption and the etiology of colorectal cancer: A review of the scientific evidence from 1957 to 1991. *Nutrition and Cancer* 18:97–111.

LaRosa, J. 1992. Cholesterol and cardiovascular disease: How strong is the evidence? *Clinical Cardiology* 15(Suppl 3):III2–III9.

Lefferts, L. 1990. Water: Treat it right. *Nutrition Action Health Letter* 17:5–7.

Lichtenstein, A. 1993. Trans fatty acids, blood lipids, and cardiovascular risk: Where do we stand? *Nutrition Review* 51:340–43.

Liebman, B. 1993. The ultra mega vita guide. *Nutrition Action Newsletter* 20 (January/February): 7–9.

Liebman, B. 1994. The heart health-E vitamin? *Nutrition Action Health Letter* 21:8–10.

Liebman, B. 1995. Dodging cancer with diet. *Nutrition Action Health Letter.* 22 (January/February): 4–7.

Machlin, L., and J. Sauberlich. 1994. New views on the function and health effects of vitamins. *Nutrition Today* 29:25–29.

Marwick, C. 1990. International conference gives boost in including omega fatty acids in diet. *Journal of the American Medical Association* 263:3153–54.

Matkovic, V., and J. Ilich. 1993. Calcium requirements for growth: Are current recommendations adequate? *Nutrition Reviews* 51:171–80.

McCarron, D., et al. 1990. Dietary calcium and chronic diseases. *Medical Hypotheses* 31:265–73.

Mela, D. 1992. Nutritional implications of fat substitutes. *Journal of the American Dietetic Association* 92:472–76.

Miller, N. 1990. Raising high density lipoprotein cholesterol. *Biochemical Pharmacology* 40:403–10.

Mufti, S. 1992. Alcohol acts to promote incidence of tumors. *Cancer Detection and Prevention* 16:157–62.

Newberne, P., and M. Locniskar. 1990. Roles of micronutrients in cancer prevention: Recent evidence from the laboratory. *Progress in Clinical Biology Research* 346:119–34.

Notelovitz, M. 1993. Osteoporosis: Screening, prevention, and management. *Fertility and Sterility* 59:707–25.

Reed, D. 1993. Which risk factors are associated with atherosclerosis? *Circulation* 87 (Suppl II):II-54–II-55.

Renaud, S., and M. De Lorgeril. 1992. Wine, alcohol, platelets, and the French paradox for coronary heart disease. *The Lancet* 339:1523–25.

Rheinstein, P. 1993. Update on food labeling. *American Family Physician* 47:979–82.

Ripsin, C., et al. 1992. Oat products and lipid lowering. *Journal of the American Medical Association* 267:3317–25.

Rolls, B., and D. Shide. 1992. The influence of dietary fat on food intake and body weight. *Nutrition Reviews* 50:283–90.

Rose, D. 1990. Dietary fiber and breast cancer. *Nutrition and Cancer* 13:1–8.

Rose, D., and J. Connolly. 1992. Dietary fat, fatty acids and prostate cancer. *Lipids* 27:798–803.

Rosenberg, I. 1992. Maximizing peak bone mass: Calcium supplementation increases bone mineral density in children. *Nutrition Reviews* 50:335–37.

Rush, D. 1994. Periconceptional folate and neural tube defect. *American Journal of Clinical Nutrition* 59:511S–515S.

Schardt, D. 1993. Do or diet. Treating disease with food. *Nutrition Action Health Letter* 20 (July/August): 1, 5–7.

Schardt, D. 1993. The problem with protein. *Nutrition Action Health Letter* 20 (June): 1, 5–7.

Schardt, D. 1994. Phytochemicals: Plants against cancer. *Nutrition Action Health Letter* 21 (April): 1, 9–11.

Schoonderwoerd, K., and H. Stam. 1992. Lipid metabolism of myocardial endothelial cells. *Molecular and Cellular Biochemistry* 116:171–79.

Schwartz, C., et al. 1993. A modern view of atherogenesis. *American Journal of Cardiology* 71:9B–14B.

Scrimshaw, N. 1990. Nutrition: Prospects for the 1990s. *Annual Review in Public Health* 11:53–68.

Scrimshaw, N. 1991. Iron deficiency. *Scientific American* 265:46–52.

Shankar, S., and E. Lanza. 1991. Dietary fiber and cancer prevention. *Hematology/Oncology Clinics of North America* 5:25–36.

Shapira, D. 1990. Alcohol abuse and osteoporosis. *Seminars in Arthritis and Rheumatism* 19:371–76.

Sherman, A. 1992. Zinc, copper, and iron nutriture and immunity. *Journal of Nutrition* 122:604–9.

Sies, H., et al. 1992. Antioxidant functions of vitamins: Vitamins E and C, beta-carotene, and other carotenoids. *Annals of the New York Academy of Sciences* 669:7–20.

Simopoulos, A. 1990. The relationship between diet and hypertension. *Comprehensive Therapy* 16:25–30.

Slavin, J. 1990. Dietary fiber: Mechanisms or magic on disease prevention? *Nutrition Today* 25 (November/December): 9–13.

Slavin, J. 1992. Dietary fiber and cancer update. *Contemporary Nutrition* 17(8): 1–2.

Snodgrass, S. 1992. Vitamin neurotoxicity. *Molecular Neurobiology* 6:41–73.

Stam, J., et al. 1990. Vitamins and lung cancer. *Lung* 168:1075–81.

Stern, J., and M. Hermann-Zaidins. 1992. Fat replacements: A new strategy for dietary change. *Journal of the American Dietetic Association* 92:91–93.

Suh, I., et al. 1992. Alcohol use and mortality from coronary heart disease: The role of high-density lipoprotein cholesterol. *Annals of Internal Medicine* 116:881–87.

Sweeten, M., et al. 1990. Lean beef: Impetus for lipid modifications. *Journal of the American Dietetic Association* 90:87–92.

Thom, S. 1993. Nutritional management of diabetes. *Nursing Clinics of North America* 28:97–112.

Trachtenbarg, D. 1990. Treatment of osteoporosis. What is the role of calcium? *Postgraduate Medicine* 87:263–66.

Wattenberg, L. 1990. Inhibition of carcinogenesis by naturally occurring and synthetic compounds. *Basic Life and Science* 52:155–66.

Welsh, S., et al. 1992. Development of the food guide pyramid. *Nutrition Today* 27 (November/December): 12–23.

Willett, W. 1990. Epidemiologic studies of diet and cancer. *Progress in Clinical Biology Research* 346:159–68.

Willett, W., and D. Hunter. 1993. Diet and breast cancer. *Contemporary Nutrition* 18:(3,4)1–4.

Wood, P. 1994. Physical activity, diet and health: Independent and interactive effects. *Medicine and Science in Sports and Exercise* 26:838–43.

Wynder, E., et al. 1992. Breast cancer—the optimal diet. *Advances in Experimental Medicine and Biology* 322:143–53.

Young, V., et al. 1990. Assessment of protein nutritional status. *Journal of Nutrition* 120:1496–1502.

Young, V., and Pellett, P. 1994. Plant proteins in relation to human protein and amino acid nutrition. *American Journal of Clinical Nutrition (Supplement)* 59:1203S–1212S.

Ziegler, R. 1991. Vegetables, fruits, and carotenoids and the risk of cancer. *American Journal of Clinical Nutrition* 53:251S–219S.

Specific Studies

Abdalla, D., et al. 1992. Low density lipoprotein oxidation by stimulated neutrophils and ferritin. *Atherosclerosis* 97:149–59.

Ascherio, A., et al. 1994. Trans-fatty acids intake and risk of myocardial infarction. *Circulation* 89:94–101.

Assmann, G., et al. 1993. High density lipoproteins, reverse transport of cholesterol, and coronary artery disease. *Circulation* 87:III-28–III-34.

Bairati, I., et al. 1992. Double-blind, randomized, controlled trial of fish-oil supplements in prevention of recurrence of stenosis after coronary angioplasty. *Circulation* 85:950–56.

Bonaa, K., et al. 1992. Habitual fish consumption, plasma phospholipid fatty acids, and serum lipids: The Tromso study. *American Journal of Clinical Nutrition* 55:1126–34.

Bostick, R., et al. 1993. Calcium and colorectal epithelial cell proliferation: A preliminary randomized, double-blinded, placebo-controlled clinical trial. *Journal of the National Cancer Institute* 85:132–41.

Centers for Disease Control. 1992. Annual and New Year's Day alcohol-related traffic fatalities—United States, 1982–1990. *Journal of the American Medical Association* 267:214–15.

Eicholzer, M., et al. 1992. Inverse correlation between essential antioxidants in plasma and subsequent risk to develop cancer, ischemic heart disease and stroke respectively: A 12 year follow-up of the Prospective Basel Study. *EXS* 62:398–410.

Flaten, H., et al. 1990. Fish-oil concentrate: Effects on variables related to cardiovascular disease. *American Journal of Clinical Nutrition* 52:300–306.

Hansen, J., et al. 1993. Inhibition of exercise-induced shortening of bleeding time by fish oil in familial hypercholesterolemia (type IIa). *Arteriosclerosis and Thrombosis* 13:98–104.

Hunter, D., et al. 1993. A prospective study of the intake of vitamins C, E, and A and the risk of breast cancer. *New England Journal of Medicine* 329:234–40.

Jackson, R., et al. 1992. Does recent alcohol consumption reduce the risk of acute myocardial infarction and coronary death in regular drinkers? *American Journal of Epidemiology* 136:819–24.

Jenkins, D., et al. 1993. Effect on blood lipids of very high intakes of fiber in diets low in saturated fat and cholesterol. *New England Journal of Medicine* 329:21–26.

Jorens, P., et al. 1992. Vitamin A abuse: Development of cirrhosis despite cessation of vitamin A. A six-year clinical and histopathologic follow-up. *Liver* 12:381–86.

Kahn, R., et al. 1990. Oat bran supplementation for elevated serum cholesterol. *Family Practitioner Research Journal* 10:37–46.

Kim, I., et al. 1993. Vitamin and mineral supplement use and mortality in a US cohort. *American Journal of Public Health* 83:546–50.

Knekt, P., et al. 1994. Antioxidant vitamin intake and coronary mortality in a longitudinal population study. *American Journal of Epidemiology* 139:1180–89.

McKenney, J., et al. 1994. A comparison of the efficacy and toxic effects of sustained- vs immediate-release niacin in hypercholesterolemic patients. *Journal of the American Medical Association* 271:672–77.

Micozzi, M., et al. 1990. Carotenoid analyses of selected raw and cooked foods associated with a lower risk for cancer. *Journal of the National Cancer Institute* 82:282–85.

Ornish, D., et al. 1990. Can lifestyle changes reverse coronary heart disease? The lifestyle heart trial. *Lancet* 336:129–33.

Reid, I., et al. 1993. Effect of calcium supplementation on bone loss in postmenopausal women. *New England Journal of Medicine* 328:460–64.

Resnicow, K., et al. 1991. Diet and serum lipids in vegan vegetarians: A model for risk reduction. *Journal of the American Dietetic Association* 91:447–53.

Rimm, E., et al. 1993. Vitamin E consumption and the risk of coronary heart disease in men. *New England Journal of Medicine* 328:1450–56.

Salonen, J., et al. 1992. High stored iron levels are associated with excess risk of myocardial infarction in Eastern Finnish men. *Circulation* 86:1036–37.

Schapira, D., et al. 1990. The value of current nutrition information. *Preventive Medicine* 19:45–53.

Singh, R., et al. 1990. Dietary modulators of blood pressure in hypertension. *European Journal of Clinical Nutrition* 44:319–27.

Smith-Schneider, L., et al. 1992. Dietary fat reduction strategies. *Journal of the American Dietetic Association* 92:34–38.

Squires, R., et al. 1992. Low-dose, time-release nicotinic acid: Effects in selected patients with low concentrations of high-density lipoprotein cholesterol. *Mayo Clinic Proceedings* 69:855–60.

Srikumar, T., et al. 1992. Trace element status in healthy subjects switching from a mixed to a lactovegetarian diet for 12 months. *American Journal of Clinical Nutrition* 55:885–90.

Stampfer, M., et al. 1993. Vitamin E consumption and the risk of coronary disease in women. *New England Journal of Medicine* 328:1444–49.

Suter, P., et al. 1992. The effect of ethanol on fat storage in healthy subjects. *New England Journal of Medicine* 326:983–87.

Vatten, L., et al. 1990. Frequency of meat and fish intake and risk of breast cancer in a prospective study of 14,500 Norwegian women. *International Journal of Cancer* 46:12–15.

Wannamethee, G., and A. Shaper. 1992. Alcohol and sudden cardiac death. *British Heart Journal* 68:443–48.

Warner, J., et al. 1989. Combined effects of aerobic exercise and omega-3 fatty acids in hyperlipidemic persons. *Medicine and Science in Sports and Exercise* 21:498–505.

Watts, G., et al. 1992. Effects on coronary artery disease of lipid-lowering diet, or diet plus cholestyramine, in the St. Thomas' Atherosclerosis Regression Study (STARS). *Lancet* 339:563–69.

West, D., et al. 1989. Dietary intake and colon cancer: Sex- and anatomic site specific associations. *American Journal of Epidemiology* 130:883–94.

Willett, W., et al. 1993. Intake of trans fatty acids and risk of coronary heart disease among women. *Lancet* 341:581–85.

Wood, R., et al. 1993. Effect of butter, mono- and polyunsaturated fatty acid-enriched butter, trans fatty acid margarine, and zero trans fatty acid margarine on serum lipids and lipoproteins in healthy men. *Journal of Lipid Research* 34:1–10.

7

WEIGHT CONTROL THROUGH PROPER NUTRITION AND EXERCISE

Key Terms

aminostatic theory
android-type obesity
basal metabolic rate (BMR)
behavior modification
body image
Body Mass Index (BMI)
brown fat
caloric concept of weight control
cellulite
creeping obesity

energy balance
essential fat
fat patterning
glucostatic theory
gynoid-type obesity
hunger center
hypothalamus
lean body mass
lipostatic theory
long-haul concept

metabolic rate
metabolic syndrome
morbid obesity
negative energy balance
obesity
positive energy balance
resting energy expenditure
 (REE)
satiety center
set-point theory

spot reducing
storage fat
subcutaneous fat
syndrome X
Thermic effect of exercise (TEE)
Thermic effect of food (TEF)
very low-Calorie diets (VLCD)
visceral fat
waist:hip ratio (WHR)
weight cycling

Key Concepts

■ Although the ultimate cause of obesity is a positive energy balance, the underlying cause is not known but probably involves the interaction of multiple genetic and environmental factors.

■ Excess body fat is associated with a variety of chronic diseases and impaired health conditions, including coronary heart disease, diabetes, high blood pressure, and several forms of cancer.

■ Body composition may be classified as consisting of two components: lean body mass, which is about 70 percent water, and body fat.

■ All techniques currently used to measure body composition are prone to error; even the underwater weighing technique, the so-called gold standard, may be in error by 2 to 2.5 percent.

■ Although there are no methods that predict exactly what your ideal or healthy weight should be, some normal ranges of body fat percentage, or weight, appear to be related to better health.

■ Weight control is based upon energy balance, or caloric balance; a negative energy balance decreases body weight; a positive energy balance increases body weight.

■ Energy expenditure in humans represents the sum of the basal, resting, and exercise metabolic rates.

The latter is the most effective means for increasing energy output during a weight-control program.

■ The caloric deficit (caloric intake minus caloric expenditure) may be used to predict body-weight losses on a long-term basis. One pound of body fat equals approximately 3,500 Calories.

■ For the overweight individual who desires to lose body weight without the guidance of a physician, the recommended maximal loss is two pounds per week; however, one pound per week may be a more achievable and sustainable goal.

■ To be effective, a diet for reducing body weight should be low in Calories, high in nutrients, appeal to your taste, fit into your life-style, and be lifelong.

■ The basic principles underlying an exercise program for weight control are the same as those for prevention of coronary heart disease. Large muscle activities must be included at fairly intense levels; duration and frequency are increasingly important.

■ Exercise can increase energy expenditure considerably, but in order to lose body fat through exercise, one should think in terms of months, not days.

■ Behavior modification techniques can be effective in helping to implement a diet-exercise program for weight control.

■ Rapid loss of body weight, which may occur during the early stages of dieting, is primarily due to body-water changes; the rate at which weight loss occurs will slow down as your body weight decreases because body fat stores are then the prime source of weight loss.

■ Under strict medical supervision, a very-low-Calorie diet may be an effective method for weight loss in the morbidly obese; however, it is not a recommended technique for the average individual trying to lose excess pounds because it may be associated with a variety of health risks if not used properly.

■ For several reasons, weight loss may not occur in the early stages of an exercise program; however, body composition changes may be favorable, i.e., a decrease in body fat and an increase in fat-free mass.

■ A comprehensive weight-control program involves a balanced low-Calorie diet, an aerobic exercise program, and appropriate behavior modification.

■ For those who want to gain weight, a weekly increase of one pound is a sound approach; however, the weight gain should be primarily muscle tissue and not body fat.

■ Adequate rest and sleep, increased caloric intake, and a proper resistance-training program should be effective in helping to increase lean body mass.

INTRODUCTION

The human body is a remarkable food processor. As an adult, you may consume over a ton of food per year and still not gain or lose a pound of body weight. You are constantly harnessing and expending energy through the intricacies of your bodily metabolism in order to remain in energy balance. To maintain a given body weight, your energy input must balance your energy output. However, sometimes the energy-balance equation becomes unbalanced, and your normal body weight will either increase or decrease.

The term **body image** refers to the mental image we have of our own physical appearance, and it can be influenced by a variety of factors, including how much we weigh or how that weight is distributed. Relative to our appearance, body weight appears to be a major concern of many Americans. Research has revealed that about 40 percent of adult men and 55 percent of adult women are dissatisfied with their current body weight. Similar findings have also been reported at the high school and even the elementary school level, primarily with female students. At the college level, a study by Drewnowski and Yee found that 85 percent of both male and female first-year students desired to change their body weight, probably because of the proverbial "freshman fifteen"—the fifteen pounds or so gained during the freshman year due to life-style changes. The primary cause of this concern is the value that American society, in general, assigns to physical appearance. Thinness is currently an attribute that females desire highly. Males generally desire muscularity. The vast majority of individuals who want to change their body weight do it for the sake of appearance; most want to lose excess body fat, while a smaller percentage of individuals actually want to gain weight.

However, our body weight may also exert a significant impact upon our health. Recent estimates suggest that a significant proportion of adults, adolescents, and children in the United States are carrying too much body fat for optimal health and the problem appears to be increasing. A recent report by Kuczmarski and others, for the National Center for Health Statistics, indicated that the percentage of adults who are overweight increased from one-fourth to one-third of the population over the past decade, and experts note that obesity among children is increasing at an even faster rate. Indeed, the Public Health Service has stated in *Healthy People 2000* that one of its major health objectives for the year 2000 is to decrease the proportion of adults and children who are significantly overweight, or obese.

By medical definition, **obesity** is an accumulation of fat beyond that considered to be normal for the age, sex, and body type of a given individual. As shall be noted in chapter 11, it is one of the major health problems in the United States and is associated with over twenty-six known health conditions, including coronary heart disease, hypertension, diabetes mellitus, and several types of cancer. Although overall obesity is a major risk factor, **fat patterning** (the location of the fat in different body regions) may have significant implications for the development of certain diseases, as shall be noted below. Additionally, since body image is a contributing factor to self-esteem, being overweight may also negatively affect mental health, particularly during childhood and adolescence.

Because it may have a multitude of causes, obesity is a complex medical problem. Some causes may be genetic in nature, such as hormonal imbalances or impaired metabolism that predispose some individuals to accumulate more body fat. One theory proposes a "thrifty gene" that may predispose some individuals to store body fat more efficiently than other individuals, while another theory suggests a "sweet tooth" gene may predispose individuals to crave foods rich in sugar and fat. Other causes may be environmental in nature, such as the presence of fattening foods in the home or low levels of physical activity.

Morbid obesity is a severe case of obesity that usually has a strong genetic basis and often begins early in life, possibly because a child has inherited a thrifty gene or some other predisposition, such as a greater number of fat cells. The morbidly obese are the ones who need to lose weight for health reasons, but are generally unsuccessful. This type of obesity poses major health risks to the individual and may be difficult to treat, for the major function of fat cells is to convert what is eaten into fat and store it. Thus, the more fat cells an individual has, the greater the ability to accumulate fat and the greater the chances of developing severe obesity. Such cases of obesity may merit medical attention, including hospitalization involving the use of surgery, drugs, or starvation-type diets. It should be noted, however, that the success rate in the treatment of severe obesity is relatively low; 95 to 99 percent of those individuals who lose weight regain it within a year or two because this type of obesity is a chronic condition that needs continuous care.

Most individuals do not have a genetic predisposition to obesity, but may still accumulate excessive body fat. No one is immune to obesity. This increase in body fat, sometimes referred to as **creeping obesity** because it gradually sneaks up on us, is usually attributed to environmental factors such as low levels of physical activity and increased food intake, particularly dietary fat (fig. 7.1). In this type of obesity, the cells appear to increase in size rather than in number, and the adverse effects on health increase with increasing fatness as recently documented by Willett and his associates. Creeping obesity underlies the cause of the "freshman fifteen" and the fact that the average American aged 25–30 increased body weight by 10 pounds over the past 7 years according to the National Institutes of Health. Fortunately, programs to control creeping obesity have greater chances for success since many of the environmental factors that contribute to its development can be effectively modified.

Although not as major a health problem as obesity, a small percentage of the population is underweight and may have a difficult time gaining weight. Many of these individuals may desire to increase their body weight in order to improve their appearance or athletic performance. Although such increases in body weight usually have few specific health benefits related to disease prevention, such improvements may help foster an enhanced body image and/or self-concept that may improve the psychological health of an individual.

With proper knowledge and a strong desire, almost anyone can design a diet-exercise program to achieve a desirable weight goal. For those who are currently at a desirable body weight, this chapter will provide you with the knowledge to maintain your current body weight, an important health goal since in obesity, prevention is more

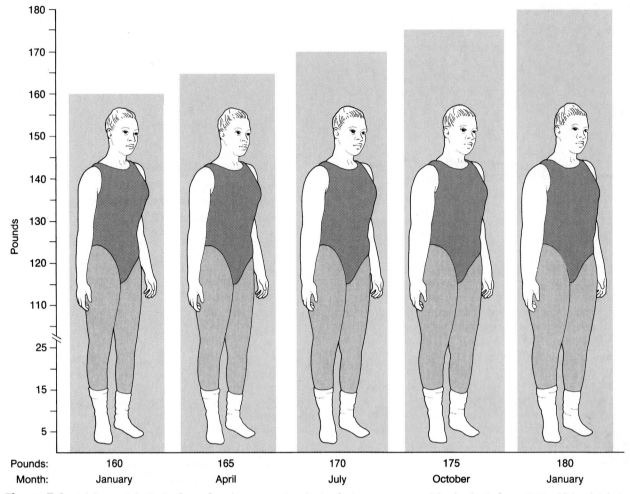

| Pounds: | 160 | 165 | 170 | 175 | 180 |
| Month: | January | April | July | October | January |

Figure 7.1 *Adult-onset obesity is often referred to as creeping obesity, for it creeps up on adults slowly. As few as 200 additional Calories per day above normal requirements would result in a gain of approximately 20 pounds of body fat in one year.*

effective than treatment. For those who desire to lose weight, the three basics of a comprehensive weight-control program are provided: (1) a dietary regimen stressing balanced nutrition with a reduced caloric (energy) intake; (2) an aerobics exercise program to increase energy expenditure; and (3) a behavioral modification approach to help implement diet and exercise changes in your life-style. For those who desire to gain weight, a diet-exercise program consistent with a Positive Health Life-style is provided.

Occasionally, some individuals who initiate a weight-control program to improve their appearance or health become overzealous and may actually use weight-control methods that can be harmful. They do not need to lose weight, but continue to try to do so. Concern with weight loss may become an obsession, particularly so with females, leading to disordered eating practices, a topic that is discussed in chapter 10. In attempts to increase muscularity, males may use various drugs, such as anabolic steroids, which as noted in chapter 9 can adversely affect health.

This chapter discusses the nature of body composition, the determination of desirable body weight, the basic principles of weight control, the roles of diet, exercise, and behavior modification in maintaining and losing body weight, and principles of gaining body weight

Body Composition
Major Body Components
We all have heard the expression "You are what you eat." In general, this is true. Our body takes the fifty or so nutrients we obtain in our food and rearranges them to form our body tissues. Although various minerals constitute a small portion of your body weight, the vast majority of body weight consists of four elements—carbon, oxygen, hydrogen, and nitrogen. These elements are the structural basis of your body stores of carbohydrate, protein, fat, and water. To understand body composition and how one loses or gains body weight, you should understand how these substances are stored in the body. Figure 7.2 provides a general overview.

Minerals
As noted in the last chapter, your body uses over twenty-five different minerals to function effectively. About 3 to 4 percent of your body is composed of minerals, primarily the calcium, phosphorus, and other minerals in your bone tissue.

Carbohydrate
The body contains about a pound of carbohydrate, stored primarily in the muscles and liver. About 3 pounds of water are stored with this carbohydrate.

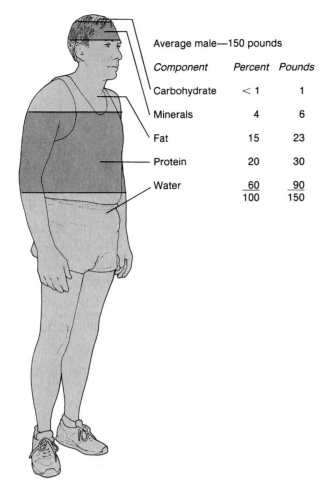

Average male—150 pounds

Component	Percent	Pounds
Carbohydrate	< 1	1
Minerals	4	6
Fat	15	23
Protein	20	30
Water	60	90
	100	150

Figure 7.2 *The majority of body weight is water, while varying amounts of fat, protein, and carbohydrate make up the solid tissues. Body weight losses or gains may result from changes in any of these components.*

Protein

Protein is the major structural component of all body tissues. Your muscles, bones, liver, heart, blood, and other tissues have a high protein content. Protein tissues hold substantial amounts of water.

Fat

Body fat is classified as either essential or storage. **Essential fat** is necessary in body structures such as the brain, nerve tissue, bone marrow, heart, and cell membranes. Adult females have additional essential fat associated with their reproductive processes, primarily the fat in breast tissue. **Storage fat** is basically a depot for excess energy. Some fat, known as deep **visceral fat,** is stored deep in the body, particularly in the abdominal area. Another major storage site is the adipose tissue cells just under the skin, known as **subcutaneous fat.** When this latter type of fat is separated by connective tissue into small compartments, it gives a dimpled, waffle-like look to the skin and is known as **cellulite.** Although cellulite is primarily fat, research from Italy has shown that cellulite contains greater amounts of proteoglycans (a protein and carbohydrate compound) that attract water, which may augment the dimpled, unsightly appearance.

Table 7.1 Percentages of Body Weight Attributable to Body Fat and Lean Body Mass

	Adult Male		Adult Female	
Total Body Fat	15		26	
Essential fat		3		15
Storage fat		12		11
Lean Body Mass	85		74	
Muscle		43		36
Bone		15		12
Other tissues		27		26
	100	100	100	100

Water

The greatest percentage of the body's weight is water—approximately 60 percent of the weight of the average adult. Some water is found in all tissues; it is very high in some tissues (blood) and very low in others (bone). Water content in protein-type tissues, such as muscle, is high (about 72 percent); it is low (about 10 percent) in fat-type tissue.

Scientists usually divide the body into four components—water, bone tissue, protein tissues, and fat. For our purposes, we will condense body composition into two components, body fat and lean body mass. Body fat is the total amount of fat in the body. **Lean body mass** primarily consists of the muscles and bones and other body organs such as the heart, liver, and kidneys. Table 7.1 presents approximate percentages of body weight partitioned as body fat and lean body mass, although these percentages may vary tremendously among individuals.

Body composition may be influenced by a number of factors such as age, sex, diet, and exercise. Age effects are significant during the developmental years while muscle and other body tissues are being formed. Also, muscle mass may decrease during adulthood due to physical inactivity, and body fat normally increases as one ages. There are minor differences in body composition between boys and girls up to the age of puberty, but at this age the differences become fairly great. In general, beginning at puberty, the female deposits more fat, while the male develops more muscle tissue. Diet can affect body composition over a short period, such as in acute water restriction and starvation, but its main effects are seen over a long period. For example, chronic overeating may lead to increased body fat stores. Conversely, a sound exercise program may help build muscle and lose fat.

Techniques for Measuring Body Composition

When doing exacting research, scientists use a variety of highly sophisticated techniques to determine bone mass, water content, protein content, and fat content in the body. Table 7.2 provides a broad overview of various techniques. Techniques such as dual photon/dual energy X-ray absorptiometry (DPA; DEXA) magnetic resonance imaging (MRI), underwater weighing, and others may be used to get a fairly

Table 7.2 Techniques Used to Determine Body Composition

Measurement Technique	Component Measured
Anthropometry	Measures body segment girths to predict body fat.
Bioelectrical impedance analysis (BIA)	Measures resistance to electric current to predict body water content, lean body mass, and body fat.
Computed tomography (CT)	X-ray scanning technique to image body tissues. Useful in determining subcutaneous and deep fat to predict body fat percentage. Used also to calculate bone mass.
Dual energy X-ray absorptiometry (DEXA)	X-ray technique at two energy levels to image body fat. Used also to calculate bone mass.
Dual photon absorptiometry (DPA)	Beam of photons passes through tissues, differentiating soft tissues and bone tissues. Used to predict body fat and calculate bone mass.
Infrared interactance	Infrared light passes through tissues, and interaction with tissue components used to predict body fat.
Magnetic resonance imaging (MRI)	Magnetic field and radio-frequency waves are used to image body tissues similar to CT scan. Very useful for imaging deep abdominal fat.
Neutron activation analysis	Beam of neutrons passes through the tissues, permitting analysis of nitrogen and other mineral content in the body. Used to predict lean body mass.
Skinfold thicknesses	Measures subcutaneous fat folds to predict body fat content and lean body mass.
Total body electrical conductivity (TOBEC)	Measures total electrical conductivity in the body, predicting water and electrolyte content to estimate body fat and lean body mass.
Total body potassium	Measures total body potassium, the main intracellular ion, to predict lean body mass and body fat.
Total body water	Measures total body water by dilution techniques to predict lean body mass and body fat.
Ultrasound	High frequency ultrasound waves pass through tissues to image subcutaneous fat and predict body fat content.
Underwater weighing (Densitometry)	Underwater weighing technique based on Archimedes principle to predict body density, body fat, and lean body mass.

accurate measure of the various components in the body. However, since such techniques are relatively expensive and time-consuming, more practical methods have been devised.

In recent years, the measurement of body fat has become very popular in fitness and wellness centers. The most commonly used methods to determine body composition include skinfold techniques, girth measurements, and bioelectrical impedance analysis (BIA). Skinfold and girth techniques attempt to predict your body fat from subcutaneous fat measures, while BIA is used to measure total body water content that is then used to predict body fat percentage.

It is important to note that all techniques currently used to measure body fat are only estimates and are prone to error. Such errors are usually expressed as standard errors of measurement or estimates. Without going into the statistics of standard errors, look at the following example. Let us suppose you go into a fitness center, they do a BIA for you, and the computer says you have 20 percent body fat. In the computer is a formula predicting your body fat based upon your estimated body water content; these formulae typically have a standard error of about 3 percent. This means that your body fat is *probably* within one standard error of your prediction, or a 70 percent probability that it is somewhere between 17 and 23 percent; it may actually be lower than 17 or higher than 23, but

less likely to be so. Thus, do not think of body fat determinations as precise measures, but only a possible range associated with the standard error of measurement. Even the underwater weighing technique, sometimes referred to as the "gold standard" in body fat measurement, has a standard error of approximately 2 percent. Measurement of body composition is not an exact science. The review by Martin and Drinkwater is particularly informative for the interested reader.

In the next section we look at how you can determine a desirable weight for yourself. One method is based upon body fat percentage. Let us look at the technique most commonly used to determine body composition in most college and university fitness classes—the skinfold technique. Since a major portion of the storage fat is contained just under the skin, various skinfold measures have been used to predict body fat (fig. 7.3). The skinfold measures are inserted into a formula to estimate the percent of body fat. Care must be taken to use a formula appropriate for your age and sex and one that uses a variety of body sites, since fat may be distributed unevenly on your body, e.g., you may have little fat on your arms but a good deal at your waist. Most skinfold techniques have a standard error of approximately 3 percent.

Probably the best application of the skinfold technique is to have yourself measured periodically to see if you are

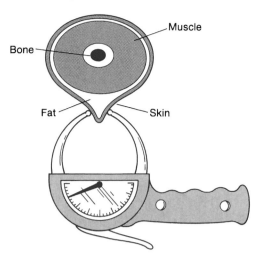

Figure 7.3 A schematic drawing showing the skinfold of fat that is pinched up away from the underlying muscle tissue.

losing body fat, particularly when you are on a weight-loss program. Simply keep a sum of skinfold thicknesses from selected body sites. Since the skinfold technique is rather practical, Laboratory Inventory 7.1 may be used to provide you with an approximation of your body fat percentage. Keep in mind that the percentage value has a standard error of approximately 3 percent.

Another important practical technique involves measurement of body girths (circumferences), particularly the girth of the waist and hip. As shall be noted below, the ratio of the waist girth to the hip girth may be an important indicator of disease risk. Laboratory Inventory 7.2 provides a means to determine this ratio.

Simpler methods may also be used to determine if you are too fat. Probably the least complicated and most revealing is the mirror test, as proposed by the late Jean Mayer, an internationally renowned authority on nutrition and obesity. He suggests that you look at yourself, nude, in a full-length mirror using both a front and side view. If you study yourself objectively, this is usually all the evidence you need. Most of us have a pretty good idea of how we would like our bodies to look, and this test offers us a guide to our desirable physical appearance, at least as far as body-weight distribution is concerned. Exceptions to this suggestion are individuals who are obsessed with thinness and may suffer from a condition known as *anorexia nervosa.* Such individuals seem to believe they are always too fat, even though they are extremely thin. This topic is covered further in chapter 10.

Healthy Body Weight

Although we may have a good idea of how much we want to weigh relative to our physical appearance, there does not appear to be any sound evidence to indicate exactly how much any given individual should weigh for optimal health. However, some guidelines are available. Using either the relationship of body weight to height or the percent of body fat, there

are ranges of values that appear to be normal for most of the healthy population. These are often referred to as ideal or desirable body weights, but a more recent term is healthy body weight. Those individuals who exceed the upper or lower levels of these ranges may be subject to more health problems than if they were in the normal range. Although excessively underweight individuals may be more prone to certain health problems than those with normal weight, the major concern is with individuals who exceed the upper ranges of normal, for this is the more common problem in the United States.

Excessive body fat by itself is a major health risk factor for both men and women; fat patterning, or where it is carried on the body, may increase that risk. Classifications of different types of obesity based upon regional fat distribution have been proposed, the most popular differentiation being the android versus the gynoid types (see figure 7.4). **Android-(male) type obesity** is characterized by accumulation in the abdominal region—particularly the intraabdominal region—of deep, visceral fat, but also of subcutaneous fat. Android-type obesity is also known by other terms, such as central, upper-body, or lower-trunk obesity, and is often referred to as the apple-shape obesity. **Gynoid-(female) type obesity** is characterized by fat accumulation in the gluteal-femoral region—the hips, buttocks, and thighs. It is also known as lower-body obesity and is often referred to as pear-shape obesity. Both types of obesity have a strong genetic component. The android-type obesity is increasingly being recognized as causing a greater health risk than obesity itself, and the presence of excess abdominal fat, even in the absence of overall obesity, also increases health risks. Several mechanisms are under study, including different hormone patterns in the blood and dissimilar biochemical functions of the android and gynoid fat cells. Whatever the underlying mechanism, epidemiological data have shown that android-type obesity is associated wit hyperinsulinemia, insulin resistance, hypercholesteremia, hypertriglyceridemia, diabetes, and hypertension, all risk factors for coronary heart disease, and often referred to as the **metabolic syndrome** or **syndrome X.** Android-type obesity is also associated with increased risk of some forms of cancer, such as breast and endometrial cancer in women. Although android-type obesity occurs primarily in males, Folsom and others recently noted it is also a major risk factor for mortality in women as well.

Obtaining a desirable body weight with proper fat distribution is a primary health objective. There are a number of ways to predict an optimal or desirable body weight. The following sections deal with four different, but related, approaches to determination of a desirable body weight or body fat distribution. The first uses the standard height-weight charts, the second is also based upon the height-weight relationship, the third is based upon body fat percentage, and the fourth is based on the ratio of waist to hip girth. It might be a good idea to try all four approaches. If there is general agreement, you may have a fairly good idea whether or not you are at an increased health risk due to excessive body weight. Laboratory Inventory 7.2 covers all four approaches.

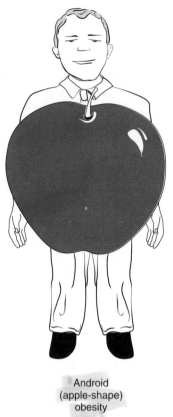

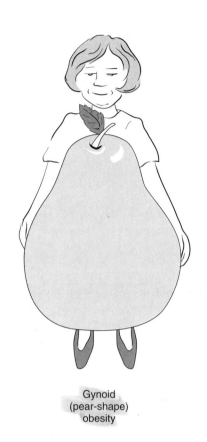

Android
(apple-shape)
obesity

Gynoid
(pear-shape)
obesity

Figure 7.4 *Male (android) and female (gynoid) type obesity.*

Height-Weight Table Approach

One of the most used, and often abused, methods of determining a desirable body weight has been the height-weight tables developed by life insurance companies. Height and weight charts are based on measurements obtained from large populations of people. The data obtained are then treated statistically, and the values that tend to cluster toward the midpoint (the mean or median) are considered to be normal, average, or desirable. Unfortunately, these tables reveal nothing about body composition. Two individuals may be exactly the same height and weight, hence classified as having normal body weight, but the distribution of their body weight might be so different that one individual could possibly be considered obese while the other might be considered very muscular.

Nevertheless, even with this limitation, height-weight tables may be a practical screening device and a useful guide to a desirable body weight, particularly if body frame size is part of the table. Probably the most popular height-weight charts are those developed by the Metropolitan Life Insurance Company in 1959. Although newer tables have been released by Metropolitan Life, the American Heart Association and other health organizations recommend that Americans continue to use the 1959 version.

Laboratory Inventory 7.2 (Method A) serves as a guide to determine a desirable body weight based on the Metropolitan Life Insurance Company height-weight tables. Tables of desirable height and weight for both men and women, as well as a table to predict body frame size as small, medium, or large, are included in Laboratory Inventory 7.2 on pages 233–237. Although the data in these tables are based on a select portion of the population—insurance policyholders—they have broad general application to the general public for screening purposes.

Body Mass Index (BMI) Approach

Another approach, the **Body Mass Index (BMI),** was developed by the National Center for Health Statistics and is an index of the relationship of weight to height. Since the BMI uses the metric system, you need to determine your weight in kilograms and your height in meters. The formula is:

$$\text{BMI} = \frac{\text{Body weight in kilograms}}{(\text{Height in meters})^2}$$

Multiplying your body weight in pounds by 0.454 will give you your weight in kilograms. Multiplying your height in inches by 0.0254 will give you your height in meters. Let's look at an example of a woman who weighs 132 pounds and is 5′5″ (65 inches) tall.

Weight in kilograms: $132 \times 0.454 = 60$
Height in meters: $65 \times 0.0254 = 1.651$

$$\frac{60}{(1.651)^2} = \frac{60}{2.726} = 22.01$$

A BMI range of 20 to 25 is considered normal; a suggested desirable range for females is 21.3 to 22.1 and for males is 21.9 to 22.4. BMI values above 27.8 for men and 27.3 for

Table 7.3 Ratings of Body Fat Percentage Levels

Rating	Males (Ages 18–30)	Females (Ages 18–30)
Athletic	6–10%	10–15%
Good	11–14%	16–19%
Acceptable	15–18%	20–25%
Too Fat	19–24%	26–29%
Obese	25% or over	30% or over

Keep in mind that these are approximate values. The athletic category may apply particularly to athletes who compete in events where excess body fat may be a disadvantage, such as gymnastics, ballet, and long-distance running. Others should strive for the good or acceptable levels, even those individuals between ages 30 and 50.

women have been associated with increased incidence rates for several health problems, including high blood pressure and diabetes. The American Dietetic Association, in their position statement on nutrition and physical fitness, classified individuals with a BMI greater than 30 as obese and those with a BMI greater than 40 as morbidly obese and in need of prompt medical attention.

Laboratory Inventory 7.2 (Method B) may be used to determine a desirable body weight using the BMI as a guide.

Body Fat Percentage Approach

Although the height-weight and BMI approaches may be useful for screening procedures, they do not directly assess body composition. Thus, someone who is very muscular with a low percent of body fat, such as a professional football player, may be classified as obese by either of these methods.

If you believe the height-weight or BMI approach is not appropriate for you, and if you have available to you a method of determining your body fat percentage, then this approach to calculation of your desirable body weight is preferable. Perusal of research literature reveals a number of recommended normal body fat percentage levels. The values presented in table 7.3 represent a consolidation of a number of studies. Use it as a guide to get your body fat percentage at least to the "good" or "acceptable" level. But, keep in mind that there is some error associated with all methods used to predict body fat.

However, athletes may desire lower body fat levels. Some male athletes function effectively at 5 to 8 percent body fat, and some elite male marathon runners have been reported to have less then 5 percent body fat. Many female athletes who compete in endurance sports also are reported to have low levels of body fat, about 10 to 12 percent. If you compete in a sport where excess body fat may be detrimental to your performance, it may be important to keep the percent low while still maintaining good strength and cardiovascular endurance levels.

Once you have determined your body fat percentage (either by Laboratory Inventory 7.1 or another appropriate technique), consult Laboratory Inventory 7.2 (Method C) to determine your desirable body weight.

The Waist:Hip Ratio

As noted previously, fat deposits in the abdominal area may increase health risks. Although expensive imaging techniques,

such as MRI, are necessary to measure deep visceral fat, a practical screening technique is available. A measure of regional fat distribution is the **waist:hip ratio (WHR),** which is the abdominal or waist girth (measured by a flexible tape at the narrowest section of the waist as seen from the front) divided by the gluteal or hip girth (measured at the largest circumference including the buttocks). This ratio is also known as the abdominal:gluteal ratio or the android:gynoid ratio. As a measure of regional fat distribution, an increased risk of coronary heart disease in males is associated with a WHR greater than 0.90–0.95, while women are at increased risk with a WHR ratio greater than 0.80–0.85. Laboratory Inventory 7.2 (Method D) provides you the opportunity to determine your waist:hip ratio.

Basic Principles of Weight Control

The vast majority of individuals interested in body weight control are really interested in body *fat* control. Body fat is nature's primary way of storing energy in the human body for future use. In essence, body fat control is human energy control. In order for you to maintain your current body weight, you must be in **energy balance.** You must expend as much energy through your daily activities as you consume in your daily diet.

In other words, energy output must equal energy input. During the growth and development years of childhood and adolescence, energy input predominates slightly, creating a positive energy balance and growth of body mass. As the adolescent enters young adulthood, the major growth processes are just about complete, and energy input and output must equalize. An individual loses weight if output predominates—a condition of **negative energy balance.** If input is greater, a **positive energy balance** exists, and the individual gains weight. For example, the input of an extra doughnut (125 Calories) per day, if not balanced by an increased energy expenditure of 125 Calories, can lead to an increase of about 13 pounds of body weight in a year. Thus, the key principle to all weight-control programs is proper energy balance (fig. 7.5).

The Calorie

Although there are a number of ways to express energy, the most common term is the *Calorie.* The Calorie is used as the unit for measuring energy requirements in the 1989 RDA; it is the way we express the energy content of the foods we eat and is one means to express the energy expenditure of physical activity. Thus, energy balance and caloric balance are synonymous.

A calorie is a measure of heat. One small calorie represents the amount of heat needed to raise the temperature of 1 gram of water 1 degree Celsius; it is sometimes called the *gram calorie.* A large Calorie, or kilocalorie, is equal to 1,000 small calories. It is the amount of heat needed to raise 1 kilogram of water (1 liter) 1 degree Celsius. In human nutrition, the kilocalorie is the main expression of energy. It is usually abbreviated as kcal, kc, C, or capitalized as Calorie. Throughout this book, Calorie refers to the kilocalorie. You may also see food energy expressed in kilojoules. You can calculate the

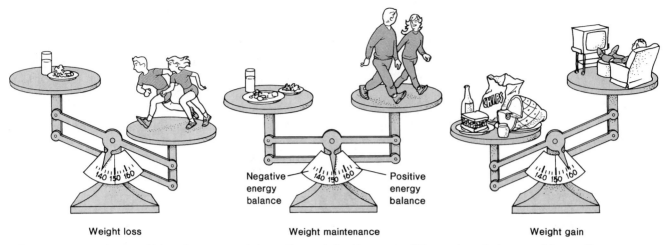

Figure 7.5 *Weight control is based upon energy balance. Too much food input or too little exercise output can result in a positive energy balance or weight gain. Decreased food intake or increased physical activity can result in a negative caloric balance or weight loss.*

caloric equivalents by dividing the number of kilojoules by 4.2, although dividing more easily by 4.0 will provide a good approximation. For example, a food portion with 200 kilojoules would equal about 50 Calories (200 ÷ 4).

According to the principles underlying the First Law of Thermodynamics, energy may be equated from one form to another. Thus, the Calorie, which represents heat energy, may be equated to other forms, such as the mechanical energy utilized during work (as in exercise). This concept is expanded later in this chapter when we discuss the role of exercise in weight control, but first let us look at how the human body expends energy through its metabolic activities.

Metabolism

Metabolism is life. Human metabolism represents the sum total of all physical and chemical changes that take place within the body. The transformation of food to energy, the formation of new compounds such as hormones and enzymes, the growth of bone and muscle tissue, the breakdown of body tissues, and a host of other physiological processes are parts of the metabolic process.

Metabolism involves two fundamental processes, anabolism and catabolism. Anabolism is a building-up process, or assimilation. Complex body components, such as muscle tissue, are synthesized from the basic nutrients. Catabolism is the tearing-down process, or disassimilation. This involves the disintegration of body compounds, such as fat, into energy. The body is constantly using energy to build up and tear down substances within the cells. Certain automatic body functions such as contraction of the heart, breathing, secretion of hormones, and the constant activity of the nervous system also are consuming energy. The **metabolic rate** reflects how rapidly the body is using its energy stores. This rate can vary tremendously depending upon a number of factors—the most influential one being exercise.

The **basal metabolic rate (BMR)** represents the energy necessary for basic life functions. Other than during sleep, it is the lowest level of energy expenditure. The determination of the BMR is a clinical procedure conducted in a laboratory or

Table 7.4	Estimation of the Daily Basal Metabolic Rate
Adult Male	**Adult Female**
BMR estimate = 1 Calorie/kg body weight/hour	BMR estimate = 0.9 Calorie/kg body weight/hour
Example:	Example:
154 pound male	121 pound woman
154 pounds × 0.454 = 70 kg	121 pounds × 0.454 = 55 kg
70 kg × 1 Calorie = 70 Calories/hour	55 kg × 0.9 Calories = 49.5 Calories/hour
70 × 24 hours = 1,680 Calories/day	49.5 × 24 hours = 1,188 Calories/day
Rounded BMR estimate = 1,700 Calories/day	Rounded BMR estimate = 1,200 Calories/day

Estimates are appropriate for young adults, age twenty to thirty. BMR normally decreases with increasing age, about 10 percent per decade.

hospital setting. In the average individual, approximately 60 to 75 percent of the total daily energy expenditure is accounted for by the BMR. There are several ways to estimate the BMR. Whichever method is used, keep in mind that the value obtained is an estimate. In order to get a truly accurate value, a standard BMR test is needed. However, the formula in table 7.4 may give you a good approximation of your daily BMR.

The resting metabolic rate (RMR) is slightly higher than the BMR. It represents the BMR plus small amounts of additional energy expenditure associated with previous muscular activity. According to the National Research Council, the BMR and RMR differ by less than 10 percent. Consequently, although there are some fine differences in the two terms, they are often used interchangeably. Additionally, the National Research Council uses the term **resting energy expenditure (REE)** to account for the energy processes at rest; REE and RMR are also considered to be equivalent terms. The REE accounts for approximately 70 percent or more of the daily energy expenditure. A technique for calculating your REE is part of Laboratory Inventory 7.3.

A significant elevation of the metabolic rate occurs after ingestion of a meal and it is referred to as dietary-induced thermogenesis (DIT), or more recently as the **thermic effect of**

food (TEF). This elevation is usually highest about one hour after a meal and lasts for about four hours, and it is due to the energy necessary to absorb, transport, store, and metabolize the food consumed. The greater the caloric content of the meal, the greater the TEF effect. Also, the type of food ingested may affect the magnitude of the TEF. Protein and carbohydrates significantly increase the TEF, whereas the effect of fat is minimal. The normal increase in the REE due to TEF from a mixed meal of carbohydrate, fat, and protein is about 8–10 percent.

The exercise metabolic rate (EMR) represents the energy expenditure during physical exercise. The EMR is known more appropriately as the **thermic effect of exercise (TEE).** In the sedentary individual, the EMR accounts for approximately 10–15 percent of the daily energy expenditure, primarily through light exercise activities such as walking, climbing stairs, and lifting various objects. However during moderate to heavy exercise, the EMR may be ten to twenty times greater than the RMR and may be a key factor in weight-control programs. In physically active persons, the EMR may account for 30 percent or more of the daily energy expenditure.

Figure 7.6 represents the interaction of the REE, TEF, and TEE in total daily energy expenditure.

Body Weight Regulation

As noted previously, you may eat over a ton of food in a year and yet not gain one pound of body weight. In order for this to occur, your body must possess an intricate regulatory system that helps to balance energy intake and output. The regulation of human energy balance is complex. At the present time, we do not appear to know the exact physiological mechanisms whereby body weight is maintained relatively constant over long periods of time, but some information is available relative to both energy intake and energy expenditure.

Appetite regulation in relation to energy needs involves a complex interaction of numerous physiological factors including the appetite centers in the brain, feedback from peripheral centers outside the brain, metabolism of ingested foods, and hormone actions (fig. 7.7). Environmental conditions, such as the home environment, also influence food intake. These factors may interact to regulate the appetite on a short-term basis (daily basis) or on a long-term basis (keeping the body weight constant for a year).

The control of the appetite appears to be centered in the **hypothalamus,** part of the brain that controls a variety of physiological processes via several centers theorized to regulate appetite. A **hunger center** may stimulate eating behavior. A **satiety center,** when stimulated, will inhibit the hunger center. It has been theorized that a number of factors influence the function of these centers and their ability to control food intake. The following may be involved in one way or another.

1. Stimulation of several senses like taste and smell. We are all aware of how these factors may stimulate or depress our appetites.

2. An empty or full stomach. An empty stomach may stimulate the hunger center by various neural pathways, whereas a full stomach may stimulate the satiety center or inhibit the hunger center.

3. Receptors in the hypothalamus, liver, or elsewhere that may be able to monitor blood levels of various nutrients. In regard to this, three theories have been proposed centered on the three energy nutrients. The **glucostatic theory** suggests that food intake is related to changes in the levels of blood glucose. A fall will stimulate appetite, whereas an increased blood-glucose level would decrease appetite. The **lipostatic theory** suggests a similar mechanism for fats, as does the **aminostatic theory** for amino acids, or protein. These nutrients may affect the activity of various neurotransmitters that influence hunger and satiety.

4. Changes in body temperature. A thermostat in the hypothalamus may respond to an increase or decrease in body temperature and either, respectively, inhibit or stimulate the feeding center.

5. Secretions of hormones. A number of different hormones in the body have been shown to affect feeding behavior, including insulin, thyroxine, and several others, particularly a number of peptides produced in the intestines that can function as hormones or neurotransmitters.

Although all of the above may be involved in the physiological regulation of food intake, the other side of the energy-balance equation is energy expenditure, or metabolism. Exercise is one way to increase energy expenditure; however, the vast majority of energy expended by the body on a daily basis is accounted for by the REE. Changes in the REE may be involved in the regulation of body weight. Several mechanisms have been proposed.

1. Brown fat. **Brown fat,** which is distinct from the white fat that comprises most fat tissue in the body, is found in small amounts around the neck and chest areas. It has a high rate of metabolism and releases energy in the form of heat. Activity of the brown fat tissue may be increased or decreased under certain conditions, such as after a meal or exposure to the cold. This activity is referred to as nonshivering thermogenesis. Research with animals indicates that low levels of brown fat are associated with a higher incidence of obesity. The amount of brown fat in humans appears to be small, but according to Stock, even 50 grams could influence energy turnover by 10–15 percent in humans. Its role in the etiology of obesity is being studied.

2. Hormones. Hormones from the thyroid and adrenal glands may increase or decrease and affect energy metabolism accordingly. Triiodothyronine, a hormone from the thyroid gland, may be involved in the stimulation of brown adipose tissue. Hormones such as epinephrine also may increase the activity of certain enzymes and thus increase energy expenditure. Decreases in hormonal activity may depress energy metabolism.

The human body has developed a number of physiological systems, called feedback systems, to regulate most body processes. Feedback systems controlling body weight may

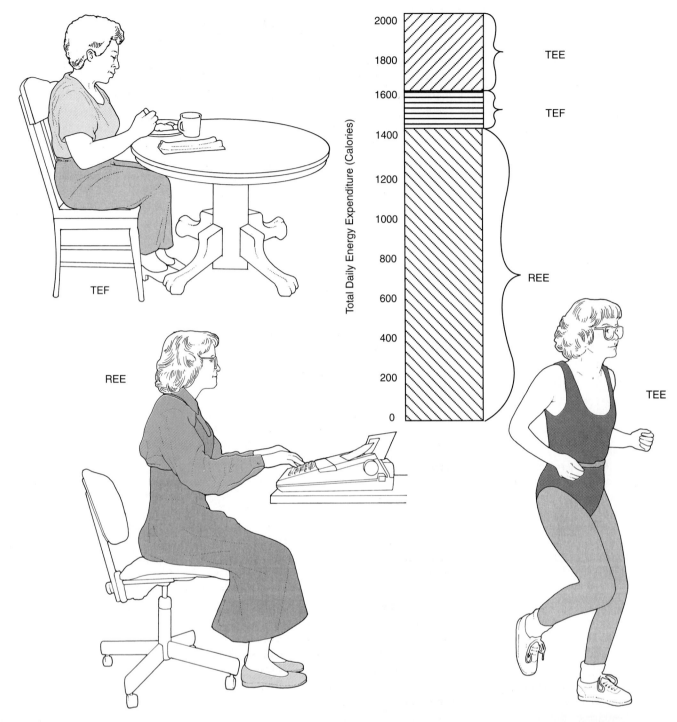

Figure 7.6 *Total daily expenditure of 2,000 Calories for an average-sized female (121 pounds). REE is the resting energy expenditure, TEF represents the thermic effect of food, and TEE is the thermic effect of exercise. In this figure, REE is 70 percent, TEF is 10 percent, and TEE is 20 percent of the daily energy expenditure.*

operate on both a short-term and long-term basis. For example, as the stomach expands while eating a meal, nerve impulses are sent from receptors in the stomach wall to the hypothalamus to help suppress food intake on a short-term basis. On a long-term basis the **set-point theory** of weight control is a proposed feedback mechanism. This theory proposes that your body is programmed to be a certain weight, or a set point. If you begin to deviate from that set point, your

body will make physiological adjustments to return you to normal, often referred to as adaptive thermogenesis. Although developed primarily with rats and still only a theory, the set-point theory does involve the interaction of those factors cited above, such as a glucostat and lipostat, which may influence energy intake and expenditure in humans. For example, when individuals go on a starvation-type diet, the REE decreases in an attempt to conserve body energy stores. The body recognizes that

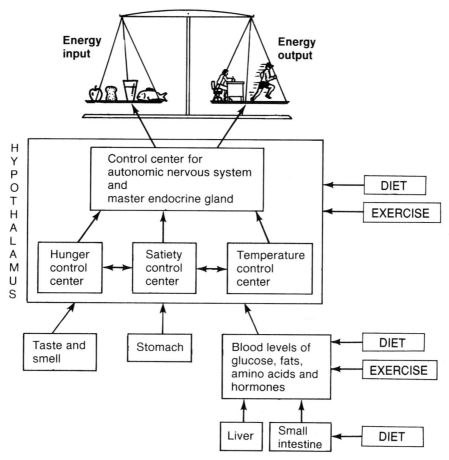

Figure 7.7 *Basic control mechanisms for body weight. The control of food intake (energy intake) and resting metabolism (energy output) is governed primarily by the hypothalamus. The numerous control centers in the hypothalamus are influenced by feedback from the body, such as the blood concentrations of glucose and other nutrients. In turn, food intake and energy expenditure may influence the hypothalamus. For example, exercise will stimulate the hypothalamus, which will result in the secretion of several hormones by the endocrine glands in the body. The effects of exercise will also influence the temperature control center and the blood levels of several nutrients, which will in turn influence the hypothalamus.*

it is being deprived of energy intake and slows down the rate of energy output. When subjects are overfed in experiments, the REE increases as does the TEF. Moreover, there is usually also a significant decrease in voluntary food intake, an indication that some metabolic change has depressed the appetite. A recent study by Leibel and others found that attempts by humans to maintain a body weight either above or below the usual body weight were associated with compensatory changes in REE. Thus, the set-point theory may be the reason whereby most people maintain their usual body weight throughout life. The interested reader is referred to the review by George Bray on the nutrient approach to obesity.

Although the set point is an important theory, and although a variety of factors interact to help regulate body weight, weight control is ultimately based upon energy balance, or Calorie control.

Caloric Concept of Weight Control

The **caloric concept of weight control** is relatively simple. If you take in more Calories than you expend, you gain weight, a positive energy balance. If you expend more than you take in, you lose weight, a negative energy balance. To maintain your body weight, caloric input and output must be equal. As

far as we know, human energy systems are governed by the same laws of physics that rule all energy transformations. The First Law of Thermodynamics is as pertinent to us in the conservation and expenditure of our energy sources as it is to any other machine. Since a Calorie is a unit of energy and can neither be created nor destroyed, Calories we consume must either be expended or conserved in the body. Since no substantial evidence is available to disprove the caloric theory, it is still the physical basis for body-weight control.

Keep in mind, however, that total body weight is made up of different components; those notable in weight-control programs are body water, protein, and fat stores, the three major body components affecting weight. Changes in these components may bring about body-weight fluctuations that would appear to be contrary to the caloric concept. You may lose 5 pounds in an hour, but it will be water weight. Starvation techniques may lead to rapid weight losses, but a good proportion of the weight loss will be in glycogen stores and body-protein stores, such as muscle mass, and the associated water bound with glycogen and protein. In programs to lose body weight, we usually desire to lose excess body fat. Certain dietary and exercise techniques may help to maximize fat losses while minimizing protein losses. The metabolism of human energy

Table 7.5	Approximate Daily Caloric Intake Needed to Maintain Healthy Body Weight

Activity Level	Calories per Pound
1. Very sedentary (movement restricted, such as patient confined to house)	13
2. Sedentary (most Americans, office job, light work)	14
3. Moderate activity (weekend recreation)	15
4. Very active (meet ACSM standards for vigorous exercise three times/week)	16
5. Competitive athlete (daily vigorous activity in high-energy sport)	17+

sources is complex. Although the caloric theory is valid relative to body-weight control, one must be aware that weight changes will not always be in line with caloric input and output, and that weight losses may not be due to body fat loss alone. These concepts are explored later in this chapter.

Since the caloric concept is a sound basis for weight control, you may ask, "How many Calories do I need daily in order to maintain my body weight?" This depends upon a number of factors, notably age, body weight, sex, genetic variations in the REE, and physical activity levels. The caloric requirement per pound of body weight is very high during the early years of life when a child is developing and adding large amounts of body tissue. The Calorie/pound requirement decreases throughout the years from birth to old age. Body weight influences the total amount of daily Calories you need but does not influence the Calorie/pound level. A large individual simply needs more total Calories to maintain body weight. Up to the age of eleven or twelve, the caloric needs of boys and girls are similar in terms of Calories/pound body weight. After puberty, however, males need more Calories/pound, probably due to their greater percentage of muscle tissue. Because REE appears to be genetically determined, individual variations in the REE may either increase or decrease daily caloric needs, depending on whether they are above or below normal. Physical activity levels above resting may have a very significant impact upon caloric needs, in some cases adding 1,000 to 1,500 or more Calories to the daily energy requirement. All of these factors make it difficult to make an exact recommendation relative to daily caloric needs, but some guidelines are available.

The Food and Nutrition Board of the National Research Council presents the following average caloric needs for the adult male and female, aged nineteen to fifty: males, 2,900 Calories; females, 2,200 Calories. On the average, males would need about 17 Calories for every pound of body weight, while the corresponding figure for females would be 16 Calories.

Table 7.5 represents some figures from the American Heart Association that may be a more appropriate guide for those who want to lose some extra body fat, since it provides information relative to activity level. The Calories allocated per pound are slightly less than those advocated by the National Research Council. For example, a sedentary individual who weighs 170 pounds needs approximately 2,380 Calories per day (170×14) simply to maintain body weight. To lose or gain weight, the caloric intake must be adjusted downward or upward. Keep in mind that these figures are approximations, and actual daily caloric needs may vary somewhat. However, they do offer an estimate of daily caloric needs and may be useful in starting a weight-control program. For a more detailed approach to determining your daily caloric needs, consult Laboratory Inventory 7.3, which will guide you in determining your daily levels of physical activity.

If you decide to lose weight without the guidance of a physician, the recommended maximal loss value for adults is 2 pounds/week. Since there are 3,500 Calories in a pound of body fat, this necessitates a deficit of 7,000 Calories for the week, or 1,000 Calories/day. For growing children, the general recommendation is about 1 pound/week, or a 500 Calorie deficit/day. Weight losses may not parallel the caloric deficit incurred during the early stages of a weight-reduction program because of water losses. Hence, the 2-pound limit may be adjusted upward somewhat during that time period. However, it is important to note that a slower rate of weight loss, about one pound per week, may be a more realistic, achievable, and sustainable goal for sedentary individuals starting a long-term weight loss program.

Laboratory Inventory 7.4 presents a method to determine the caloric deficit needed to lose excess body fat.

Comprehensive Weight-Control Programs

In a recent conference relative to methods for voluntary weight loss and control, the National Institutes of Health noted that the fundamental principle of weight loss or control is a commitment to changes in life-style. A properly designed diet and exercise program, complemented by appropriate behavior modification techniques, as discussed in the following three sections, represent the three major components of a successful weight control program for individuals with mild obesity. Those with more severe cases may need additional education and skills, social support, and continued professional assistance in order to maintain a stable healthy body weight. Some guidelines are presented in chapter 12 for individuals who may consider enrolling in commercial weight loss programs.

The Role of Diet in Weight Control

As you are probably aware, there are literally hundreds of different diet plans available to help you lose weight. Hardly a month goes by without a leading magazine revealing a new miracle diet or an entertainment personality writing a diet book that makes the best seller list.

Some of these diet plans may satisfy the criteria for a safe and effective weight-reduction diet. On the other hand, many of these diets may be nutritionally deficient and potentially hazardous to your health. An analysis of eleven popular diets revealed deficiencies in one or more of several key nutrients. Formula diets sold over the counter, such as Slender®

and Slim·Fast®, may be low in some essential nutrients and may be dangerous if used as the only source of nutrition. Low-carbohydrate/high-protein diets such as the early Dr. Atkins diets are generally high in fat and cholesterol. Food-combination diets, such as the Beverly Hills Diet, that claim that various food combinations help burn fat, are usually un-balanced, being low in protein, vitamins, and minerals. Single food diets such as the rice diet or the bananas-and-milk diet are deficient in key nutrients. Diets suggested to contain a special weight-reducing formula or fat-burning enzyme, such as the grapefruit diet, are generally ineffective, for such for-mulae or enzymes do not exist. Very low-Calorie diets, such as the Rotation Diet, also may be unbalanced in nutrient con-tent but may possibly be effective under medical supervision, as discussed later in this chapter.

In general, avoid diets that promise fast and easy weight losses. There is no fast and easy dietary method to lose excess body fat that is effective in the long run. If you have questions concerning the safety or effectiveness of any published diet, ob-tain information from a dietician at a local hospital or univer-sity or from a local branch of the American Dietetic Associa-tion. However, if you know some basic principles, you should be able to evaluate the value of most diet plans yourself.

Highly recommended diets are based upon sound nutri-tion principles and are also designed to satisfy personal food tastes. Research with dieters has shown that any safe, effec-tive, and realistic weight-reduction diet should adhere to the following principles:

1. It should be low enough in Calories to create an appropriate negative caloric balance, yet sufficient enough to supply all nutrients essential to normal body functions.

2. It should contain a wide variety of foods that appeal to your taste and help to prevent hunger sensations between meals.

3. It should be easily adaptable to your current life-style and readily obtainable, whether you eat most of your meals at home or in restaurants.

4. It should be a lifelong diet, one that will satisfy the previous three principles once you attain your desired weight.

In addition, foods should be selected that adhere to the princi-ples of healthy eating discussed in chapter 6.

General Dietary Guidelines

As for the diet itself, there are a variety of helpful suggestions that may help in the battle against Calories.

1. The key principle is to select foods with high nutrient density—low Calorie, high-nutrient foods from across the six food exchanges. Learn what foods are low in Calories in each of the food exchanges and incorporate those palatable to you in your diet. Some points relative to selection of proper foods in the food exchanges are presented below. Learn to substitute low-Calorie foods for high-Calorie ones. Avoid refined, processed foods as much as possible and include more natural, unrefined products in your diet. If you buy convenience foods,

select those that are low in Calories and fat. The key to a lifelong weight-maintenance diet is your knowledge of sound nutritional principles and the application of this knowledge to the design of your personal diet.

2. Reduce the amount of fat in the diet. Dietary fat appears to play several roles in the development of obesity in some individuals. First, it appears to stimulate the appetite, thereby leading to an increase in caloric intake. Second, dietary fat appears to be stored as fat more efficiently than either carbohydrate or protein, even if the caloric intake is similar; this is especially true in individuals who have lost weight and may be one of the most important reasons that they regain weight so readily. Your body actually needs to expend more energy to convert carbohydrate or protein into body fat. Third, dietary fat may also be stored preferentially as body fat in the abdominal region, which may increase health risks. Suggestions for reducing dietary fat are included in the following guidelines, but you may wish to review chapter 6 for additional information.

   In order to reduce the amount of fat in your diet, you may wish to count the total grams of fat you eat each day. A general recommendation is to keep your daily total fat intake to 30 percent or less of your total caloric intake. To calculate the total grams of fat you may eat per day when 30 percent of the Calories are derived from fat, simply drop the last 0 from your caloric intake and divide by 3. For example, a 2,100 Calorie diet would contain 70 grams of fat (2,100 = 210 ÷ 3 = 70).

   Once individuals adapt to a low-fat diet, they may actually prefer it because high fat meals are digested more slowly, possibly leading to indigestion and some gastrointestinal distress. You may wish to get the fat content to a lower percentage, such as 20 percent. Table 7.6 presents the formula and some calculations for different caloric intake levels and percentages of dietary fat intake.

3. Reduce the amount of simple refined sugars in the diet. This may be accomplished by restricting the amount of sugar added directly to foods and limiting the consumption of highly processed foods that may add substantial amounts of high-Calorie sweeteners. If you desire sweets, choose products with artificial sweeteners. In a recent review, F. Xavier Pi-Sunyer noted that substitution of artificial sweeteners, such as aspartame, for sugar has been shown to reduce caloric intake without leading to an increased consumption of other foods.

   In many cases, simply reducing the fat and sugar content in the diet will save substantial numbers of Calories and may be all that is needed. Did you know that fat and sugar together account for nearly 60 percent of the Calories in the average American diet? That represents 3 out of every 5 Calories. Table 7.7 provides some examples of how to save Calories via simple substitutions of comparable foods containing less fat or sugar.

Table 7.6 Calculation of Daily Fat Intake in Grams

Daily Caloric Intake	30% Fat Calories (Maximal Grams)	20% Fat Calories (Maximal Grams)	10% Fat Calories (Maximal Grams)
1,000	33	22	11
1,200	40	26	13
1,500	50	33	16
1,800	60	40	20
2,000	66	44	22
2,200	73	49	24
2,500	83	55	28

To use this table, determine the number of Calories per day in your diet and the percent of dietary Calories you want from fat, and then find the grams of fat you may consume daily. For example, if your diet contains 2,200 Calories, and you desire to consume only 20 percent of your daily Calories as fat, then you could consume 49 grams of fat.

Table 7.7 Simple Food Substitutions to Save Calories

Instead of	Select	To Save This Many Calories
1 croissant	1 plain bagel	35
1 whole egg	2 egg whites	50
1 ounce cheddar cheese	1 ounce mozzarella (skim)	30
1 ounce regular bacon	1 ounce Canadian bacon	100
3 ounce tuna in oil	3 ounces tuna in water	60
1 cup regular ice cream	1 cup fat-free frozen dessert	150
1 ounce turkey bologna	1 ounce turkey breast	50
1 cup premium ice cream	1 cup ice milk	140
1 cup whole milk	1 cup skim milk	60
1 ounce potato chips	1 ounce pretzels	90
1 can regular cola	1 can diet cola	150
1 tbsp. mayonnaise	1 tbsp. mustard	80

4. Milk-exchange products are excellent sources of protein but may contain excessive Calories unless fat is removed. Use nonfat or skim milk, low-fat cottage cheese, fat-free cheese, low-fat yogurt, and nonfat dried milk instead of their high-fat counterparts like whole milk, sour cream, and powdered creamers.

5. The meat-exchange products are sources of high-quality protein and many other nutrients but may contain excessive fat Calories. Use leaner cuts of meat, such as beef eye of round, flank steak, pork tenderloin, or 96 percent fat-free hamburger. Fish, chicken, turkey, and eggs are excellent low-Calorie meat exchanges, although egg yolks are very high in cholesterol and contain all of the fat in the egg. Trim away excess fat; broil or bake your meats to let the fat drip away. If you eat in fast-food restaurants, select foods that are low in fat such as baked fish, grilled chicken breasts, or lean meat. Avoid the high-fat foods normally containing 40–60 percent fat Calories.

6. The starch/bread exchanges are high in vitamins, minerals, and fiber. Use whole-grain breads, cereals, brown rice, oatmeal, beans, bran products, and starchy vegetables for dietary fiber, which helps curb hunger. Limit the use of processed grain products that add fat and sugar. Eat pasta with low-Calorie tomato sauce. Substitute products low in fat, such as bagels, for those high in fat, like croissants.

7. Foods in the fruit exchange are high in vitamins and fiber. Select fresh whole fruits or fruits canned in their own juices. Avoid those in heavy sugar syrups. Limit the intake of dried fruits, which are high in Calories. Eat at least one citrus fruit daily.

8. The vegetable-exchange foods are low in Calories yet high in vitamins, minerals, and fiber. Select dark green leafy and yellow-orange vegetables daily. Low-Calorie items like carrots, radishes, and celery are highly nutritious snacks for munching. Many of these vegetables are listed as free exchanges in Appendix A because they contain fewer than 20 Calories per serving. Fruits and vegetables may provide bulk and a sensation of fullness to the diet without excessive Calories.

9. Use lesser amounts of high-Calorie fat exchanges like salad dressings, mayonnaise, butter, margarine, and cooking oil. Do not prepare foods in fats. Use nonstick cooking utensils. If necessary, substitute low-Calorie dietary versions instead, or those containing fat substitutes. Many fat-free products are currently available and may decrease total fat and caloric intake if used judiciously within a healthful diet.

10. Beverages other than milk and juices should have no Calories. Fluid intake should remain high, for it helps create a sensation of satiety during a meal. Water is the recommended fluid, although diet drinks and unsweetened coffee and tea may be used sparingly. Consult the free food list in Appendix A.

11. Limit your intake of alcohol. It is high in Calories and zero in nutrient value. One gram of alcohol is equal to seven Calories, almost twice the value of protein and carbohydrate. For 100 Calories in a shot of gin you receive zero nutrient value, but for the same amount of Calories in approximately two ounces of chicken breast you get nearly one-third of your RDA in protein and substantial amounts of iron, zinc, niacin, and other vitamins. If you desire alcohol, select light varieties of wine and beer. Substitution of a light beer for a regular beer will save about 50 Calories. Try the nonalcoholic beers, which contain even fewer Calories.

12. Instead of two or three large meals a day, eat five or six smaller ones. Use low-Calorie, nutrient-dense foods for snacks. Research has shown that this may help control sensations of hunger between meals and may help in other ways, possibly by minimizing the release of insulin, which assists in the storage of fat in the body.

13. Cook and serve only small portions of food for meals. The temptation to overeat may be removed. Other behavior modification techniques discussed later can help you modify your diet.

14. If you consume fewer than 1,200 Calories per day, consider taking a simple one-a-day vitamin-mineral

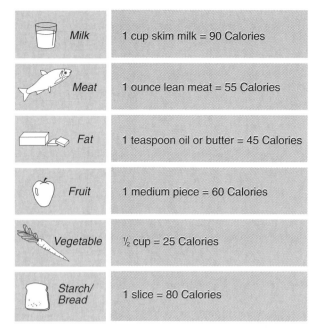

	Milk	1 cup skim milk = 90 Calories
	Meat	1 ounce lean meat = 55 Calories
	Fat	1 teaspoon oil or butter = 45 Calories
	Fruit	1 medium piece = 60 Calories
	Vegetable	½ cup = 25 Calories
	Starch/Bread	1 slice = 80 Calories

Figure 7.8 *Knowledge of the various food exchanges and their caloric values can be very helpful in planning a diet. With a little effort, you can learn to estimate the caloric value of most basic foods.*

tablet with no more than 100 percent of the RDA for each nutrient. Diets containing fewer than 800 Calories per day should be supervised by medical personnel.

15. Once you have attained your desired weight, a good set of scales would be most helpful. Keeping track of your weight on a day-to-day basis will enable you to decrease your caloric intake for several days once you notice your weight beginning to increase again. Short-term prevention is more effective than long-term treatment. The dietary habits you acquire during the Calorie-counting phase of your diet will help you during these short-term prevention periods.

Your Personal Diet

The key to your personal diet is nutrient density, the selection of low-Calorie, high-nutrient foods. As mentioned previously, low-Calorie foods must be selected wisely. For our purposes, the Exchange List System is used as the means to select low-Calorie foods. In ascending order, the caloric content of one serving from each of the six lists follows. A basic example of each is highlighted in figure 7.8.

1 vegetable exchange	= 25 Calories
1 fat exchange	= 45 Calories
1 fruit exchange	= 60 Calories
1 starch/bread exchange	= 80 Calories
1 meat exchange	= 55–100 Calories
Lean	= 55 Calories
Medium fat	= 75 Calories
High fat	= 100 Calories
1 milk exchange	= 90–150 Calories
Skim	= 90 Calories
Lowfat	= 120 Calories
Whole	= 150 Calories

The Food Exchange Lists may be found in Appendix A. Study these lists carefully to get an appreciation for the number of Calories in the foods you eat. Knowledge of the Exchange Lists enables you to substitute one low-Calorie food for another in your daily menu. As you become familiar with the caloric content of various foods, it becomes easier to select those that are low in Calories and high in nutrient value. Pay particular attention to the fat exchanges and foods that include fat exchanges, such as whole-milk products and high-fat meats. It requires a little effort in the beginning phases of a diet to learn the Calories in a given quantity of a certain food exchange, but once learned and incorporated into your lifestyle, it is a valuable asset to possess when trying to lose weight. Knowledge, however, is not the total answer; your behavior should reflect your knowledge. For example, you may know that regular milk contains 60 more Calories per glass than skim milk, but if you cannot develop a taste for skim milk, the advantage of your knowledge is lost. One strategy is to begin first with a switch to 2% lowfat milk, change to 1% lowfat milk, and eventually drink skim milk.

Table 7.8 presents a suggested meal plan adapted from a model developed by the Committee on Dietetics of the Mayo Clinic. It is based upon the Food Exchange System. The total caloric values are close approximations for a three-meal pattern. If you decide to include snacks such as a fruit in your diet, then remove each snack from one of the main meals. The beverages, other than milk and fruit juice, should contain no Calories. Although only seven meal plans are listed (1,000, 1,200, 1,500, 1,800, 2,000, 2,200, and 2,500 Calories), you may adjust values by simply adding or subtracting the caloric value for a given food exchange.

After you have determined the number of Calories you need daily, select the appropriate diet plan from table 7.8. To help implement your diet plan and keep track of the food exchanges you eat on a daily basis, design a 3″ × 5″ card for the number of food exchanges in your daily diet (see table 7.9). As you consume an exchange at each meal, simply cross it off on the card. Make a new card each day. The model in table 7.9 is for 1,500 Calories; total exchanges are obtained from table 7.8. An example of a 1,500 Calorie diet based on the Food Exchanges system is presented in table 7.10.

Keep in mind that this is not a rigid diet plan. At the minimum, you should have two skim milk exchanges, five lean meat exchanges, four starch/bread exchanges, two vegetable exchanges, and two fruit exchanges. Once you have guaranteed these minimum requirements, you may do some substitution among the various exchanges so long as you keep the total caloric content within range of your goals. For example, you may delete two starch/bread exchanges (160 Calories) and substitute one skim milk and one lean meat (145 Calories). You may also shift a limited number of the exchanges from one meal to another. If you prefer a more substantial breakfast and a lighter lunch, simply shift some of the exchanges from lunch to breakfast. A recommended plan is to eat some of your daily food as snacks, so you may eat five or six small meals a day.

Laboratory Inventory 7.5 may be used as a guide to developing your own personal diet plan.

Approximate Daily Caloric Intake

	1,000	1,200	1,500	1,800	2,000	2,200	2,500
Breakfast							
Milk, skim	1	1	1	1	1	1	1
Meat, lean	1	1	2	2	2	3	3
Starch/bread	1	1	2	3	3	3	3
Fruit	1	1	1	1	2	2	2
Fat	0	½	½	1	1	2	2
Beverage	1	1	1	1	1	1	1
Lunch							
Milk, skim	1	1	1	1	1	1	2
Meat, lean	2	2	2	3	3	3	4
Starch/bread	2	2	2	2	2	3	3
Vegetable	1	1	1	2	2	2	2
Salad	1	1	1	1	1	1	1
Fruit	1	2	2	2	2	2	2
Fat	½	½	½	2	2	2	2
Beverage	1	1	1	1	1	1	1
Dinner							
Milk, skim	0	0	0	0	1	1	1
Meat, lean	2	2	3	3	3	3	4
Starch/bread	1	2	2	3	3	4	4
Vegetable	1	2	2	2	2	2	2
Salad	1	1	1	1	1	1	1
Fruit	0	0	1	1	2	2	2
Fat	½	1	1	1	1	1	2
Beverage	1	1	1	1	1	1	1
Totals							
Milk, skim	2	2	2	2	3	3	4
Meat, lean	5	5	7	8	8	9	11
Starch, bread	4	5	6	8	8	10	10
Vegetable	2	3	3	4	4	4	4
Salad	2	2	2	2	2	2	2
Fruit	2	3	4	4	6	6	6
Fat	1	2	2	4	4	5	6
Beverage	3	3	3	3	3	3	3

Key points:
1. *Caloric values:*

Milk exchange, skim	*= 90*
Meat exchange, lean	*= 55*
Fruit exchange	*= 60*
Vegetable exchange	*= 25*
Starch/Bread exchange	*= 80*
Fat exchange	*= 45*
Beverage	*= 0*
Salad	*= 20*

2. *See Appendix A for a listing of foods in each exchange. Note the following:*
   a. *Foods other than milk, such as yogurt, are included in the milk exchange.*
   b. *The meat list includes foods such as eggs, cheese, fish, and poultry; select those from the lean meat exchange; low-fat products, like beans and peas, may be considered as meat substitutes.*
   c. *Some starchy vegetables are included in the bread list.*
3. *Foods should not be fried or prepared in fat unless you count the added fat as a fat exchange. Broil or bake foods instead.*
4. *Low-Calorie vegetables like lettuce and radishes should be used in the salads. Use only small amounts of very low-Calorie salad dressing.*
5. *Beverages should contain no Calories.*

The Role of Exercise in Weight Control

Humans are meticulously designed for physical activity, yet our modern mechanical age has eliminated many of the opportunities we once had to incorporate moderate physical activity as a natural part of our lives. The regulation of food intake was never designed to adapt to the highly mechanized conditions in

Daily Meal Plan	1,500 Calories
Milk exchange, skim	(2) 1 2
Meat exchange, lean	(7) 1 2 3 4 5 6 7
Fruit exchange	(4) 1 2 3 4
Vegetable exchange	(3) 1 2 3
Salad	(2) 1 2
Starch/bread exchange	(6) 1 2 3 4 5 6
Fat exchange	(2) 1 2
Beverage	(3) 1 2 3

today's society. Hence, the combination of overeating and inactivity has led to increasing levels of overweight and obesity.

It is generally recognized that prevention of obesity, or excess body weight, is more effective than treatment. Most people do not become overweight overnight; they accumulate an extra 70 to 150 Calories per day that, over time, leads to excess fat tissue. A daily exercise program could easily counteract the effect of these additional Calories (see fig. 7.9). Dr. Jean Mayer, the late international authority on weight control, has reported that no single factor is more frequently responsible for the development of obesity than lack of physical exercise.

Although it will take some time for exercise to produce significant weight loss, all health professionals recommend exercise as an important component of a comprehensive weight control program. It may take weight off slowly, but the weight loss is primarily body fat, and exercise is effective for decreasing body fat stored in the abdominal region. Exercise has also been shown to be very effective as a means to maintain weight loss once a desirable body weight has been attained, and some investigators believe that this is one of the critical factors in preventing weight regain. A large body of knowledge substantiates the point that exercise can help reduce and control body weight. The purpose of this section is to explore the different mechanisms whereby increased levels of physical activity may help to lose body fat.

Exercise and the Metabolic Rate

For most Americans, the vast majority of daily energy expenditure, about 80–90 percent, is accounted for by the resting energy expenditure (REE) and the thermic effect of food (TEF), while only about 10–20 percent of the daily Calories are accounted for by thermic effect of exercise (TEE), usually by light exercise such as walking or climbing stairs. In typical sedentary individuals, these forms of light exercise are a form of unstructured physical activity, not part of a planned exercise program, but simply activities involved in their normal life-style. Most sedentary individuals even attempt to reduce this amount of exercise in their daily lives by parking as close as possible to the store or by taking an elevator to the second floor.

Increasing the level of the REE or TEE will help to expend Calories. An acute bout of exercise will, of course, increase the TEE, but a sound exercise training program may also exert some significant effects on the REE, and simple changes in daily habits may increase energy expended via the TEE.

Table 7.10 A 1,500-Calorie Diet Based upon the Food Exchange System*

Exchange	Number of Servings	Calories per Serving	Total Calories	Food Selected
Breakfast				
Meat, lean	2	55	110	1 ounce lean ham and 1
Fat	½	25	25	ounce diet cheese
Starch/bread	2	80	160	melted on 2 pieces whole-grain toasted bread
Fruit	1	60	60	4 ounces orange juice
Beverage	1	0	0	1 cup coffee with noncaloric sweetener
Lunch				
Milk, lowfat	1	120	120	8 ounces plain lowfat yogurt
Fruit	1	60	60	with cut-up fresh fruit added
Meat	2	55	110	Turkey sandwich with 2
Starch/bread	2	80	160	ounces turkey breast on whole-grain bun
Vegetable	1	25	25	1 carrot
Salad	1	20	20	Lettuce with
Fat	½	25	25	low-Calorie dressing
Beverage	1	0	0	Diet cola
Dinner				
Milk, skim	1	90	90	½ cup ice milk
Meat	3	55	165	3 ounces broiled fish
Starch/bread	2	80	160	1 baked potato
Vegetable	2	25	50	1 cup steamed broccoli
Salad	1	20	20	Cucumbers
Fat	1	45	45	Small amount of margarine for potato and low-Calorie dressing for salad
Fruit	2	60	120	1 banana cut up on ice milk
Beverage	1	0	0	Iced tea

*This is an example of a one-day diet. Can you think of appropriate substitutes for each of the food exchanges to change the diet in order to get a wider variety of foods over a 5–7 day period?

200-Calorie milkshake =

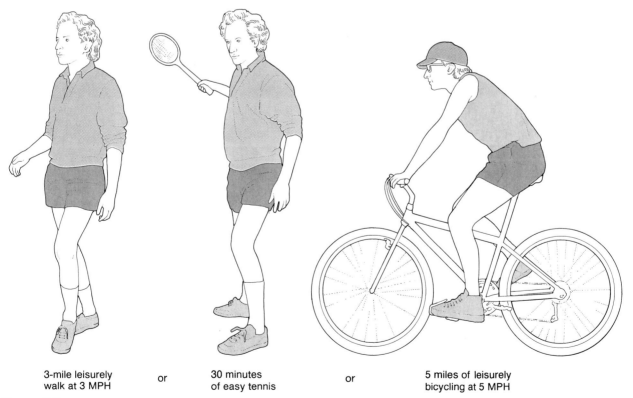

3-mile leisurely walk at 3 MPH   or   30 minutes of easy tennis   or   5 miles of leisurely bicycling at 5 MPH

Figure 7.9   *It is very easy to consume 200 additional Calories per day, which can lead to an increase of about 2 pounds of body fat per month. However, increased physical activity may help to expend these Calories.*

Of all the factors that influence the REE, the change in body composition may be one way we may help alter it. Decreasing the amount of body fat and increasing lean body mass (muscle tissue) may increase the REE. This effect may be due to the increased activity levels of muscle tissue as compared to fat tissue, or the increased ratio of body surface area to body weight. Some research has suggested that exercise programs help increase the REE or at least prevent it from decreasing, particularly in overweight individuals who attempt to lose weight with very low-Calorie diets.

The TEE may be increased or decreased, depending on average daily activities. Sitting burns up fewer Calories than standing; standing uses fewer Calories than walking, and so on. Simply changing the nature of your daily sedentary activities by incorporating more light exercise tasks, such as walking to the store and climbing the stairs to your class or office, will increase the REE to a TEE level. Make such activities a natural part of your daily routine. One suggestion is to take three to five miniwalks of 5–10 minutes during the day. Increasing your REE to a TEE by only 50 Calories per day, which could be done by incorporating about one mile of walking in your daily schedule, would account for an energy equivalency of 5 pounds of body fat loss in one year.

Some research has shown that the REE may remain elevated during the recovery period following exercise and account for additional caloric expenditure beyond that expended during exercise. Following high-intensity exercise, the REE may remain elevated for several hours and use a total of 20 to 70 Calories more than would be used at rest. Exercising on a daily basis, this additional benefit could account for up to a loss of an extra quarter to half pound of body fat per month. However, following low-intensity exercise, the effect is not as great; studies report about 5 to 20 additional total Calories are expended during the recovery period. A recent study looked at nine different combinations of exercise intensity and duration, ranging from 20 minutes at 30 percent $\dot{V}O_{2MAX}$ to 80 minutes at 70 percent $\dot{V}O_{2MAX}$. The higher levels of exercise intensity generally elicited a higher REE in the postexercise recovery period, accounting for up to 70 additional Calories used in the recovery period of up to eight hours.

Increasing the TEE, however, is the most effective means to increase daily caloric expenditure and should be a major component of a weight-control program. For example, while the average person may expend only about 60–70 Calories per hour during rest, this value may range from 300 to 1,000 Calories per hour during sustained activity such as aerobic walking, running, swimming, or bicycling, the number of Calories burned being dependent on the intensity of the exercise.

Many of these Calories that you burn are fat Calories. During aerobic exercise, fat is one of the preferred fuels. It is mobilized from the body's fat cells to supply energy to the muscle cells. (See fig. 7.10.) During training, your body actually adapts and during exercise derives a greater proportion of its energy from fat; although the total number of Calories you expend jogging a mile will not change, more of them will come from fat stored in your body. Hence, body fat stores are reduced.

The most important factor affecting the TEE is the intensity or speed of the exercise. In order to move faster, your muscles must contract more rapidly and, hence, consume proportionately more energy. However, other factors may affect the total caloric expenditure during exercise. First, if you plan to cover a set distance, the nature of the activity is critical; swimming a mile expends more Calories than running the same distance, and running a mile expends more Calories than bicycling. Second, the efficiency of movement in some activities modifies the number of Calories expended; a beginning swimmer wastes a lot of energy, while one who is more efficient may swim a set distance with less effort, hence consuming fewer Calories. Third, the individual with a greater body weight burns more Calories for any given amount of work where the body has to be moved, as in walking, jogging, or running. It simply takes more energy to move a heavier load. Now we do not recommend that you become less skilled or gain body weight in order to burn more Calories during exercise. In fact, the opposite is true: try to become more efficient so that the exercise task may become more enjoyable.

Exercise Programs

As your are probably aware, there are a number of different exercise programs available to lose body weight. Perusal of the daily newspaper reveals numerous advertisements for weight-reduction programs sponsored by various commercial physical-fitness businesses. Resistance training with sophisticated equipment, slimnastic exercises, aerobic dancing, and special exercise apparatus are a few of the approaches often advertised as the best means to quickly lose body fat. The truth is that you do not need any special apparatus or any specially designed program. The design of an exercise program to lose body fat is based upon the same principles underlying an aerobic exercise program as discussed in chapter 3. Aerobic exercises to lose body fat should involve large muscle groups, should be rhythmic and continuous in motion, should be enjoyable, and should be properly designed relative to exercise intensity and especially to duration and frequency.

Intensity

The higher the intensity of the exercise, the more Calories you expend. Per unit of time, walking uses fewer Calories than jogging, which uses fewer Calories than fast running. Simply put, it costs you more energy to move your body weight at a faster pace. However, there is an optimal intensity level for each person depending on how long the exercise will last. You can run at a very high intensity for 200 yards, but you certainly could not maintain that same fast pace for 2 miles. Thus, intensity and duration are interrelated. Table 7.11 presents levels of caloric expenditure per minute for an average-sized adult male and female, illustrating the effect of exercise intensity on caloric expenditure per minute.

In order to facilitate the determination of the energy cost (in Calories) of a wide variety of physical activities, Appendix C has been developed. It is a composite table of a wide variety of individual reports in literature. When using this appendix, keep the following points in mind.

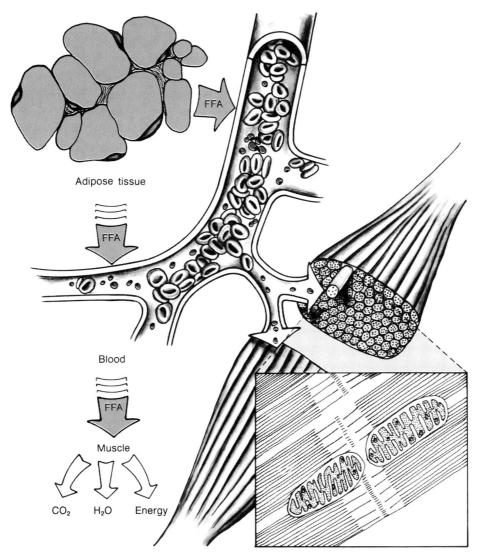

Figure 7.10 *Exercise helps to release fat (free fatty acids) from the adipose tissues. The fat then travels by way of the bloodstream to the muscles, where the free fatty acids are oxidized to provide the energy for exercise. Thus, exercise is an effective means to reduce body fat.*

1. The figures are approximate and include the resting metabolic rate. Thus, the total cost of the exercise includes not only the energy expended by the exercise itself, but also the amount you would have used anyway during the same period of time. Suppose you ran for 1 hour and the calculated energy cost was 500 Calories. During that same time at rest you may have expended 75 Calories, so the net cost of the exercise is 425 Calories.

2. The figures in the table are only for the time you are performing the activity. For example, in an hour of basketball, you may only exercise strenuously for 35 to 40 minutes, as you may take time-outs and may rest during foul shots. In general, record only the amount of time that you are actually moving during the activity.

3. The figures may give you some guidelines to total energy expenditure, but actual caloric costs might vary somewhat due to such factors as skill level, environmental factors (biking against the wind or up hills), and so forth.

Table 7.11 Caloric Expenditure per Minute at Varying Rates of Metabolism*

Level of Intensity	Caloric Expenditure per Minute	
	Male (155 pounds)	Female (120 pounds)
Basal metabolic rate	1.0	0.9
Sitting and writing	2.0	1.5
Walking at 2 m.p.h.	3.3	2.5
Walking at 3 m.p.h.	4.2	3.3
Running at 5 m.p.h.	9.4	7.3
Running at 10 m.p.h.	18.8	14.5
Running at 15 m.p.h.	29.3	22.5
Running at 20 m.p.h.	38.7	29.8

*Based on an average-sized male and female

4. Not all body weights could be listed, but you may approximate by going to the closest weight listed.

5. There may be small differences between men and women, but not enough to make a marked difference in the total caloric value for most exercises.

Table 7.12 Classification of Physical Activities Based upon Rate of Energy Expenditure*

Light Mild Aerobic Exercise (<7 Calories/Min)

Badminton, social	Dancing, mild square	Nautilus weight training
Baseball	Golf	Swimming (20–25 yards/min)
Bicycling (5–10 m.p.h.)	Horseback riding	Walking (2–4 m.p.h.)

Moderate to Heavy Aerobic Exercise (8–12 Calories/Min)

Badminton, competitive	Handball, moderate	Soccer
Basketball	Paddle ball	Squash
Bicycling (11–14 m.p.h.)	Racquetball	Swimming (30–50 yards/min)
Circuit weight training, vigorous	Rope skipping (60–80 r.p.m.)	Tennis, competitive
Dancing, aerobic	Running (5–6 m.p.h.)	Volleyball, competitive
Field hockey	Skiing, cross-country (4–6 m.p.h.)	Walking (4.5–5.5 m.p.h.)

Maximal Aerobic Exercise (>13 Calories/Min)

Bicycling (15–20 m.p.h.)	Running (7–9 m.p.h.)	
Calisthenics, vigorous	Skiing, cross-country (7–9 m.p.h.)	
Handball, competitive	Swimming (55–70 yards/min)	
Rope skipping (120–140 r.p.m.)	Walking (5.6–6.0 m.p.h.)	

*Calories per minute based upon a body weight of 70 kg, or 154 pounds. Those weighing more or less will expend more or fewer Calories, respectively, but the level of the exercise will be the same. The actual amount of Calories expended may also depend on a number of other factors, depending on the activity. For example, bicycling into or with the wind will increase or decrease, respectively, the energy cost.

Source: M. H. Williams, Nutritional Aspects of Human Physical and Athletic Performance. Charles C Thomas, 1985.

Appendix C is useful to determine which types of activities may be of appropriate intensity for your weight-control program. You may wish to blend those activities with higher caloric expenditure per minute into your life-style. Chapter 3 also lists exercises that expend large amounts of Calories. As a general guide for your perusal, table 7.12 provides a classification of physical activities based upon the rate of energy expended, expressed in Calories per minute.

A common myth contends that in order to burn fat, you must exercise at a lower intensity. It is true that at lower intensities you do derive a greater percentage of your energy from fat than when exercising at higher intensities, but your total calorie expenditure is also lower. At higher exercise intensities you will derive a lower percentage of your energy output from fat, but the total energy expenditure will be greater and you will still burn about the same amount of fat Calories as you would exercising at the lower intensity. If you want to burn Calories to lose body fat, your objective should be to burn the greatest total Calories possible within the time frame you have to exercise. As an example, suppose an athletic female had 30 minutes to exercise and ran at 50 percent of her $\dot{V}O_{2MAX}$, running 10-minute miles and deriving 50 percent of her energy from fat. She would cover 3 miles, expending about 300 total Calories at an energy cost of 100 Calories per mile. About 150 of these total Calories would be derived from fat. If she was able to run at 75 percent of her $\dot{V}O_{2MAX}$, running 7.5-minute miles and deriving 33 percent of her energy from fat, she would cover 4.5 miles, expending 450 total Calories, 150 of which would still be fat Calories. However, she has expended a total of 450 versus 300 Calories, which will lead to a greater weight loss or permit her to consume an additional 150 Calories in her daily diet. But, if she has unlimited time, she may be able to exercise longer at the lower exercise intensity and eventually burn more total Calories.

Duration

Probably the most important factor in total energy expenditure is the duration of an exercise. In swimming, bicycling, running, or walking, distance is the key. For example, running a mile costs the average-sized individual about 100 Calories. Five miles would approximate 500 Calories. If you run 1 mile a day, it will take over 1 month to lose 1 pound of fat, whereas if you run 5 miles a day, the time span would shorten to about 1 week. Thus, if the purpose of the exercise program is to lose weight, stress the duration concept.

One of the key points about the duration concept is the notion of distance traveled rather than time. For example, an hour of tennis and an hour of running are both good exercises. However, the runner expends considerably more Calories in an hour than the tennis player because the activity involved in running is continuous. The tennis player has a number of rest periods in which energy expenditure is lower. Consequently, at the end of an hour's activity, the runner may have expended two to three times more Calories than the tennis player.

A major reason many adults do not use exercise as a weight-loss mechanism is that their level of physical fitness is so low they cannot sustain a moderate level of exercise intensity for very long. However, keep in mind that, as you continue to train, your body will begin to adapt, so that in time your exercise period may be prolonged.

Many individuals have a major misconception of the duration concept that may deter them from initiating an exercise program for weight control. They believe that exercise is a poor means to lose body weight because it expends so few Calories. For example, they have heard that one has to jog about 35 miles to lose a pound of body fat. Since the average person uses approximately 100 Calories per mile, and since 1 pound of body fat contains about 3,500 Calories, there is some truth to that statement. However, you must look at the

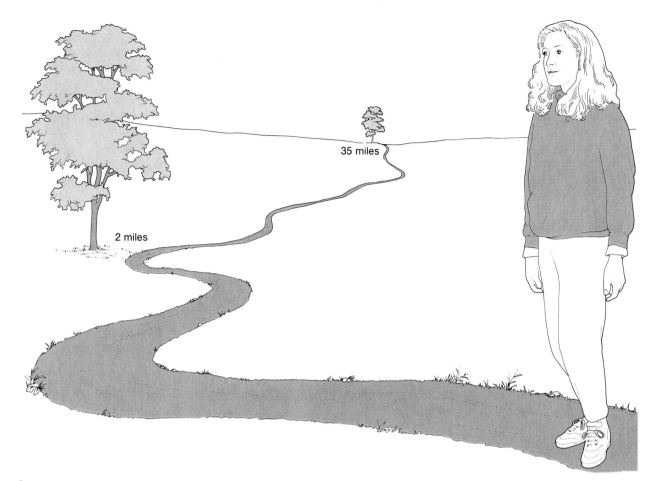

Figure 7.11 *To lose body fat by exercising, you must look at the long-haul concept of weight control. The average-weight individual needs to jog about 35 miles to burn off one pound of body fat. This would be nearly impossible for most of us to do in one day. At 2 miles per day, however, it could be done in about 2½ weeks—and at 5 miles per day, in only 1 week. Even though it takes time, an exercise program is a very effective approach to reduce excess body fat.*

2 miles

35 miles

long-haul concept of weight control (fig. 7.11). Jogging about 2 miles daily would expend about 6,000 Calories in a month, accounting for almost 2 pounds of body fat. Over a year, the weight loss may be substantial.

Frequency

Frequency of exercise complements duration and intensity. Frequency of exercise refers to how often you participate each week. As would appear obvious, the more often you exercise, the greater the total weekly caloric expenditure. In general, three to four times per week is satisfactory, provided duration and intensity are adequate, but six to seven times would just about double your caloric output. A daily exercise program is recommended, possibly alternating activities to help prevent overuse injuries, as discussed in chapter 3.

Walking, Running, Swimming and Bicycling

In general, activities that use the large-muscle groups of the body and are performed in a continuous manner expend the greatest number of Calories. Intensity and duration are the two key determinants of total energy expenditure. Activities in which you are able to exercise continuously at a fairly high

intensity for a prolonged period of time maximize your caloric loss. As discussed in chapter 3, this may encompass a wide variety of different physical activities, but those that have become increasingly popular include walking, jogging, running, swimming, and bicycling. A few general comments are in order relative to these modes of exercising.

As a general rule, the caloric cost of running a given distance does not depend on the speed. It will take a longer time to cover the distance at a slower speed, but the total caloric cost will be similar to that expended at a faster speed. Thus, it is your choice. You can exercise at a higher intensity for a shorter period of time, or at a lower intensity for a longer period of time, so long as the distance is covered. However, walking is more economical than running and, hence, you generally expend fewer Calories for a given distance walking than you do running. This does not hold true, however, if you walk vigorously at a high speed. At high walking speeds, you may expend more energy than if you jogged at the same speed. Fast, vigorous walking, known as aerobic walking, can be an effective means to expend Calories. (See table 7.12.)

In recent years, many individuals have utilized small weights in conjunction with their walking programs, usually carrying them in their hands. A number of research studies have reported that this technique, particularly if the arms are swung vigorously through a wide range of motion during walking, may increase the energy expenditure about 5 to 10 percent or higher above unweighted walking at the same speed. Such exercises may benefit the cardiovascular system, but they may also exaggerate the blood pressure response to exercise and should be used with caution by individuals with blood pressure problems. The hand weights may also increase the impact forces of landing and may be uncomfortable to carry. Since some researchers have noted that simply walking a little faster without weights will have the same effect on energy cost, this may be a good alternative. Nevertheless, at any given walking speed, hand weights will increase energy expenditure, but not as greatly as that suggested by many manufacturers of these products.

You can calculate the approximate caloric expenditure for running a given distance by either of the following formulas:

Caloric cost = 1 C/kg body weight/kilometer

Caloric cost = .73 C/pound body weight/mile

If you are an average-sized male of about 154 pounds (70 kg) or an average-sized female of about 121 pounds (55 kg), you burn about the following amounts of Calories for running either a kilometer or a mile.

	Average Male	*Average Female*
Kilometer	70 Calories	55 Calories
Mile	112 Calories	88 Calories

Slow, leisurely walking uses about half this number of Calories per mile, while rapid aerobic walking, about 5.6 miles per hour, would use about the same number of Calories.

Due to water resistance, swimming takes more energy to cover a given distance than does either walking or running. Although the amount of energy expended is dependent somewhat on the type of swimming stroke used and the ability of the swimmer, swimming a given distance takes about four times as much energy as running. For example, swimming a quarter-mile is the energy equivalent of running a mile. Other forms of water exercises, such as jogging or calisthenics in waist-deep water, may help burn Calories.

Bicycling takes less energy, approximately one-third the cost, to cover a given distance in comparison to running on a level surface. The energy cost of bicycling depends on a number of factors such as body weight, the type of bicycle, hills, and body position on the bike (such as a streamlined position to reduce air resistance). When air resistance is high, the energy cost of bicycling increases exponentially.

Resistance Training

Research has suggested that resistance training be incorporated in a weight-loss program, for such training may help stimulate the development of lean body mass and possibly help minimize the decrease in the REE, which is often observed in weight-loss programs that primarily use dieting alone. Thus, a weight-training program, as outlined in chapter 4, may complement an aerobic exercise program in facilitating loss of excess body fat and maintaining or increasing lean body mass.

Spot Reducing

Spot reducing, using local isolated exercises in an attempt to deplete local fat deposits, does not appear to be effective. One study actually biopsied fat tissue to determine whether sit-ups would reduce fat in the abdominal area. Subjects did a total of 5,000 sit-ups over a 27-day period, and this localized exercise did not preferentially reduce the adipose cell size in the abdominal area.

The current viewpoint suggests that reduction of body fat is most likely to occur from fat deposits throughout the body, not from specific areas, regardless of the exercise format. Although both large muscle activities and local isolated muscle exercises may both be beneficial in reducing fat stores, the former is recommended because the total caloric expenditure is larger. However, localized exercises may help increase muscle tone in specific muscle groups.

The Role of Behavior Modification in Weight Control

When breaking any well-established habit, self-discipline, or willpower, is the key. The most important component of a weight-control program is you. You must want to lose weight and you must take the major responsibility for achieving your goals. You must be convinced that reduced body weight will enhance your life, and you must establish this goal as a high priority. According to a recent report by the National Institutes of Health, you have to make life-style changes in order to successfully lose body fat and keep it off.

One of the key components of a successful weight-control program is the need to identify and modify behaviors that contribute to the weight problem. The subject of human behavior development and change is very complex, but psychologists note that three factors are generally involved—the physical environment, the social environment, and the personal environment. For the person with a weight problem, a refrigerator brimming with food (physical environment), a family that consumes high-Calorie snack food around the house (social environment), and an acquired taste for sweet foods (personal environment) may trigger behaviors that make it very difficult to maintain a proper body weight.

As noted in chapter 1, a model often used to explain the development or modification of health behaviors, such as a proper diet and exercise program for weight control, involves three steps—knowledge, values, and behavior. First, proper knowledge is essential. Although there are substantial scientific data regarding the health risks of obesity, there exists a considerable amount of misinformation relative to the roles of nutrition and exercise in weight control, so you need to possess accurate information to implement an appropriate plan. Second, the health implications of this knowledge may help you develop a set of personal values, or attitudes, toward a specific health behavior. If you perceive excess body fat as a threat to your personal physical or psychological health, you are more likely to initiate behavioral changes. Third, your health behavior should reflect the knowledge you acquired and the values you developed so that you develop reasonable goals and implement a weight loss program.

Behavior modification is a technique often used in psychological therapy to elicit desirable behavioral changes. The rationale underlying behavior modification is that many behavioral patterns are learned via stimulus-response conditioning; for example, a stimulus in your environment such as a commercial break in a television program elicits a response of a mad dash to the refrigerator. Because such responses are learned, they also may be unlearned. For a discussion of a comprehensive program conducted by a behavioral psychologist, the reader is referred to the review by Brownell and Kramer. Relative to a self-designed program of weight control, behavior modification is used primarily to reduce or eliminate physical or social stimuli that may lead to excessive caloric intake or decreased physical activity. George Bray, an international authority on obesity treatment, has noted that the most important component of any weight-control program is the associated behavior modification through which the individual learns new ways to deal with old problems.

Both long-range and short-range realistic goals need to be established. A long-range goal may be to lose 40 pounds over six months, whereas a short-range goal would be to lose about 1 to 2 pounds per week. A long-range goal may also include a large number of behavioral changes to achieve the 40-pound weight loss, but the number of changes would be phased in gradually on a short-term basis. Do not expect to make all recommended behavioral changes overnight.

Identifying and Modifying Eating and Exercise Behaviors

One of the first steps in a behavior-modification program is to identify those physical and social environmental factors that may lead to problem behaviors. Keep a diary of your daily activities for a week or two to help you identify some behavioral patterns that may contribute to overeating and extra body weight. The following are some of the factors that might be recorded each time you eat, along with a brief explanation of their possible importance. You should also record your daily physical activity.

1. Type of food and amount. This may be related to the other factors. For example, do you eat high-Calorie foods during your snacks?
2. Meal or snack. You may find yourself snacking four or five times a day.
3. Time of day. Do you eat at regular hours or have a full meal just before retiring at night?
4. Degree of hunger. How hungry were you when you ate—very hungry or not hungry at all? You may be snacking when not hungry.
5. Activity. What were you doing while eating? You may find TV watching and eating snack foods are related.
6. Location. Where do you eat? The office or school cafeteria may be the place you eat a high-Calorie meal.
7. Persons involved. Whom do you eat with? Do you eat more when alone or with others? Being with certain people may trigger overeating.
8. Emotional feelings. How do you feel when eating? You might eat more when depressed than when happy, or vice versa.
9. Exercise. How much walking, stair climbing, or regular exercise do you get? Do you ride when you could possibly walk? How much time do you just sit?

Recording this information may make you aware of the physical and social circumstances under which you tend to overeat or be physically inactive. This awareness may be useful to help implement behavioral changes that may make weight control easier. The following suggestions are often helpful:

Foods to eat:

1. Use low-Calorie foods for snacks.
2. Plan low-Calorie, high-nutrient meals.
3. Preplan your food intake for the entire day.
4. Eat foods that have had minimal or no processing.

Food purchasing:

1. Do not shop when hungry.
2. Prepare a shopping list and do not deviate from it.
3. Buy only those foods that are low in Calories and high in nutrient value.
4. Buy natural foods as much as possible.
5. Buy low-fat or fat-free alternatives.

Food storage:

1. Keep high-Calorie food out of sight and in sealed containers or cupboards.
2. Have low-Calorie snacks like carrots and radishes readily available.

Food preparation and serving:

1. Buy foods that need some type of preparation.
2. If possible, do not add fats or sugar in preparation; bake, broil, steam or microwave foods.
3. Prepare only small amounts.
4. Do not use serving bowls on the table.
5. Put the food on a small plate.

Location:

1. Eat only in one place, such as the kitchen or dining area.
2. Avoid food areas such as the kitchen or a snack table at a party.
3. Avoid restaurants where you are most likely to buy high-Calorie items.

Restaurant eating:

1. When eating out, select low-Calorie items.
2. Request that items by prepared without fat.
3. Have condiments like butter, mayonnaise, and salad dressing served on the side. Use sparingly.

Methods of eating:

1. Eat slowly; chew food thoroughly, and drink water between bites.
2. Eat with someone, for conversation can slow down the eating process.
3. Cut food into small pieces.
4. Do not do anything else while eating, such as watching TV.
5. Relax and enjoy the meal.
6. Eat only at specific times.
7. Eat only until pleasantly satisfied, not stuffed.
8. Spread your Calories over the day, eating small amounts more often.

Activity:

1. Walk more. Park the car or get off the bus some distance from work.
2. When possible, use the stairs instead of the elevator.
3. Take a brisk walk instead of a coffee-donut break.
4. Get involved in activities with other people, preferably physical activities that will burn Calories.
5. Avoid sedentary night routines.
6. Start a regular aerobic exercise program.

Mental attitude:

1. Recognize that you are not perfect and that relapses may occur.
2. Deal positively with your relapse; put it behind you and get back on the program.
3. Put reminders on your refrigerator door or telephone.
4. Reward yourself for sticking to your plans.

Self-discipline and self-control:

1. Establish weight loss as a high priority.
2. Think about this priority before eating.

For the interested reader, the books by Dusek and the Mahoneys provide an in-depth coverage of behavior modification for weight-control purposes. Many of the commercial, medically oriented weight-loss centers as well as organizations such as Weight Watchers International also may be sources of information.

Special Considerations in Weight Control

The preceding sections in this chapter offer a number of suggestions to help you lose body fat, primarily by a decrease in

Table 7.13 Approximate Number of Days Required to Lose Body Fat for a Given Caloric Deficit

Daily Caloric Deficit	To Lose 5 Pounds	To Lose 10 Pounds	To Lose 15 Pounds	To Lose 20 Pounds	To Lose 25 Pounds
100	175	350	525	700	875
200	87	175	262	350	438
300	58	116	175	232	292
400	44	88	131	176	219
500	35	70	105	140	175
600	29	58	87	116	146
700	25	50	75	100	125
800	22	44	66	88	109
900	19	39	58	78	97
1,000	17	35	52	70	88
1,250	14	28	42	56	70
1,500	12	23	35	46	58

energy intake through dieting and an increase in energy expenditure through exercise. However, your body-weight losses may often be different from what you expect them to be. Thus, it is important for you to understand what may be happening in your body so you do not become discouraged during periods when you are not losing body weight but are still dieting and exercising. This section deals with predicting your body-weight losses, the variation in the rate of weight loss during different phases of your program, and a comparison of the values of dieting versus exercise.

Prediction of Weight Loss

The human body is compartmentalized into body fat and lean body mass. Because of this, it is difficult to predict exactly how much body weight one will lose on any given diet, but an approximate value may be obtained. Remember, weight loss may reflect decreases in body fat, body water, or muscle mass.

For our purposes, we will use the value of 3,500 Calories to represent 1 pound of body fat loss. In order to lose 1 pound of body fat, you must create a 3,500 Calorie deficit. Thus, you must be aware of both your caloric intake and your caloric expenditure. The caloric intake reflects your dietary restrictions, while your caloric expenditure involves your resting energy expenditure and your normal activities, including exercise. Laboratory Inventory 7.4 presents some guidelines to create a deficit of 1,000 Calories per day, but this may be adjusted to other levels, such as 500, 700, 1,200, and so forth.

Table 7.13 illustrates the importance of the caloric deficit in determining the rapidity of weight loss by dieting. The higher the deficit, the faster you lose weight. You should recall, though, that no more than 2 pounds per week should be lost without medical supervision. Also, if you want to maintain a constant caloric deficit, you will have to decrease your caloric intake as you lose body weight. This point is discussed further in the following section.

Although these prediction methods are good for the long run, daily body-weight changes may not coincide with daily caloric deficits. The rate of weight loss may vary considerably during different stages of your program.

Rate of Body-Weight Losses

The rate at which you lose weight may vary somewhat during different phases of your weight-control program and may be partially dependent on the method you use to lose weight—diet or exercise.

Dieting and Rate of Weight Loss

If you start a diet with a significant caloric deficit, say 1,000 Calories/day, it would normally take about 3½ days to lose 1 pound of body fat. However, body-weight loss would be more rapid during the first several days, possibly totaling as much as 3 to 4 pounds. A large percentage of this weight loss would be due to a decrease in body carbohydrate and water stores. When you restrict your food intake, the body draws on its reserves to meet its energy needs. These reserves consist of both fat and carbohydrate stores, but much of the carbohydrate, stored as liver and muscle glycogen, could be used up in a day or so. Since each gram of glycogen is stored with about 3 grams of water, a significant weight loss could occur. For example, 300 grams of glycogen along with 900 grams of water stored with it, would account for a loss of 1,200 grams, or 1.2 kg; this would equal over 2½ pounds alone. About 70 percent of the weight loss during the first few days of a reduced-Calorie diet is due to body water losses. About 25 percent comes from body fat stores and 5 percent from glycogen and protein tissue. It is important to keep in mind that rather large fluctuations in daily body weight (2 to 3 pounds) are not due to rapid changes in body fat or lean body mass; these fluctuations are due primarily to body water changes.

Since water has no Calories, caloric loss during the first phase of your weight-control program does not need to total 3,500 in order to lose 1 pound of weight. You may lose 1 pound of body weight with a deficit of only about 1,200 Calories, since 70 percent of the weight loss is water. The 1,200 Calories are mostly from body fat, with a small amount from body protein. However, by the end of the second week of dieting, water loss may account for only about 20 percent of body-weight loss; 1 pound of weight loss will now cost you approximately 2,800 Calories. At the end of the third week, water losses are minimal. The energy deficit needed to lose 1 pound of body weight is now about 3,500 Calories. In essence, as you continue your diet, weight losses cost you more Calories since less body water is being lost. At the end of 3 weeks, you can still be losing weight, but at a much slower rate than during the early stages.

Another factor also slows down the rate of weight loss. As you lose weight, you need fewer Calories to maintain your new body weight. Let's take an example. Suppose you weigh 200 pounds, and from table 7.5 you see that you need 15 Calories/pound body weight to maintain your weight. At 200 pounds this represents 3,000 Calories/day (200 × 15). However, if your weight drops to 180 pounds after dieting for 2 months, you would need only 2,700 Calories (180 × 15) to maintain your weight, a difference of 300 Calories per day.

If you want to continue to have a standard caloric deficit, then you will have to adjust your caloric intake as you lose weight. Suppose at 200 pounds you wanted to have a daily caloric deficit of 1,000 Calories. Your diet should then contain about 2,000 Calories/day (3,000 − 1,000). However, once you are down to 180 pounds, your diet should now include only 1,700 Calories/day (2,700 − 1,000). If you did not adjust your diet from 2,000 Calories, then the daily deficit would only be 700 Calories/day, not the standard 1,000 you wanted. Weight loss would continue, but at a slower rate.

You should realize that the rate of weight loss decreases as a natural consequence of your diet, but the weight you are losing is now primarily body fat. To keep a standard caloric deficit may also require an additional reduction in caloric intake. Knowledge of these factors may help you through the latter stages of a diet designed to attain a set weight goal.

Very Low-Calorie Diets **Very low-Calorie diets (VLCD)** are defined technically as those containing fewer than 800 Calories, most commonly about 400–500 Calories, and are often referred to as modified fasts. In some medical institutions, total fasting programs are used. VLCD and other fasting programs should be used only after a thorough medical examination. Such programs are usually designed for individuals with substantial levels of obesity. The American Dietetic Association (ADA), in a position statement on VLCD, has noted that such diets should be regarded as being only one part, usually the first phase, of a comprehensive weight-management program. The ADA has also noted that VLCD are generally regarded as being safe and effective in inducing rapid weight loss in very obese patients if supervised by a physician and a registered dietician. However, the ADA and others state that there may be some contraindications to the use of VLCD, for a variety of complications may arise, including headaches, nausea, constipation, loss of libido, kidney stones, gallbladder disease, hypoglycemia, anemia, fatigue, cardiac arrhythmias, and even death. Because of these possible complications, one should be cautious to select a VLCD program that is supervised by qualified medical health professionals, for as Garrow has noted, "nutritional counselors" for some commercially available VLCD programs may not be as expert as suggested in advertisements.

VLCD are not recommended for the individual who is not obese but simply wants to lose 15–20 pounds, nor for the individual who is not under medical supervision, not only because of the possible adverse health consequences noted above, but also because they may be counterproductive to the ultimate goal of long-term weight loss. For one, these diets do not conform to the general principles of a sound diet mentioned earlier in this section. Moreover, research has revealed that VLCD may lead to a decreased resting energy expenditure because of a number of mechanisms, including a decrease in total body weight (including a significant amount of lean body mass), a decreased TEF related to the small amount of food consumed, and a decreased level of spontaneous physical activity throughout the day because of fatigue. In some studies, the REE decreased by 15–20 percent in the first week of a VLCD. In essence, your body is recognizing that it is being starved and will attempt to conserve body stores of energy by reducing energy output. It should be noted, however, that several studies with obese subjects have revealed that although the REE decreased on a short-term basis, it recovered partially following a long-term maintenance diet phase, when the caloric intake was adjusted to maintain the desired weight. Overall, although VLCD may be safe and effective for promoting short-term weight loss, they are not very satisfactory in long-term maintenance of weight loss and fare no better than other dietary approaches.

Weight Cycling   Not all studies are in agreement, but one of the problems associated with VLCD may be the loss of lean body mass. VLCD are usually low in carbohydrates, so a good proportion of the weight lost during these diets is protein, primarily from muscle tissue, which is catabolized to produce glucose for the brain. If you go off the diet and resume normal eating, the protein tissue is not readily replaced, so the extra Calories are likely to be converted to fat. Moreover, resumption of normal eating habits may lead to binge eating, episodes in which large amounts of Calories are consumed. A vicious cycle may develop, with repeated bouts of weight loss followed by weight gain, leading to increased amounts of body fat at the same body weight. An individual who engages in this **weight cycling,** also known as the yo-yo syndrome, may start out at 200 pounds with 30 percent body fat and, after several cycles, eventually return to the same weight but at 35 percent body fat. However, more current research with both animals and humans suggests this may not be the case, and Prentice and others concluded, in a recent review, that weight cycling exerts no adverse effects on body composition. Earlier research had also suggested that obese subjects who repeatedly lose and gain weight are at an increased risk for cardiovascular disease compared to obese subjects whose weight remains stable. Not all data are in agreement however, and a recent meta-analysis indicated weight cycling may not increase health risks as previously believed and should not deter individuals from attempting to lose weight. Nevertheless, the debate over the health risks of weight cycling continues.

Exercise and Rate of Weight Loss

Many individuals are disappointed during the early stage of an exercise program because they do not lose weight very rapidly. Unless they understand what is happening in their body, the results on the scale may convince them that exercise is not an effective means to reduce weight, and they may quit exercising altogether. Let's look at several reasons that an individual may not lose weight during the early stages of a weight-reduction program, and also why it becomes more difficult to lose weight after some weight loss has occurred.

When a sedentary individual begins a daily exercise program, the body reacts to the exercise stress and changes so it can more easily handle the demands of exercise:

1. The muscles may increase in size because of hypertrophy of the muscle cells. The increased protein will hold more water.

2. Certain structures within the muscle cell that process oxygen (mitochondria), along with numerous enzymes involved in oxygen use, will increase in quantity.

3. Energy substances in the cell will increase, particularly glycogen, and will bind water.

4. The connective tissue will toughen and thicken.

5. The total blood volume may increase. An increase of approximately 500 milliliters, or about a pound, has been recorded in one week.

At the same time, body fat stores begin to diminish as fat is used as a source of energy for exercise. Overall, there is an increase in the lean body mass and body water and a decrease in body fat. These changes may counterbalance each other and the individual may not lose any weight. However, although little or no weight is lost during these early phases, the body composition changes are favorable. Body fat is being lost (see fig. 7.12).

Once these adaptive changes have occurred (usually in about a month), body weight should decrease in relationship to the number of Calories spent through exercise. Keep in mind that weight loss is slow on an exercise program, but if you can build up to an exercise energy expenditure of about 300 Calories per day, about 2½ pounds per month will be exercised away.

After several months you may begin to notice that your body weight has stabilized even though you continue to exercise and have not reached your weight goal. Part of the reason may be due to your lower body weight. If you look at Appendix C, you can see that the less you weigh, the fewer Calories you burn for any given exercise. If you have been doing the same amount of exercise all along, you may now be at the body weight where your energy output is matched by your energy input in food; your body weight has stabilized. In addition you may be more skilled, and hence more efficient in your physical activity. Fewer Calories may then be expended for any given amount of time. However, this is usually true only of activities that involve a skill factor. It can be highly significant in swimming, but not as great in jogging.

In summary, your body weight may not change during the early stages of an exercise program; it may then begin to drop during a second stage and plateau at the third stage. If you are aware of these possible stages, your adherence to an exercise program may be enhanced. Also, if you desire to lose more weight by exercise during the third stage, the amount of exercise must be increased.

One last point should be made before leaving this section. A very rapid weight loss may occur during exercise. Some individuals have lost as much as 10 to 12 pounds in an hour or so. As you probably suspect, this weight loss may be attributed to body water losses. This is particularly evident while exercising in warm or hot weather. The weight loss is temporary; under normal food and water intake, the body water content will return to normal within a day. In the heat of summer, you may occasionally see individuals training

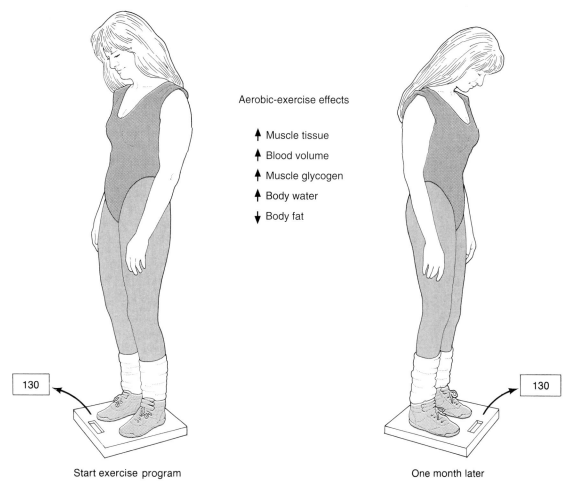

Aerobic-exercise effects

↑ Muscle tissue
↑ Blood volume
↑ Muscle glycogen
↑ Body water
↓ Body fat

130

130

Start exercise program

One month later

Figure 7.12 *Body weight may not change much during the beginning phases of an aerobic exercise program. However, body composition may change. The exercise stimulates an increase in muscle tissue, blood volume, and muscle glycogen stores, which tend to increase weight. Body fat is reduced, but the increases in the other components can balance out the fat losses with no net loss of body weight. Eventually, body weight begins to drop as the exercise program is continued.*

with heavy sweat clothes or a rubberized suit. The reason often given is to lose more body weight. They will lose more body weight, but again it will be body water and will be regained as soon as they drink fluids. In this regard, the technique is worthless. Moreover, it may predispose the individual to unusually high heat stress and may cause severe medical problems.

Dieting Versus Exercise for Weight Control

By now you may be wondering which is better for weight control—diet or exercise. Most major health-related organizations such as the American Dietetic Association (ADA) and the American College of Sports Medicine (ACSM) recommend a comprehensive weight-control program that involves both a dietary and an exercise regimen and supportive behavioral modification techniques. The principles of developing such a program have been presented earlier in this chapter.

Dieting alone or exercise alone may be effective means to reduce body fat, but both techniques have certain advantages

and disadvantages and it appears that the advantages of one technique help to counterbalance the disadvantages of the other. Dieting will contribute to a negative caloric balance and may help produce a rapid weight loss during the early stages of the program. However, some of this weight loss will be lean body mass, such as muscle tissue; moreover, very low-Calorie diets may lead to decreases in the REE. On the other hand, exercise usually results in a slower rate of weight loss. But, as noted previously, exercise mobilizes fatty acids from the adipose tissue and thus produces greater proportions of body fat loss than dieting. Weight loss by exercise alone can help preserve the lean body mass and the REE; when diet and exercise are combined to lose weight, some loss in lean body mass occurs, but exercise minimizes the loss and the decrease in the REE seen with diet alone. As noted previously, in addition to aerobic exercise, resistive exercise training may be a valuable adjunct to a weight-loss program as a means to help maintain lean body mass. Several recent studies in men, women, and adolescents have shown that weight loss via dieting and exercise will preferentially decrease fat from the abdominal area. A combined diet-exercise program may help to reduce

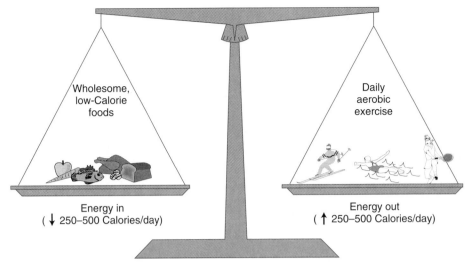

Figure 7.13 *The most effective weight-reduction program involves both dieting and exercise. Mild caloric restriction and an aerobic exercise program can be effectively combined to lose 1–2 pounds per week.*

gynoid-type obesity, but the pear-shape figure appears to be more resistant to change compared to the apple type. Dieting and exercise may also interact to maximize other health benefits. For example, weight loss by dieting helps decrease total cholesterol, but HDL-cholesterol (the good cholesterol) may also fall. Exercise helps to increase HDL-cholesterol and may help to prevent the decline seen with dieting alone.

Exercise complements dieting in other ways. For example, exercise may be used to curb the appetite at an appropriate time. Exercise raises the body temperature and stimulates the secretion of several hormones (notably adrenalin) in the body; both of these conditions, it has been hypothesized, depress the appetite for a short time afterwards. If you exercise before a meal, your food intake may be reduced considerably. Try it and see if it works for you. If you have the facilities available, a good 30 minutes of exercise may be an effective substitute for a large lunch. You may lose Calories two ways, expending them through exercise and replacing the large lunch with a low-Calorie nutritious snack. Although exercise may be an effective means to suppress the appetite on a short-term basis, it may not be as effective on a long-term basis. Thus, it may help curb your appetite at lunch, but unless you are cautious you may increase your caloric intake above normal at dinner.

A dietary reduction of 500 Calories per day along with an exercise energy expenditure of 500 Calories per day, could lead to approximately 2 pounds of weight loss per week—the maximal amount recommended unless under medical supervision. The removal of 500 Calories from the typical American diet could be done immediately by removing some excess sugar and fat, but it may take a month or more before you may be able to exercise enough to use 500 Calories daily. By following the principles for developing an aerobic exercise program outlined in chapter 3, you should be able to reach that exercise level safely (fig. 7.13).

Once you have reached the body-weight level you want, a proper exercise program will help keep you there. It is generally recognized that prevention of obesity or excess body weight is more effective than treatment. Most people do not become overweight overnight, but rather accumulate an extra 75 to 150 Calories per day, which over time will lead to excess fat tissue. A daily exercise program could easily counteract the effect of these additional Calories. In three recent reviews, King and Tribble, Phinney, and Safer all indicated that exercise exerted a strong influence on long-term preservation of weight loss. For those who like to eat but not gain weight, exercise is the intelligent alternative.

Changing your diet by reducing Calories, saturated fats, and cholesterol, by eating more nutritious foods, and by initiating and continuing a good aerobic endurance exercise program are considered to be several of the most important components of a Positive Health Life-style. These life-style changes complement each other nicely, both for helping you maintain a proper body weight and for prevention of other health problems noted previously.

Gaining Body Weight

The major focus of this chapter has been on how to lose or maintain body weight. However, a small segment of the population (less than 10 percent) is considerably underweight for one reason or another. Both males and females may suffer from psychological problems associated with a poor body image if they are too skinny. For example, although the current social attitude stresses leanness in females, some degree of curvature is desirable. Also, most males desire a muscular body because it is, well, masculine. Research with college-aged males revealed an improved body image and self-concept following a resistance-training program designed to increase muscle mass.

The energy balance equation, as you may recall, is the basis for weight control. A negative caloric balance results in a weight loss, preferably a loss of body fat and not lean body mass. A positive caloric balance results in a weight gain. In order to increase your body weight and still be in accord with

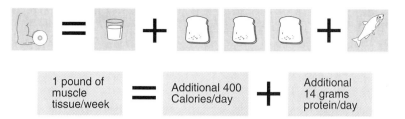

Figure 7.14 *In order to add a pound of muscle tissue per week, you need to consume approximately 400 additional Calories and 14 grams of additional protein per day. A weight-training program is an essential part of a muscle-building program. One glass of skim milk, three slices of whole wheat bread, and one ounce of lean meat provide the necessary Calories and about 24 grams of protein.*

a Positive Health Life-style, the weight gain should be lean body mass and not body fat. As diet and exercise are the two mechanisms to create a weight loss, they are also the main means to increase body weight. The diet must be higher in Calories and still conform to healthful eating, while the exercise program should be one designed to increase muscle mass.

Before looking at dietary and exercise principles to gain body weight, the cause of being underweight in the first place should be determined because numerous factors may be involved. Heredity may be an important factor, as your parents' genetic material may have predisposed their children toward leanness. For example, a high basal metabolic rate may have been acquired through your parents. Medical problems could adversely affect food intake and digestion, so a physician should be consulted to rule out nutritional problems caused by organic disease, hormonal imbalance, or inadequate absorption of nutrients. Social pressures, such as the strong desire of a teenage girl to have a slender body, could lead to undernutrition—an extreme example is anorexia nervosa, discussed in chapter 10. Emotional problems also may affect food intake. In many cases, food intake is increased during periods of emotional crisis, but the appetite may also be depressed in some individuals for long periods. Economic hardships may reduce food purchasing power, so some individuals simply may sacrifice food intake for other life necessities.

Being considerably underweight, such as 10 percent below the standard height-weight tables or a Body Mass Index below 19, may be considered a symptom of malnutrition or undernutrition. It is important to determine the cause before prescribing a treatment. Our concern here is with the individual who does not have any of these medical, psychological, social, or economic problems, but who simply cannot create a positive energy balance because of excess energy expenditure or insufficient energy (Calorie) intake. Caloric intake has to be increased, and the output has to be modified somewhat.

Dietary and Exercise Considerations for Gaining Body Weight

If you decide to initiate a weight gaining program, the following guidelines may help you develop an effective program to maximize your gains in muscle mass and keep body-fat increases relatively low.

1. Have an acceptable purpose for the weight gain. The desire for an improved physical appearance and body image may be reason enough. For athletes, increased muscle mass may be important for a variety of sports, particularly if strength and power are improved.

2. Calculate your average Calorie and protein needs daily. The key to gaining weight is to create a positive energy balance; if you accumulate an additional 3,500 Calories, then about 1 pound of body fat will be formed. But you are interested in increasing your muscle mass, not your body fat content. Muscle tissue consists of about 70 percent water, 22 percent protein, and the remainder primarily fat and carbohydrate. The total caloric value of muscle tissue is only about 700 to 800 per pound, but extra energy is needed to help synthesize the muscle tissue. It is not known exactly how many additional Calories are necessary to form 1 pound of muscle tissue in human beings, nor is it known in what form these Calories have to be consumed. However, literature suggests that approximately 2,500 to 3,000 additional Calories are necessary to synthesize 1 pound of body protein. This averages out to an additional 400 Calories per day in order to gain a pound of muscle tissue per week. Laboratory Inventory 7.3 will help you determine your daily energy expenditure now and may be used in conjunction with Laboratory Inventory 7.6 to determine your daily caloric intake necessary for a weight gain of about 1 pound per week. If you have already completed Laboratory Inventory 7.3, and if you already are doing both aerobic and resistance exercise training, all you need to do is add about 400 to 500 Calories per day to your daily caloric needs.

   Besides increasing your caloric intake, you may also need to assure that you are obtaining sufficient protein in your diet. Let us calculate how much protein is needed for someone undertaking a weight-gaining program to add one pound of muscle tissue per week (fig. 7.14). One pound of muscle is equal to 454 grams, but only about 22 percent of this tissue, or about 100 grams (454 × .22), is protein; the remainder is primarily water (with a small amount of lipids and carbohydrates). If we divide 100 grams by 7 days, we would need approximately 14 grams of protein per day above our normal protein requirements, if we are in protein balance. Fourteen grams of protein can be obtained in such small amounts of food as two glasses of milk or about two ounces of meat, fish, cheese, or poultry. The RDA for protein is 0.8 grams per kilogram body weight. For a 70 kg male, this would be 56 grams of protein per day (0.8×70 kg). Adding 14 grams would come to a total of 70 grams of protein per day. However, some research suggests that protein requirements may increase to about 1.2 to 1.6 grams per kilogram body weight for individuals initiating a resistance training program designed to increase muscle mass. For our 70 kg male, this would approximate 84 to 112 grams of protein per day. The average American diet contains approximately 100 grams of protein per day, which is probably enough to meet the protein requirements for someone attempting to gain body weight, even in the early stages of resistance training. For individuals of smaller or larger body size, their caloric intakes would vary accordingly and would satisfy protein requirements.

Laboratory Inventory 6.1 will provide you with data relative to the protein content of your diet.

3. Keep a three- to seven-day record of what you normally eat. Laboratory Inventory 6.1 will provide you with appropriate data if you expand it to three or seven days, and as noted, computerized dietary analysis will facilitate completion of this laboratory. If your daily caloric and protein intake is less than your energy needs calculated above, this may be the reason why you are not gaining weight.

4. Check your living habits. Do you get enough rest and sleep? If not, you may be burning more energy than the normal individual. Smoking increases your metabolic rate almost 10 percent and may account for approximately 200 Calories per day. Caffeine in coffee and soft drinks also increases the metabolic rate for several hours. Getting enough rest and sleep and eliminating smoking and caffeine will help decrease your energy output.

5. Set a reasonable goal within a certain time period. In general, about 1 pound per week is a sound approach once you have acquired some basic strength training. However, weight gaining is difficult for some individuals and may occur at a slower rate. Specific goals may also include muscular hypertrophy in various parts of the body.

6. Adjust your diet. Before you initiate changes in your diet to gain weight, you should review the major points in chapter 6. The basic principles of nutrition are as relevant to those attempting to gain weight as they are to those who desire to maintain or lose weight. The major adjustments to the diet include an increased caloric intake and assurance that you are obtaining adequate amounts of dietary protein.

In order to increase your caloric intake, follow the basic recommendations for food selection from the Exchange Lists as presented in the last two chapters, and then simply increase the amount of food you eat. After you have calculated your caloric needs from Laboratory Inventory 7.6, consult table 7.8 for the number of servings from each Exchange List. For example, if you need 3,600 Calories per day, simply double the number of exchanges from the 1,800 Calorie diet. This will provide you with the additional Calories you need, yet give you a balanced diet across the food groups.

As with losing weight, the Food Exchange System may serve as the basis for a sound weight-gaining diet. Foods must be selected that are high in nutrient value and high in calories. Total fat, saturated fat, and cholesterol intake should be minimized. The following suggestions may be helpful for those trying to gain weight:

- Milk exchange. Drink 1% or 2% milk instead of skim milk. This will add 15 to 30 Calories per glass. Prepare milk shakes with dry milk powder and supplement with fruit. Add low-fat cheeses to sandwiches or snacks. Eat yogurt supplemented with fruit. The milk exchange is high in protein.
- Meat exchange. Increase your intake of lean meats, poultry, and fish. Legumes such as beans and dried peas are high in protein and Calories and low in fat. Use nuts, seeds, and limited amounts of peanut butter for snacks. The meat exchange is also high in protein.
- Starch/bread exchange. Increase your consumption of whole-grain products. Pasta and rice are nutritious side dishes that provide adequate Calories. Starchy vegetables like potatoes are also nutritious sources of Calories. Breads and muffins can possibly be supplemented with fruits and nuts. Whole-grain breakfast cereals can provide substantial Calories and even make a tasty dessert or snack with added fruit. The starch/bread exchange is high in complex carbohydrates and contains about 15 percent of its Calories as protein.
- Fruit exchange. Add fruit to other food exchanges. Drink more fruit juices, which are high in both Calories and nutrients. Dried fruit such as apricots, pineapple, dates, and raisins make excellent high-Calorie snacks.
- Vegetable exchange. Use fresh vegetables like broccoli and cauliflower as snacks with melted low-fat cheese or a nutritious dip.
- Fat exchange. Try to minimize the intake of saturated fats, using monounsaturated and polyunsaturated fats instead. Salad dressings and margarine added to vegetables can increase their caloric content.
- Beverages. Milk and juices are nutritious and high in Calories. Some liquid supplements are available commercially and may contain 300 to 400 Calories with substantial amounts of protein. However, check the label for fat and sugar content.
- Snacks. Eat three balanced meals per day; supplement the meals with two or three snacks. Dried fruit, nuts, and seeds are excellent snacks. Some of the high-Calorie, high-nutrient liquid meals on the market also make good snacks; although convenient, they are relatively expensive.

Table 7.14 A High-Calorie Diet Based on the Food Exchange System

Exchange		Calories
	Breakfast	
Milk	8 ounces 2% milk	120
Meat	1 poached egg	80
	2 ounces lean ham	110
Starch/bread	2 slices whole wheat toast	160
Fruit	8 ounces of orange juice	120
Other	1 tablespoon jelly	50
	Mid-morning Snack	
Fruit	8 ounces apricot nectar	160
Starch/bread	2 slices whole wheat	160
Meat	1 tablespoon peanut butter	100
	Lunch	
Milk	8 ounces 2% milk	120
Meat	4 ounces lean sandwich meat	220
Starch/bread	2 slices whole wheat	160
	2 granola cookies	100
Fruit	1 banana	120
Vegetable	1 order french fries	300
	Afternoon Snack	
Fruit	¼ cup raisins	120
	Dinner	
Milk	8 ounces 2% milk	120
Meat	5 ounces chicken breast	275
Starch/bread	2 slices whole wheat bread	160
Fruit	1 piece apple pie	350
Vegetable	1 cup peas	160
	1 sweet potato, candied	300
	Evening Snack	
Fruit	½ cup dried peaches	210
Milk	8 ounces 2% milk with banana	240
Total		4,015

From Melvin H. Williams, Nutrition for Fitness and Sport, *3rd ed. Copyright © 1992 Wm. C. Brown Publishers, Dubuque, Iowa. All Rights Reserved. Reprinted by permission.*

Table 7.14 presents an example of a high-Calorie diet plan based upon the Food Exchange System. It consists of three main meals and three snacks and totals about 4,000 Calories with 160 grams of protein (16 percent of the Calories). It is also high in carbohydrate which may increase insulin release, facilitating amino acid transport into the muscle to help promote protein synthesis. Carbohydrate also spares the use of protein as an energy source. Alternate foods may be substituted from the food exchange list presented in Appendix A. This suggested diet provides the necessary nutrients, Calories, and protein essential to increased development of muscle mass and yet less than 30 percent of the Calories are derived from fat. The total number of Calories can be adjusted to meet individual needs as calculated in Laboratory Inventory 7.6.

From a health standpoint, probably the most important consideration in developing a high-Calorie diet is to keep the fat content, particularly saturated fat, as low as feasible. If there is a history of heart disease in the family or if an individual is known to have high blood lipid levels, then diets with increased levels of fat may be contraindicated. Individuals with kidney

problems may also have difficulty processing high-protein diets due to the increased need to excrete urea. Any person initiating such a weight-gaining program should be aware of his or her medical history.

Selection of food for a weight-gaining diet, if done wisely, can satisfy the criteria for healthful nutrition. Foods high in complex carbohydrates with moderate amounts of protein and a low fat content are able to provide substantial amounts of Calories and nutrients and yet minimize health risks associated with the typical American diet. To gain weight wisely, continue to eat healthful foods, but just more of them.

7. Start a resistance exercise training program, but also include some aerobic exercise in your weekly regimen. In order to stimulate the development of muscle mass during a weight-gaining program, you need to exercise with weights. Proper resistance-training programs, particularly if used in conjunction with a high-Calorie diet, may be designed to produce increases in body weight through increased muscle mass and some loss of body fat. Although exercise does cost Calories, the amount expended during resistance training is relatively small. In any resistance-training workout, the amount of time actually spent lifting the weights is not great enough to use substantial numbers of Calories. For example, in an hour workout, only about 10 to 15 minutes may be involved in actual exercise, the remaining time being recovery between exercises. Although resistance-training can be a high-intensity exercise, the duration is usually short, which limits the number of Calories used (usually in the range of 200 to 250 per workout).

Although resistance-training is primarily recommended as a means to gain muscle mass, body weight, and strength, it may also confer some other physiological benefits as well. Accumulating evidence suggests that both the traditional and circuit types of weight training may increase $\dot{V}O_{2MAX}$ and improve cardiovascular efficiency both at rest and during exercise. Studies also have reported improvement in several risk factors associated with coronary heart disease, such as increased levels of HDL_2 cholesterol and improved glucose tolerance. These findings are contrary to the belief that resistance-training does not confer any health benefits comparable to aerobic exercise; it does, but just not as much.

Therefore, it still appears to be prudent health behavior to incorporate some aerobic exercise into your life-style, even when trying to gain weight. To be sure, aerobic-exercise programs do consume more Calories, so you would have to balance the expenditure with increased food intake. However, the expenditure does not need to be excessive in order to get a beneficial training effect. For example, running 2 to 3 miles about four days per week would provide you with an adequate training effect for your heart, but it would only cost you about

200 to 300 Calories per day. This 200- to 300-Calorie expenditure could be replaced easily by consuming two glasses of orange juice or similar small amounts of food.

To design your resistance-training program, simply follow the principles discussed in chapter 4. The basic program described in that chapter covers most of the major muscle groups in the body. If you desire to incorporate an aerobics component in your workout, you may wish to develop a program of circuit aerobics, which involves alternating aerobic and resistance-training exercises in order to achieve both aerobic and muscular benefits.

8. Use a good cloth or steel tape to take body measurements before and during your weight-gaining program. Be sure you measure at the same points about once a week. Those body parts measured should include the neck, upper and lower arm, chest, abdomen, hips, thigh, and calf. This is to ensure that body weight gains are proportionately distributed. You should look for good gains in the chest and limbs; the abdominal and hip girth increase should be kept low because that is where the fat is more likely to be stored.

In summary, adequate rest, increased caloric intake, and a proper resistance training program may be very effective as a means to gain the right kind of body weight. Commercial protein supplements, including individual amino acids, have not been found to be effective as a means to enhance muscle growth. Although some individuals have successfully used anabolic steroids in order to gain muscle mass, the use of drugs may pose some rather serious short-term and long-term health consequences. A discussion of anabolic steroids is presented in chapter 9, which is about risky health behaviors.

References
Books

American Diabetes Association and American Dietetic Association. 1986. *Exchange lists for meal planning.* Chicago: American Dietetic Association and American Diabetes Association.

Bouchard, C., et al. 1994. *Physical activity, fitness, and health.* Champaign, Ill.: Human Kinetics.

Brownell, K., et al., eds. 1992. *Eating, body weight and performance in athletes: Disorders of modern society.* Philadelphia, Pa.: Lea & Febiger.

Cooper, K. 1982. *The aerobics program for total well-being.* New York: M. Evans.

Dusek, D. 1989. *Weight management: The fitness way.* Boston: Jones and Bartlett Publishers.

Fleck, S., and W. Kraemer. 1988. *Designing resistance training programs.* Champaign, Ill.: Life Enhancement Publications.

Food and Nutrition Board. National Research Council. 1989. *Recommended dietary allowances.* Washington, D.C.: National Academy of Sciences.

Hunt, S., and J. Groff. 1990. *Advanced nutrition and human metabolism.* St. Paul: West Publishing.

Logue, A. 1986. *The psychology of eating and drinking.* New York: W. H. Freeman.

Lohman, T., et al. 1988. *Anthropometric standardization reference manual.* Champaign, Ill.: Human Kinetics Books.

Mahoney, M., and K. Mahoney. 1970. *Permanent weight control: The total solution to the dieter's dilemma.* New York: Norton.

National Research Council. 1989. *Diet and health: Implications for reducing chronic disease risk.* Washington, D.C.: National Academy Press.

Shils, M., et al. 1994. *Modern nutrition in health and disease.* Philadelphia: Lea & Febiger.

Simopoulos, A., ed. 1992. *Metabolic control of eating, energy expenditure and the bioenergetics of obesity.* Basel, Switzerland: Karger.

Stamford, B., and P. Shimer. 1990. *Fitness without exercise.* New York: Warner Books.

U.S. Department of Health and Human Services. Public Health Service. 1991. *Healthy people 2000.* Washington, D.C.: U.S. Government Printing Office.

Williams, M. 1995. *Nutrition for fitness and sport.* Dubuque, Iowa: Brown & Benchmark Publishers.

Yates, A. 1991. *Compulsive exercise and the eating disorders.* New York, N.Y.: Brunner/Mazel.

Reviews

Ailhaud, G., et al. 1992. A molecular view of adipose tissue. *International Journal of Obesity* 16:S17–S21.

Ainsworth, B. 1993. Compendium of physical activities: Classification of energy costs of human physical activities. *Medicine and Science in Sports and Exercise* 25:71–80.

American College of Sports Medicine. 1983. Proper and improper weight loss programs. *Medicine and Science in Sports and Exercise* 15:ix–xiii.

American College of Sports Medicine. 1990. ACSM position stand: The recommended quantity and quality of exercise for developing and maintaining cardiorespiratory and muscular fitness in healthy adults. *Medicine and Science in Sports and Exercise.* 22:265–74.

American Dietetic Association. 1989. Position of the American Dietetic Association: Optimal weight as a health promotion strategy. *Journal of the American Dietetic Association* 89:1814–17.

American Dietetic Association. 1990. Position of the American Dietetic Association: Very-low-Calorie weight-loss diets. *Journal of the American Dietetic Association* 90:722–26.

American Dietetic Association. 1992. Position of the American Dietetic Association: Fat replacements. *ADA Reports* 91:1285–88.

American Heart Association Scientific Council. 1992. Position statement on exercise. Benefits and recommendations for physical activity programs for all Americans. *Circulation* 86:340–44.

American Institute of Nutrition. 1994. Report of the American Institute of Nutrition (AIN) steering committee on healthy weight. *Journal of Nutrition* 124:2240–43.

Ashwell, M. 1992. Why do people get fat: Is adipose tissue guilty? *Proceedings of the Nutrition Society* 51:353–65.

Atkinson, R. 1992. Treatment of obesity. *Nutrition Reviews* 50:338–45.

Bartels, R. 1992. Weight training. How to lift-and eat-for strength and power. *Physician and Sportsmedicine* 20 (March): 233–34.

Berdanier, C., and M. McIntosh. 1991. Weight loss—weight regain. A vicious cycle. *Nutrition Today* 26 (September/October): 6–12.

Berggren, R. 1990. Liposuction. What it will and won't do. *Postgraduate Medicine* 87:187–95.

Bjorntorp, P. 1992. Abdominal fat distribution and the metabolic syndrome. *Journal of Cardiovascular Pharmacology* 20:S26–S28.

Blair, S. 1993. Evidence for success of exercise in weight loss and control. *Annals of Internal Medicine* 119:702–6.

Bouchard, C. 1991. Heredity and the path to overweight and obesity. *Medicine and Science in Sports and Exercise* 23:285–91.

Bray, G. 1991. Treatment for obesity: A nutrient balance/nutrient partition approach. *Nutrition Reviews* 49:33–45.

Bray, G. 1993. The nutrient balance approach to obesity. *Nutrition Today* 28 (May/June): 13–18.

Brownell, K., and F. Kramer. 1989. Behavioral management of obesity. *Medical Clinics of North America* 73:185–202.

Calles-Escandon, J., and E. Horton. 1992. The thermogenic role of exercise in the treatment of morbid obesity: A critical evaluation. *American Journal of Clinical Nutrition* 55:533S–537S.

Campaigne, B. 1990. Body fat distribution in females: Metabolic consequences and implications for weight loss. *Medicine and Science in Sports and Exercise* 22:291–97.

Ciliska, D. 1993. Women and obesity. Learning to live with it. 1993. *Canadian Family Physician* 39:145–52.

Clark, N. 1991. How to gain weight healthfully. *Physician and Sportsmedicine* 19 (September): 53–54.

Clark, N. 1994. Are you a slow burner? Set your metabolism in motion. *Physician and Sportsmedicine* 22 (January): 33–36.

Convertino, V. 1991. Blood volume: Its adaptation to endurance training. *Medicine and Science in Sports and Exercise* 23:1338–48.

Czajka-Narins, D., and E. Parham. 1990. Fear of fat: Attitudes towards obesity. *Nutrition Today* 25 (January/February): 26–32.

Dattilo, A. 1992. Dietary fat and its relationship to body weight. *Nutrition Today* 27 (January/February): 13–19.

Dattilo, A., and P. Kris-Etherton. 1992. Effects of weight reduction on blood lipids and lipoproteins: A meta-analysis. *American Journal of Clinical Nutrition* 56:320–28.

de Groot, L. 1995. Reduced physical activity and its association with obesity. *Nutrition Reviews* 53:11–13.

Donnelly, J., et al. 1991. Diet and body composition: Effect of very low calorie diets and exercise. *Sports Medicine* 12:237–49.

Donnelly, J. 1995. What research says about the treatment of obesity with exercise. *Research Consortium Newsletter* 17 (Winter): 3.

Dudley, G. 1988. Metabolic consequences of resistive-type exercise. *Medicine and Science in Sports and Exercise* 20:S158–S161.

Everhart, J. 1993. Contributions of obesity and weight loss to gallstone disease. *Annals of Internal Medicine* 119:1029–35.

Fisher, M., and P. Lachance. 1985. Nutrition evaluation of published weight-reducing diets. *Journal of the American Dietetic Association* 85:450–54.

Forbes, G. 1992. Exercise and lean weight: The influence of body weight. *Nutrition Reviews* 50:157–61.

Foreyt, J., and G. Goodrick. 1992. Potential impact of sugar and fat substitutes in American diet. *Monograph of the National Cancer Institute* 12:99–103.

Foreyt, J., and G. Goodrick. 1993. Weight management without dieting. *Nutrition Today* 28 (March/April): 4–9.

Garrow, J. 1989. Very low-calorie diets should not be used. *International Journal of Obesity* 13 (Supplement 2): 145–47.

Goodrick, G., and J. Foreyt. 1991. Why treatments for obesity don't last. *Journal of the American Dietetic Association* 91:1243–47.

Grodner, M. 1992. "Forever dieting": Chronic dieting syndrome. *Journal of Nutrition Education* 24:207–10.

Grubbs, L. 1993. The critical role of exercise in weight control. *Nurse Practitioner* 18:20–26.

Harris, R. 1990. Role of set-point theory in regulation of body weight. *FASEB Journal* 4:3310–18.

Hill, J., et al. 1993. Obesity treatment: Can diet composition play a role? *Annals of Internal Medicine* 119:694–97.

Houtkooper, L. 1986. Nutritional support for muscle weight gain. *National Strength Coaches Association Journal* 8:62–63.

Hyman, F., et al. 1993. Evidence for success of caloric restriction in weight loss and control. *Annals of Internal Medicine* 119:681–87.

Institutes of Food Technologists' Expert Panel on Food Safety and Nutrition. 1993. Human obesity. *Contemporary Nutrition* 18 (Number 7,8): 1–4.

James, W., et al. 1990. Metabolism and nutritional adaptation to altered intakes of energy substrates. *American Journal of Clinical Nutrition* 51:264–69.

King, A., and D. Tribble. 1991. The role of exercise in weight regulation in nonathletes. *Sports Medicine* 11:331–49.

Kirkland, L., and R. Anderson. 1993. Achieving healthy weights. *Canadian Family Physician* 39:157–62.

Kromhout, D. 1992. Dietary fats: Long-term implications for health. *Nutrition Reviews* 50:49–53.

Kushner, R. 1993. Body weight and mortality. *Nutrition Reviews* 51:127–36.

Leibel, R. 1992. Fat as fuel and metabolic signal. *Nutrition Reviews* 50:12–16.

Lucas, C., et al. 1993. Medically supervised weight loss. *Medicine, Exercise, Nutrition, and Health* 2:284–98.

Martin, A., and D. Drinkwater. 1991. Variability in the measures of body fat. Assumption or technique? *Sports Medicine* 11:277–88.

Mela, D. 1992. Nutritional implications of fat substitutes. *Journal of the American Dietetic Association* 92:472–76.

Miller, W. 1991. Clinical symposium: Obesity: Diet composition, energy expenditure, and treatment of the obese patient. *Medicine and Science in Sports and Exercise* 23:273–97.

Munnings, F. 1993. Strength training. Not only for the young. *Physician and Sportsmedicine* 21 (April): 133–40.

Munnings, F. 1994. Syndrome X. *Physician and Sportsmedicine* 22 (August): 63–66.

National Institutes of Health. 1992. Methods for voluntary weight loss and control. Technology Assessment Conference Statement. *Nutrition Today* 50 (July/August): 27–33.

National Task Force on the Prevention and Treatment of Obesity. 1993. Very low-calorie diets. *Journal of the American Medical Association* 270:967–74.

National Task Force on the Prevention and Treatment of Obesity. 1994. Weight cycling. *Journal of the American Medical Association* 272:1196–1202.

Pera, V., et al. 1992. Current treatment of obesity: A behavioral medicine perspective. *Rhode Island Medicine* 75:477–81.

Perri, M., et al. 1993. Strategies for improving maintenance of weight loss. Toward a continuous care model of obesity management. *Diabetes Care* 16:200–209.

Petersmarck, K. 1992. Building consensus for safe weight loss. *Journal of the American Dietetic Association* 92:679–80.

Phinney, S. 1992. Exercise during and after very-low-calorie dieting. *American Journal of Clinical Nutrition* 56:190S–194S.

Pi-Sunyer, F. X. 1987. Exercise effects on caloric intake. *Annals of the New York Academy of Science* 499:94–103.

Pi-Sunyer, F. X. 1990. Effect of the composition of the diet on energy intake. *Nutrition Reviews* 48:94–105.

Pi-Sunyer, F. X. 1991. Health implications of obesity. *American Journal of Clinical Nutrition* 53:1595S–1603S.

Pi-Sunyer, F. X. 1994. The fattening of America. *Journal of the American Medical Association* 272:238–39.

Poehlman, E. 1989. A review: Exercise and its influence on resting energy metabolism in man. *Medicine and Science in Sports and Exercise* 21:515–25.

Prentice, A., et al. 1992. Effects of weight cycling on body composition. *American Journal of Clinical Nutrition* 56:209S–216S.

Ravussin, E., and C. Bogardus. 1990. Energy expenditure in the obese: Is there a thrifty gene? *Infusionstherapie* 17:108–12.

Robison, J., et al. 1993. Obesity, weight loss, and health. *Journal of the American Dietetic Association* 93:445–49.

Rolls, B. 1991. Effects of intense sweeteners on hunger, food intake, and body weight: A review. *American Journal of Clinical Nutrition* 53:872–78.

Rolls, B., and D. Shide. 1992. The influence of dietary fat on food intake and body weight. *Nutrition Reviews* 50:283–90.

Roubenoff, R., and J. Kehayias. 1991. The meaning and measurement of lean body mass. *Nutrition Reviews* 49 (June): 163–72.

Safer, D. 1991. Diet, behavior modification, and exercise: A review of obesity treatments from a long-term perspective. *Southern Medical Journal* 84:1470–74.

Saris, W. 1993. The role of exercise in the dietary treatment of obesity. *International Journal of Obesity* 17:S17–S21.

Schlicker, S., et al. 1994. The weight and fitness status of United States children. *Nutrition Review* 52:11–17.

Seidell, J., et al. 1989. Overweight: Fat distribution and health risks. Epidemiological observations. A review. *Infusionstherapie* 16:276–81.

St. Jeor, S., et al. 1993. Obesity: Workshop III. *Circulation* 88:1391–96.

Stefanick, M. 1993. Exercise and weight control. *Exercise and Sport Sciences Review* 21:363–96.

Stock, M. 1989. Thermogenesis and brown fat: Relevance to human obesity. *Infusionstherapie* 16:282–84.

Stoll, B., and G. Secreto. 1992. New hormone-related markers of high risk to breast cancer. *Annals of Oncology* 3:435–38.

Stricker, E., and J. Verbalis. 1990. Control of appetite and satiety: Insights from biologic and behavioral studies. *Nutrition Reviews* 48:49–56.

Swinburn, B., and E. Ravussin. 1993. Energy balance or fat balance? *American Journal of Clinical Nutrition* 57:766S–771S.

Telch, C., and W. Agras. 1993. The effect of a very low calorie diet on binge eating. *Behavior Therapy* 24:177–93.

Vogel, J., and K. Friedl. 1992. Body fat assessment in women. *Sports Medicine* 13:245–69.

Wadden, T. 1993. Treatment of obesity by moderate and severe caloric restriction. Results of clinical research trials. *Annals of Internal Medicine* 119:688–93.

Wadden, T., and A. Stunkard. 1985. Social and psychological consequences of obesity. *Annals of Internal Medicine* 103:1062–67.

Weingarten, H. 1992. Determinants of food intake: Hunger and satiety. In *Eating, body weight, and performance in athletes: Disorders of modern society,* eds. K. Brownell, et al. Philadelphia, Pa.: Lea & Febiger.

Westover, S., and R. Lanyon. 1990. The maintenance of weight loss after behavioral treatment. A review. *Behavior Modification* 14:123–37.

Wilmore, J. 1992. Body weight and body composition. In *Eating, body weight, and performance in athletes: Disorders of modern society,* eds. K. Brownell, et al. Philadelphia, Pa.: Lea & Febiger.

Wilmore, J. 1994. Exercise, obesity, and weight control. *Physical Activity and Fitness Research Digest* 1 (May): 1–8.

Wurtman, J. 1993. Depression and weight gain: The serotonin connection. *Journal of Affective Disorders* 29:183–92.

York, D. 1990. Metabolic regulation of food intake. *Nutrition Reviews* 48:64–70.

Zierath, J., and H. Wallberg-Henriksson. 1992. Exercise training in obese diabetic patients. *Sports Medicine* 14:171–85.

Specific Studies

Abadie, B. 1990. Physiological responses to grade walking with wrist and hand-held weights. *Research Quarterly for Exercise and Sport* 61:93–95.

Atkinson, R., et al. 1992. Combination of very-low-calorie diet and behavior modification in the treatment of obesity. *American Journal of Clinical Nutrition* 56:199S–202S.

Ballor, D., and E. Poehlman. 1992. Resting metabolic rate and coronary-heart-disease risk factors in aerobically and resistance-trained women. *American Journal of Clinical Nutrition* 56:968–74.

Bernhauer, E., et al. 1989. Exercise reduces depressed metabolic rate produced by severe caloric restriction. *Medicine and Science in Sports and Exercise* 21:29–33.

Bouchard, C., et al. 1990. The response to long-term overfeeding in identical twins. *New England Journal of Medicine* 322:1477–82.

Brodie, D., and R. Eston. 1992. Body fat estimations by electrical impedance and infra-red interactance. *International Journal of Sports Medicine* 13:319–25.

Busetto, L., et al. 1992. Assessment of abdominal fat distribution in obese patients: Anthropometry versus computerized tomography. *International Journal of Obesity* 16:731–36.

Cabanac, M., and J. Morrissette. 1992. Acute, but not chronic, exercise lowers body weight set-point in male rats. *Physiology and Behavior* 52:1173–77.

Chesley, A., et al. 1992. Changes in human muscle protein synthesis after resistance exercise. *Journal of Applied Physiology* 73:1383–88.

Clark, R., et al. 1993. Prediction of percent body fat in adult males using dual energy x-ray absorptiometry, skinfolds, and hydrostatic weighing. *Medicine and Science in Sports and Exercise* 25:528–35.

Colvin, R., and S. Olson. 1983. A descriptive analysis of men and women who have lost significant weight and are highly successful at maintaining the loss. *Addictive Behaviors* 8:287–95.

DeBusk, R., et al. 1990. Training effects of long versus short bouts of exercise in healthy subjects. *American Journal of Cardiology* 65:1010–13.

Drewnowski, A., and D. Yee. 1987. Men and body image: Are males satisfied with their body weight. *Psychosomatic Medicine* 49:626–34.

Eckerson, J., et al. 1992. Validity of bioelectrical impedance equations for estimating fat-free weight in lean males. *Medicine and Science in Sports and Exercise* 24:1298–1302.

Eston, R., et al. 1992. Effect of very low calorie diet on body composition and exercise response in sedentary women. *European Journal of Applied Physiology* 65:452–58.

Folsom, A., et al. 1993. Body fat distribution and 5-year risk of death in older women. *Journal of the American Medical Association* 269:483–87.

Forbes, G. 1990. The abdomen:hip ratio. Normative data and observations on selected patients. *International Journal of Obesity* 14:149–57.

Forbes, G. 1991. Exercise and body composition. *Journal of Applied Physiology* 70:994–97.

Foster, G., et al. 1990. Controlled trial of the metabolic effects of a very low-calorie diet: Short- and long-term effects. *American Journal of Clinical Nutrition* 51:167–72.

Frey-Hewitt, B., et al. 1990. The effect of weight loss by dieting or exercise on resting metabolic rate in overweight men. *International Journal of Obesity* 14:327–34.

Fricker, J., et al. 1992. Underreporting of food intake in obese "small eaters." *Appetite* 19:273–83.

Hoie, L., et al. 1993. Reduction of body mass and change in body composition on a very low calorie diet. *International Journal of Obesity* 17:17–20.

Howley, E., and M. Glover. 1974. The caloric costs of running and walking one mile for men and women. *Medicine and Science in Sports* 6:235–37.

Jackson, A., et al. 1988. Reliability and validity of bioelectric impedance in determining body composition. *Journal of Applied Physiology* 64:529–34.

Jeffery, R., et al. 1992. Weight cycling and cardiovascular risk factors in obese men and women. *American Journal of Clinical Nutrition* 55:641–44.

Kaminsky, L., and M. Whaley. 1993. Differences in estimates of percent body fat using bioelectrical impedance. *Journal of Sports Medicine and Physical Fitness* 33:172–77.

Kanaley, J., et al. 1993. Differential health benefits of weight loss in upper-body and lower-body obese women. *American Journal of Clinical Nutrition* 57:20–26.

Kendall, A., et al. 1991. Weight loss on a low-fat diet: Consequence of the imprecision of the control of food intake in humans. *American Journal of Clinical Nutrition* 53:1124–29.

Kirkwood, S., et al. 1990. Spontaneous physical activity is a major determinant of 24-hour sedentary energy expenditure. *Medicine and Science in Sports and Exercise* 22:S49.

Kirschner, M., et al. 1990. Androgen-estrogen metabolism in women with upper body versus lower body obesity. *Journal of Clinical and Endocrinological Metabolism* 70:473–79.

Kissileff, H., et al. 1990. Acute effects of exercise on food intake in obese and nonobese women. *American Journal of Clinical Nutrition* 52:240–45.

Klesges, R., et al. 1993. Effects of television on metabolic rate: Potential implications for childhood obesity. *Pediatrics* 91:281–86.

Kohrt, W., et al. 1993. Insulin resistance in aging is related to abdominal obesity. *Diabetes* 42:273–81.

Kreitzman, S., et al. 1992. Glycogen storage: Illusions of easy weight loss, excessive weight regain, and distortions in estimates of body composition. *American Journal of Clinical Nutrition* 56:292S–293S.

Kuczmarski, R., et al. 1994. Increasing prevalence of overweight among U.S. adults. *Journal of the American Medical Association* 272:205–11.

Kune, G., et al. 1990. Body weight and physical activity as predictors of colorectal cancer risk. *Nutrition and Cancer* 13:9–17.

Lee, I., and R. Paffenbarger, Jr. 1992. Change in body weight and longevity. *Journal of the American Medical Association* 268:2045–49.

Leenen, R., et al. 1992. Visceral fat accumulation in obese subjects: Relation to energy expenditure and response to weight loss. *American Journal of Physiology* 263:E913–919.

Leibel, R., et al. 1995. Changes in energy expenditure resulting from altered body weight. *New England Journal of Medicine* 332:621–28.

Lemon, P., et al. 1992. Protein requirements and muscle mass/strength changes during intensive training in novice bodybuilders. *Journal of Applied Physiology* 73:767–75.

Levy, A., and A. Heaton. 1993. Weight control practices of U.S. adults trying to lose weight. *Annals of Internal Medicine* 119:661–66.

Lissner, L., et al. 1991. Variability of body weight and health outcomes in the Framingham population. *New England Journal of Medicine* 324:1839–44.

Lotti, T., et al. 1990. Proteoglycans in so-called cellulite. *International Journal of Dermatology* 29:272–74.

Marin, P., et al. 1992. The morphology and metabolism of intraabdominal adipose tissue in men. *Metabolism* 41:1242–48.

Mattes, R. 1993. Fat preference and adherence to a reduced-fat diet. *American Journal of Clinical Nutrition* 57:373–81.

Maughan, R. 1993. An evaluation of a bioelectrical impedance analyzer for the estimation of body fat content. *British Journal of Sports Medicine* 27:63–66.

Miller, W., et al. 1993. Successful weight loss in a self-taught, self-administered program. *International Journal of Sports Medicine* 14:401–5.

Mole, P., et al. 1989. Exercise reverses depressed metabolic rate produced by severe caloric restriction. *Medicine and Science in Sports and Exercise* 21:29–33.

Newman, B., et al. 1990. Nongenetic influences of obesity on other cardiovascular disease risk factors: An analysis of identical twins. *American Journal of Public Health* 80:675–78.

Pamuk, E., et al. 1992. Weight loss and mortality in a national cohort of adults, 1971–1987. *American Journal of Epidemiology* 136:686–97.

Peterson, S., et al. 1989. The influence of high-velocity circuit resistance training on $\dot{V}O_{2max}$ and cardiac output. *Canadian Journal of Sport Sciences* 14:158–63.

Poehlman, E., et al. 1992. Resting energy metabolism and cardiovascular disease risk in resistance-trained and aerobically trained males. *Metabolism* 41:1351–60.

Prineas, R., et al. 1993. Central adiposity and increased risk of coronary artery disease mortality in older women. *Annals of Epidemiology* 3:35–41.

Quaade, F., and A. Astrup. 1989. Initial very low calorie diet (VLCD) improves ultimate weight loss. *International Journal of Obesity* 13 (Supplement 2): 107–11.

Rattan, S., et al. 1989. Maintenance of weight loss with recovery of resting metabolic rate following 8 weeks of very low calorie dieting. *International Journal of Obesity* 13 (Supplement 2): 189–92.

Ravussin, E. 1993. Energy metabolism in obesity. Studies in the Pima Indians. *Diabetes Care* 16:232–38.

Roberts, S., et al. 1993. Energy expenditure, aging and body composition. *Journal of Nutrition* 123:474–80.

Rodin, J., et al. 1992. Weight cycling and fat distribution. *International Journal of Obesity* 14:303–10.

Roust, L., and M. Jensen. 1993. Postprandial free fatty acid kinetics are abnormal in upper body obesity. *Diabetes* 42:1567–73.

Rutherford, J., et al. 1993. Genetic influences on eating attitudes in a normal female twin population. *Psychological Medicine* 23:425–36.

Schapira, D., et al. 1990. Abdominal obesity and breast cancer risk. *Annals of Internal Medicine* 112:182–86.

Schapira, D., et al. 1991. Estimate of breast cancer risk reduction with weight loss. *Cancer* 67:2622–25.

Schutz, Y., et al. 1989. Failure of dietary fat intake to promote fat oxidation: A factor favoring the development of obesity. *American Journal of Clinical Nutrition* 50:307–14.

Sedlock, D., et al. 1989. Effect of exercise intensity and duration on postexercise energy expenditure. *Medicine and Science in Sports and Exercise* 21:662–66.

Serdula, M., et al. 1993. Weight control practices of U.S. adolescents and adults. *Annals of Internal Medicine* 119:667–71.

Shake, C., et al. 1993. Predicting percent body fat from circumference measurements. *Military Medicine* 158:26–31.

Sorensen, T., and A. Stunkard. 1993. Does obesity run in families because of genes? *Acta Psychiatrica Scandinavica* 370:67–72.

Staten, M. 1991. The effect of exercise on food intake in men and women. *American Journal of Clinical Nutrition* 53:27–31.

Stout, J., et al. 1994. Validity of percent body fat estimations in males. *Medicine and Science in Sports and Exercise.* 26:632–36.

Strain, G., et al. 1992. Food intake of very obese persons: Quantitative and qualitative aspects. *Journal of the American Dietetic Association* 92:199–203.

Suter, P., et al. 1992. The effect of ethanol on fat storage in healthy subjects. *New England Journal of Medicine* 326:983–87.

Swanson, C., et al. 1993. Relation of endometrial cancer risk to past and contemporary body size and body fat distribution. *Cancer Epidemiology, Biomarkers and Prevention* 2:321–27.

Sweeney, M., et al. 1993. Severe vs moderate energy restriction with and without exercise in the treatment of obesity: Efficiency of weight loss. *American Journal of Clinical Nutrition* 57:127–34.

Tremblay, A., et al. 1990. Effect of intensity of physical activity on body fatness and fat distribution. *American Journal of Clinical Nutrition* 51:153–57.

Tucker, L., 1987. Effect of weight training on body attitudes: Who benefits most. *Journal of Sports Medicine and Physical Fitness* 27:70–78.

Tucker, L., and G. Friedman. 1989. Television viewing and obesity in adult males. *American Journal of Public Health* 79:516–18.

van der Kooy, K., et al. 1993. Effect of a weight cycle on visceral fat accumulation. *American Journal of Clinical Nutrition* 58:853–57.

van der Kooy, K., et al. 1993. Waist-hip ratio is a poor predictor of changes in visceral fat. *American Journal of Clinical Nutrition* 57:327–33.

Wade, A., et al. 1990. Muscle fibre type and aetiology of obesity. *Lancet* 335:805–8.

Webb, P. 1985. Direct calorimetry and the energetics of exercise and weight loss. *Medicine and Science in Sports and Exercise* 18:3–5.

Westerterp, K., et al. 1992. Long-term effect of physical activity on energy balance and body composition. *British Journal of Nutrition* 68:21–30.

White, J. 1991. Women: Weight loss decreases cancer risk. *Physician and Sportsmedicine* 19 (December): 52–54.

Wilcosky, T., et al. 1990. Obesity and mortality in the Lipid Research Clinics Program Follow-Up Study. *Journal of Clinical Epidemiology* 43:743–52.

Willett, W., et al. 1995. Weight, weight change, and coronary heart disease in women. *Journal of the American Medical Association* 273:461–65.

Williams, P., et al. 1990. Changes in lipoprotein subfractions during diet-induced and exercise-induced weight loss in moderately overweight men. *Circulation* 81:1293–1304.

Yoshioka, K., et al. 1992. Brown adipose tissue thermogenesis and metabolic rate contribute to the variation in obesity among rats fed a high fat diet. *Japanese Journal of Physiology* 42:673–80.

8

STRESS-REDUCTION TECHNIQUES

Key Terms

assertiveness	homeostasis	progressive relaxation	stress management
autogenic relaxation	hypoglycemia	self-actualization	stressor
Benson's relaxation response	imagery	self-empowerment	stress response
caffeine	inverted-U hypothesis	self-esteem	trait anxiety
distressors	mantra	state anxiety	Transcendental Meditation
endorphins	negative addiction	stress	(TM)
eustressors	pituitary gland		

Key Concepts

- Although most of the stressors our ancient ancestors faced are no longer with us (such as the threat of wild animals), our bodies still retain the physiological response to stress that can be evoked by other threats, such as threats to our esteem.

- Both physical and mental stressors may evoke the stress response in which the body prepares for action by increasing muscular tension, increasing heart rate and blood pressure, and eliciting other physiological responses to help counteract the stressor.

- The stress response evolved as a normal reaction to stress and was vital in the survival of the fittest, but the constant physiological actions of the stress response, particularly in individuals with trait anxiety, may create a predisposition to certain health problems.

- There are a variety of means to assess the tendency toward trait anxiety. One of the more practical means is a self-assessment questionnaire.

- There exists a wide variety of procedures to help manage stress, ranging from passive techniques, such as meditation, to active techniques, such as physical exercise. You should experiment to find those most appropriate for you.

- Relaxation is a motor skill and needs to be learned, just like tennis. In order to be maximally effective, it must be practiced and perfected like any other motor skill.

- One of the first steps in reducing stress is to try to remove the cause of the stress, which may be psychological, environmental, or dietary.

- A breathing exercise that concentrates upon a slow, deep inhalation followed by a slow, deep exhalation is one of the simplest ways to induce a state of relaxation.

- The major passive relaxation techniques involve meditation, imagery, and autogenic relaxation. Active techniques include progressive relaxation training and aerobic exercise.

- Research has shown that both passive and active relaxation techniques may be helpful as stress management procedures.

INTRODUCTION

Abraham Maslow, a psychologist who has written extensively about motivation and personality development, has proposed a theory of motivation and behavior based upon a hierarchy of human needs. The hierarchy, in order from the lowest level to the level of **self-actualization,** is presented in table 8.1. Individuals who achieve self-actualization possess high but not exaggerated levels of **self-esteem,** an objective respect and favorable impression of oneself. According to Maslow, the ultimate goal for most individuals is to become self-actualized. In general, Maslow has characterized self-actualized individuals as being realistically oriented, autonomous, independent, creative, democratic, spontaneous, not self-centered, having an air of detachment and a need for privacy, accepting themselves and the world for what they are, having a sincere appreciation of people, and experiencing deep, emotional, intimate relationships with a few specially loved people. In general, Maslow has noted that you must satisfy your needs at a lower level before you can concentrate on achieving satisfaction at the next highest level. Thus in order to become self-actualized, your needs at the lower four levels must be fulfilled first.

In prehistoric times, hunger, thirst, and danger were primary drives for human behavior. The quest for food, water, and safety was ever present. Man would often risk his life for food. In other words, basic physiological needs took precedence over safety needs. In order to satisfy the needs at the first two levels, the human body had to be prepared for action, to fight for food or to run to safety, whatever the case happened to be. Throughout history, then, the human body developed a basic physiological response whenever some need, such as safety, became great enough. This physiological response was designed to mobilize the body reserves for immediate activity (fig. 8.1). It was a beneficial response because it helped make the caveman run faster or fight more vigorously. Once the threat to safety was removed, so too was the basic physiological response.

For most of us in our modern society, hunger and thirst are no longer major needs driving our behavior, and although safety is still a concern, it is not as much a problem as it was in prehistoric times. However, the potential for the basic physiological response to these needs remains with us. All of us can remember having been frightened by a sudden movement in the dark and recall such obvious body reactions as a pounding heart, tightened musculature, and sweating palms. An anticipated danger activated this physiological response; later, just walking by a dark alley or into a dark room may elicit the same response. In essence, a threat of danger elicits a response similar to that elicited by the actual danger. More is said about this basic physiological response in the next section, but it is sufficient to realize that our thoughts, anticipating the threat of danger, may activate a physiological response even though an actual need for safety is not present.

Although hunger is a major problem for a segment of our population, and although personal safety is an increasing concern, for most of us our basic physiological and safety needs are satisfied by the benefits of modern society. Thus, the major drives for behavior originate in the next two levels—the needs for belongingness and love and for esteem. Most of us want to belong to a loving family, have friends, share a special love with someone, and achieve some degree of

---

Table 8.1 Maslow's Hierarchy of Needs Involved in Human Motivation

Self-actualization needs
Esteem needs
Belongingness and love needs
Safety needs
Basic physiological needs

---

success and recognition in our vocations and avocations. If we perceive a threat in these areas, we may still experience the same basic physiological responses we would if exposed to some actual danger. A classic example is the pounding heart, tightened musculature, sweating palms, and dry mouth that often occur before delivering a speech to a group of your peers. You may feel that your speech will be a failure, and this is a threat to your need for esteem.

Although there are some obvious threats to personal safety in our external environment, it is important to realize that many of the threats we experience today are internally generated. They originate in our minds as perceived threats to our needs for fulfillment in love and esteem and may impose a stress upon our bodies that may eventually be harmful to our health. We live in an Age of Anxiety. Current estimates suggest that nearly 30 million Americans suffer from various symptoms associated with such mental stress, most commonly anxiety and depression, and a recent Centers for Disease Control survey revealed one of every three Americans feels troubled at least one day a month.

All of us experience stress and the accompanying mild anxiety or depression from time to time and have developed our own coping mechanisms. However, for some individuals, the inability to cope with excessive stress leads to a life without joy and may even result in tragic consequences. For example, suicide is the third leading cause of death among young people aged fifteen to twenty-four. The Public Health Service has noted that stress identification and control should be an integral component of a total health program, for stress-related health problems may be costing Americans $200 billion yearly. One of the major risk-reduction objectives of the Public Health Service, listed under Mental Health in the national report *Healthy People 2000,* is to decrease the proportion of people aged eighteen and over who report experiencing significant levels of stress but who do not take steps to reduce or control their stress. The ultimate health objective is to reduce levels of stress-related chronic diseases and suicide.

The purpose of this chapter is threefold:

1. To discuss the basic physiological response to stress and to relate it to possible medical problems

2. To determine if you are prone to stress

3. To discuss various means that may be utilized to prevent or reduce stress levels ▪

Effects of Stress on the Body

Before we look at the actual effects that stress may cause in the body—the stress response—let us briefly discuss the general causes of stress. A **stressor** is anything in life that causes the stress response in any given individual. Stressors may be physical in nature (bodily pains or exercise) or may be mental

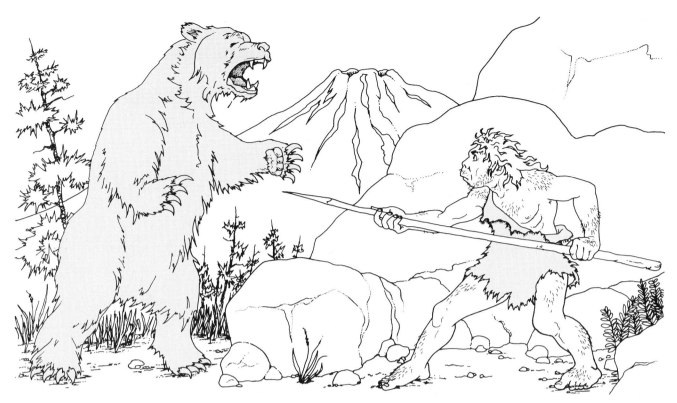

From the origin of life, humans developed a physiological response to stress that prepared the body for action—to fight or take flight. This physiological response to stress helped in the survival of the fittest, but may be a cause of several major health problems if a prolonged response occurs in our modern stressful society.

Figure 8.1

or emotional in nature and affect the mind (worrying about an examination, a speech, or a first date). Stressors may be good **(eustressors),** positive life events such as beginning college, or bad **(distressors),** negative life events, such as flunking out of college. The key point is that both physical and mental stressors, and both eustressors and distressors, may elicit a similar stress response in the body. It is important to note, however, that research has suggested that eustressors do not generally cause illness in individuals with high self-esteem but may in individuals with low self-esteem, possibly because positive life events may be perceived by the individual with low esteem to be inconsistent with his or her self-perception and thus actually cause distress.

From a medical viewpoint, the stressor is the cause, and **stress** is the physiological response (the stress response) the body makes to any stressor. Most of us associate other terms with the feelings of stress, such as strain, tension, and anxiety. These three terms are often used interchangeably to characterize the stress response.

The **stress response** is the mechanism whereby the body prepares to help counteract a stressor. The stressor may be external and be perceived by our senses, such as seeing a vicious dog coming at us while jogging; it may be internal, such as a change in our blood chemistry, e.g., decreased blood glucose. Both external and internal stressors stimulate the hypothalamus, a key control area in the brain that helps regulate **homeostasis,** the normal functioning of our internal environment. The hypothalamus regulates homeostasis by two major

pathways—the nervous system and the endocrine system. Genetics may influence the specific stress response in an individual, possibly by inherited patterns of neurotransmitter or hormone production in the brain areas that regulate emotions.

The hypothalamus contains various clusters of nerve cells, called centers, that respond to specific stimuli. As noted in the last chapter, there are centers for such basic physiological stimuli as hunger, thirst, and temperature. The hypothalamus also receives stimuli from the areas of the brain that control human emotions and, thus, contains centers that respond to such emotional feelings as pleasure, rage, and aggression. When any of these hypothalamic centers are activated by appropriate stimuli, a particular response is generated.

The hypothalamic centers stimulate the sympathetic nervous system. The primary function of the sympathetic nervous system is the maintenance of normal homeostasis; it affects almost all organs and glands in the body, including the heart and blood vessels. By activating the sympathetic nervous system, the hypothalamus is able to rapidly mobilize the body for action. The hypothalamus also exerts significant control over the **pituitary gland,** the so-called master gland of the endocrine system. The pituitary gland, in turn, exerts a significant effect upon many of the other endocrine glands in the body concerned with homeostasis, particularly the adrenal gland. The interaction of these three glands is often referred to as the hypothalamic-pituitary-adrenal axis, which we will encounter again in chapter 10 when we discuss potential risks associated with excessive exercise in females. Thus, by regulating the

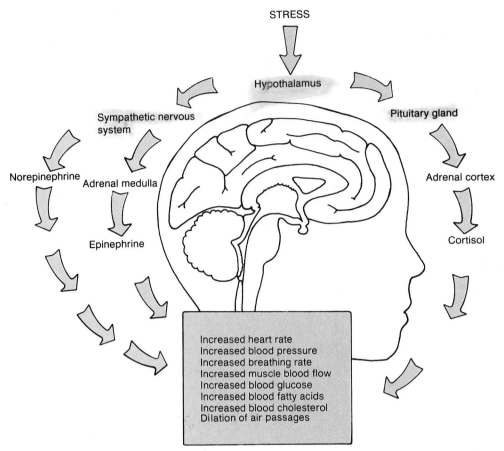

STRESS

Hypothalamus

Sympathetic nervous system

Pituitary gland

Norepinephrine

Adrenal medulla

Adrenal cortex

Epinephrine

Cortisol

Increased heart rate
Increased blood pressure
Increased breathing rate
Increased muscle blood flow
Increased blood glucose
Increased blood fatty acids
Increased blood cholesterol
Dilation of air passages

Figure 8.2 *The hypothalamus responds to physical or mental stress by stimulating the sympathetic nervous system and the pituitary gland; both may cause a number of physiological effects throughout the body.*

activities of both the sympathetic nervous system and the pituitary gland, the hypothalamus can control the state of homeostasis in the body and activate the stress response when stimulated by an appropriate stressor. An overview of the hypothalamic control mechanism is presented in figure 8.2.

The response to stress is complex and may vary in different individuals, but the major effect of the stress response is the mobilization of the cardiovascular system to meet anticipated energy needs. In essence, the heart rate is increased and the heart pumps more forcefully with each beat. The blood flow to some parts of the body is increased, while it is decreased to others. Blood pressure is increased. Muscular tension is increased throughout the body, preparing the individual for rapid activation of muscle strength and power. Stress proteins are produced by body cells, although their physiological significance is not currently known. Blood levels of both glucose and free fatty acids increase, providing fuel for body tissues. This stress response is the body's way of preparing for activity and has been instrumental in the preservation of the human species throughout history. Thus, the stress response is natural and is beneficial when an actual danger is encountered. When the danger is gone, the stress response fades away. However, the stress response may lead to certain health problems if it persists for a prolonged period of time. Let us explore the stress response a little further by looking at the concepts of state and trait anxiety.

State and Trait Anxiety and Your Health

Any situation may be a stressor for any one individual at any given time. **State anxiety** refers to any situational stressor that evokes the stress response. It is usually temporary and fades away when the stressor is removed. What may be a stressor for one individual may not be for another. The different moods we experience each day are examples of state anxiety. For example, John may be very muscular and possess a great deal of upper body strength, but he may not have good public speaking ability; Paul may possess excellent public speaking skills but have low levels of upper body strength. Climbing a 20-foot rope in gym class would be a major stressor for Paul; an oral book report in English class would evoke the stress response in John. The stress response will usually disappear when these tasks are completed.

As mentioned earlier, the stress response is not considered to be an inappropriate body response. As a matter of fact, a little bit of stress may be necessary to obtain optimal levels of performance. Figure 8.3 illustrates the **inverted-U hypothesis** relative to stress, arousal, and performance. In certain activities, such as giving a speech or participating in some athletic events, too little stress may result in a lower level of arousal and, hence, an individual will not key up sufficiently to perform at an optimal level. On the other hand, too much stress may destroy performance, as forgetting your speech or being

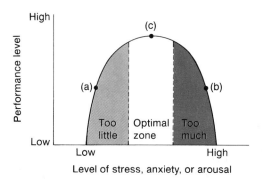

Figure 8.3 *The inverted-U theory suggests that there is an optimal level of stress or anxiety that improves performance (c). Too little stress (a) does not provide sufficient motivation for the task; too much stress (b) may disrupt performance.*

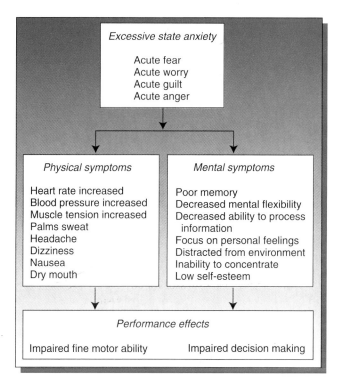

Figure 8.4 *Excessive state anxiety may elicit various bodily reactions that may impair physical and mental performance.*

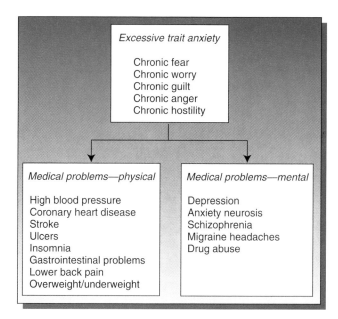

Figure 8.5 *Excessive trait anxiety over a period of time may be a contributing factor to a host of physical and mental health problems.*

too nervous in a sport that requires precision. Thus, there appears to be an optimal level of stress and arousal that results in optimal performance; these appear to be dependent upon the individual and the type of task to be performed.

The key point is that an excessive stress response during a situation of state anxiety may be disruptive to performance. A schematic of excessive state anxiety is presented in figure 8.4. In essence, an excessive stress response can create both physical and mental alterations that detract from optimal performance levels.

As is noted later in this chapter, many of the stress reduction techniques may be helpful in reducing the magnitude of the stress response during conditions of state anxiety.

In contrast to state anxiety, which is considered to be a temporary condition, **trait anxiety** represents a general disposition of an individual to psychological stressors. It is more permanent and is associated with one's personality. Individuals who possess trait anxiety have a feeling of being threatened and are very prone to feelings of worry and guilt.

Hans Selye has conducted extensive research relative to the effects of excessive constant stress, or distress, on health. Selye developed a theory of stress based on three phases—the alarm phase, the adaptation phase, and the exhaustion phase. The alarm phase is the stress response discussed previously; it prepares the body for action. In state anxiety it is transitory. However, in trait anxiety it persists, and the body has to adapt to this response in the second phase. Some of these adaptations, such as high blood pressure, are harmful to the health. If they persist, they may lead to a third stage, the exhaustion stage, and may have severe health consequences.

Trait anxiety may cause physical and mental symptoms identical to those caused by excessive state anxiety. Many of these symptoms may persist and lead to other more severe health problems. Figure 8.5 presents a broad overview of some of the medical problems that may occur in certain individuals following prolonged trait anxiety. These medical problems may be directly caused by the effect of chronic psychological stressors upon nervous and endocrine functions in the body or indirectly caused through overeating and physical inactivity responses to the imposed stress. In particular, the stress response to chronic anger and hostility has been associated with increased health risks. Selye's theory of stress suggests that almost any disease may be caused by the chronic excessive emotional stress response present in individuals with trait anxiety. In some cases, a decreased stress response will lead to illness. In a recent review, Plowman identified over thirty-five diseases associated with impaired regulation of the stress response, including alcoholism, anorexia, cancer, cardiovascular disease, diabetes, low back pain, migraine headaches, obesity, and suicide.

As with state anxiety, various relaxation techniques may be helpful in reducing, or possibly reversing, the adverse effects of chronic stress response in individuals with trait anxiety.

Your Stress Profile

There are a number of different ways that have been used to evaluate stress levels in an individual: measuring muscle tension by electromyographic techniques, voice analysis, certain blood tests for stress markers, and psychological interview techniques. However, several of the most practical techniques developed involve self-assessment inventories, in which an individual responds to some form of questionnaire designed to provide a general predisposition toward stress. Laboratory Inventory 8.1 is a very simple instrument to help evaluate your stress level, particularly state anxiety, on a daily basis. Laboratory Inventory 8.2 is more detailed and is related to trait anxiety. It has four parts: measuring your vulnerability to stress from being frustrated; measuring your vulnerability to stress from being overloaded; testing for type A, or compulsive, time-urgent behavior; and evaluating how well you cope with stress in your life.

If the results of these Laboratory Inventories suggest you are under stress, methods to help reduce stress (presented in the next section) should be of interest to you. Passive relaxation techniques, such as breathing exercises and meditation, may be very useful in helping to reduce the stress response in cases of state anxiety, but you may need to develop a more comprehensive stress-reduction program if you are prone to trait anxiety.

If you continue to experience deep anxiety or depression, seek out resources in your university or community, such as the student counseling center or community mental health centers, for professional advice.

Methods to Reduce Stress

Now that you have a general idea of what stress is, how it may affect the body, and whether or not you have a general tendency toward trait anxiety, what can you do to eliminate or minimize the adverse psychological and physical health effects of excessive acute or chronic stress? The general term for dealing with stress is known as **stress management.** In some cases, the stress level may be increased in a given individual in order to obtain an optimal performance level. A number of special motivational techniques have been developed for that purpose. However, for our purposes, we are interested in those stress-management techniques that may reduce stress levels and their possible adverse effects on our mental and physical functioning.

A wide variety of techniques have been utilized to help reduce both state and trait anxiety, ranging on a continuum from

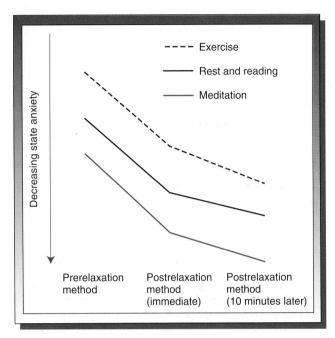

Figure 8.6 *A variety of relaxation techniques have been successful in reducing state anxiety. Exercise, quiet reading, and meditation have been equally effective in reducing state anxiety.*

active techniques such as strenuous exercise to very passive techniques such as meditation. In general, these two techniques, plus others on the continuum, have been shown to be equally effective in reducing stress. (See figure 8.6.) A number of theories have been advanced in attempts to explain how the stress-reduction techniques work, but no major consensus of opinion appears to have been reached. For example, it has been suggested that exercise and meditation produce chemical changes in the brain by influencing the release of various neurotransmitters, induce neuromuscular relaxation, train the parasympathetic nervous system, or provide a distraction—all of which may produce a relaxing effect on the mind and body. Some of these possible methods of stress reduction are integrated into the following discussion.

There are many techniques for dealing with stress. The techniques described in the following list have been utilized and found to be effective in many individuals. Not all techniques work with all people. Become familiar with each technique and find which one works for you. An aerobic exercise program is advocated for other health benefits above and beyond the beneficial effects it may have as a means to reduce stress. If your aerobic exercise program helps to reduce your stress levels, that is all the better. However, one or more of the other techniques, such as meditation or breathing exercises, may be very useful additions to your stress-reduction program.

Space does not permit a full detailed discussion of each stress-reduction technique, but a basic explanation and/or example of each method is presented. For those desiring an expanded coverage, *Comprehensive Stress Reduction* by J. Greenberg and *Controlling Stress and Tension* by D. Girdano,

Table 8.2 Possible Psychological and Situational Stressors in the Lives of College Students

Time Constraints

Job/sports/school conflicts
Deadlines for course projects
Quality study time for tests

Personal Relationships Conflicts

Roommates
Parents
Instructors
Employer
Spouse, fiancé, boyfriend/girlfriend

College Concerns

Money for tuition, books, supplies
Academic performance

Future Plans

Major course of study
Employment opportunities
Acceptance into graduate school

G. Everly, and D. Dusek are highly recommended. *Stress Map,* by E. Orioli, provides a personalized guide to stress management. The common techniques are

1. Removing the stressor
2. Rest and sleep
3. Breathing
4. Meditation
5. Imagery
6. Autogenic training
7. Progressive relaxation training
8. Active exercises

It is important to realize that some relaxation techniques are motor skills that need to be learned. In order to effectively use such techniques as breathing exercises, meditation, autogenic training, and progressive relaxation training, they must be practiced and perfected as must any other motor skill.

Removing the Stressor

Behind every stress response there is a cause, or stressor. The first step in any stress-reduction program should be an attempt to remove this stressor. In order to remove the stressor, you must first be able to identify it. Table 8.2 lists some of the possible psychological or situational stressors in the life of a college student. In some cases you may not be able to identify the cause of your stress since it may be the result of deep-seated and subconscious feelings of insecurity and distrust. In such cases, professional psychological help may be necessary to identify and remove these ingrained psychological causes.

There are three general classes of stressors: psychological, environmental or situational, and dietary.

Psychological Stressors

Some identifiable psychological causes may be manifestations of the deep-seated causes noted previously and may include such traits as excessive wants and desires, excessive drive and ambition, expectations of perfection from others, inability to

make decisions, and low self-esteem, or negative thoughts about oneself. Volumes of books have been written about how to remove psychological stressors and become the person you want to be. The following general suggestions may help eliminate the most common psychological causes of stress.

1. Free yourself of worry and guilt. Both of these are useless emotions and may prevent you from being yourself. If you feel you have committed a wrongdoing, admit it and resolve to change the behavior. A good book to help you achieve this objective is *Your Erroneous Zones* by Dr. Wayne Dyer. Becoming more assertive helps remove feelings of guilt as you recognize the fact that you don't always have to conform to others' expectations. Worrying may be diminished by concentrating on the present, by enjoying the pleasures of where you are and who you are with now. Be content in the fact that the future will bring more pleasant experiences.

2. Become more assertive. **Assertiveness** is simply honest communication and should not be confused with aggressiveness. You are assertive when you express your feelings and desires in a straightforward manner; you are aggressive when you demand your desires or express your feelings with undertones of threats and intimidation. Recognize that you have certain basic rights of assertiveness, such as the right to be treated with respect, to say no and not feel guilty, to act in ways to promote your self-respect, to express your feelings, to show your emotions, to change your mind, to ask for what you want, to make mistakes, and to feel good about yourself. You also have the responsibility not to violate the assertive rights of others. To become more assertive, take a class in assertiveness training or consult an appropriate book such as *The Assertiveness Option: Your Rights and Responsibilities* by Patricia Jakubowski and Arthur Lange.

3. Free yourself of hostility and anger. Hostility is characterized by unfriendly behavior, often accompanied by anger, strong feelings of displeasure provoked by real or imagined wrongs. Occasionally, almost everyone becomes hostile or gets angry, but the anger is normally short-lived. Chronic hostility and anger may be devastating not only to your social relationships, but also to your physical health. Becoming angry frequently because of many common daily occurrences, such as slow movement in the express checkout lane at the supermarket or rude drivers on the highway, may lead to a prolonged stress response and related health problems. Hostility in individuals is affected by both genetic and environmental factors. Deep-seated hostility may necessitate professional counseling, but several stress reduction techniques may help many of us defuse our hostility and anger. Learning assertiveness and practicing the Optimist's Creed will help reduce hostility. Breathing techniques, discussed below, have also been shown to be helpful. Take a deep breath and count to ten is wise advice when confronted with a situation which normally makes you angry. Laughter also modifies your breathing,

especially deep laughing, a form of forced exhalation. Learn to laugh for laughter may help reduce hostility and anger. Find humor in various aspects of your life, even yourself. Learn to laugh at yourself when you make foolish errors (but also learn to correct those errors). Watch cartoons and funny movies. Go to a comedy club. If you can, learn to laugh during stressful times. Other techniques discussed below, particularly meditation, are recommended to help reduce hostility and anger. For those who want more detailed information, an excellent book recently available is *Anger kills: Seventeen strategies for controlling the hostility that can harm your health* by Redford and Virginia Williams.

4. Empower yourself. **Self-empowerment** means to give power or authority to yourself. In his classic *The Power of Positive Thinking,* the late Norman Vincent Peale noted that in solving personal problems the most important point is to realize that the power to solve them correctly is inherent within you, but you must develop an emotional and spiritual plan. Freeing yourself of guilt, worry, anger and hostility, becoming assertive, and thinking positively will help empower you to remove many of the psychological stressors in your life. Although somewhat dated, Peale's book contains advice still relevant to dealing with the current Age of Anxiety.

5. Be cheerful and kind to others. Remember the commandment, "Do unto others as you would have them do unto you." Do at least one random act of kindness daily, such as waving to children in a school bus or bringing freshly picked flowers to someone at work. In this regard "The Optimist's Creed" may be a helpful reminder. Make a copy of it and put it near your mirror or on the refrigerator door and review it every morning.

The Optimist's Creed
Promise Yourself—

To be so strong that nothing can disturb your peace of mind.

To talk health, happiness, and prosperity to every person you meet.

To make all your friends feel there is something in them.

To look at the sunny side of everything and make your optimism come true.

To think only of the best, to work only for the best, and to expect only the best.

To be just as enthusiastic about the success of others as you are about your own.

To forget the mistakes of the past and press on to the greater achievements of the future.

To wear a cheerful countenance at all times and to give every living creature you meet a smile.

To give so much time to the improvement of yourself that you have no time to criticize others.

To be too large for worry, too noble for anger, too strong for fear, and too happy to permit the presence of trouble.

Environmental or Situational Stressors

Environmental or situational causes of stress may be many and varied. Too many unsolved problems and too many difficult responsibilities may be sources of worry and constant stress. Often this type of stress is a matter of disorganization and a lack of priorities. Learn time-management skills, to take time during the week to establish priorities; decide what is worth your immediate attention and what is not. Set daily, weekly, or long-term goals that focus upon the most important issues and tasks. Make a priority list and give yourself credit as you check off each accomplishment. Five term papers or reports may seem mind-boggling when you think of doing them all at once; they will be much less stressful if you set daily and weekly goals to research and write them. A set routine, guided by realistic goals, will help eliminate the stressful effects of disorganization. Learn also how to say no to additional responsibilities that will overburden you in the first place.

Your relationships with others at work, home, or school may also be situational stressors. Constant problems with your superiors at work, your roommate, or your college instructor may induce a stress response. A good approach to these types of problems is assertiveness. Honestly communicating your feelings and desires may help resolve the problem. If not, then other solutions, such as finding a new job, or changing roommates or instructors should be tried, if feasible. If these solutions are not possible, various professional resources, such as a Student Counseling Center, may be able to provide assistance.

Noise and overcrowding may also be situational stressors. Finding a quiet place where you can be alone—which is necessary for some of the relaxation techniques discussed later in this chapter—will effectively reduce this stressor temporarily. If a noise bothers you, such as a stereo in the dorm room next door while you are attempting to study, be assertive and express your desires. Find ways to avoid the stress of overcrowding if it bothers you; drive to work or school a little earlier to avoid the morning traffic rush.

Another situational stressor is boredom, which may lead to depression. The basic cure is to have a life full of meaning and purpose. Develop a variety of interests, join clubs, become involved in community projects, or take up new recreational activities. Research with college students has shown that involvement in college activities decreases symptoms of depression, increases feelings of health and fitness, and may enhance class attendance (which may also have a positive effect on course grades). Also learn to entertain yourself, to feel content being alone once in a while with a good book. An active mind deters boredom.

Even the weather may be a stressor to some. We all know how depressing a prolonged bout of cold, rainy, cloudy weather may be, but most of us find alternative activities to compensate because it is a good time to study or concentrate on other indoor activities. Some individuals, particularly in the northern parts of the United States, suffer from seasonal

Table 8.3 How to Deal with Test Anxiety

1. **Prepartion is the key**

   Start early, from the first day of the course. Outline your text, and organize your notes into meaningful areas of study for each test, including the midterm and final. By mastering the material throughout the course, you will be well prepared and confident for each test, as well as the final exam. Confidence is the key factor in preventing stress anxiety.

2. **Work on skills that enhance your ability to take tests**

   Memory skills, such as the use of mnemonic devices to recall lists of important items, can help you retain information more effectively. Test-taking skills for different types of tests, such as multiple choice or essay, may also be learned. Learn concentration skills, how to avoid distractions while studying; this will help you also when you concentrate on taking the test. Check with your office of student services; often courses on study techniques and test taking are offered to students free of charge. The university wants to keep you as a customer.

3. **Some key points to taking the exam**

   a. Eat lightly, if at all, prior to an exam. A heavy meal in your stomach may make you drowsy. Take a brisk walk instead; it will help relax you and stimulate blood flow.

   b. Be prepared. Have all of the pencils, paper, and other equipment you need. Have backup batteries for your calculator.

   c. Dress in a relaxed and comfortable manner.

   d. Go to the room where the test is to be taken days or hours in advance. If tension develops, plan to combat it with a stress-reduction technique.

   e. If you feel tense during the exam, use some of the relaxation techniques discussed below, such as breathing exercises or autogenic relaxation. Feelings of stress in the neck and upper back may be relieved by the stretching exercises suggested in figures 5.17 and 5.18 on page 98.

   f. Think positive! You have prepared for the exam, so expect to do well. A positive, relaxed mind is more effective than one filled with the stress of test anxiety.

affective disorder (SAD), or prolonged anxiety or depression thought to be caused by the decreased amount of sunshine and daylight during the winter months. Some of the stress reduction techniques discussed below may help reduce the effects of SAD, but professional assistance including light therapy may be necessary for some individuals.

The control of environmental stressors is dependent upon your individual situation, but if they are daily sources of stress for you, take action to reduce or eliminate them. For example, table 8.3 provides some approaches to reduce test anxiety.

Dietary Stressors

Certain substances in the diet, particularly drugs, may be stressors for some individuals. **Caffeine,** a natural stimulant, is found in coffee, tea, colas, and chocolate. Not everyone reacts the same way to caffeine, but it can cause nervousness and sleeplessness, particularly if consumed in large amounts. If caffeine appears to be an excessive stimulant in your diet, reduce your intake by switching to decaffeinated coffee, tea, and colas, the primary source of caffeine in most diets. Caffeine is

also found in certain over-the-counter drugs like aspirin, so be sure to check the labels. Although not a dietary source, nicotine in cigarettes is also a stimulant and may cause a stress response in some individuals. Alcohol, a depressant drug, may possibly help reduce some forms of stress when consumed in moderation but may actually contribute to stress when consumed in excess. These drugs may have other adverse health effects and will be discussed further in chapter 9.

Too much refined carbohydrate, such as table sugar, may create transient periods of **hypoglycemia,** or low blood sugar, in some persons. This may be accompanied by feelings of weakness and lethargy and may be stressful to some individuals. Shifting to the type of diet suggested in chapter 6 will help reduce the amount of refined carbohydrate you consume and thus reduce this potential dietary cause of stress.

Stress may affect your nutritional status in a variety of ways, such as an increase in your serum cholesterol and an increased use of some vitamins important to the immune system. A diet based on the nutritional principles presented in chapter 6 is one of your best defenses against several of the adverse metabolic effects of stress in your body.

Rest and Sleep

No extensive discussion of rest and sleep is offered here. However, recognize that adequate rest and sleep are necessary to avoid fatigue, a possible stressor. Take about 15 to 30 minutes each day and earmark it as a quiet time to rest. A short nap, closing your eyes and putting your feet on the desk, or quiet meditation may eliminate mental fatigue and restore vigor and enthusiasm for the task at hand.

A great deal has been written about the importance of sleep and the relative importance of various phases of sleep, such as deep sleep and dream sleep. There is no consensus about how much sleep we need, but a ballpark figure is about 6 to 8 hours of restful sleep per night. Probably the best guideline as to whether or not you have had enough sleep is if you feel rested when you awaken. A well-rested body and mind is an important weapon against stress.

Although exercise is a very important component of a healthy life-style, exercise late in the evening may affect sleep. The small elevation in the metabolic rate and increased body temperature following exercise may make it more difficult for some individuals to fall asleep. If you face this problem, try to exercise earlier in the day or evening, adjusting the time so that there is no interference with your sleep processes.

Breathing Exercises

One of the simplest ways to induce a state of relaxation is a breathing exercise. This technique may be particularly useful when you encounter a stressor, as in cases of state anxiety. Learn to use it on a regular basis throughout the day.

Breathing exercises for relaxation purposes should concentrate on a slow, deep inhalation followed by a slow, deep exhalation. The following steps illustrate a basic breathing exercise.

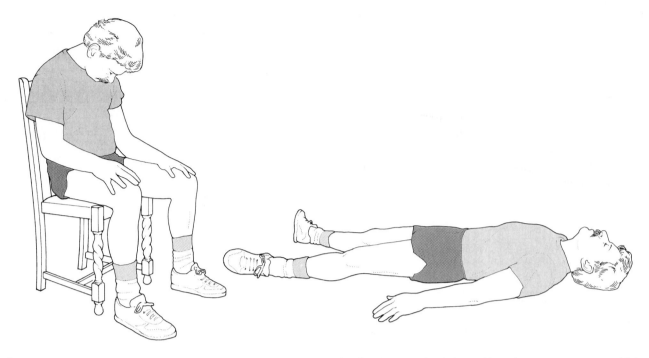

Figure 8.7 *In all passive relaxation exercises it is important to assume a relaxed position. For the sitting position, place your arms on your thighs, spread your fingers, let your head hang forward gently, and relax all of your muscles. For the lying position, use a bed or the floor and spread your legs, letting your feet roll to the outside. Your arms should be away from the side of your body, palms down and fingers spread. You may wish to have a pillow or rolled towel placed under your neck, under the lower curve in your back, and under your knees and elbows for support.*

1. Assume a comfortable position, either sitting or lying on your back. Close your eyes throughout the exercise (fig. 8.7).

2. Inhale slowly and deeply through the nose. (You may inhale through the mouth if it is uncomfortable to inhale through the nose.) As you inhale, slowly count mentally from one to five to ensure that you do not rush your breathing. Both your stomach and your chest should expand considerably. You may place your hands on both to check their outward and upward motions. Focus your mind on the act of inhalation.

3. Once you have reached a full inhalation, hold that position for about 3 seconds and think to yourself, "My body is very calm and relaxed."

4. Exhale slowly through both the nose and mouth and again mentally count down from five to one. Concentrate upon expelling as much air as you possibly can. As you exhale, concentrate on the image of tension fleeing your body. If you are alone, an alternate approach is to close your mouth and emit the sound OM. Make a long OOOOMMMMMM and vibrate the MMMMMM inside your skull.

5. You may combine breathing and stretching. Stretch your arms overhead toward the ceiling as you inhale deeply. Then exhale slowly as you lower your arms to your side.

Try it! Do you feel calmer and more relaxed? Do you feel less tension in your muscles? This technique may not reduce all of your stress, but it is simple to use and may be effective in many cases. Other changes in breathing that focus on exhalation, even a long sigh, may induce a sense of relaxation. Mirthful laughter, which is a form of exhalation, actually has been shown to reduce levels of stress hormones. Laugh more; it's good for you.

Meditation

Meditation was introduced to the United States as **Transcendental Meditation (TM)** in the late 1960s by Maharishi Mahesh Yogi. In TM, each student is given a **mantra,** a particular word or sound to be used during the meditation session. For example, the OM sound in the breathing exercises could be a mantra. During the 20-minute meditation session, the student should concentrate solely on the mantra and eliminate all other distractions from his or her mind.

Dr. Herbert Benson studied TM and published his findings in a book entitled *The Relaxation Response.* The resultant meditation technique is known as **Benson's relaxation response.**

To practice meditation, the following guidelines may be helpful.

1. Find a quiet area. Sit quietly in a comfortable position with your eyes closed.

2. Do several repetitions of the breathing exercise discussed previously to start the relaxation process.

3. Think about your body and let all of your muscles relax. Let yourself go limp.

4. Choose a mantra that has little significance to you, such as the number *one.* Concentrate on the mantra. You may associate the mantra with your breathing, mentally picturing the word *one* as you inhale and exhale. Do not think, feel, hear, or see anything but your mantra. Repeat it over and over again in your mind. Do not dwell on distracting thoughts; always return to your mantra.

5. After about 20 minutes, open your eyes, sit quietly for a minute or two as you phase out the mantra, make a fist with both hands and say to yourself, "I am totally awake, alert, and refreshed." Beginners may start with a 5-minute session, increasing to 20 minutes once or twice per day.

Imagery

Imagery for relaxation purposes involves the mental visualization of feelings that are relaxing to you. The basic principles of the meditation technique apply, but instead of a mantra, you think of a relaxing scene, such as sinking into a soft cloud with the sun warming your whole body. Thoughts that convey feelings of floating, warmth, or heaviness of the body (such as sinking into a soft surface) are key points in imagery.

To practice imagery, simply follow the instructions for the meditation procedure noted above, substituting your mental image for the mantra.

Autogenic Relaxation Training

Autogenic means self-generating. In **autogenic relaxation,** you use a form of self-hypnosis to bring about specific body sensations associated with the state of relaxation. Autogenic training is closely associated with meditation and imagery. Quietness and feelings of warmth and heaviness are important components.

A basic autogenic relaxation technique follows. You may wish to tape-record the phrases so you can listen and relax even more. Some excellent relaxation tapes are also available commercially.

1. Assume a comfortable position seated or lying in a quiet area. Close your eyes.

2. Practice a few repetitions of the breathing exercises to induce the relaxation process.

3. Remove all distracting thoughts from your mind, repeating to yourself three times "I am totally relaxed and feel good about myself."

4. Progressively relax parts of your body by creating a feeling of warmth or heaviness. You may start at the top of your body and work down, or vice versa.

Slowly repeat in your mind each of the following phrases *three times* as you progressively move down the body. For example, think "My head and neck feel heavy. My head and neck feel heavy. My head and neck feel heavy."

My head and neck feel heavy.
My shoulders feel heavy.
My right arm feels heavy.
My left arm feels heavy.
My chest feels heavy.
My abdomen feels heavy.
My right leg feels heavy.
My left leg feels heavy.
My head and neck feel warm and calm.
My shoulders feel warm and calm.
My right arm feels warm and calm.
My left arm feels warm and calm.
My chest feels warm and calm.
My abdomen feels warm and calm.
My right leg feels warm and calm.
My left leg feels warm and calm.
My breathing is calm.
My heart rate is calm.
I am totally relaxed and feel good about myself.

As with meditation and imagery, end the session by saying to yourself, "I am totally awake, alert, and refreshed."

Progressive Relaxation Training

Dr. Edmund Jacobson, in his book *Progressive Relaxation,* describes **progressive relaxation** as a technique for reducing muscular tension through a series of exercises designed to teach muscle awareness and relaxation. Muscles in various parts of the body are tensed or stretched and then consciously relaxed. Jacobson theorizes that an anxious mind cannot exist in a relaxed body, so relaxing the muscles will reduce stress. Progressive relaxation can be practiced in a fashion similar to those already mentioned for about 20 minutes per day. Once you have mastered this technique, it may be utilized when you feel excessive muscular tension during moments of mental or emotional stress. For example, if you are taking a test and feel tension beginning to develop in the back of your neck, isolate those muscles, tense them, and then consciously relax them.

Jacobson utilized over two hundred exercises in his full program. The following technique is one of the most often used adaptations. In essence, you contract and relax various muscle groups, moving progressively from the lower part to the upper part of the body. There are three levels of muscle contraction—maximal, half-strength, and very light.

1. The first step is to assume a relaxed position lying on your back. Put a small pillow or some support under your neck or knees if needed. Your legs should be straight, your arms should be at your side, and your eyes should be closed. Let your body go limp.

2. Practice a few repetitions of the breathing exercises to induce the relaxation response.

3. Remove any distracting thoughts from your mind. Say to yourself, "I am completely relaxed."

4. For each of the following muscle actions, use this procedure:

   a. Take a deep breath. Contract the muscles as hard as possible and hold for 5 seconds. Concentrate on the muscular tension you have developed. After 5 seconds, slowly release the contraction and relax the muscles as you exhale slowly. After you have exhaled, concentrate on the full state of relaxation in that muscular area of the body.

   b. Repeat **a,** but utilize only about one-half of your maximal strength.

   c. Repeat **a,** but utilize only a very light amount of muscular force.

   As you perform **a, b,** and **c,** be aware of the different sensations during tension and relaxation. Learn the feeling of muscular relaxation and reduced muscular tension.

5. Do the following muscular contractions and movements in sequence, developing the force slowly. Try to isolate the contraction to that body part. Try not to contract other muscle groups.

   a. Curl just your toes in your right foot.

   b. Curl just your toes in your left foot.

   c. Bend your right foot upward toward your face as far as possible.

   d. Bend your left foot upward toward your face as far as possible.

   e. Extend the right foot downward as far as possible.

   f. Extend the left foot downward as far as possible.

   g. Tense your upper right leg.

   h. Tense your upper left leg.

   i. Tense your buttocks, squeezing in.

   j. Tense your stomach muscles by flattening your lower back against the floor.

   k. Bring your shoulders as far forward as possible, keeping your head and elbows in place.

   l. Push your shoulders back as far as possible, trying to pull your shoulder blades together.

   m. Spread the fingers on your right hand.

   n. Spread the fingers on your left hand.

   o. Make a fist with your right hand.

   p. Make a fist with your left hand.

   q. Bring your head forward, chin to chest, as far as possible.

   r. Push your head back against the mat.

   s. Open your mouth as wide as possible.

   t. Pucker your lips.

   u. Clench your teeth.

   v. Wrinkle your forehead.

   w. Press your eyes tightly closed.

This relaxation technique is a motor skill to be learned, but with practice you should be able to isolate most of these muscular movements. You may even develop your own

exercises and incorporate them into your routine. For a more detailed discussion of this procedure, consult Jacobson's book, *Progressive Relaxation.*

If you find, however, that this procedure creates tension due to its active nature, you may wish to stay with some of the more passive procedures described earlier.

Active Exercise

As mentioned previously, exercise in itself can be a stressor. However, it may also be a very effective means to reduce stress. Not all individual studies find that exercise reduces stress, but in a recent review of 159 studies dealing with exercise and anxiety reduction, Landers and Petruzzello indicated that over 80 percent of the studies supported the finding that aerobic exercise induced a mild to moderate reduction in both state and trait anxiety and psychological indicators of stress. For state anxiety, the beneficial effects began almost immediately after the exercise bout and continued for 2 hours. To help reduce trait anxiety, aerobic training must persist for at least 10 weeks. Other reviews by Morgan and Raglin support these findings, noting that a chronic exercise training program may help improve self-esteem, mental health, and well-being. The beneficial emotional effects of exercise training have been reported primarily for young and middle-aged individuals, and although Brown notes an association between exercise and mental well-being in the elderly, he indicates more research is needed to confirm the beneficial effect.

It should be noted that exercise is no more effective than other techniques, such as meditation, relaxation training, or even quiet rest, as a means to reduce anxiety. All may be equally effective. However, as noted in previous chapters, exercise may confer additional health benefits.

Various types of exercise programs may help reduce stress. Tai Chi (slow, precise body movements accompanied by meditation) has been shown to reduce state anxiety. Stretching exercises also may be used to induce relaxation and are part of several relaxation techniques discussed above. Yoga is a form of stretching exercise program that has been shown to improve mood by decreasing anger, tension, and depression.

A recommended type of exercise program is one that is aerobic in nature. The guidelines presented in chapter 3 are appropriate for determining the intensity, duration, and frequency of such an exercise program. You may also attempt to learn to meditate while exercising aerobically. Exercise in an isolated area, away from noise and traffic (a park or nature trail [fig. 8.8]). If you are running, start slowly and build up to a comfortable pace. Think about your breathing and your body movements; they should blend together in a relaxed, comfortable synchrony. Look around you as you run, and take in the beauty of your surroundings. Breathe in on one footstep, and exhale on the next two or three. As you continue to run, think about the muscles in various parts of your body, such as your neck, shoulders, and arms, and relax them. As you relax your body, turn your thoughts inward and think peaceful thoughts about your environment or about something that is pleasing to you. Do not create stress by reviewing arguments in your mind or by thinking about how much work

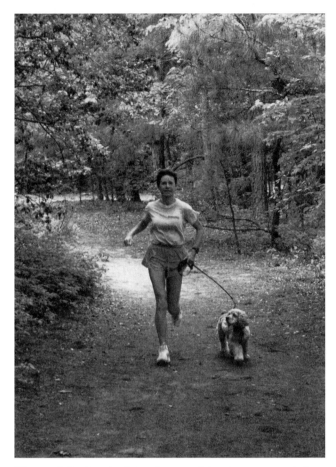

Figure 8.8 *Running in a quiet, peaceful environment may help to reduce stress.*

you have to do later. Learning to relax and meditate while you exercise may help reduce some of the stress-producing effects of the exercise itself.

You may ask the question, If exercise is a stressor, how can it possibly reduce stress? We can look at the answer from two viewpoints—reducing state anxiety and reducing trait anxiety.

A single bout of aerobic exercise twenty minutes or more, has been shown to decrease state anxiety. One theory is that the exercise may simply be a diversion, freeing your mind from the stressors contributing to state anxiety. Another theory suggests that the feeling of accomplishment—taking the time and effort to do something for your body—is a key factor. An accompanying theory to accomplishment is one of expectation. Exercise may be a placebo to enhance your self-esteem because you expect some benefits from it, for example to lose excess body fat or become more physically fit. Still another theory suggests that exercise reduces muscular tension and induces a state of muscular relaxation by increasing body temperature. Finally, there may be some chemical changes that occur in the brain during exercise that may reduce stress levels. Some earlier research suggested that naturally produced tranquilizers in the brain called **endorphins** may be involved, but research is equivocal at the present and there appears to be more evidence against than for this theory. Recent findings suggest that other chemicals in the brain, which act as stimulants, may be involved. Possibly all of these factors are involved in one way or another, but whatever the cause, aerobic exercise does appear to reduce state anxiety. Try it the next time you feel stressed.

The major theory underlying the reduction of trait anxiety by chronic exercise training centers around the effects such training may have on the body. The physical development that occurs (decreased body weight and better appearance) and the physiological changes that make you feel better enhance the way you feel about yourself. The feelings brought by personal accomplishment of long-range exercise goals (such as completing a 10-kilometer race or a marathon) also improve your self-concept. The improvements in self-confidence and self-esteem are critical to the reduction of trait anxiety. Moreover, the beneficial physiological adaptations in the body to chronic exercise training, such as increased efficiency of the heart, may provide increased resistance to the stress of exercise and reduce the effect of other stressors, such as emotional stressors.

It is important to note, however, that exercise may become a major source of stress, particularly if you overexercise, or overtrain. Adherence to the principles and guidelines in chapter 3 will help you develop an optimal exercise program so that exercise will be a positive factor in your Positive Health Lifestyle. However, for some individuals who become obsessive about competition and winning or who set unreasonable goals for themselves, exercise may become a negative factor, a **negative addiction.** They may begin to need more and more exercise in order to continue to achieve a feeling of accomplishment or well-being. This addiction to exercise is not necessarily harmful or undesirable in itself, providing it does not become so obsessive or compulsive that you begin to sacrifice your job, family, and friends. Another possibility resulting from negative addiction is an increased chance of injury from overtraining. Overtraining may actually be counterproductive to stress management, for if you become injured and cannot run, you may go through withdrawal symptoms that may lead to anxiety and depression. Overtraining may also impair the immune system, predisposing you to infections such as the common cold. Overtraining has also been associated with the chronic fatigue syndrome, a condition in which you may feel tired all the time, have a frequent sore throat, experience headaches, or do not sleep well. Finally, excessive exercise may interact with unhealthy eating practices and contribute to several health problems in females, a topic covered in more detail in chapter 10.

A properly designed aerobic exercise program can produce many beneficial physiological and psychological effects. In order to do so, however, the program must be within your capacity so you are not overstressed. It must not lead to staleness and chronic fatigue or injuries, and it must not become obsessive. Moderation is the key.

In summary, there are a number of different ways to reduce stress levels. A good aerobic exercise program may be all that you need. If aerobic exercise is not enough, incorporate one or more of the other relaxation techniques, such as meditation or progressive relaxation training, into your Positive Health Life-style. Combined with positive life-style behaviors in diet and exercise, stress management may help decrease heart disease, according to Dean Ornish, an investigator with the Lifestyle Heart Trial.

References

Books

Allen, R. 1983. *Human stress: Its nature and control.* Minneapolis: Burgess Publishing Company.

Benson, H. 1975. *The relaxation response.* New York: William Morrow and Company.

Bouchard, C., et al., eds. 1994. *Physical activity, fitness, and health.* Champaign, Ill.: Human Kinetics.

Charlesworth, E., and R. Nathan. 1984. *Stress management: A comprehensive guide to wellness.* New York: Atheneum.

Dyer, W. 1976. *Your erroneous zones.* New York: Funk and Wagnalls.

Editors of Rodale Press. 1988. *Take control of your life: A complete guide to stress relief.* Emmaus, Pa.: Rodale Press.

Franks, D., ed. 1994. *The academy papers: Physical activity and stress. Quest 46.* Champaign, Ill.: Human Kinetics.

Girdano, D., et al. 1990. *Controlling stress and tension.* Englewood Cliffs, N.J.: Prentice-Hall.

Greenberg, J. 1996. *Comprehensive stress management.* Dubuque, Iowa: Brown & Benchmark Publishers.

Jacobson, E. 1956. *Progressive relaxation.* Chicago: University of Chicago Press.

Jakubowski, P., and A. Lange. 1978. *The assertiveness option: Your rights and responsibilities.* Champaign, Ill.: Research Press.

Morgan, W. P., and S. Goldston, eds. 1987. *Exercise and mental health.* New York: Hemisphere Publishing Corporation.

Orioli, E. 1991. *Stress map. The ultimate stress management, self-assessment and coping guide developed by ESSI systems.* New York: Newmarket Press.

Padus, E. 1986. *The complete guide to your emotions and your health.* Emmaus, Pa.: Rodale Press.

Peale, N. V. 1952. *The power of positive thinking.* New York: Prentice-Hall.

Rice, P. 1987. *Stress and health: Principles and practice for coping and wellness.* Monterey, Calif.: Brooks/Cole.

Selye, H. 1956. *The stress of life.* New York: McGraw-Hill.

United States Department of Health and Human Services, Public Health Service. 1991. *Healthy people 2000: National health promotion and disease prevention objectives.* Washington, D.C.: U.S. Government Printing Office.

Williams, R., and V. Williams. 1993. *Anger kills: Seventeen strategies for controlling the hostility that can harm your health.* New York: Harper.

Reviews

Bennett, P., and D. Carroll. 1990. Stress management approaches to the prevention of coronary heart disease. *British Journal of Clinical Psychology* 29:1–12.

Berger, B. 1994. Coping with stress: The effectiveness of exercise and other techniques. *Quest* 46:100–119.

Blass, E., et al. 1989. Stress-reducing effects of ingesting milk, sugars, and fats. A developmental perspective. *Annals of the New York Academy of Sciences* 575:292–305.

Brown, D. 1992. Physical activity, aging, and psychological well-being: An overview of the research. *Canadian Journal of Sport Sciences* 17:185–93.

Consumers Union. 1995. Does stress kill? *Consumer Reports on Health* 7:73–76.

DeBenedette, V. 1988. Getting fit for life: Can exercise reduce stress? *Physician and Sportsmedicine* 16 (June): 185–200.

Dishman, R. 1994. Biological psychology, exercise, and stress. *Quest* 46:28–59.

Dubovsky, S. 1990. Generalized anxiety disorder: New concepts and psychopharmacologic therapies. *Journal of Clinical Psychiatry* 51 (Supplement): 3–10.

Dyment, P. 1993. Frustrated by chronic fatigue? *Physician and Sportsmedicine* 21 (November): 47–54.

Eppley, K., et al. 1989. Differential effects of relaxation techniques on trait anxiety: A meta-analysis. *Journal of Clinical Psychology* 45:957–74.

Everly, G., and H. Benson. 1989. Disorders of arousal and the relaxation response: Speculations on the nature and treatment of stress-related diseases. *International Journal of Psychosomatics* 36:15–21.

Farah, M. 1989. The neural basis of mental imagery. *Trends in Neurosciences* 12:395–99.

Franks, D. 1994. What is stress? *Quest* 46:1–7.

Gelderloos, P., et al. 1991. Effectiveness of the transcendental meditation program in preventing and treating substance misuse: A review. *International Journal of the Addictions* 26:293–325.

Jevning, R., et al. 1992. The physiology of meditation: A review. A wakeful hypometabolic integrated response. *Neuroscience and Biobehavioral Reviews* 16:415–24.

LaFontaine, T., et al. 1992. Aerobic exercise and mood. *Sports Medicine* 13:160–70.

Landers, D. 1994. Performance, stress, and health: Overall reaction. *Quest* 46 (February): 123–35.

Landers, D., and J. Petruzzello. 1994. Physical activity, fitness, and anxiety. In *Physical activity, fitness, and health,* eds. C. Bouchard, et al. Champaign, Ill.: Human Kinetics.

Martinsen, E. 1990. Benefits of exercise for the treatment of depression. *Sports Medicine* 9:380–89.

Martinsen, E. 1990. Physical fitness, anxiety, and depression. *British Journal of Hospital Medicine* 43:194–99.

McCubbin, J. 1993. Stress and endogenous opioids: Behavioral and circulatory interactions. *Biological Psychology* 35:91–122.

Meier, K. 1994. Physical activity and stress: The road not taken and the implications for society. *Quest* 46:136–45.

Morgan, W. 1994. Physical activity, fitness and depression. In *Physical activity, fitness, and health,* eds. C. Bouchard, et al. Champaign, Ill.: Human Kinetics.

Newsholme, E., et al. 1991. A biochemical mechanism to explain some of the characteristics of overtraining. *Medicine and Sports Science* 32:79–93.

Petruzzello, S., et al. 1991. A meta-analysis on the anxiety-reducing effects of acute and chronic exercise. *Sports Medicine* 11:143–82.

Plowman, S. 1994. Stress, hyperactivity, and health. *Quest* 46:78–99.

Polivy, J. 1994. Physical activity, fitness, and compulsive behaviors. In *Physical activity, fitness, and health,* eds. C. Bouchard, et al. Champaign, Ill.: Human Kinetics.

Raglin, J. 1990. Exercise and mental health. Beneficial and detrimental effects. *Sports Medicine* 9:323–29.

Ransford, C. 1982. A role for amines in the antidepressant effect of exercise: A review. *Medicine and Science in Sports and Exercise* 14:1–10.

Schatz, M. 1994. Stressed out? Breathe easier with relaxation exercises. *Physician and Sportsmedicine* 22 (November): 87–88.

Schneiderman, N., et al. 1989. Biobehavioral aspects of cardiovascular disease: Progress and prospects. *Health Psychology* 8:649–76.

Sonstroem, R., and W. Morgan. 1989. Exercise and self-esteem: Rationale and model. *Medicine and Science in Sport and Exercise* 21:329–37.

Stevens, M. 1993. Tension-type headaches. *American Family Physician* 47:799–806.

Thoren, P., et al. 1990. Endorphins and exercise: Physiological mechanisms and clinical applications. *Medicine and Science in Sports and Exercise* 22:417–28.

Wichman, S., and D. Martin. 1992. Exercise excess. Treating patients addicted to fitness. *Physician and Sportsmedicine* 20 (May): 193–200.

Williams, R., et al. 1993. Behavior change and compliance: Keys to improving cardiovascular health. *Circulation* 88:1406–7.

Specific Studies

Anda, R., et al. 1993. Depressed affect, hopelessness, and the risk of ischemic heart disease in a cohort of U.S. adults. *Epidemiology* 4:285–94.

Berger, B., and D. Owen. 1992. Mood alteration with yoga and swimming: Aerobic exercise may not be necessary. *Perceptual and Motor Skills* 75:1331–43.

Berk, L., et al. 1989. Neuroendocrine and stress hormone changes during mirthful laughter. *American Journal of Medical Sciences* 298:390–96.

Brown, J., and K. McGill. 1989. The cost of good fortune: When positive life events produce negative health consequences. *Journal of Personality and Social Psychology* 57:1103–10.

Brown, S., et al. 1992. Aerobic exercise in the psychological treatment of adolescents. *Perceptual and Motor Skills* 74:555–60.

Carlson, C., et al. 1990. Muscle stretching as an alternative relaxation training procedure. *Journal of Behavioral Therapy and Experimental Psychiatry* 21:29–38.

Crocker, P., and C. Grozelle. 1991. Reducing induced state anxiety: Effects of acute aerobic exercise and autogenic relaxation. *Journal of Sports Medicine and Physical Fitness* 31:277–82.

de Geus, E., et al. 1993. Regular exercise and aerobic fitness in relation to psychological make-up and physiological stress reactivity. *Psychosomatic Medicine* 55:347–63.

Desharnais, R., et al. 1993. Aerobic exercise and the placebo effect: A controlled study. *Psychosomatic Medicine* 55:149–54.

Dua, J., and L. Hargreaves. 1992. Effect of aerobic exercise on negative affect, positive affect, stress, and depression. *Perceptual and Motor Skills* 75:355–61.

Edinger, J., et al. 1993. Aerobic fitness, acute exercise and sleep in older men. *Sleep* 16:351–59.

Gelderloos, P., et al. 1990. Transcendence and psychological health: Studies with long-term participants of the transcendental meditation and TM-Sidhi program. *Journal of Psychology* 124:177–97.

Hassmen, P., et al. 1993. Psychophysiological responses to exercise in type A/B men. *Psychosomatic Medicine* 55:178–84.

Helmers, K., et al. 1993. Hostility and myocardial ischemia in coronary artery disease patients: Evaluation by gender and ischemic index. *Psychosomatic Medicine* 55:29–36.

Jacobs, G., and J. Lubar. 1989. Spectral analysis of the central nervous system effects of the relaxation response elicited by autogenic training. *Behavioral Medicine* 15:125–32.

Jin, P. 1992. Efficacy of Tai Chi, brisk walking, meditation, and reading in reducing mental and emotional stress. *Journal of Psychosomatic Research* 36:361–70.

Kabat-Zinn, J., et al. 1992. Effectiveness of a meditation-based stress reduction program in the treatment of anxiety disorders. *American Journal of Psychiatry* 149:936–43.

Lockett, D., and J. Campbell. 1992. The effects of aerobic exercise on migraine. *Headache* 32:50–54.

Maroulakis, E., and Y. Zervas. 1993. Effects of aerobic exercise on mood of adult women. *Perceptual and Motor Skills* 76:795–801.

McCubbin, J., et al. 1992. Aerobic fitness and opiodergic inhibition of cardiovascular stress reactivity. *Psychophysiology* 29:687–97.

McGowan, R., et al. 1993. Beta-endorphins and mood states during resistance exercise. *Perceptual and Motor Skills* 76:376–78.

Norris, R., et al. 1990. The effects of aerobic and anaerobic training on fitness, blood pressure, and psychological stress and well-being. *Journal of Psychosomatic Research* 34:367–75.

Orcutt, J., and L. Harvey. 1991. The temporal patterning of tension reduction: Stress and alcohol use on weekdays and weekends. *Journal of Studies on Alcohol* 52:415–24.

Ornish, D., et al. 1990. Can lifestyle changes reverse coronary heart disease? The lifestyle heart trial. *Lancet* 336:129–33.

Raglin, J., and W. Morgan. 1987. Influence of exercise and quiet rest on state anxiety and blood pressure. *Medicine and Science in Sports and Exercise* 19:456–63.

Raglin, J., et al. 1993. State anxiety and blood pressure following 30 min of leg ergometry or weight training. *Medicine and Science in Sports and Exercise* 25:1044–48.

Reifman, A., and C. Dunkel-Schetter. 1990. Stress, structural social support, and well-being in university students. *Journal of American College Health* 38:271–77.

Rejeski, W., et al. 1992. Acute exercise: Buffering psychosocial stress responses in women. *Health Psychology* 11:355–62.

Scherwitz, L., et al. 1992. Hostility and health behaviors in young adults: The CARDIA Study. Coronary artery risk development in young adults study. *American Journal of Epidemiology* 136:136–45.

Shadel, W., and R. Mermelstein. 1993. Cigarette smoking under stress: The role of coping expectancies among smokers in a clinic-based smoking cessation program. *Health Psychology* 12:443–50.

Siegler, I., et al. 1992. Hostility during late adolescence predicts coronary risk factors at mid-life. *American Journal of Epidemiology* 136:146–54.

Somervell, P., et al. 1989. Psychologic distress as a predictor of mortality. *American Journal of Epidemiology* 130:1013–23.

Sonstroem, R., et al. 1991. Test of structural relationships within a proposed exercise and self-esteem model. *Journal of Personality Assessment* 56:348–64.

Stein, P., and R. Motta. 1992. Effects of aerobic and nonaerobic exercise on depression and self-concept. *Perceptual and Motor Skills* 74:79–89.

Thayer, R. 1987. Energy, tiredness, and tension effects of a sugar snack versus moderate exercise. *Journal of Personality and Social Psychology* 52:119–25.

Veale, D., et al. 1992. Aerobic exercise in the adjunctive treatment of depression: A randomized controlled trial. *Journal of the Royal Society of Medicine* 85:541–44.

Wynd, C. 1992. Relaxation imagery used for stress reduction in the prevention of smoking relapse. *Journal of Advanced Nursing* 17:294–302.

C   H   A   P   T   E   R

9

▼▼▼

HEALTH EFFECTS OF HIGH-RISK BEHAVIORS

Key Terms

acquired immunodeficiency
   syndrome (AIDS)
addiction
alcohol
alcoholism
anabolic steroids
blood alcohol content (BAC)
caffeine
carbon monoxide
chlamydia
cirrhosis
cocaine

crack
delta-9-tetrahydrocannabinol
   (THC)
drug abuse
emphysema
ethanol
ethyl alcohol
fetal alcohol effects (FAE)
fetal alcohol syndrome (FAS)
genital herpes
genital warts

gonorrhea
habituation
health risk management
human immunodeficiency
   virus (HIV)
human papilloma virus (HPV)
ice
marijuana
methamphetamine
nicotine
passive smoking

pelvic inflammatory disease
   (PID)
proof
sexually transmitted diseases
   (STDs)
smokeless tobacco
substance abuse
syphilis
tar
urethritis
vaginitis

Key Concepts

■ Individual life-styles may involve activities that are classified as high-risk health behaviors incompatible with a Positive Health Life-style. Moderation in behavior or use of substitute behaviors may help reduce the associated health risks.

■ Although the use of some drugs brings a transitory sense of pleasure, they also are dangerous to one's health. There are other ways to derive pleasure from life that actually enhance your health.

■ Alcohol is the number-one drug problem in the United States. Although progress is being made to reduce alcohol abuse, the problem is still massive and is actually increasing among the young.

■ There is the same amount of alcohol in one 12-ounce bottle of beer, one 4-ounce glass of wine, and 1.25 ounces of 40 percent (80 proof) liquor. All of these are considered as one drink.

■ In the average individual, one drink will raise the blood alcohol content (BAC) to a level of 0.025.

■ Alcohol is metabolized primarily by the liver, but its acute effect is felt mainly in the brain and can range on a continuum from mild euphoria to death. Chronic excess alcohol consumption is associated with a significant number of diseases.

■ Consumption of alcohol in moderation, approximately the equivalent of one to three drinks per day for the average-sized adult, may be compatible with a Positive Health Life-style.

■ For some individuals, such as those who will be driving, those with a family history of alcoholism, and women who are pregnant, abstinence is the best policy.

■ If you use alcohol, it should enhance your general sense of well-being and your social interactions; if used in excess, it may pose a threat to your immediate safety or future health.

■ In general, moderate consumption of caffeine or coffee, about the equivalent of two to three cups per day, is not

considered to pose any serious health risks to the healthy individual. Pregnant women may be advised to limit caffeine intake.

■ Cigarette smoking is recognized as the single most important preventable cause of death in our society; those who smoke are at twice the risk for premature death prior to the age of sixty-five compared to those who do not smoke.

■ Cigarette smoke contains three major substances that may adversely affect health: nicotine, an addictive drug; tar, a yellowish-brown mass of over 4,000 chemicals; and carbon monoxide, a toxic gas.

■ Although cigarette smoking is recognized as a major contributing factor to the development of lung cancer and other diseases of the lungs, its role as a major factor in the development of coronary heart disease results in greater mortality. Even second-hand smoke increases health risks.

■ The number of former smokers in the United States is now almost equal to the number of current smokers, for millions of Americans have successfully quit the habit. If you do smoke, do your body a favor. Quit!

■ The use of smokeless tobacco (snuff and chewing tobacco) is associated with a significantly increased risk of developing oral cancer.

■ Marijuana is a psychoactive drug that can cause either stimulating or depressing effects. Regular use may adversely affect the health of the lungs similar to cigarette smoking and impair psychomotor skills associated with driving an automobile similar to alcohol.

■ Cocaine is a highly addictive drug whose use may lead to a variety of health problems, including death. The Public Health Service (PHS), in *Healthy People 2000*, recommends that individuals should not even consider experimentation with the use of cocaine or crack.

■ Methamphetamine in the form of ice is a powerful stimulant, but, like cocaine, it possesses a major risk for addiction and adverse effects on physical and mental health.

■ Anabolic steroids provide an effective means to increase muscle mass and strength, but the potential health risks associated with their use, such as liver damage, cancer, and heart disease, far outweigh any potential benefits.

■ The use of illegal drugs may lead to arrest, conviction, and a criminal record that may limit future career opportunities of the college student.

■ Women who desire to become pregnant or who are pregnant should abstain from using any drug unless under the advice and supervision of an attending physician. The potential health threat to the unborn child is too great.

■ More and more Americans are contracting sexually transmitted diseases (STDs), primarily vaginitis, genital warts, genital herpes, chlamydia, gonorrhea, syphilis, and AIDS.

■ Each STD may be associated with an increased risk for other health problems, and several of the infecting viruses have been linked with genital cancer, principally cancer of the cervix.

■ Early diagnosis and treatment of STDs is critical to prevent further health complications. STDs can be cured with appropriate medical treatment with the exception of genital herpes and AIDS, although some drugs are used to treat these latter two diseases.

■ The current belief is that those who become infected with the HIV will eventually develop AIDS and die, but adopting components of a Positive Health Life-style, such as exercise and stress management, may help them cope better psychologically.

■ Abstinence is the only truly safe sex, although other sexual practices and the use of a condom may help reduce the risk of contracting STDs or AIDS.

INTRODUCTION

Life is full of risks! A risk may be defined as a hazard or a dangerous chance, and every day you confront a variety of hazards or take somewhat dangerous chances, thus exposing yourself to the chance of injury or loss. Although many of the daily activities you do are associated with various risks, you do them because they are either a necessity or convenience of modern living. Driving an automobile is not an absolute necessity in contemporary society, but it provides a convenient means to accomplish many of your daily responsibilities. Every time you drive an automobile you increase your risk of injury, but you can minimize the risk by adhering to safe and courteous driving practices, obeying traffic regulations, and buckling up for safety. If you take a dangerous chance, say exceeding the speed limit or not using a seat belt, you increase your risk of injury above normal.

You also engage in various risky endeavors because they bring you enjoyment and pleasure. For example, some of you may actually pay money to strap two boards to your feet and shoot down a snow-covered mountain at 30–40 miles per hour. This activity will certainly increase your risk of injury but it may be highly pleasurable if you possess appropriate skiing skills and safety equipment.

Whether you incur increased health risks daily out of necessity, convenience, or pleasure, you can minimize those risks through the use of appropriate, prudent health behaviors. Chapter 1 introduced the concept of risk factors in relation to disease, and in succeeding chapters, strategies believed to be prudent health behaviors to reduce various risks associated with the development of acute health problems or chronic diseases were discussed. If you began to practice these prudent health behaviors, you were learning **health risk management,** reducing the risk to a level compatible with good health. For example, you may have previously consumed substantial amounts of high-fat foods because you enjoyed the taste, particularly that of premium ice cream, but you learned that a diet high in total fat and saturated fat may increase the risk associated with the development of several chronic diseases, including obesity. However, you also learned that a healthy diet does contain some fat, and by keeping track of your dietary fat intake you could incorporate an occasional high-fat food, even premium ice cream, in your diet. You may also have learned to use and enjoy an appropriate substitute, such as frozen fat-free yogurt. Thus, you have learned to experience the pleasure and enjoyment of a given activity while minimizing the risk to your health.

As noted in previous chapters, many life-style behaviors may be incompatible with good health, and thus are risky behaviors, such as physical inactivity, an unbalanced diet, excess body fat, and high stress levels. If you have progressed to this point in the text, you should possess adequate knowledge and skills to implement a total exercise program, a healthy diet, and appropriate stress management techniques to help minimize the health risks associated with these life-style behaviors.

In this chapter we shall focus on two broad categories of life-style behaviors that are often referred to as high-risk behaviors: substance abuse and unsafe sex practices that transmit disease. Space limitations prevent a detailed discussion of all substances whose use is abused and of all sexually transmitted diseases, so we shall highlight those substances,

primarily drugs, and diseases targeted by the Public Health Service (PHS) in *Healthy People 2000: National Health Promotion and Disease Prevention Objectives* as being major health threats to Americans. The PHS has classified these major health threats into four categories: alcohol and other drugs, tobacco, HIV infection, and sexually transmitted diseases.

Substance abuse and sex are most commonly used to derive pleasure, but both can carry substantial health risks. There are various prudent health behaviors to reduce these risks to manageable levels, but the techniques may vary. We may apply the approaches to modification of the high-fat diet noted previously to substance abuse and decide that moderation in use may be an acceptable behavior for some substances, whereas finding a healthful substitute may be more appropriate for others ▪

Substance Abuse

Health professionals use the collective term **substance abuse** when referring to the use of certain substances or behaviors in ways that are detrimental to the physical, psychological, or social health of the user or to the health of others. Since the term is rather imprecise and could encompass a large number of substances and behaviors, the National Research Council (NRC) developed an operational definition of substance abuse to help remove the ambiguity. In essence, the NRC categorized substance abuse into the four areas exerting a significant negative impact upon the health of our nation. Overeating is one area of substance abuse, primarily because it may lead to obesity and related health problems, as discussed in chapter 7. The other three areas of substance abuse are alcohol abuse, cigarette smoking, and drug abuse. Alcohol and cigarettes are two separate entities, but **drug abuse** usually refers to the recreational use of illegal drugs or to the misuse of prescription drugs. Examples include the two main recreational drugs, cocaine and marijuana, narcotics such as heroin, analgesics such as Darvon®, tranquilizers such as Valium®, stimulants such as amphetamines, and hallucinogens such as LSD. *Drug abuse* and *substance abuse* are normally considered to be synonymous terms.

The first section of this chapter will focus on alcohol, cigarette smoking, and drug abuse, particularly those substances whose abuse has been targeted for reduction by the PHS in *Healthy People 2000*. Specific substances covered include alcohol, caffeine, tobacco, smokeless tobacco, marijuana, cocaine, methamphetamine in the form of ice, and anabolic steroids. Most of the substances, with the exception of caffeine, have been targeted for reduction by the PHS. It is also important to note that most of these drugs may be addicting.

Addiction, a term derived from the Latin verb "addicere," means to bind a person to one thing or another. This binding may occur for a variety of reasons, but, in general, the individual usually receives some pleasure or sense of well-being from a particular experience (related to the use of one thing or another) that tends to reinforce the repetition of that experience.

In the health profession, addiction is usually interpreted to involve a sequence of three stages as the individual repeats some particular experience. First, the individual develops a tolerance to the experience so that increasing amounts may be needed to provide gratification. Second, the individual becomes *dependent* upon the experience to derive pleasure and may go to great sacrifice to repeat it. Third, the individual will suffer both physical and psychological withdrawal symptoms if deprived of the experience for a period of time. **Habituation** is a term closely associated with addiction: however, with habituation the individual experiences only psychological withdrawal symptoms, not physical ones. Addiction or habituation to any of the substances in this chapter may increase the risk of health problems. The American Psychiatric Association, in its *Diagnostic and Statistical Manual of Mental Disorders,* has developed specific criteria for identification of substance dependence and abuse in general, as well as for specific substances, such as alcohol, marijuana, cocaine, etc., and also covers some adverse health effects. Laboratory Inventory 9.1 may be used as a general guide to determine whether you may have a substance-abuse problem.

Prevention and treatment of substance abuse are complex problems, but a current model focuses on the total well-being of the individual rather than simply targeting the specific substance being abused. Wellness education centering on exercise, proper nutrition, stress management, smoking cessation, health risk management, and spirituality is sound preventive medicine, but is increasingly being recognized as a very sound approach for treatment as well. Exercise is an important component of many substance abuse treatment programs. As noted in chapter 1, exercise may be considered a medicine. Researchers from Sweden suggest that exercise may complement psychological and psychiatric treatment by stimulating the release of endorphins (natural opiates) in the body during exercise. The endorphin may be a therapeutic substitute for various drugs, such as alcohol, and possibly replace a negative addiction with a positive one.

Alcohol and Health

Alcohol has existed from earliest times, and almost all societies include a traditional alcoholic beverage as part of their culture. It is an integral part of many celebrations such as parties, birthdays, and weddings, and other social gatherings such as conventions and sport events. Drinking is considered to be a rite of passage on many college campuses. Alcohol is a big business. The alcohol industry spends over one billion dollars each year in advertising. Much of this advertising, particularly for beer, is targeted for the young adult, creating a positive view of alcohol by associating it with sex, sports, recreation, and good times.

In the United States alone, more than 120 million people consume alcohol in one form or another on a regular basis, primarily as a social beverage for its mood-modifying effects. The vast majority of adults use alcohol in a rational manner, but a significant proportion, approximately one out of every ten drinkers (10 percent), experiences some alcohol-related problem. People of all ages, races, religions, socioeconomic statuses, and educational backgrounds experience alcohol-related problems. Unfortunately, alcohol consumption is prevalent in adolescents. About 50 percent of all high

school juniors and seniors are drinkers, and more than 3 million teenagers (aged fourteen to seventeen) have problems with alcohol. One survey even noted that about 30 percent of the nation's nine-year-olds feel peer pressure to drink.

Alcohol is a drug, and it is the major drug problem in the United States. The health problems associated with alcohol abuse are numerous and varied, ranging on a scale from headaches to homicide. In this regard, the Public Health Service, in *Healthy People 2000* expressed the primary objectives as decreasing fatalities from alcohol-related motor vehicle accidents, decreasing the mortality rate from cirrhosis of the liver, decreasing the number of birth defects due to alcohol, decreasing the number of heavy drinkers, particularly among high school and college students, and holding the line against increases in per capita consumption of alcohol. Recent progress reports of *Healthy People 2000* have suggested that adults are adopting more reasonable drinking habits and alcohol-related motor vehicle accidents have declined, but the problem is still massive. Moreover, efforts to curtail excess drinking in teenagers and young adults have failed, and alcohol-related problems actually are increasing in these age groups. Conflicting messages from society and alcohol product advertising may be involved in this failure.

Alcohol is a legal drug for those over twenty-one. Used in moderation it may add pleasure to our lives; used in excess it may lead to serious health consequences. The purpose of this section is to provide you with some basic knowledge so you can make a rational decision relative to the role alcohol will play in your life.

Common Dietary Sources

The **alcohol** produced for human consumption is **ethyl alcohol, or ethanol.** It is a transparent, colorless liquid derived from the fermentation of sugars in fruits, vegetables, and grains. Although classified legally as a drug, alcohol is a component of many common beverages served throughout the world. In the United States, alcohol is consumed mainly as a natural ingredient of beer, wine, and liquors. Although the alcohol content may vary in different types, in general, beer is about 4 to 5 percent alcohol, wine is about 12 to 14 percent alcohol, and typical bar liquor (whiskey, rum, gin, vodka) is about 40 to 45 percent alcohol. The term **proof** is a measure of the alcohol content in a beverage and is double the percentage; an 86-proof bottle of whiskey is 43 percent alcohol, while a 150-proof bottle of Caribbean rum is 75 percent alcohol.

One drink of alcohol is the equivalent of one-half ounce of pure ethyl alcohol or the equivalent of about 13 to 14 grams of alcohol. The following amounts of beer, wine, and liquor, illustrated in figure 9.1, contain approximately equal amounts of alcohol and are classified as one drink:

12 ounces (one bottle) of beer
4 ounces (one wine glass) of wine
1.25 ounces (one jigger or shot glass) of liquor

Technically, alcohol may be classified as a food because it provides energy, one of the major functions of food. Alcohol contains about 7 Calories per gram, almost twice the

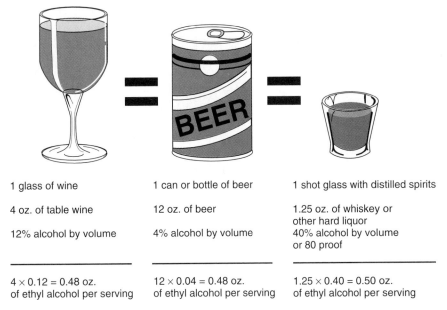

1 glass of wine

4 oz. of table wine

12% alcohol by volume

4 × 0.12 = 0.48 oz.
of ethyl alcohol per serving

1 can or bottle of beer

12 oz. of beer

4% alcohol by volume

12 × 0.04 = 0.48 oz.
of ethyl alcohol per serving

1 shot glass with distilled spirits

1.25 oz. of whiskey or
other hard liquor
40% alcohol by volume
or 80 proof

1.25 × 0.40 = 0.50 oz.
of ethyl alcohol per serving

Note: Of course, the above calculations would not apply if a wine cooler or a dessert wine were consumed in place of table wine, if a higher alcohol content beer or a "lite beer" were drunk instead of regular beer, and if higher proof distilled spirits were used in place of 80-proof liquor.

Figure 9.1 Alcohol equivalencies and drinking.

Table 9.1 Energy Content of Typical Alcoholic Beverages

| Beverage | Amount | Carbohydrate | | Alcohol | | Total |
		Grams	Calories	Grams	Calories	Calories
Beer, regular	12 ounces	13	52	13	91	150
Beer, light	12 ounces	4	16	11	77	96
Beer, nonalcoholic	12 ounces	12	48	1	7	55
Beer, alcohol free	12 ounces	12	48	0	0	48
Wine, table	4 ounces	4	16	12	84	100
Liquor, (80 proof)	1.25 ounces	0	0	14	98	100

The small discrepancies in the calculation of total Calories for beer and liquor may be attributed to a small protein content in beer and some energy value and trace amounts of carbohydrate in liquor.

value of an equal amount of carbohydrate or protein. Beer and wine also contain some carbohydrate, a source of additional Calories. In general, a bottle of regular beer has about 150 Calories, while a 4-ounce glass of wine or a shot glass of liquor contains about 100 Calories. Table 9.1 provides an approximate analysis of the caloric content of common alcoholic beverages and nonalcoholic beer.

In general, the Calories found in beer, wine, and liquor are empty Calories. Although wine and beer contain trace amounts of protein, vitamins, and minerals, liquor is void of any nutrient value. Alcohol may have a certain value to us as a social beverage, but its value as a food and source of nutrients is extremely limited.

Metabolism and Function of Alcohol

About 20 percent of the alcohol ingested may be absorbed by the stomach; the remainder passes on to the intestine for absorption. The absorption is rapid, particularly if the digestive tract is empty. The alcohol enters the blood and is distributed to the various tissues, being diluted by the water content of the body. A small portion of the alcohol, about 3 to 10 percent, is excreted from the body through the breath, urine, or sweat, but the majority is metabolized by the liver, the organ that metabolizes other drugs. As the blood circulates, the liver of an average adult male will metabolize about 8–10 grams of alcohol per hour, or slightly less than the amount of alcohol in one drink.

Although alcohol is derived from the fermentation of carbohydrates, it is metabolized in the body like fat. The liver helps to convert the metabolic by-products of alcohol into fatty acids, which may be stored in the liver or transported into the blood. Several other compounds, such as lactate, acetate, and acetaldehyde, may also be released into the blood. These products may eventually be utilized for energy and converted into carbon dioxide and water. A schematic of alcohol metabolism is presented in figure 9.2.

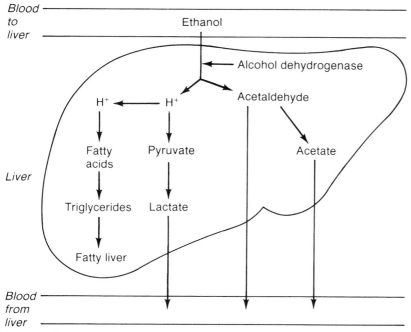

Figure 9.2 *Simplified metabolic pathways of ethanol (alcohol) in the liver. Hydrogen ions are removed from ethanol as it is converted to acetaldehyde, which may be released to the blood for transport to other tissues. The excess hydrogen ions may combine with fatty acids to form triglycerides or with pyruvate to form lactate. Excess accumulation of triglycerides may lead to the development of a fatty liver.*

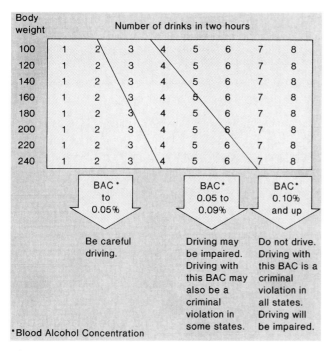

Figure 9.3 *Estimated blood alcohol concentrations with number of drinks over a one-hour period. The actual BAC may depend on other factors, such as the amount of food in the stomach. The effects on the brain may be influenced by mood, fatigue, or use of other medications.*

As noted above, the liver in a 150-pound male can metabolize less than one-half ounce of alcohol per hour. This rate may vary, being less in smaller individuals and more in larger individuals. Thus, consumption of alcohol at a rate greater than one drink per hour will result in an accumulation of alcohol in the blood; this is measured as the **blood alcohol content (BAC)** in grams per 100 milliliters of blood. For the average male, one drink will result in a BAC of about 0.025; four drinks in an hour would lead to a BAC of approximately 0.10. However, since alcohol is usually consumed over time, some of it is metabolized by the liver or excreted by the kidneys or lungs, so the BAC is reduced somewhat. Figure 9.3 provides an approximate BAC that could occur by drinking over a two-hour period, along with some guidelines for driving an automobile.

Alcohol affects all cells in the body. Many of these effects may have significant health implications. For example, laboratory research has shown that, in a test tube, alcohol and acetaldehyde could cause changes in DNA, the genetic material in body cells, comparable to changes elicited by carcinogens. Alcohol may suppress the immune system in various ways. Alcohol also may generate free radicals when metabolized in the liver. Other constituents in alcoholic beverages, particularly nitrosamines in beer, may be carcinogenic. These findings could be related to the increased risk in those who drink of certain forms of cancer, such as cancer of the esophagus, colon, rectum, pancreas, and liver, and breast cancer in women.

Alcohol also has a direct toxic effect on the intestinal walls; it tends to impair the absorption of vitamins such as thiamin (B_1). In addition, alcohol affects liver metabolism in several ways. It may interfere with the metabolism of other drugs, increasing the effect of some and lessening the effect of others. In excess, alcohol may also lead to the accumulation of fat in the liver and eventual destruction of liver cells. Fat may also accumulate in the adipose cells.

However, the most immediate effects of alcohol are on the brain; often these effects are paradoxical. Although alcohol

Table 9.2 Typical Effects of Increasing Blood Alcohol Content

Number of Drinks* Consumed in Two Hours	Blood** Alcohol Level	Typical Effects
2–3	.02–.04	Reduced tension, relaxed feeling, relief from daily stress
4–5	.06–.09	Impaired judgment, a high feeling, impaired fine motor ability and coordination
6–8	.11–.16	Legally drunk, slurred speech, impaired gross motor coordination, staggering gait
9–12	.18–.25	Loss of control of voluntary activity, erratic behavior, impaired vision
13–18	.27–.39	Stuporous, total loss of coordination
19 and above	>.40	Coma, depression of respiratory centers, death

*One drink = 12 ounce regular beer
4 ounce wine
1.25 ounce liquor

**BAC based on body weight of 160 pounds (72.6 KG). The BAC will increase proportionally for individuals weighing less (such as a 120-pound female) and will decrease proportionally for individuals weighing more (such as a 200-pound football player). For example, four to five drinks in two hours could lead to a BAC of 0.08–0.12 in a 120-pound individual.*

is a depressant, a small amount often exerts a stimulating effect, because it may release some of the normal inhibitory control mechanisms in the brain. For the most part, however, alcohol acts as a depressant, and the effects on the brain are dose dependent. The effects occur in a hierarchical fashion related to the development of the brain. In general, alcohol first affects the higher brain centers. With increasing dosages, lower levels of brain function become depressed with subsequent disturbance of normal functions. This hierarchy of brain functions, from higher levels to lower levels, and some of the functions affected by alcohol may be generalized as follows:

Thinking and reasoning—Judgment
Perceptual-motor responses—Reaction time
Fine-motor coordination—Muscles of speech
Gross-motor coordination—Walking
Visual processes—Double vision
Alertness—Sleep, coma
Respiratory control—Respiratory failure, death

The BAC is the major factor controlling the effect of alcohol on the brain and, as noted previously, may be determined from the number of drinks consumed. However, a variety of factors may influence the effects of alcohol consumption upon the brain, such as body size, amount of food in the digestive tract, an individual's state of mind, level of tolerance developed, and for women, even the phase of their menstrual cycle. In general, however, the symptoms listed in table 9.2 may be typical.

Alcohol and a Positive Health Life-Style

The acute effects of alcohol consumption have been noted above, and the implications these effects may have upon the immediate health status of the individual, primarily increased susceptibility to accidents, are fairly well established. In general, the more you drink during a single bout, the more prone you are to acute health problems. This same relationship also holds true relative to the development of health problems associated with the chronic use of alcohol.

Individual consumption of alcohol in the United States ranges on a continuum from abstinence to alcoholism. In adults, approximately 10 percent of the population abstain from alcohol consumption, 20 percent are infrequent drinkers, 35 percent are light drinkers, 25 percent are moderate drinkers, and 10 percent are heavy drinkers. In one classification system, light drinkers are those who consume 1 to 9 grams of alcohol per day (less than one drink), moderate drinkers are those who consume 10 to 34 grams per day (about one to three drinks), and heavy drinkers are those who consume more than 34 grams per day (more than three drinks). It is interesting to note that in the United States, the 10 percent of the heavy drinkers account for nearly 50 percent of the alcohol consumed.

Those who abstain will, of course, not have any health problems associated with alcohol, while those who are heavy drinkers are most prone to alcoholism and related health disorders. There is some controversy relative to the health implications of those who are light or moderate drinkers.

If you do drink, you may wish to complete Laboratory Inventory 9.2, which may help you evaluate whether or not you may have a problem with alcohol.

Abstinence If you want to avoid health problems associated with alcohol, abstinence is the best approach. As shall be noted, there are actually some possible health benefits associated with alcohol consumption in moderation, but health authorities caution that these potential benefits are not sufficient cause to start drinking if you currently abstain. For those who have a family history of alcohol problems, abstinence is probably the best policy for there appears to be some genetic or familial predisposition towards alcoholism. For those who do drink, abstinence is advised under certain conditions. As noted previously, the acute effects of excessive alcohol consumption include impairment of both motor coordination and judgment—two factors that are extremely important in the safe operation of an automobile. At the least, being arrested for drunk driving may have serious social and personal consequences. At the worst, alcohol is involved as a cause of nearly one-half of all automobile fatalities—nearly 25,000 deaths per year in the United States alone. As the saying goes, "Don't drink and drive!" Figure 9.3 may provide you with some useful guidelines.

Drinking should be minimized in individuals with certain health conditions, such as liver disease, peptic ulcers, and gout, for alcohol may aggravate these problems, and it should

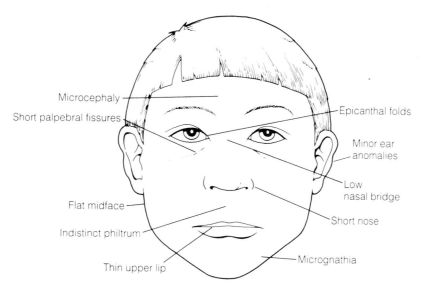

Figure 9.4 *Common facial characteristics of children with Fetal Alcohol Syndrome (FAS). Features labeled on the left are seen frequently; those on the right are less specific to this syndrome.*

Labels: Microcephaly, Short palpebral fissures, Flat midface, Indistinct philtrum, Thin upper lip, Epicanthal folds, Minor ear anomalies, Low nasal bridge, Short nose, Micrognathia

also be minimized for those taking certain medications, such as aspirin or nonsteroidal anti-inflammatory agents (ibuprofen) because alcohol may promote gastrointestinal bleeding.

Women who drink should abstain during pregnancy. The **Fetal Alcohol Syndrome (FAS)** refers to the effects upon the development of a fetus if a mother consumes alcohol while pregnant. The child is multihandicapped and may experience retardation in growth and mental development as well as facial birth defects (see figure 9.4). Some FAS features may disappear with time, but many still remain in late childhood and adolescence. **Fetal alcohol effects (FAE)** may be observed in children when the full-blown FAS syndrome is not present. FAE children are easily distracted and have poor attention spans. Both FAS and FAE are associated with learning disorders in children and possible speech defects. Fortunately, both are totally preventable. Most cases of FAS are associated with women who drink heavily; however, as little as one to two drinks per day, particularly in the first months of pregnancy, have been associated with premature infants and FAE. At the present time, safe amounts of alcohol during pregnancy have not been determined. Thus, the safest approach is abstinence.

Moderation   There is some controversy as to whether or not light to moderate drinking, the equivalent of about one to three drinks per day, poses a significant health hazard. Most of the research data is epidemiological in nature, although some experimental studies in the laboratory and with humans have been conducted.

On the negative side, the previously mentioned effects of alcohol on damage to the DNA in the cell nucleus may occur at an alcohol concentration equivalent to one to two drinks and thus may be involved in the development of certain cancers. Although the possible link between alcohol intake and breast cancer is being debated and continues to be studied, there is increasing evidence supporting a positive relationship between the two. There are more than a dozen epidemiological studies that have shown a link between alcohol consumption and breast cancer in women, even with as little as one drink per day. One reviewer noted a relative risk of 1.4, an increased risk of 40 percent, for development of breast cancer in women who consumed the equivalent of two drinks per day. A recent review has noted that although more research needs to be conducted in this area, women who are at high risk for breast cancer, such as those whose mothers have had breast cancer, those who are obese, those who have had few children, or those who have had their first child past the age of twenty-five, should abstain or limit their alcohol intake. One of the leading researchers studying the link between diet and cancer, Walter Willett, noted that of all dietary factors, an increased risk among women who consume alcohol is probably the best established dietary risk for breast cancer. Willett also notes this risk may possibly be greatest during adolescence and early adulthood when the breast is more susceptible to cancer risk factors, and suggests women should possibly reduce alcohol consumption earlier in life.

Individuals on medication should be aware of drug-alcohol interactions. Since alcohol may interfere with oral medications taken by diabetics, intake should be limited. If you take medication on a regular basis, consult your physician to determine any potential harmful effects.

Other research has shown that three or more drinks per day increase the risk of developing high blood pressure and may increase blood lipid levels. Some individuals may experience heart arrhythmias following alcohol intake. Alcohol is also a significant source of Calories, about seven per gram, and may be a contributing factor to obesity. All of these conditions are risk factors for coronary heart disease (CHD).

On the positive side, some epidemiological research has shown that moderate consumption of alcohol (one to three beers or glasses of wine per day) is associated with a lesser chance of developing CHD. Many studies support a J-shaped relationship, indicating that moderate intake of alcohol may reduce the risk of CHD below that of abstainers. This finding is consistent even when other interfering variables have been controlled, such as diet, exercise, and former drinkers now being abstainers. The mechanism is not known, but one theory is that the relaxant effect of alcohol may help reduce emotional stress, a risk factor associated with CHD. Another theory has focused upon the effect of alcohol to raise HDL cholesterol, the form of cholesterol that protects against the development of CHD (see discussion on page 245). Studies have consistently shown that alcohol consumption is associated with increased levels of total HDL cholesterol, HDL_2 cholesterol, HDL_3 cholesterol, apolipoprotein A-1, and a decreased total cholesterol:HDL cholesterol ratio, all serum lipid profiles which are thought to help prevent CHD. Alcohol is believed by some to affect various enzymes in the liver that may affect HDL metabolism. Additionally, alcohol consumption has been associated with increased eicosanoid production, particularly a prostacyclin that may cause vasodilation and inhibit platelet aggregation (clotting ability), and increased levels of enzymes that break down clots, all factors which may protect against the development of CHD.

With some of the exceptions noted above, health professionals generally support the viewpoint that alcohol consumed in moderation, along with a balanced diet, should not pose any health problem to the average, healthy individual.

Heavy Drinking   Although drinking in moderation may confer some small health benefits, heavy alcohol consumption is a different matter. In the United States, according to Burke, one of every ten deaths is alcohol-related and the health-care economic costs approximated $150 billion in 1995. There is an increased non-coronary heart disease mortality with heavy alcohol consumption resulting in a higher overall mortality rate for heavy drinkers. As noted in the discussion above, alcohol is involved in a high percentage of automobile injuries and fatalities and is also a key factor in other accidental deaths, such as boating accidents and falls in the home. Aggressive behavior is also positively associated with alcohol intake, which contributes to increased risk for sexual abuse, suicide, and homicide. Chronic heavy drinking also increases the risk for various cancers. By exacerbating the effects on the gastrointestinal tract, excess alcohol intake increases the relative risk of cancer of the mouth, esophagus, colon, and rectum. The relative risk for breast cancer also increases markedly with increases in alcohol intake. Additionally, other health problems are associated with heavy drinking, such as osteoporosis, hypertension, and some forms of stroke. Also, as noted earlier, alcohol is high in Calories, and when consumed in excess of energy needs may be readily stored as fat, leading to obesity.

One of the major body organs affected by alcohol is the liver. Even with a balanced diet high in protein, consuming six drinks a day for less than a month has been shown to cause significant accumulation of fat in the liver. If continued over the years, the liver cells degenerate. Eventually the damaged liver cells are replaced by nonfunctioning scar tissue, a condition known as **cirrhosis.** As liver function deteriorates, fat, carbohydrate, and protein metabolism are not regulated properly; this has possible pathological consequences for other body organs such as the kidney, pancreas, and heart.

Alcohol abuse is the major drug problem in the United States, posing a problem for one out of every ten drinkers. It is also a major problem on college campuses. A recent news conference by the U.S. Surgeon General revealed that over 40 percent of college students engage in heavy drinking, that they consume more alcohol than any other beverage, that they spend more on alcohol than on books, and that alcohol was a factor in over 20 percent of college dropouts. Academic achievement is inversely related to alcohol consumption in college, that is, the more alcohol one drinks, the lower the grade point average. As elsewhere in society, excessive use of alcohol on college campuses has been associated with increased aggressive behavior and is directly related to the incidence rate of sexual abuse, suicide, and homicide. Although males have been most likely to be involved in heavy drinking, particularly weekly binge drinking, more females are drinking heavily. A recent report indicated that 30 percent of college women said they drink to get drunk.

Excessive intake of alcohol may lead to a disorder known as **alcoholism,** a condition whose etiology is unknown but probably is related to a variety of physiological, psychological, and sociological factors. The National Council on Alcoholism suggests that there is no pat definition for alcoholism; it may be evidenced by a variety of behaviors. The number of behaviors exhibited by the drinker may be related to various stages in the progression towards alcoholism. Laboratory Inventory 9.1, a questionnaire developed by the National Council on Alcoholism, provides for an assessment of some of these behaviors.

The physical, psychological, and social health hazards of alcoholism have been well documented; anyone with such a problem should seek professional help.

Recommendations   How does alcohol fit into a Positive Health Life-style? As noted in chapter 1, the key to a Positive Health Life-style is personal choice based upon proper knowledge. This brief section has provided you with some knowledge to make an informed decision. The references at the end of this chapter may provide you with more in-depth reading. For many individuals, alcohol is one of the pleasures of life. If you do drink, the following general recommendations are advisable.

Drink moderately. A guideline for moderate drinking that has persisted over the years was developed by an English physician, F. E. Anstie, in the nineteenth century and is known as Anstie's Rule or Anstie's Limit. In essence, no more than 0.5 ounce per 50 pounds body weight should be consumed per day. That averages out to be about one drink for each 50 pounds you weigh, or a maximum of about three drinks per day. However, some researchers recommend no more than one to two drinks per day. As noted above, you should not drink at all under certain conditions, such as pregnancy.

To minimize the increase in the blood alcohol content and its adverse effects, eat some food before or while you drink, particularly food that is high in protein and has some fat. Alternate an alcoholic beverage with one containing little to no alcohol, such as the wide variety of no-alcohol and low-alcohol beers or wines available or the fashionable mineral waters concocted into a "mocktail."

Know your capacity and do not exceed it. Nurse your drinks by drinking slowly. Set a definite limit on how many drinks you will have; keep track and don't exceed it. Remember, your body can metabolize less than one drink per hour.

Do not drink alcohol if you are taking other drugs that may also be depressants or cause drowsiness, such as certain cold medications.

Do not drive after drinking and do not let your friends do so either. If you plan to drink more than normal, arrange to have a designated driver.

Your use of alcohol should enhance your general sense of well-being and should not interfere with your social interactions with other individuals. Your behavior should not become disruptive or socially unacceptable.

If you use alcohol to relax and unwind, or to cope with academic pressures, find an alternative, such as exercise. It not only may help reduce stress; it may also counteract some of the adverse effects of alcohol. Contrary to alcohol, exercise may help to decrease blood triglycerides, decrease high blood pressure, improve glucose tolerance, and burn Calories. Exercise also helps to increase HDL cholesterol.

Caffeine, Coffee, and Health

Caffeine is a naturally-occurring compound in many of the foods and beverages that we consume every day, such as coffee, tea, colas, and chocolate. Yet caffeine is legally classified as a drug and has some powerful physiological and metabolic effects on the human body. A normal therapeutic dose of caffeine may range from 100–300 milligrams. Some approximate amounts in beverages, chocolate, and medications are presented in table 9.3.

In general, caffeine is a central nervous system stimulant that will increase alertness, but it also stimulates heart function, blood circulation, and release of epinephrine (adrenaline) from the adrenal gland. Epinephrine, also a stimulant, augments these effects and also, in conjunction with the caffeine, stimulates a wide variety of tissues. As a matter of fact, caffeine was used extensively in diet pills because it would increase the resting metabolic rate about 8–12 percent, but its use was discontinued for this purpose because of potential for abuse.

Because caffeine is a powerful stimulant and because it is most commonly consumed as coffee, the health effects of both caffeine and coffee have been studied extensively, and whether or not either one is harmful to health has been one of the most hotly-debated questions over the past twenty years.

Table 9.3 Caffeine Content in Common Beverages, Foods, and Medications

Beverages (6 ounces)	Milligrams of Caffeine
Coffee, regular	100–150
Coffee, instant	60–80
Coffee, decaffeinated	6–12
Cola drinks	15–30
Tea, black	25–40
Chocolate (per ounce)	
Syrup	10–15
Milk chocolate	5–6
Medications (per tablet)	
Stimulants (Vivarin®)	200

Since the early 1970s, a number of epidemiological studies have linked coffee or caffeine consumption with the development of a variety of health problems, including heart disease, high serum cholesterol, high blood pressure, pancreatic cancer, fibrocystic breast disease (painful lumps in the breast tissue), infertility in the female reproductive system, and for pregnant women, the possibility of lower birth height and weight, birth defects, or spontaneous abortion. Conversely, other epidemiological studies have shown no relationship between coffee or caffeine consumption and these health problems. Investigators have looked at a variety of factors, including different sources of caffeine such as coffee versus tea, regular coffee versus decaffeinated coffee, and even the method of preparing coffee, such as filtered versus boiled.

Several recent reviews have investigated the relationship between coffee consumption and serum lipid levels, noting an inconsistency in the results of most studies. Some studies have shown that both caffeinated and decaffeinated coffee may raise serum cholesterol, but others have reported no effects. In some cases where the cholesterol levels rose, the authors noted the increases were of little clinical significance. Boiled coffee, a common method of preparation in Northern European countries, may contain a lipoid fraction that raises serum cholesterol more so than filtered coffee, the most common preparation method in the United States. Based on these conflicting data, reviewers indicate that our state of knowledge is too limited to draw any conclusions regarding the effect of coffee or caffeine on serum lipid levels.

Coffee or caffeine may pose some problems to some individuals. Abstainers, or those who consume little caffeine, may experience nervousness, irritability, headaches, or insomnia with moderate doses, although long-term consumption of coffee leads to the development of tolerance and reduction of these "coffee nerves" symptoms. Caffeine may potentiate the hormonal response to stress. Some susceptible individuals experience heart arrhythmias following caffeine consumption, while others experience gastric distress due to increased secretion of acids in the stomach. Thus, individuals with such cardiovascular and gastrointestinal problems should avoid caffeine or use naturally-decaffeinated beverages. Moreover, the association between caffeine and fibrocystic breast disease and problems during pregnancy continues to be investigated. Also, massive doses of caffeine may be fatal; although rare, death may result from overdosing on caffeine-containing diet or stimulant pills.

In general, however, the conclusion of most reviewers and health organizations appears to suggest that moderate coffee or caffeine consumption poses few major health risks to the average American. For example, in 1988, the office of the U.S. Surgeon General reported that evidence of the relationship between coffee and heart disease was too weak to warrant recommending a reduction of coffee consumption. The American Heart Association stated that moderate coffee consumption does not appear to be harmful, while the American Cancer Society concluded that coffee does not increase the risk of cancer. It is also noteworthy that the PHS, in *Healthy People 2000,* does not target caffeine or coffee as a health risk.

Overall, physicians and other reviewers generally recommend moderation in coffee or caffeine consumption for regular consumers of these products, which usually is translated as approximately two to three 6-ounce cups of coffee per day, or about 200–300 milligrams of caffeine. It may be prudent for women who are pregnant or nursing to lower this amount or to abstain.

Finally, caffeine may confer some possible health benefits. It may diminish drowsiness, increase alertness, and promote clearer thinking, all factors that may contribute to safer automobile operation under certain conditions.

Cigarette Smoking and Health

Currently there are over 60,000 scientific articles written about the relationship between smoking and disease which have supported the contention of the United States Public Health Service that cigarette smoking is the most important single preventable cause of death in our society. Approximately 25 percent of the population over the age of seventeen, or nearly 50 million people, smoke on the average of one and a half packs of cigarettes per day, totaling over 600 billion cigarettes annually. The adverse health effects associated with this magnitude of cigarette smoking are pervasive. The number of deaths associated with cigarette smoking averages over 1,000 per day, or over 420,000 per year (20 percent of all deaths), including 2,000 children who die before the age of one because their mothers smoked during pregnancy. One third of all cancer deaths, over 100,000 per year, are attributed to cigarette smoking. It is also a major risk factor for coronary heart disease. The health-care costs associated with the treatment of problems caused by cigarette smoking have been estimated to be approximately 50 to 65 billion dollars per year in the United States alone.

The ultimate goal established by C. Everett Koop, a former surgeon general, is to make the United States a smokeless society by the year 2000. Major health objectives in *Healthy People 2000* include the reduction of the proportion of adults, children, and pregnant women who smoke to less than 15 percent of the population, and to decrease exposure of children to passive smoking. The goal is to develop the viewpoint in our society that smoking is no longer considered to be a normal, acceptable behavior. The Public Health Service has reported that progress has been made toward that goal, such as decreasing the percentage of adults and children who smoke and passage of laws prohibiting smoking in public places. However, Bartecchi and others recently noted that cigarette smoking has stopped declining in the United States. The magnitude of the problem is still enormous and much remains to be done.

In this section, we shall address several aspects related to the use of tobacco, primarily focusing upon cigarette smoking, namely the physiological effects of smoking on the human body, disease processes associated with such effects, and guidelines to avoid starting smoking or to stop smoking if you currently smoke.

Physiological Effects of Tobacco Use

Tobacco contains over 4,000 different compounds, many of which may modify human physiology. The three major substances in cigarette smoke include nicotine, tar, and carbon monoxide.

Nicotine is a drug, a powerful stimulant. In large doses (over 60 milligrams) it is a potent poison; in small doses, it may elicit a mild, stimulating effect. Although a typical cigarette contains about 20–30 milligrams of nicotine, only about 10 percent is absorbed into the body from cigarette smoke; this is more than enough to elicit a pharmacological effect. Since it may be absorbed directly from the lungs, its effects are rapid; it reaches the brain in about 6 seconds. The nicotine in smokeless tobacco is absorbed more slowly through the mucous membranes in the mouth.

Nicotine exerts its effects directly on the central nervous system. As a stimulant, it may create a psychological state of alertness and excitation. Nicotine also affects the hypothalamus, the center in the brain that helps to control a wide variety of physiological functions throughout the body, including an increased secretion of the hormone adrenalin from the adrenal medulla. The combined effects of hypothalamic stimulation and increased adrenalin levels result in an increased heart rate, constriction of blood vessels, and increased blood pressure. The appetite center in the hypothalamus may also be inhibited and total body metabolism may be increased; this may be why cigarette smoking at one time was advertised for its ability to keep women thin. An early advertisement stated, "Reach for a Lucky, not a sweet."

In many individuals, nicotine helps reduce stress and induce relaxation, a psychological state usually associated with the use of depressants such as alcohol, not stimulants. But larger doses of nicotine may lead to increased release of chemicals called endorphins, depressants produced naturally in the pituitary gland, an endocrine gland under the influence of the hypothalamus. Smokers claim that nicotine helps them regulate moods, control anger, reduce anxiety and stress, and provide a moderate state of euphoria.

These psychological effects of nicotine, either stimulation or relaxation, are the basic reasons that individuals continue to smoke even when they are aware of potential health risks. The Food and Drug Administration (FDA) recently investigated allegations that researchers at major tobacco companies may have manipulated cigarette recipes to increase nicotine levels. Nicotine is a legal, widely available, powerful addictive drug, and its use exhibits the triad associated with addiction. When nicotine is first used, the body reacts adversely and initially attempts to repulse its use; however, tolerance is developed rather rapidly. The individual then becomes dependent upon nicotine for the desired psychological effects. Finally, upon withdrawal, there are both physical and psychological symptoms that may take weeks or months to disappear. The Surgeon General of the United States has declared nicotine to be addictive, which has helped support the passage of legislation regulating the use of tobacco. One congressman has stated that many tobacco companies are nothing more than drug cartels, and the FDA is currently looking at labeling nicotine as a drug.

Tar is a general term that encompasses over 4,000 different chemicals found in cigarette smoke. These compounds include acids, alcohols, corrosive gases, and a host of others. The average smoker, at a pack and a half a day, inhales these compounds into the lungs approximately 100,000 times per year. When the hot smoke cools in the lungs, these chemicals solidify into a brownish-yellow, sticky mass. A number of these chemicals, such as tobacco-specific nitrosamines, are carcinogens capable of initiating tumor development. Recent research has found that some tar extracts may induce strand breaks in DNA, which may explain some carcinogenic effects of cigarette smoking. Other substances in tobacco are promoters that help the tumor grow at a faster rate.

Carbon monoxide is a poisonous gas resulting from incomplete combustion of materials in tobacco. It has a tremendous ability to combine with hemoglobin in the blood; when it does, it reduces the ability of hemoglobin to transport oxygen to the tissues. Such an effect not only would impair aerobic endurance capacity in athletes but also would place an additional stress on the heart, an organ almost totally dependent on oxygen for energy production.

These effects are also noted with **passive smoking,** the inhalation by a nonsmoker of the sidestream smoke from the burning tip of a cigarette, also known as second-hand smoke or environmental tobacco smoke.

Tobacco Use and Your Health

Tobacco has recently been labeled the number one culprit in causing death in the United States. Individuals who smoke are at twice the risk of premature death prior to the age of sixty-five compared to individuals who do not smoke. Epidemiological studies have indicated that the decrease in life expectancy associated with lifelong smoking is 7–18 years. The two major chronic diseases associated with cigarette smoking are coronary heart disease (CHD) and lung cancer, although there are a variety of other health problems associated with cigarette smoking and smokeless tobacco. Some of these adverse health effects are due to direct contact between the chemicals in tobacco and the affected tissue, while other health effects are caused by physiological responses in other body tissues.

The use of cigarettes involves the oral cavity (mouth, cheek, and gums), the trachea, and bronchial passageways to the lungs, and is associated with an increased risk for cancer in the oral cavity, probably due to direct contact of mucous membrane tissues with carcinogenic chemicals. It is interesting to note that some research has revealed that the use of both alcohol and cigarettes will lead to a synergistic effect regarding the development of oral cancer. Although epidemiological research has shown that each may contribute individually to the development of oral cancer, the effect is significantly elevated in individuals who both smoke and drink; in some studies the relative risk was in excess of 100, an amazing 10,000 percent increased risk for developing oral cancer in those who both smoke cigarettes and drink alcohol. On the way to the lungs, irritants in cigarette smoke will initiate the action of cilia, little hairlike projections lining the airways, to help repel them from the body. However, in a short time, this cilia defense mechanism is paralyzed, and the body attempts to remove these irritants by the cough reflex. Chronic coughing and bronchitis (inflammation of the bronchial tubes) eventually result. Irritants and chemicals may also affect the larynx (the voice box) and lead to laryngitis or, in prolonged smoking, laryngeal cancer.

In the lungs, the tar eventually leads to the breakdown of the elastic fibers in the alveoli, the tiny sacs where the gases are exchanged, and reduces the lung surface area. This condition, known as **emphysema** (a chronic obstructive pulmonary disease, or COPD), makes breathing extremely difficult, especially with any mild degree of exertion.

As is well known, the carcinogens in cigarette smoke are associated with a very significant risk for lung cancer in individuals who have smoked for years. These carcinogens may also contribute to the development or promotion of cancers in other organs of the body, including leukemia. Some of these pathological effects of cigarette smoking on the lungs are highlighted in figure 9.5.

Although a direct cause-and-effect relationship has not been determined, epidemiological research shows a consistent relationship between cigarette smoking and CHD. This relationship may be due to the physiological effects of nicotine and other chemicals in the body that increase the risk for atherosclerosis. For example, cigarette smoking has been shown to cause changes in the blood lipid levels, increasing triglycerides and total cholesterol while decreasing HDL cholesterol, a lipid profile more prone to atherosclerosis. Smoking may also increase fibrinogen levels in the blood, thus increasing the potential for the more rapid formation of clots that may block the coronary blood vessels that nurture the heart. These factors also underlie the increased incidence of cerebral stroke seen with tobacco use (see fig 9.6).

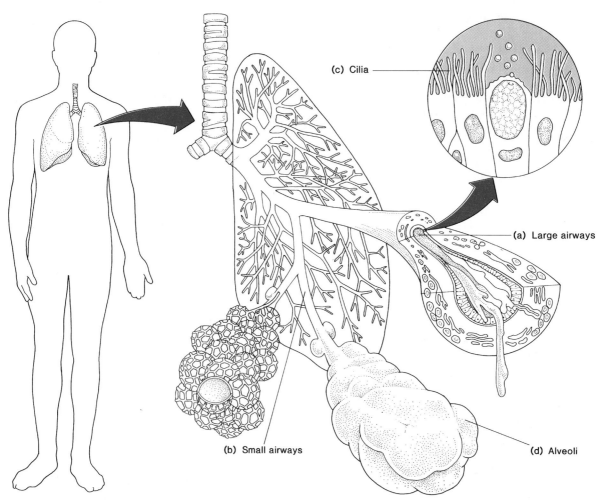

Figure 9.5 *The pathophysiologic effects of cigarette smoke on the pulmonary system. (a) Effects on airways—modest increase in mucous secretion, which leads to increased cough and sputum production in smokers (large airways). (b) Initial response is inflammation with associated ulceration and narrowing of the airways (small airways). (c) Effects on ciliary clearance—cigarette smoke produces structural and functional abnormalities in the airway ciliary system. Chronic bronchitis in smokers and ex-smokers is characterized by an impairment of ciliary clearance. (d) Effects on lung parenchyma—increased numbers of inflammatory cells are found in the lungs of cigarette smokers, causing structural abnormalities in the alveoli.*

Cigarette smoking may also cause abnormal heart rhythms that may trigger a heart attack. The increased blood pressure and secretion of adrenalin caused by nicotine will increase the oxygen demand of the heart muscle at the same time carbon monoxide decreases the oxygen supply. In cases of compromised circulation to the heart, such as in atherosclerosis, the heart may not be able to meet its oxygen needs and thus will lose its functional ability, resulting in a heart attack. Some of the pathological effects of cigarette smoking on the cardiovascular system are presented in figure 9.6. Although the effects of smoking on cardiovascular health may be seen in both men and women, research has shown that women who smoke and use oral contraceptives are at a tenfold greater risk for a heart attack compared to women who neither smoke nor use oral contraceptives.

Women who smoke while pregnant also expose their unborn child to increased risk. In general, such women have a greater number of miscarriages, stillbirths, premature births, and children with low body weights at birth. More of these children also die within the first year of life, probably due to increased respiratory problems and the associated Sudden Infant Death Syndrome.

Passive smoking, the inhalation of second-hand smoke, by nonsmokers may also lead to similar health problems. For example, lung cancer is more prevalent in those exposed to passive smoking. In a recent review, the Consumers Union indicated passive smoking increased the risk of lung cancer by 20–40 percent, possibly because the sidestream smoke (smoke that curls off the end of a smoldering cigarette) contains higher concentrations of several human carcinogens than mainstream smoke (smoke inhaled by the smoker). Additionally, a coalition of health agencies, including the American Heart Association, the American Lung Association, and the American Cancer Society, noted that second-hand smoke was a significant factor in cardiovascular deaths each year. Also, children of parents who smoke experience more cases of chronic coughing, bronchitis, and laryngitis. After reviewing the epidemiological data, Glantz and Parmley concluded that passive smoking

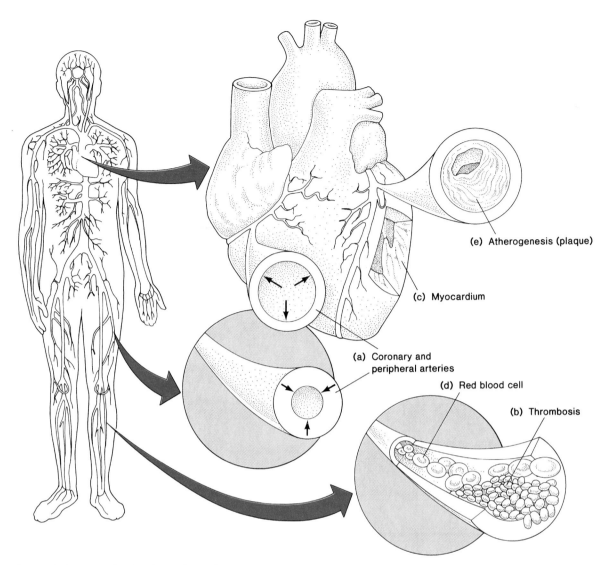

Figure 9.6 *The pathophysiologic effects of cigarette smoke on the cardiovascular system. (a) Sympathomimetic effects of nicotine—acute cardiovascular responses with each cigarette smoked include increased systolic blood pressure, increased diastolic blood pressure, increased heart rate, increased cardiac output, and increased coronary blood flow. Another sympathomimetic effect is vasoconstriction of peripheral arteries. (b) Effects favoring thrombosis include increased platelet aggregation, increased platelet adhesiveness, decreased platelet survival, increased plasma fibrinogen, decreased clotting time, increased blood viscosity, and increased hematocrit. (c) Effects on electrical stability of the myocardium include nicotine lowering the ventricular fibrillation threshold. (d) Effects on oxygen transport/utilization include carbon monoxide from cigarette smoke that binds to hemoglobin and reduces oxygen transport. (e) Effects favoring atherogenesis—decreased high density lipoprotein cholesterol, increased low density lipoprotein cholesterol, increased total serum cholesterol, and increased free fatty acids. Carbon monoxide may increase endothelial permeability in the arterial wall, favoring lipid deposition.*

is the third leading preventable cause of death in the United States today, behind active smoking and alcohol; according to government figures, passive smoking causes over 45,000 deaths due to coronary heart disease and 3,000 deaths due to lung cancer annually.

A summary of the major adverse health effects of cigarette smoking is presented in table 9.4. Fortunately, most of these conditions attributed to the use of tobacco are preventable. If you don't smoke, don't start! Avoid passive smoke. If you do smoke, stop!

Cigarette Smoking and a Positive Health Life-Style

Needless to say, cigarette smoking is incompatible with a Positive Health Life-style. The evidence is overwhelming that cigarette smoking confers significant health risks. But if you are young, some subtle pressures exist that are designed to get you to start or to continue smoking.

The cigarette industry is a megabusiness, as evidenced by the use of over 600 billion cigarettes annually in the United States alone. However, the general trend to preventive medicine in the United States is toward healthier life-styles, and as part of this trend, many individuals have stopped using cigarettes. In fact, there are now almost as many former smokers as there are current smokers. This, of course, is bad for the cigarette business. Therefore, in order to attract more customers, they have marketed their product more and more to the young, using images of youth, vitality, sex (Slim and

Table 9.4 Summary of Increased Health Risks Associated with Cigarette Smoking

Pulmonary

Decreased lung function
Chronic coughing and sputum production
Asthma
Chronic Obstructive Pulmonary Disease (COPD)
    Emphysema
    Chronic bronchitis

Cardiovascular

Decreased HDL cholesterol
Increased total and LDL cholesterol
Increased serum triglycerides
Platelet adhesiveness
Synergistic interaction with hypertension and high blood cholesterol
Synergistic action in women who use oral contraceptives
Atherosclerosis, both coronary and peripheral
Arrhythmias and cardiac sudden death
Chronic heart disease
Cerebrovascular disease (stroke)

Cancers

Lung
Oral cavity
Larynx
Esophagus
Gastric
Kidney
Bladder
Pancreas

Pregnant women

Fetal injury
Premature birth
Low birth weight
Sudden Infant Death Syndrome (SIDS)

Others

Osteoporosis
Peptic ulcers

Sassy; Joe Camel), and even sports and fitness (the Virginia Slims Tennis Tournament). Such advertising, along with the ever-present peer pressure among the young, is very persuasive.

Research suggests that very few people start smoking after age twenty. If you have resisted such pressures to start smoking or if you have started but have stopped and are currently a nonsmoker, great! Continue to do so! The following information is primarily for those who do smoke or for nonsmokers who may want to get a friend or relative to stop. If you are a smoker and want to improve your health, you must decide to quit.

Suggestions to Help You Quit Smoking   One of the first things you might do is find out why you smoke. Carry a small notepad or card with you, and put a rubber band around your pack of cigarettes. Take one full day; every time you light up, use the rubber band as a reminder to jot down the time, the place, and why you are smoking, i.e., pleasure, urge, habit, or any other feeling. Reviewing this list may provide you with some insight into why you smoke. You should also complete Laboratory Inventory 9.3, "Why Do You Smoke?" There are a variety of reasons that people smoke, and this inventory assesses your behavior in relation to the six most common reasons: (1) a sense of stimulation, (2) the satisfaction of handling things, (3) a sense of well-being or pleasurable feelings, (4) a reduced sensation of stress or tension, (5) a psychological craving, or (6) a habit. It also provides you with guidelines to deal with these reasons in your quest to stop smoking, many of which will be discussed.

Also determine if you really want to quit; Laboratory Inventory 9.4 will help you in this regard. Research has shown that individuals with intrinsic motivation to quit are more likely to be successful compared to those whose motivation is extrinsic in nature, such as being told to by a physician. If you do want to quit, there are a number of different approaches to use, but there is no one best way. You may have to use a trial-and-error approach to find which one is best for you, but the following general suggestions have been helpful to many former smokers. If you fail, try again or try a new method. Never stop trying to quit. One technique may be successful for you.

1. Motivate yourself. The desire to quit must be within yourself. Develop self-efficacy, a self-awareness that you have the capacity to change an unhealthy behavior. One way to do this is to consider the benefits of quitting. One of the primary benefits is improved health, including short-term benefits such as decreased coughing and long-term benefits as noted previously. Other benefits accrue as well.

   You will save money. At $1.50 per pack, an average smoker will save nearly $840 per year. (And in some areas of the country, cigarettes cost as much as $2.00 per pack or more.)

   Your clothes and your house will smell better. Keep a butt jar (a jar filled with your old cigarette butts) and smell it occasionally to remind you of the unpleasant odor associated with smoking.

   Food will taste better. Smoking dulls the sense of taste.

   You will not have to worry about offending a nonsmoker with irritating sidestream smoke.

2. Quit cold turkey. Set a definite quit date. Use your willpower to avoid a substance harmful to your health. Does a four-inch cigarette have the power to control you? Quit today and put your last pack of cigarettes somewhere visible and use it as a symbol of your superior willpower. Research has shown that about 90 percent of nonsmokers have done it on their own, many using the cold turkey technique. Intrinsic motivation is an important factor to success. Practice positive thinking—just do it!

3. Quit in phases. If you cannot quit cold turkey, gradually taper your use of cigarettes in phases. Make a written contract with yourself or with a friend. Post it on your refrigerator door, noting the specific date by which you will have a cigarette-free day. A week or two is usually a good time frame. Use some of the suggestions below to help you taper your smoking. Also note the date at which you will be cigarette free for six months. Save the money you would normally spend each day on cigarettes and reward yourself with a meaningful gift.

4. Remove triggers to smoking. Various physical objects or situations may provide a stimulus to smoking. Throw away all cigarettes, preferably flushing them down the toilet, and other smoking paraphernalia such as lighters and ashtrays. If possible, avoid situations in which you normally smoke or situations revealed by your one-day record of when and where you smoke.

5. Change your smoking habits. Switch brands and hands; changing to another brand may give you a different taste and remind you each time to quit, while smoking with your opposite hand may make it seem more awkward. Plan to smoke only one cigarette per hour or every two hours; phase in longer delays over the week. Put your cigarette down between puffs and take a puff only every minute; this will lead to fewer puffs, and the cigarette will burn away.

6. Reduce the physical withdrawal symptoms. As you reduce your intake of nicotine, some physical withdrawal symptoms, such as sleepiness and irritability, may occur. The use of Nicorette gum, a prescription drug, may help dampen them somewhat through the initial stages, but it will not totally eliminate them. Nicorette gum contains nicotine, but it needs to be chewed thoroughly over thirty minutes to release the approximate equivalent of nicotine obtained from smoking one cigarette. There is also no tar or carbon monoxide associated with it. Nicotine patches applied to the skin, such as Nicoderm® and Habitrol®, are available via prescription. Decreasing dosages administered over time will help to wean you from nicotine. Intranasal sprays are also available. A recent meta-analysis of fifty-three studies has shown that nicotine replacement therapy is very effective to help stop smoking.

7. Reduce the psychological withdrawal symptoms. Although the physical withdrawal symptoms may last only several weeks, it may take months to eliminate the psychological urge to smoke. This is one of the most important periods of the smoking cessation program and why you should reward yourself after six months if you have been smoke free for that amount of time.

   After several weeks of being smoke free, some individuals have a high sense of confidence that they have beaten the smoking habit and feel that they may smoke a cigarette without harm. However, this one cigarette often triggers a return to old habits. On the other hand, if you do break down and have one cigarette after a smoke-free period, simply rededicate yourself to your smoking cessation program and begin the next day as the first smoke-free day. Most individuals try to stop several times before succeeding.

   The immediate psychological urge or temptation to smoke may be strong, but it is usually transitory and passes in about 15 minutes or so. You need to deter this urge until it passes by using some substitute behavior. If you can, take a 15-minute walk or use some of the relaxation techniques described in the last chapter. Deep breathing may be helpful, particularly the technique of

psychosmoking. Purse your lips, breathe softly and deeply to your full lung capacity, hold your breath for 10 seconds, and exhale slowly as you think of your mantra or some other symbol. You may also use a psychological technique involving negative thinking. For example, just think of cigarette smoke putting yellowish-brown tar in your lungs. In some cases a physical crutch may be helpful, such as rolling marbles, if you like the sense of handling a cigarette, or chewing gum, if you need oral gratification.

8. Eat a balanced, nutritious diet. You may want to substitute food for smoking; this may lead to a weight problem. Cigarettes help reduce the appetite, stimulate metabolism, and may modify the body weight set-point to a lower level, all factors that may underlie the fact that smokers are generally leaner than nonsmokers. Research suggests some individuals do gain weight after they stop smoking, but also note that weight gain may be prevented by proper attention to diet and exercise. Low-Calorie vegetables, such as carrot and celery sticks, may be used as oral substitutes for cigarettes. A review of the principles of sound nutrition presented in chapter 6, including the concept of quality Calories, will be helpful.

9. Start an aerobic exercise program. Exercise may be the perfect substitute for smoking. It may mimic the effects of nicotine, for exercise has been shown to elevate natural stimulants in the body as well as natural depressants or relaxants. Contrary to smoking, exercise produces beneficial effects relative to cardiovascular health, such as reducing blood triglycerides and blood pressure while raising HDL_2 cholesterol levels. Exercise may also help counteract the weight gain often seen when people stop smoking, for exercise burns Calories.

   Exercise also can fill time that may have been previously used in activities associated with smoking, such as the traditional drink after work. Moreover, by joining an exercise class or a local running club, you are more likely to associate with individuals who are nonsmokers and whose behaviors are in accord with a Positive Health Life-style.

10. Join a smoking cessation program. This may be an important consideration for those who are heavy smokers or who are extrinsically motivated. There are a variety of available programs directed by professional health counselors. Check with your local chapter of the American Lung Association or the National Cancer Society for reputable programs. Local hospitals and universities may also be good sources of information and may offer smoking cessation programs as part of a wellness program, as may workplace wellness programs. Quitting smoking is not easy. You may need professional guidance, and such programs could provide it.

11. Stay with it! As you may have noted, many of the suggestions above are components of the Positive Health Life-style, that is, exercise, good nutrition, and stress management. These life-style adjustments can provide

you with coping strategies to remain smoke-free for a lifetime. Continue to reward yourself at each yearly anniversary of the date that you stopped smoking.

12. Quit! It's worth it. Stopping smoking will improve your health. The younger you are when you quit, the better, but even if you have been smoking for 20–30 years, your health will improve after you stop.

Former chronic smokers reduce their risk of mortality to about the same level as never-smokers in about 10 years after having stopped smoking. You can succeed, as have over 50 percent of Americans who have smoked.

For a free kit to help you stop smoking, call the American Cancer Society at 1–800–ACS–2345.

Smokeless Tobacco

Smokeless tobacco exists in several forms, primarily chewing tobacco, a packed form of tobacco leaves, and snuff, a preparation of powdered tobacco. Both forms of smokeless tobacco have been popular for years among certain population groups, such as cowboys and baseball players. As the evidence accumulated implicating cigarette smoking as a major health risk, smokeless tobacco was perceived to be a safer alternative as a means to obtain the physiological and psychological effects of nicotine, for the nicotine could be absorbed by the oral mucosa, and contamination of the lungs with other harmful substances in cigarette smoke could be avoided. Abetted somewhat by advertising from manufacturers of smokeless tobacco, the use of smokeless tobacco had increased markedly, particularly among young males aged twelve to twenty-four.

Unfortunately, smokeless tobacco is not a harmless substance. Although its adverse effects are not comparable in magnitude to cigarette smoking, it does pose some serious health risks. Evidence suggests that smokeless tobacco, because of its nicotine content, may be addictive, and when its use becomes socially unacceptable or inconvenient, may possibly lead to cigarette smoking. Other data suggest similar physiological effects of smokeless tobacco comparable to those of cigarette smoking, such as decreased levels of HDL cholesterol.

However, the most serious documented threat is to oral health. Chewing tobacco and snuff are normally held in one place in the mouth, and studies with baseball players and other regular users of smokeless tobacco have shown excessive abrasion of the tooth surface, recession of the gums, destruction of both the soft and hard tissues of the teeth, and the formation of leukoplakia, white spots or patches on the mucous membranes of the tongue, cheek, or gums that have the potential to become malignant. The most serious damage usually occurs at the spot in the mouth where the smokeless tobacco is held. In one study, epithelial cells from the oral mucosa showed evidence of genetic damage due to the use of smokeless tobacco. Long-term use of smokeless tobacco is associated with increased risk of cancer of the mouth and, presumably because some individuals swallow the spittle, increased risk of cancer in the larynx, throat, and esophagus. Individuals who use smokeless tobacco need frequent oral screenings by a health-care professional. Because of these health risks, one of the objectives listed by the PHS in *Healthy People 2000* is the reduction of the proportion of males in the twelve to twenty-four age group who use smokeless tobacco on a regular basis, but even younger children should be educated relative to such health risks. A recent progress report of *Healthy People 2000* noted a small decrease in smokeless tobacco users among males aged twelve to twenty-four, which may be partly attributed to an act of Congress to ban electronic advertising of smokeless tobacco and the action of several athletic-governing bodies, such as the National Collegiate Athletic Association, banning smokeless tobacco use in both practices and competition. Nevertheless, much has yet to be done to reach the target goal set for the year 2000.

Smokeless tobacco users have the same problems stopping as do cigarette smokers. Comparable to the advice for those who smoke, those who use smokeless tobacco should quit. The suggestions listed for smoking cessation are applicable. Since most users are young males, who generally do not like to be controlled by others, such as parents, focusing on self-efficacy may be a good approach, i.e., learning that nicotine may be able to control them. Nicotine replacement therapy may also be effective during the early phases of withdrawal.

Marijuana

Marijuana (marihuana) contains the shredded, dried leaves, flowers, and stems from the plant *Cannabis sativa*. *Cannabis sativa* contains over 400 different chemical entities, 60 of these cannabinoids. But of all of these chemicals, only **delta-9-tetrahydrocannabinol (THC)** has psychoactive properties in significant amounts. The amount of THC in marijuana may vary but has become increasingly concentrated over the years as plants were cultivated for their psychoactive characteristics. The flower portion of the plant contains more THC, so the content of THC varies with the ratio of flowers to leaves; a typical marijuana cigarette with 1.5 percent THC contains about 20 milligrams of THC, which is enough to elicit a psychoactive effect. Hashish, which is the resin from the female flowers, has a THC content of approximately 10 percent.

The use of marijuana for medicinal purposes and for its psychoactive effects has a long history, having been used over 2,000 years ago by the Chinese and in the early Grecian era. Although marijuana possesses a variety of medicinal properties, the most promising therapeutic role of THC involves its antiglaucoma activity. Its use as a social drug gradually evolved westward, being used by the Aztec Indians in Mexico as part of their culture and eventually gravitated to the United States, where it was declared an illegal drug in 1937. Marijuana consumption was relatively limited until the counterculture revolution of the 1960s, but now its use as a social drug is firmly established and is considered to be a major illicit drug problem in the United States and other Western countries. Among adults in the United States, marijuana is the illegal drug of choice. Although surveys among high school students have shown a significant drop in marijuana use for over a decade, a recent survey from the University of Michigan reported a sharp rise in marijuana use in this population group, although it is still very significantly lower than that of the early 1980s.

Marijuana is usually smoked, but it may be incorporated in baked foods, such as chocolate cookies, and taken orally. Smoking marijuana leads to a rapid absorption of THC by the lungs, and THC appears in the blood within minutes of smoking. The peak physiological and subjective effects occur within approximately 30 minutes and may last 2–4 hours. The increase in plasma levels seen with oral ingestion is more delayed, taking 30–120 minutes to reach their peak. THC is very soluble in lipids, rapidly entering the brain and adipose tissues. Once in the adipose tissue, THC may be released gradually into the circulation, which may be related to the psychoactive effects sometimes observed hours later than the acute psychoactive period. The terminal half-life of THC is in the range of 24–36 hours, but its metabolites may be present in the urine for 4–10 days after a single cigarette and for weeks after cessation of chronic use.

Marijuana, like alcohol, may elicit both stimulant and depressant effects. Marijuana primarily affects the central nervous system. Although its mechanisms of action are poorly understood, it has been hypothesized to influence the activity of numerous brain neurotransmitters, such as norepinephrine, serotonin, dopamine, and endorphins, either increasing or decreasing their production or uptake by various parts of the brain that may influence mood and behavior. Marijuana is recognized as a psychoactive drug, but the behavioral responses to marijuana are influenced by a variety of factors such as personality, expected outcomes, preexisting mood, setting in which it is consumed, and previous use. The dosage of THC also exerts a significant effect upon behavioral responses, as do related factors such as time used for smoking, puff duration, volume inhaled, and the time of holding the breath after smoking.

Marijuana is used primarily for its potential to induce euphoria and a sense of calm and relaxation. Several of the key investigators studying the psychoactive effects of marijuana, such as Martin and Dewey, noted that the data generally indicate that THC exerts a relatively nonselective, complex mixture of excitatory and depressant effects on the central nervous system. The specific effects may be related to the multitude of possible effects on the neurotransmitters in the brain and may also be dose dependent, the excitatory, euphoric effects being more associated with lower doses and the depressive effects with higher ones. Dewey noted that the behavioral changes at low doses are characterized by a unique mixture of depressant and stimulatory effects. At higher doses, depression predominates but is often preceded by a stimulation effect. However, it has not been possible to establish the concentration of THC at its site of action that is necessary to produce a given pharmacological effect.

Because the use of marijuana increased markedly in the 1960s, its effect on health has been studied extensively, from both physical and psychological perspectives. Although experts note that occasional use of marijuana does not appear to be harmful to physical health, they do note that it exerts some alteration in almost every biological system in the body and that the state of knowledge is too limited to rule out the possibility that THC may produce adverse health effects on various body organs. They offer the caveat that at one time alcohol and tobacco were considered to be safe. Moreover, experts caution that regular use of marijuana may be associated with several physical health problems similar to those found with tobacco smoking. In particular, smoking marijuana may lead to impaired lung function, possibly leading to bronchospasm and bronchitis. Marijuana cigarettes also deposit more tar in the lungs than tobacco, and the carbon monoxide increase in the blood could decrease oxygen transport and pose problems to those with impaired cardiovascular function. Other health problems noted in regular users include impairment of cell-mediated immunity and decreased levels of testosterone, the latter being related to decreased sperm production and gynecomastia, or the development of female breast appearance in males. Another potential danger results from the spraying of marijuana plants with defoliants in attempts to eradicate the source; if such plants make it to the marketplace, carcinogens may be present.

Several of the psychological effects elicited by marijuana may induce some adverse behavioral responses. Possible adverse behavioral manifestations include panic attacks, paranoia, anxiety, lethargy, drowsiness, distortion of visual perception, and decreases in attention span, concentration, and memory. Marijuana has been studied extensively in relation to its effects upon psychomotor skills. Although researchers noted high levels of variability among subjects relative to the effects of marijuana, complex reaction time (tasks involving quick responses to multiple stimuli) was consistently impaired. Several other reviews have also noted, in general, that marijuana or THC elicited significant decrements on a wide variety of psychomotor measures, including impaired driving ability. Moreover, some studies reported impairment in psychomotor performance 24 hours after smoking marijuana. It should also be noted that although both alcohol and marijuana may impair psychomotor performance, the combination of the two social drugs appears to lead to increased deterioration of basic psychomotor skills, not to mention impaired driving ability.

Marijuana seems firmly established as another social drug in Western countries, regardless of its current legal status. The major health concern is with the young, for marijuana use may elicit an amotivational syndrome, characterized by apathy and loss of motivation. Additionally, any drug that is used on a regular basis to alter reality may be detrimental to psychosocial maturation. Thus, the risk-reduction objectives in *Healthy People 2000* are targeted to the young, those aged twelve to twenty-five, and aim not only to decrease the proportion of young people who use marijuana, but also to create the perception in the minds of young people that the regular use of marijuana is physically and psychologically harmful.

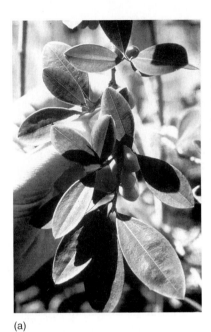

(a)

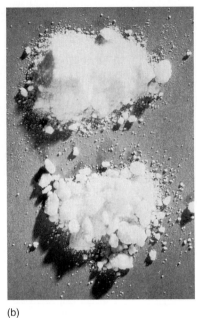

(b)

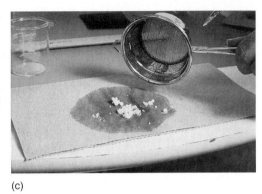

(c)

Figure 9.7 (a) *Coca plant from which cocaine is extracted.* (b) *Cocaine, a white crystalline powder (cocaine hydrochloride).* (c) *Crack, the most addictive form of cocaine, appears as white gravel, slivers of soap, or tiny chunks known as "crack rocks."*

Cocaine

Cocaine is an alkaloid derivative of the coca plant, *Erythroxylon coca,* which grows extensively in the northern countries of South America. Cocaine may be obtained by chewing the plant leaves, a tradition among Andean Indians, but it is also prepared from the plant for medicinal and social purposes in several ways. The leaves may be soaked in an organic solvent to produce a thick paste, which is then refined into cocaine as a white, crystalline powder. Prepared as a street drug, cocaine is adulterated with a variety of compounds that look like the real thing, including sugars such as lactose, other stimulants such as caffeine, and anesthetics such as benzocaine; various street terms include coke and snow. Cocaine may also be free-based, or converted chemically with heat and baking soda, into a more potent form known as **crack,** which looks like small lumps or shavings of soap but has the texture of porcelain. Cocaine may be inhaled or "snorted" into a nostril, injected into muscles or veins, or prepared as a paste and mixed with tobacco or marijuana for smoking. Crack is already in a form to be smoked. (See fig. 9.7.)

Cocaine is used primarily because it elicits a sense of exhilaration. The stimulating effect of cocaine has been known for centuries. In the sixteenth century, Spanish conquistadors in Peru reported tremendous feats of endurance by native Indians who chewed coca leaves constantly, the cocaine being absorbed through the oral mucosa. Incidentally, the Inca civilization in Peru used cocaine as their currency. In the nineteenth century, cocaine was extracted from the coca leaves and utilized in several beverages consumed daily throughout Europe and the United States, such as therapeutic elixirs, wines, and even sodas. For example, an early advertisement stated, in part, that Coca-Cola contains the valuable tonic and nerve stimulant properties of the coca plant and cola nuts.

Sigmund Freud was an early advocate, indicating that cocaine increased his vitality and capacity for work. However, when its potential for addiction was discovered, the use of cocaine was eliminated from compounds designed for everyday consumption.

Cocaine may affect the body in several ways, either locally or systemically. Locally, it is used medicinally as a topical anesthetic, primarily for the respiratory system, because it prevents transmission of pain impulses along nerve fibers and at nerve endings. Systemically, cocaine stimulates both the central and sympathetic nervous systems, leading to euphoria, mood enhancement, and a decreased sensation of fatigue. Cocaine also affects the heart, either directly or via the sympathetic nervous system, resulting in increased heart rate and blood pressure, vasoconstriction of the left coronary artery, and decreased blood flow to the heart muscle. The effects of cocaine or crack use may occur rapidly, within 1–2 minutes after smoking or injection and 5–10 minutes after snorting. The drug is metabolized rapidly in the body, and the half-life is relatively short, about 20–40 minutes, although metabolites may be detected in the urine for several days.

Although at one time cocaine was believed to be a wonder drug, eliciting powerful, stimulating effects on the body but thought to have no adverse side effects, such is not the case. Cocaine and crack are hazardous drugs for, as noted in table 9.5, both possess a high potential for abuse and addiction, particularly crack. People use cocaine or crack for different reasons: some use it out of curiosity, some to overcome depression, some for escape, some only for recreational purposes in various social situations, and some because they are addicted. Recent surveys indicated that although cocaine use is decreasing (although not among frequent users), there are still 3.4 million Americans who use cocaine occasionally. If

Table 9.5 Cocaine: Crack

Cocaine use has been one of the fastest growing drug problems in modern America. Perhaps the most alarming aspect of the cocaine epidemic was the sudden availability of this central nervous system stimulant in a cheap but potent form called crack or rock. Crack is a purified form of cocaine that is smoked.

Crack is inexpensive to try. Crack is available for as little as $10. As a result, the drug is affordable to many new users, including high school and even elementary school students.

Crack is easy to use. It is sold in pieces resembling small white gravel or soap chips and is sometimes pressed into small pellets. Crack can be smoked in a pipe or put into a cigarette. Because the visible effects disappear within minutes after smoking, it can be used at almost any time during the day.

Crack is extremely addictive. Crack is far more addictive than heroin or barbiturates. Because crack is smoked, it is quickly absorbed into the bloodstream. It produces a feeling of extreme euphoria, peaking within seconds. The desire to repeat this sensation can cause addiction within a few days.

Crack can lead to crime and severe psychological disorders. Many youths, once addicted, have turned to stealing, prostitution, and drug dealing in order to support their compulsive use of cocaine. Prolonged use can produce violent behavior and psychotic states similar to schizophrenia.

Crack is deadly. Cocaine in any form can cause cardiac arrest (stoppage of heart function) and death by interrupting the brain's control over the heart and respiratory system.

Source: Adapted from William J. Bennett, What Works: Schools without Drugs, 8, 1986. U.S. Department of Education.

we compare the risk-reduction objectives for alcohol, marijuana, and cocaine in *Healthy People 2000,* the PHS wants Americans to *decrease excess consumption* of alcohol, to *decrease the regular use* of marijuana, but to *not even experiment once or twice* with cocaine, primarily because cocaine may be so addictive. A vicious cycle may lead to addiction. The initial psychological effects, intense pleasure for about 30 minutes, are followed by depression, anxiety, or sadness, which then leads to a craving for more.

Aside from the potential for addiction, other serious health consequences may result from both acute and chronic use of cocaine or crack. As has been evidenced a number of times, in rock music stars and even in highly-fit college and professional athletes, even the single or occasional use of cocaine may be fatal. Because of the effects on the heart noted above, cocaine may increase the oxygen needs of the heart while simultaneously decreasing the oxygen supply, a condition that may induce a heart arrhythmia (an aberrant conduction of nerve impulses in the heart) that may lead to sudden death. A fatal dose may be obtained easily from street drugs, whose purity and potency may be unknown. Chronic effects include severe damage to nasal tissue and the septum wall between nasal cavities due to snorting, liver toxicity, anorexia, tremors and convulsions, and symptoms of mental illness, such as paranoia, delirium, and psychoses. Individuals who inject cocaine are more prone to infections, such as hepatitis and HIV infection. Women who use cocaine while pregnant may suffer miscarriages or stillbirths, and their "cocaine babies" are prone to congenital deformities, sudden infant death syndrome, and even heart attacks.

Relative to the Positive Health Life-style, cocaine is one of those agents from which you should abstain completely. The short-term effects may be pleasurable, but the potential for long-term, adverse effects is too great to risk even experimental usage.

Methamphetamine (Ice)

One of the most popular stimulants in the 1950s and 1960s was amphetamine, a stimulant of the central nervous system that created a sense of euphoria and well-being. Amphetamines were prescribed by physicians for a variety of purposes, primarily to curb the appetite for those dieting to lose weight, but also to enhance the performance of some athletes. Although, like cocaine, first believed to be somewhat innocuous, the toxic effects of amphetamines became more evident as individuals began to become addicted. Hence, their production and distribution were controlled, and their use as a recreational drug began to decline.

One powerful version of amphetamine is **methamphetamine,** often known as speed, chemically altered to create a more rapid, powerful stimulating effect. Methamphetamine has been available for years in a powder form, methamphetamine hydrochloride, but in recent years has been processed to form a newer version in a clear crystal form known as **ice.** Ice may be smoked and creates an instant euphoria, increased alertness, and an enhanced self-esteem and sense of well-being. It is used not only for recreational purposes, but also by workaholics to maintain high energy levels throughout the day. Ice appears to have originated in Asia but has spread to Hawaii and is now a major drug problem in that state. Its use has also surfaced in major cities in southern California.

Although crack cocaine is currently more of a drug problem than ice, authorities are concerned that ice may become the major problem in the near future. For one, the stimulating effects associated with ice may last for 8–24 hours, much longer than the 30-minute excitation gained with cocaine. Moreover, methamphetamine may be synthesized from common chemicals in a crude laboratory, and its production and distribution may be even more difficult to prevent. At the present time, the use of ice in the United States is somewhat localized geographically, but the increased health problems related to its use in Hawaii indicate that it is another toxic recreational drug.

As a powerful stimulant, toxic doses of methamphetamine may overexcite the central nervous system, causing agitation, anxiety, hallucinations, epileptic-like seizures, and acute psychoses, and may also overexcite the cardiovascular system, leading to palpitations of the heart, chest pains, and possible arrhythmias. Although the cardiovascular responses are somewhat less than those associated with cocaine, death may still result from toxic doses of methamphetamine. Additionally, as with crack cocaine, health authorities are seeing increased numbers of newborns who are suffering the consequences of addicted mothers.

The use of methamphetamine as ice or any other form is counterproductive to a Positive Health Life-style.

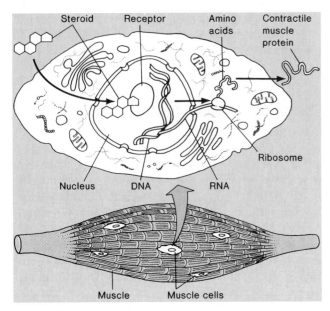

Figure 9.8 *Anabolic steroids picked up by receptors in the cell nucleus initiate the process of protein formation in such cells as muscle fibers.*

Table 9.6 Trade and Generic Names of the Most Commonly Used Anabolic Steroids in the United States

Oral Compounds

Anadrol (oxymetholone)
Anavar (oxandrolone)
Dianabol (methandienone)
Maxibolin (ethylestrenol)
Winstrol (stanozolol)

Injectable Compounds

Deca-durabolin (nandrolone decanoate)
Depo-testosterone (testosterone cypionate)
Durabolin (nandrolone phenylpropionate)
Primobolan-depot (methenolone enanthate)

Source: M. H. Williams. 1989. Beyond training: How athletes enhance performance legally and illegally. Champaign, Ill.: Human Kinetics.

Anabolic Steroids

For individuals interested in gaining body weight, primarily in the form of muscle mass, a properly designed resistance-training program (chapter 4) combined with an appropriate diet (chapter 7) is an effective approach. However, some athletes in sports such as football and bodybuilding, as well as an increasing number of nonathletes, have turned to certain drugs and hormones in attempts to maximize gains in muscle mass and strength. Testosterone, the male sex hormone, was one of the first to be used, and more recently, human growth hormone (HGH) has become more readily available through the process of genetic engineering. However, the primary choice over the past 40 years has been anabolic steroids.

Anabolic steroids, also known as anabolic/androgenic steroids, represent a class of synthetic drugs designed to mimic the effects of testosterone. Chemists rearranged the structure of the testosterone molecule in order to maximize the anabolic effects (muscle building) and minimize the androgenic effects (development of male secondary sex characteristics), but all anabolic steroids do produce some androgenic effects. Anabolic steroids may affect a variety of body cells, such as the bone marrow, to stimulate red blood cell production, and thus have some medical applications. However, the main target for most users is the muscle cell. Although the mechanism of action is not totally understood, anabolic steroids are believed to enter the cell nucleus and bind to DNA, which then promotes the generation of RNA to direct the formation of muscle proteins in the cytoplasm (see fig. 9.8). Anabolic steroids are available for oral consumption or injection. Several of the more popular anabolic steroids are listed in table 9.6.

Anabolic steroids appear to increase muscle mass and strength effectively if used in conjunction with a resistance-training program and increased caloric intake. Current estimates are that over one million Americans use anabolic steroids, including approximately 5 percent of high school students, primarily male athletes, but also about 2.5 percent of nonathletes and a small percentage of females. Nearly 500,000 high school students use anabolic steroids. Most obtain steroids on the black market; a conservative estimate is over $100 million in yearly sales.

Although anabolic steroids have been used extensively for decades, we have very little quality epidemiological data regarding their effect on health. The National Institute of Drug Abuse notes that definitive data regarding adverse health effects on the nonmedical use of anabolic steroids are lacking. Nevertheless, case studies with athletes and others self-administering steroids, observation of patients on long-term steroid therapy research, and some animal research have shown that the use of these drugs may elicit a wide variety of health problems. Because anabolic steroids are synthetic hormones, they may alter normal production and function of natural hormones in the body, for example depressing the production of testosterone and increasing the level of estradiol (female sex hormone) in males, and mimicking the effect of testosterone in females. On a short-term basis, these hormonal changes may elicit a variety of health effects that are basically cosmetic in nature. Males may experience acne, baldness, and gynecomastia (appearance of female breasts). Females may develop male secondary sex characteristics, such as growth of body and facial hair, deepening of the voice, and breast shrinkage. Changes in the reproduction system may also occur. Males may experience shrinkage of the testicles and a decrease in sperm production, while females may suffer an enlargement of the clitoris and disturbances in the menstrual cycle. More seriously, anabolic steroids may cause premature cessation of bone growth in children and adolescents. Many of these changes may be transient, but some are permanent, such as the deepened voice in females and the shortened stature of children.

Users of anabolic steroids may also experience psychological effects, such as mild personality changes like increased aggressiveness; some individuals may become extremely aggressive and hostile. Several investigators suggest that steroid use may have profound psychological effects, particularly with long-term, high-dose use. Kashkin and Kleber note that such users may have difficulty stopping despite psychological side effects and may have drug-craving withdrawal symptoms when steroids are stopped, leading to depression. Similar to cocaine addiction, a dependence upon anabolic steroids may develop.

Long-term use may also lead to serious physical health problems, such as liver problems, cardiovascular disease, and cancer. The liver is involved in catabolism of steroids, and long-term users have developed liver cancer or peliosis hepatis, a condition characterized by blood-filled sacs in the liver, which may rupture and cause serious complications or death. Users are at increased risk for atherosclerosis, the main cause of coronary heart disease and heart attacks. Steroids may retain fluids and sodium in the body, leading to high blood pressure; will decrease HDL and increase LDL; and cause some clotting abnormalities in the blood, all risk factors for atherosclerosis. Some research with bodybuilders has suggested that steroids may suppress the immune system, and animal research has revealed them to be weak carcinogens, two factors that may predispose to cancer. Recently, an All-Pro National Football League player, known for his aggressiveness, blamed his inoperable brain tumor on steroid use over the years.

Additionally, most individuals obtain these drugs illegally on the black market, where quality is not controlled, and chemical analysis has revealed some potentially hazardous constituents in these "homemade" drugs.

Because of these medical problems, in *Healthy People 2000,* the PHS has established a risk-reduction objective to decrease the use of anabolic steroids among high school seniors. To help decrease the availability, Congress has passed legislation classifying anabolic steroids as controlled substances, thus limiting their production and distribution by pharmaceutical companies. Penalties for illegal use and distribution may be severe, up to 5 years in prison and $250,000 in fines for a first offense.

The use of anabolic steroids as a means to enhance body appearance is not consistent with a Positive Health Life-style, primarily because of the potential health risks, but also because of potential legal consequences.

Legal and Illegal Drugs

In the preceding sections we have discussed seven drugs: one that is legal (caffeine), two that are legal at an appropriate age (tobacco and alcohol), and four that are illegal (marijuana, cocaine, methamphetamine, and anabolic steroids). Many young persons experiment with a variety of recreational drugs; for example, recent surveys indicate nearly 90 percent of high school seniors have experimented with alcohol, 35 percent have used marijuana, and approximately 6 percent have tried cocaine. At high school age, the use of all three drugs is illegal. Life is a series of temptations, and the temptation to use

illegal drugs is one that confronts millions of Americans. If you decide to experiment with illegal drugs, you should be aware of the following.

1. The use of illegal drugs may lead to an arrest and conviction, which may have a significant impact upon your future career. The possession, use, or sale of marijuana, cocaine, methamphetamine, or anabolic steroids may be grounds for both fines and prison sentences, some quite severe. You may have an excellent academic record, but that fact may be obscured by a criminal record when you apply for a job.

2. Since the source of many recreational drugs is not known, the strength or potency of the drug may be excessive and may result in a significant overdose with serious health consequences. The deaths of several nationally prominent athletes may be illustrative of the most severe consequence of drug overdoses.

3. Most drugs possess a high potential for addiction or habituation. Although they are taken primarily for the sense of well-being they produce, their continued use may actually be counterproductive and may lead to increased levels of stress as dependency develops. If you have a concern about drug abuse regarding yourself or a friend, you may get assistance from the National Institute of Drug Abuse Hotline [1(800)662–HELP], local community health agencies, or counselors in student services at your college or university.

4. The risks noted above far outweigh the benefits. There are other ways to derive pleasure from life, ways that will enhance your health, not impair it.

Sexually Transmitted Diseases (STDs)

Infections are caused by microorganisms, such as bacteria and viruses. At one time or another, we have all had an open wound that has become infected by bacteria, or an upper respiratory infection caused by a virus. We may become infected in a variety of ways, for bacteria and viruses may be transmitted to us by way of the air we breathe, the food we eat, the things we touch, the bugs that sting us, the animals we play with, and the humans with whom we interact. In our interactions with one another, some infections are more contagious than others. For example, we may become infected simply by breathing the airborne virus from the sneeze of an infected person, but we may need more intimate contact in order to become infected by other types of bacteria or viruses. If conditions are favorable in the body, the microorganisms will multiply and cause an infectious disease, which may elicit local signs and symptoms, may produce general symptoms throughout the body, or may produce no signs or symptoms at all.

Such is the case with **sexually transmitted diseases (STDs),** those infectious diseases that are caused almost exclusively via sexual contact, either vaginal, anal, or oral. The most predictive risk factor for contracting STDs is the number of sex partners. The infectious microorganisms may reside either on the skin or in the body fluids or secretions. The signs and symptoms of STDs may be local and confined to the point of entry or contact of the microorganism, such as the genitalia; they may be general and affect other body systems, such as the heart; or they may not exist. In any case, the infected individual is a carrier of an STD and may infect others, unknowingly if he or she has no symptoms or is unaware or unfamiliar with the symptoms of STDs. Although much progress has been made in the detection and treatment of STDs in the past, they continue to be a major health problem in the United States. More than 12 million Americans, mostly teenagers and young adults, become infected with STDs each year, not including AIDS. In a recent survey, nearly 75 percent of Americans said they did not believe they could get an STD, but the government indicates that one in four Americans will eventually get an STD.

All infections should be considered to be serious. Although a sore throat infected by streptococci may elicit only minor pain and inflammation, it may eventually lead to heart and kidney damage if left untreated. Similarly, some STDs may cause only local irritation, but others produce serious health consequences. In general, most of us practice health habits that minimize the chance of infection or infecting others and seek proper medical attention if we do get infected. These health habits are increasingly important with STDs. Knowing the signs and symptoms of STDs and seeking prompt medical attention is important, but prevention may be more critical, because for one STD there is no cure at the present time and the prognosis is death.

In this section we shall discuss the causes, symptoms, health problems, and treatment of the most common STDs, followed by a discussion of safer sex practices to help maximize prevention efforts. Individuals are often infected with several STDs at the same time. Although we shall discuss each STD separately, individuals who suspect they have contracted an STD should obtain a medical examination to determine a full diagnosis and appropriate treatment, which may involve a combination of antibiotics. Notification of others who may possibly be infected is also critical to help curb the spread of STDs.

Vaginitis

Vaginitis is an inflammation of the female vagina, which may be caused by a number of different microorganisms that may enter the vagina in different ways, such as poor personal hygiene. A parasite known as Trichomonas is transmitted primarily via sexual intercourse, causing trichomoniasis, which is classified as an STD (see fig. 9.9). Trichomoniasis is a vaginal infection with symptoms of inflammation; severe itching; pain on passing urine; and a white or yellowish discharge, sometimes with blood, possessing a strong odor. Males may be infected but have few or no symptoms; females may also be infected without symptoms. The health problems are primarily localized to the vagina or penis. Both sexual partners need treatment. A number of topical antifungal agents can be applied to the infected areas, but oral agents such as fluconazole are also helpful to cure the problem and

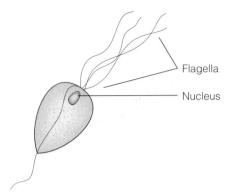

Figure 9.9 *Trichomonas vaginalis. This microscopic one-celled animal causes vaginitis and can live in the male reproductive organs.*

help prevent reinfection. Other forms of vaginitis, such as vulvovaginal candidiasis, may be treated in a similar fashion.

Genital Warts

Genital warts, also known as venereal warts, are caused by the **human papilloma virus (HPV).** A papilloma is any benign growth on the skin, including warts. Genital warts appear as small elevations on the skin, often appearing in the shape of a cauliflower, and may be soft or hard, pink, red, or yellowish. They may appear on the genitalia, in the vagina, around the anus, and on the cervix. Although they may be painless, genital warts may itch, burn, or even give off a discharge or bleed. Without treatment, they may disfigure, interfere with intercourse, obstruct the urethra, or complicate vaginal delivery in childbirth. There are seventy different types of HPV, and twenty-five may infect the genital tract. Some varieties of the HPV have been linked to increased risk of venereal cancers, particularly cancer of the cervix. To remove the warts, both partners should have a complete venereal examination. Several treatments are available, including surface medications; freezing with liquid nitrogen (cryotherapy); cauterization with heat, electricity, or chemicals; and laser surgery.

Genital Herpes

Genital herpes is one form of the infectious disease herpes simplex. It is classified as an STD and is caused by the type 2 strain of the herpes simplex virus (HSV). Facial herpes (cold sores; fever blisters) is another form of herpes simplex caused by the type 1 strain, and although facial herpes is not classified as an STD, the type 1 strain may infect the genital area. Diagnosis by examination and laboratory tests may differentiate between the two strains or differentiate genital herpes from genital warts. Some studies indicate 20 percent of young adults in the United States are infected with HSV-2, but only 60 to 70 percent exhibit symptoms.

Local signs and symptoms of genital herpes are small, painful, itching sores or blisters appearing on or around the genitalia (see fig. 9.10). Females may experience a burning sensation during urination. General symptoms may include fever and flu-like symptoms. Local signs usually appear 2 to 10 days after infection and disappear in approximately 2 to 3

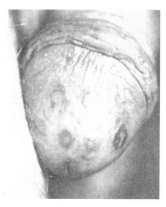

Figure 9.10 *Genital herpes. Herpes begins as small fluid-filled blisters that soon break, leaving painful, pitted spots. The surrounding area is usually inflamed and swollen.*

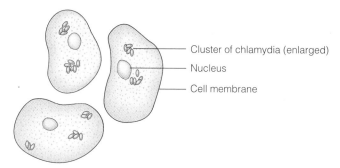

Cluster of chlamydia (enlarged)
Nucleus
Cell membrane

Figure 9.11 *Chlamydia trachomatis, currently believed to be the most prevalent sexually transmitted disease in the United States. Chlamydia, shown here in color, are oval bacterial cells found within infected human cells in the membranes lining the genital organs. If untreated, chlamydia can cause sterility.*

weeks. However, the virus may still reside in nerve endings and, although not displaying any signs or symptoms, the individual is still infected and may be contagious. An individual with herpes always puts his or her partner at risk during unprotected sex. Herpes sores may never recur after the first episode, although there may be occasional flare-ups occurring spontaneously, often in times of stress. When herpes does recur, the signs and symptoms are generally milder than the first occurrence. Although many may adapt to the fate of lifetime herpes, for many the psychological and social consequences may be devastating. Support groups are available in many communities.

Genital herpes may be especially harmful to women and the newborn. Females are at increased risk for cervical cancer and thus should have a Pap smear at least once a year. The virus also may be transmitted to the infant during birth, increasing the risk of brain damage or even death to the newborn. Pregnant women who have had herpes should inform their physician so that proper precautions may be taken, including cesarean section delivery if warranted.

Although there presently is no cure for herpes, treatment with the drug acyclovir, available in capsules or ointment, may help relieve the pain and shorten the duration of the signs and symptoms. The drug is more effective if taken early in the infective stage, so individuals with recurrent episodes should keep a 5-day supply on hand, although the drug is rather costly.

Chlamydia

Chlamydia (pronounced klə·mid′·ē·ə) is caused by a bacterium, Chlamydia trachomatis (see fig. 9.11). It is the most common STD in the United States, infecting nearly three million people annually. Because the bacterium infects the urethra of males, chlamydia is also known as nongonococcal **urethritis** (inflammation of the urethra). Other bacteria may also cause nongonococcal urethritis. The bacterium infects the cervix in women. About 10–30 percent of men and up to 80 percent of women experience no symptoms. Those most often observed in males include painful urination, a thin or creamy discharge from the penis, and possibly pain in the testicles. Females may experience a vaginal discharge, some pain or discomfort on urination, and possibly pain in the lower abdomen.

Possible health complications include sterility in both sexes, as inflammation from the infection may block the sperm ducts in males or fallopian tubes in females. In females, sterility is usually associated with **pelvic inflammatory disease (PID),** a more generalized inflammation in the pelvic region. PID may be associated with longer, heavier periods; more cramping; fever; nausea; or pain during intercourse. These symptoms are important to consider, since the initial stages of infection may be symptom free, and PID is the stage of the disease that leads to sterility. A chronic, untreated infection may also lead to systemic problems, including arthritis, inflammation of the liver, and damaged heart tissues. Women may pass the infection to babies during delivery, and the child may develop eye damage or pneumonia.

A diagnosis may be made based on examination of the urethral or vaginal discharge and on special tests. Both sex partners need treatment, and the most effective therapy is several weeks of antibiotics, primarily doxycycline. There are a number of other drugs available depending on the characteristics of the infection, and some drugs are effective against several forms of bacteria. As with drug therapy for any STD, it is important to take the full prescription, for the STD may resurface.

Gonorrhea

Gonorrhea is an inflammatory, contagious disease caused by the Neisseria gonorrhoeae bacterium, or for short, gonococcus (see fig. 9.12). The gonococcus lives in warm, moist areas of the body, primarily in the urethra and cervix, and is transmitted during sexual intercourse. The genital mucous membranes are primarily affected, although other mucous membranes in the body may also be infected. Approximately five hundred thousand new cases of gonorrhea are reported each year.

Although a small percentage of males will experience no symptoms, males generally have a burning sensation on urination and a thin, whitish discharge from the penis, which later becomes thick and creamy. Females may experience symptoms similar to chlamydia, including a slight discharge from the vagina, a mild burning sensation during urination, and abdominal pain or tenderness. However, symptoms in women may be mild and may go unnoticed. Moreover, the symptoms in both men and women may disappear within a few weeks, but the gonococcus may still be present and contagious.

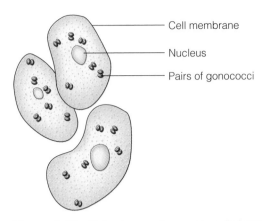

Cell membrane

Nucleus

Pairs of gonococci

Figure 9.12 *Neisseria gonorrhoeae. Also called gonococci, these pairs of bean-shaped bacteria, shown here in color, live on and inside the cells of the membranes lining the genital organs. They can also infect the eyes, throat, and rectum. In untreated cases, they can enter the blood to infect the membranes lining the heart and joints.*

Complications from untreated gonorrhea may be widespread, including PID, sterility in both males and females, arthritis, inflammation of the heart, and damage to nerve tissue. If gonorrhea is passed to the newborn in the birth process, permanent blindness may result from eye infections, although by law most states require eye treatments for all newborns.

Gonorrhea may be diagnosed by a physical examination, and laboratory tests of the penis discharge and of multiple tissue sites from the female, including the cervix, vagina, and urethra. Traditionally, penicillin was the drug of choice in the treatment of gonorrhea. However, some strains of gonococci have become penicillin resistant. The current treatment is based on the assumption that the patient is infected with a resistant strain of gonorrhea. A number of drugs are available, but the gold standard for treatment appears to be the injectable antibiotic, ceftriaxone.

Syphilis

Syphilis, one of the most dangerous of the STDs, is caused by a spiral-shaped bacterium, Treponema pallidum. It is transmitted almost exclusively by sexual intercourse but may also be transmitted via blood contact, such as kissing an infected person with a cut lip or bleeding gum, as the bacteria can enter the body through mucous membranes. Currently over one hundred thousand cases occur each year. Syphilis in newborns has soared to a record high, primarily because of the increasing number of women who are swapping sex for drugs but who receive little or no prenatal care.

Syphilis may progress through various stages. In the first stage (primary syphilis) the only symptom may be a chancre (pronounced shank·er), a reddish bump that appears where the bacteria entered the body, usually on the penis, vagina, or vulva, but also on the rectum or in the mouth. The size of the chancre may vary, from a tiny spot to a dime, and unlike herpes, it is painless and thus might go undetected. This first stage occurs anywhere from 1 to 12 weeks after contact and may last 1–5 weeks. In the second stage (secondary syphilis), which may occur any time from less than a month to about a

year after contact, symptoms may include fever; a sore throat; headaches; a rash on the chest, back, arms, and legs; infected lymph nodes; and large sores, which contain the bacteria and are a source of contagion. These symptoms generally subside in several weeks, but the rash and sores may reappear. However, the disease usually goes into a latent stage, in which the bacteria continue to multiply and infect internal organs. The final stage (tertiary syphilis) is characterized by multiple symptoms as the bacteria attack the cardiovascular and central nervous systems, including ulcers on the skin and internal organs, arthritis, pain and disability, blindness, paralysis, psychotic behavior, insanity, heart failure, and usually death. As with other STDs, the pregnant mother may pass the disease to the child at birth.

Diagnosis may be made by physical examination and laboratory tests of blood or secretions from sores, if present. Antibiotic therapy will cure syphilis, although follow-up diagnoses are recommended to ensure that the therapy has been effective.

Acquired Immunodeficiency Syndrome (AIDS)

Acquired immunodeficiency syndrome (AIDS) is caused by the **human immunodeficiency virus (HIV),** which is also known as the AIDS virus (see fig. 9.13). AIDS is also referred to as HIV disease or HIV infection, and an individual infected with HIV virus is HIV-positive. In the human body, the HIV causes no damage unless it enters a body cell. Thus, an individual may be infected with the HIV virus and be a carrier without symptoms or without developing AIDS. In general, however, the HIV binds with a receptor on one of the cells of the immune system, a type of lymphocyte (white blood cell) known as the helper T cell. The HIV impairs the immunologic function of the helper T cell, exposing the individual to a wide variety of infections. Although the HIV may cause no symptoms for years, the disease is progressive, and the final manifestation is the collection of signs and symptoms called AIDS.

Although traced back to as early as 1959, AIDS was virtually unknown until about 1980, but has now reached epidemic proportions. The World Health Organization estimated 14 million adults and 1 million children have AIDS, mostly in developing countries, and predicts there will be 30 to 40 million cases by the year 2000. The Centers for Disease Control estimate that well over 1 million Americans are infected with HIV, and that there will be approximately 400,000–500,000 cases of AIDS by the mid-1990s. Depending on the source quoted, the number of new cases of AIDS is projected to be about 50,000–70,000 annually during the 1990s, but the annual rate of increase in new cases appears to be slowing from nearly 50–60 percent in the mid-1980s to about 3 percent in the mid-1990s.

The HIV concentrates mainly in the blood, semen, and vaginal secretions. The two main means of transmitting HIV are sexual intercourse (vaginal, anal, or oral), and by an infected hypodermic needle, but it may also be transmitted in other ways by contacting the blood of an infected person. Current research suggests that AIDS cannot be transmitted by normal daily contact among individuals. Groups at high risk

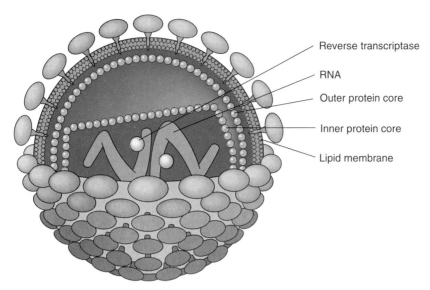

Figure 9.13 *Human immunodeficiency virus (HIV), the cause of AIDS. This virus is a retrovirus, having RNA as its genetic material. Using the enzyme reverse transcriptase, it has the ability to produce DNA from RNA. The DNA is then incorporated into the chromosomes of the virus's human host cell.*

include homosexuals (62 percent of all cases) and intravenous drug users (24 percent of all cases), but AIDS is increasing in children and heterosexual adults. Recent data indicate that the percentage of new cases of HIV is higher for heterosexuals, particularly in women, than for homosexuals. Epidemiologists also indicate that HIV infection is occurring at an earlier age. AIDS is considered to be one of the most serious health threats to face our nation.

Symptoms of AIDS may vary. Individuals may experience a milder illness known as AIDS-related complex, involving fever, chills, headache, rashes, weight loss, loss of appetite, fatigue, swollen lymph glands, white spots in the mouth, and flu-like symptoms. These symptoms may occur when the virus first begins to replicate in the body, and HIV levels increase in the blood and fluid surrounding the brain. HIV may also infect the brain and spinal cord, causing neurological symptoms such as forgetfulness, incoordination, confusion, mental disorders, and even paralysis. The current viewpoint is that although the amount of time may vary, almost all individuals infected with HIV eventually will develop full-blown AIDS. Death is the inevitable result because the weakened immune system cannot fight potentially harmful, everyday bacteria that a healthy immune system normally kills, particularly one bacterium that can cause pneumonia. In 1993, AIDS became the leading cause of death among 25–44 year olds.

Presently there is no cure or treatment for AIDS, although the search for a cure or an effective preventive vaccine is the focus of much concentrated research. Antiviral drugs such as azidothymidine (AZT) and several others may help delay the symptoms of HIV infection and may prolong the lives of AIDS victims. Other drugs such as interleukin-2, may be used to boost the immune system in HIV-positive individuals by holding the HIV virus in check, allowing the immune system to recover. However, the HIV virus has a strong capacity to mutate, and eventually sidesteps the treat-

ment. Intense research is being devoted to development of an effective vaccine. In contrast to the other STDs, prevention is the only effective treatment for AIDS. Any STD may be associated with an increased risk of HIV/AIDS so all individuals with STDs should have a serologic (blood) test for HIV. It should be noted that there are both false positives and false negatives with some screening tests, so several screenings may be needed. Knowledge that one is infected with HIV may help to prevent its spread. For those with AIDS, research has shown that a healthy life-style, such as proper weight control, stress management, spirituality, and exercise, may help psychologic well-being, but may not affect the progress of the disease. However, one current research effort is focused on individuals who are infected with HIV, but who have shown delayed onset of AIDS for 10 years or more. The study is trying to identify possible mechanisms associated with this delayed onset. If you have questions concerning AIDS, you may contact local Offices of Public Health or use the national AIDS hotline, 1(800)342–AIDS.

Safer Sex Practices

The PHS, in *Healthy People 2000,* has established risk-reduction objectives specifically for STDs and HIV infection. In general, the objectives are to decrease the proportion of Americans who become infected with syphilis, gonorrhea, chlamydia, and genital herpes and warts, and to limit the increase in the proportion of the population that will become infected with HIV. Several strategies have been proposed to achieve these general objectives, but the main focus is prevention through education, particularly among teenagers and young adults. One recommended approach is to incorporate a discussion of STDs and HIV infection in personal health education programs from fourth grade in elementary school through college.

The topics to be discussed and the sensitivity of the educational approach would be adjusted to the educational level, but the main objective would be to stress the concept of self-responsibility for personal health behaviors related to the prevention of STDs or HIV infection. Preventive education should involve other related health behaviors, such as personal hygiene and substance abuse. For example, sharing personal care objects that may contain blood of an infected person, such as a razor, toothbrush, or towel, may be a source of infection. Drug users who share needles or other drug paraphernalia risk infection. But the most effective means to reduce the magnitude of STDs and HIV infection is the use of safer sex practices.

As mentioned with drugs, such as tobacco and alcohol, abstinence is the safest way to prevent any adverse effects associated with their use. Abstinence from sexual intercourse of any kind is also the safest way to prevent STDs and HIV infection and is the only truly safe sex. Although abstinence may be feasible for some sexually mature, healthy adults, it is unlikely to be an acceptable approach for others, but some approaches are safer than others. Sexual gratification may be obtained in a number of ways by both partners without pene-

tration, such as making love fully clothed or other forms of noncoital sex. Having sex only with a partner who is mutually faithful and uninfected is a safe alternative. The risk of infection increases dramatically with multiple sex partners. For those who are sexually active, and particularly for those who practice indiscriminate sex, one specific objective in *Healthy People 2000* is to increase the number who use a condom. Although a condom is not foolproof, the latex models provide very effective protection against infection with all STDs and the HIV and should be *de rigueur* in all casual or nonmonogamous sexual encounters (see fig. 9.14). Both male and female condoms are available. Most condoms come with explicit instructions to maximize their effectiveness. Some key points are presented in table 9.7.

A healthy sexual relationship is an integral part of a Positive Health Life-style. With some of the Positive Health Life-style behaviors, you may reap benefits by practicing them yourself, such as exercising alone. Sexual relationships, however, involve a partner, so you have not only the responsibility to protect your own health but that of your partner as well. Learn to practice safer sex. The risks of not doing so far outweigh the benefits.

(a)

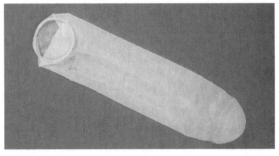

(b)

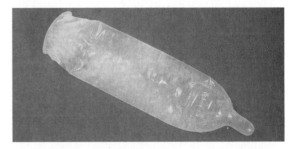

(c)

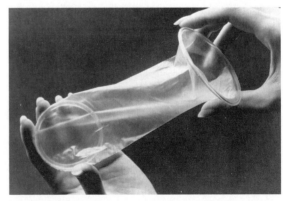

(d)

Figure 9.14 (a) Many reliable brands of condoms are readily available today. (b) Unrolled condom with plain end. (c) Unrolled condom with reservoir tip. (d) Female condom.

Table 9.7 Correct Means to Use a Condom

All Condoms

Use a new latex condom for any act of intercourse. Do not use a condom after its expiration date or if it has been damaged in any way.
Be careful when opening the condom. Do not use your teeth, fingernails, or other sharp object to open the condom wrapper because you might tear the condom inside.
Throw the used condom away in the trash. Never reuse a condom.
If the condom breaks during sex, separate from your partner and put on a new condom.

Male Condoms

Put the condom on after the penis is erect and before any sexual contact.
Hold the tip of the condom and unroll the condom all the way down the erect penis; the rolled rim should be on the outside. Leave space at the tip of the condom for semen, but make sure that no air is trapped in the condom's tip.
If additional lubrication is needed, lubricate the outside of the condom if it is not prelubricated. Use only water-based lubricants, which you can purchase at any pharmacy. Oil-based lubricants, such as petroleum jelly or baby oil, weaken the condom.
Withdraw from your partner while the penis is still erect. Hold the condom firmly to keep it from slipping off.

Female Condoms

Follow the specific instructions which accompany the condom for proper insertion techniques.
Insert the condom before sexual contact.
Insert the inner ring into the vagina just past the pubic bone, which you can feel with a curved index finger when it is inserted several inches into the vagina.
If added lubrication is desired, either lubricate the penis or the outside ring of the condom with the lubricant that normally comes packaged with the condoms.
Make sure the condom is inserted straight, not twisted.
Make sure the outside ring is outside the vagina and lies against the outside lips.
Stop if you feel the outside ring being pushed inside the vagina.
To remove the condom, twist and squeeze the outside ring to keep the sperm inside and pull out slowly. Stop if the penis begins to enter underneath or beside the sheath of the condom.

Partial Source: Using Condoms to Prevent HIV Infection and other STDs. U.S. Department of Health and Human Services, Centers for Disease Control and Prevention. HIV/NAIEP/10-93/035

References

Books

American Psychiatric Association. 1994. *Diagnostic and statistical manual of mental disorders.* (Fourth edition). DSM-IV. Washington, D.C.: APA.

Bunting, S., ed., 1995. *Annual editions: Human sexuality.* Guilford, Conn.: Dushkin Publishing Group.

Centers for Disease Control and Prevention. 1994. *Surgeon General's report to the American public on HIV infection and AIDS.* Bethesda, Md.: National Institutes of Health.

Crooks, R., and K. Baur. 1990. *Our sexuality.* Redwood City, Calif.: Benjamin/Cummings.

Ellison, R. 1993. *Does moderate alcohol consumption prolong life?* New York: American Council on Science and Health.

Kinney, J., and G. Leaton-Twichell. 1995. *Loosening the grip: A handbook of alcohol information.* St. Louis: Mosby.

Lamb, D., and M. Williams. 1991. *Ergogenic enhancement of performance in exercise and sport.* Dubuque, Iowa: Brown & Benchmark.

Leccese, A. 1991. *Drugs and society.* Englewood Cliffs, N.J.: Prentice-Hall.

McKim, W. 1991. *Drugs and behavior.* Englewood Cliffs, N.J.: Prentice-Hall.

Meeks, L., et al. 1993. *Education for sexuality and HIV/AIDS.* Blacklick, Ohio: Meeks Heit Publishing.

Nass, G., et al. 1984. *Sexual choices.* Monterey, Calif.: Wadsworth.

National Research Council. 1989. *Diet and health.* Washington, D.C.: National Academy Press.

Ornstein, R., and D. Sobel. 1989. *Healthy pleasures.* Reading, Mass.: Addison-Wesley.

Peele, S. 1989. *The meaning of addiction.* Lexington, Mass.: D. C. Heath.

Pinger, R., et al. 1995. *Drugs: Issues for today.* St. Louis: Mosby.

Ray, O., and C. Ksir. 1990. *Drugs, society, and human behavior.* St. Louis: Mosby.

United States Department of Health and Human Services. Public Health Service. 1991. *Healthy people 2000. National health promotion and disease prevention objectives.* Washington, D.C.: U.S. Government Printing Office.

Reviews

Al-Hachim, G. 1989. Teratogenicity of caffeine; a review. *European Journal of Obstetrics & Gynecology and Reproductive Biology* 31:237–47.

American Medical Association. 1990. Council on Scientific Affairs. Medical and nonmedical uses of anabolic-androgenic steroids. *Journal of the American Medical Association* 264:2923–27.

Aral, S., and K. Holmes. 1991. Sexually transmitted diseases in the AIDS era. *Scientific American* 264:62–69.

Bahrke, M., et al. 1990. Psychological and behavioral effects of endogenous testosterone levels and anabolic-androgenic steroids among males. A review. *Sports Medicine* 10:303–37.

Baker, R., and T. Jerrells. 1993. Recent developments in alcoholism: Immunological aspects. *Recent Developments in Alcohol* 11:249–71.

Barnhart, K., and S. Sondheimer. 1993. Contraception choice and sexually transmitted disease. *Current Opinions in Obstetrics and Gynecology* 5:823–28.

Bartecchi, C., et al. 1995. The global tobacco epidemic. *Scientific American* 272 (May): 44–51.

Becker, D., et al. 1993. Setting the policy, education, and research agenda to reduce tobacco use. *Circulation* 88:1381–86.

Behnke, M., and F. Eyler. 1993. The consequences of prenatal substance use for the developing fetus, newborn, and young child. *International Journal of the Addictions* 28:1341–91.

Boily, M., and R. Brunham. 1993. The impact of HIV and other STDs on human populations. Are predictions possible? *Infectious Disease Clinics of North America* 7:771–92.

Bowie, W. 1990. Approach to men with urethritis and urologic complications of sexually transmitted diseases. *Medical Clinics of North America* 74:1543–57.

Burke, T. 1988. The economic impact of alcohol abuse and alcoholism. *Public Health Reports* 103:564–68.

Camargo, C. 1989. Moderate alcohol consumption and stroke. The epidemiologic evidence. *Stroke* 20:1811–26.

Carney, O., et al. 1993. The effect of suppressive oral acyclovir on the psychological morbidity associated with recurrent genital herpes. *Genitourinary Medicine* 69:457–59.

Carson, V. 1993. Prayer, meditation, exercise, and special diets: Behaviors of the hardy person with HIV/AIDS. *Journal of the Association of Nurses in Aids Care* 4:18–28.

Cates, W., et al. 1990. Sexually transmitted diseases, pelvic inflammatory disease, and infertility: An epidemiologic update. *Epidemiologic Reviews* 12:199–220.

Centers for Disease Control. 1992. Annual and New Year's Day alcohol-related traffic fatalities—United States, 1982–1990. *Journal of the American Medical Association* 267:214–15.

Christen, A., et al. 1989. Smokeless tobacco addiction: A threat to the oral and systemic health of the child and adolescent. *Pediatrician* 16:170–77.

Christie, A., and P. Toon. 1993. Safer sexual practices. *The Practitioner* 237:901–4.

Clottey, C., and G. Dallabetta. 1993. Sexually transmitted diseases and human immunodeficiency virus. Epidemiologic synergy? *Infectious Disease Clinics of North America* 7:753–70.

Conlee, R. 1991. Amphetamine, caffeine, and cocaine. In *Ergogenics: Enhancement of performance in exercise and sport,* ed. D. Lamb and M. Williams. Dubuque, Iowa: Brown & Benchmark.

Consumers Union. 1993. How to spot and treat a drinking problem. *Consumer Reports on Health* 5:120–21.

Consumers Union. 1995. Hooked on tobacco: The teen epidemic. *Consumer Reports* 60:142–47.

Consumers Union. 1995. How reliable are condoms? *Consumer Reports* 60:320–25.

Consumers Union. 1995. Secondhand smoke. Is it a hazard? *Consumer Reports* 60:27–33.

Das, G. 1993. Cardiovascular effects of cocaine abuse. *International Journal of Clinical Pharmacology Therapy and Toxicology* 31:521–28.

Davies, K. 1990. Genital herpes. An overview. *Journal of Obstetric, Gynecologic, and Neonatal Nursing* 19:401–6.

Derlet, R., and B. Heischober. 1990. Methamphetamine: Stimulant of the 1990s? *Western Journal of Medicine* 153:625–28.

DeSchryver, A., and A. Meheus. 1990. Epidemiology of sexually transmitted diseases: The global picture. *Bulletin of the World Health Organization* 68:639–54.

Des Jarlais, D., and S. Friedman. 1994. AIDS and the use of injected drugs. *Scientific American* 270 (February): 82–88.

Dewey, W. L. 1986. Cannabinoid pharmacology. *Pharmacological Reviews* 38:151–78.

Farquhar, J. 1993. Keynote address: How health behavior relates to risk factors. *Circulation* 88:1376–80.

Flatt, J. 1992. Body weight, fat storage, and alcohol metabolism. *Nutrition Reviews* 50:267–70.

Fridinger, F., and B. Dehart. 1993. A model for the inclusion of a physical fitness and health promotion component in a chemical abuse treatment program. *Journal of Drug Education* 23:215–22.

Friedl, K. 1990. Reappraisal of the health risks associated with the use of high doses of oral or injectable androgenic steroids. *NIDA Research Monographs* 102:142–68.

Friedman, G., and A. Klatsky. 1993. Is alcohol good for your health? *The New England Journal of Medicine* 329:1882–83.

Gibbons, B. 1992. Alcohol: The legal drug. *National Geographic* 181 (February): 3–35.

Glantz, S., and W. Parmley. 1991. Passive smoking and heart disease: Epidemiology, physiology and biochemistry. *Circulation* 83:1–12.

Glantz, S., and W. Parmley. 1995. Passive smoking and heart disease. *Journal of the American Medical Association* 273:1047–53.

Graham, S., and M. Kennedy. 1990. Recent developments in the toxicology of anabolic steroids. *Drug Safety* 5:458–76.

Hart, B. 1993. Vascular consequences of smoking and benefits of smoking cessation. *Journal of Vascular Nursing* 11:48–51.

Hoffmann, D., et al. 1994. Tobacco-specific N-nitrosamines and Areca-derived N-nitrosamines: Chemistry, biochemistry, carcinogenicity, and relevance to humans. *Journal of Toxicology and Environmental Health* 41:1–52.

Hollister, L. E. 1986. Health aspects of cannabis. *Pharmacological Reviews* 38:1–20.

Hutchinson, C., and E. Hook. 1990. Syphilis in adults. *Medical Clinics of North America* 74:1389–1416.

Jackman, J., and D. Glamann. 1991. Gonococcal endocarditis: Twenty-five-year experience. *American Journal of Medical Sciences* 30:221–30.

Jaret, P. 1994. Viruses. *National Geographic* 186 (July): 58–91.

Jewett, J., and F. Hecht. 1993. Preventive health care for adults with HIV infection. *Journal of the American Medical Association* 269:1144–53.

Johnson, M. 1990. Anabolic steroid use in adolescent athletes. *Pediatric Clinics of North America* 37:1111–19.

Judson, F. 1990. Gonorrhea. *Medical Clinics of North America* 74:1353–66.

Kashkin, K., and H. Kleber. 1989. Hooked on hormones: An anabolic steroid addiction hypothesis. *Journal of the American Medical Association* 262:3166–70.

Kinghorn, G. 1993. Genital herpes: Natural history and treatment of acute episodes. *Journal of Medical Virology* Supplement 1:33–38.

Kune, G., and L. Vitetta. 1992. Alcohol consumption and the etiology of colorectal cancer: A review of the scientific evidence from 1957 to 1991. *Nutrition and Cancer* 18:97–111.

Landry, G., and W. Primos. 1990. Anabolic steroid abuse. *Advances in Pediatrics* 37:185–205.

Larrat, E., and S. Zierler. 1993. Entangled epidemics: Cocaine use and HIV disease. *Journal of Psychoactive Drugs* 25:207–21.

Lilley, L., and S. Schaffer. 1990. Human papilloma virus. A sexually transmitted disease with carcinogenic potential. *Cancer Nursing* 13:366–72.

Lombardo, J., et al. 1991. Anabolic/androgenic steroids and growth hormone. In *Ergogenics: Enhancement of exercise and sport performance,* ed. D. Lamb and M. Williams. Dubuque, Iowa: Brown & Benchmark.

Martin, B. R. 1986. Cellular effects of cannabinoids. *Pharmacological Reviews* 38:45–72.

McCormack, W. 1990. Overview: Sexually transmitted disease. *Mount Sinai Journal of Medicine* 57:187–91.

Mertz, G. 1990. Genital herpes simplex virus infections. *Medical Clinics of North America* 74:1433–54.

Mertz, G. 1993. Epidemiology of genital herpes infections. *Infectious Disease Clinics of North America* 7:825–39.

Mindel, A. 1993. Long-term clinical and psychological management of genital herpes. *Journal of Medical Virology* 1 (Supplement): 39–44.

Mitchell, R. 1993. Syphilis as AIDS? A call for research. *Medical Hypotheses* 41:115–17.

Morony, J., and M. Allen. 1994. Cocaine and alcohol use in pregnancy. *Advances in Neurology* 64:231–42.

Moss, G., and J. Kreiss. 1990. The interrelationship between human immunodeficiency virus infection and other sexually transmitted diseases. *Medical Clinics of North America* 74:1647–60.

Osborn, J. 1990. AIDS: Challenges to our health care systems. *Cleveland Clinic Journal of Medicine* 57:709–14.

Perkins, K. 1992. Metabolic effects of cigarette smoking. *Journal of Applied Physiology* 72:401–9.

Perkins, K. 1993. Weight gain following smoking cessation. *Journal of Consulting Clinical Psychology* 61:768–77.

Petty, T. 1993. Pharmacology of smoking cessation. *Monaldi Archives for Chest Disease* 48:576–79.

Pirich, C., et al. 1993. Coffee, lipoproteins and cardiovascular disease. *Wiener Klinische Wochenschrift* 105:3–6.

Pohorecky, L. 1990. Interaction of ethanol and stress: Research with experimental animals—an update. *Alcohol and Alcoholism* 25:263–76.

Public Health Service. 1993. Mortality trends for selected smoking-related cancers and breast cancer—United States, 1950–1990. *Morbidity and Mortality Weekly Report* 42:857–66.

Public Health Service. 1993. Use of smokeless tobacco among adults—United States, 1991. *Morbidity and Mortality Weekly Report* 42:263–66.

Raloff, J. 1994. The great nicotine debate. Are cigarette recipes 'cooked' to keep smokers hooked? *Science News* 145:314–17.

Regan, T. 1990. Alcohol and the cardiovascular system. *Journal of the American Medical Association* 264:377–81.

Rein, M. 1993. Sexually transmitted diseases. *Comprehensive Therapy* 19:136–44.

Reinke, L., et al. 1990. Possible roles of free radicals in alcoholic tissue damage. *Free Radical Research Communications* 9:205–11.

Rosenberg, I., ed. 1992. Regular or decaf? Coffee consumption and serum lipoproteins. *Nutrition Reviews* 50:175–78.

Rosmarin, P. 1989. Coffee and coronary heart disease: A review. *Progress in Cardiovascular Diseases* 32:239–45.

Ruegg, C., and E. Engleman. 1990. Impaired immunity in AIDS. The mechanisms responsible and their potential reversal by antiviral therapy. *Annals of the New York Academy of Sciences* 616:307–17.

Sasco, A. 1992. Tobacco and cancer: How to react to the evidence. *European Journal of Cancer Prevention* 1:367–73.

Schacter, J. 1990. Chlamydial infections. *Western Journal of Medicine* 153:523–34.

Schwartz, J. 1992. Methods of smoking cessation. *Medical Clinics of North America* 72:451–76.

Seidman, S., and R. Rieder. 1994. A review of sexual behavior in the United States. *American Journal of Psychiatry* 151:330–41.

Silagy, C., et al. 1994. Meta-analysis on efficacy of nicotine replacement therapies in smoking cessation. *Lancet* 343:139–42.

Sobel, J. 1990. Vaginal infections in adult women. *Medical Clinics of North America* 74:1573–1602.

Spitzer, W., et al. 1990. Links between passive smoking and disease: A best-evidence synthesis. *Clinical and Investigative Medicine* 13:17–42.

Steinmetz, G. 1992. The preventable tragedy: Fetal Alcohol Syndrome. *National Geographic* 181 (February): 36–39.

Stratton, P., and N. Alexander. 1993. Prevention of sexually transmitted infections. Physical and chemical barrier methods. *Infectious Disease Clinics of North America* 7:841–59.

Taylor, S., and S. Chermack. 1993. Alcohol, drugs, and human physical aggression. *Journal of Studies on Alcohol* 11:78–88.

Thoren, P., et al. 1990. Endorphins and exercise: Physiological mechanisms and clinical implications. *Medicine and Science in Sports and Exercise* 22:417–28.

Tinkle, M. 1990. Genital human papilloma virus infection. A growing health risk. *Journal of Obstetric, Gynecologic, and Neonatal Nursing* 19:501–7.

Trivedi, A., et al. 1993. Monitoring of smokeless tobacco consumers using cytogenetic endpoints. *Anticancer Research* 13:2245–49.

Viscarello, R. 1990. AIDS. Natural history and prognosis. *Obstetrics and Gynecology Clinics of North America* 17:545–55.

Waterson, E., and I. Murray-Lyon. 1990. Preventing alcohol-related birth damage: A review. *Social Science and Medicine* 30:349–64.

Watson, R. 1988. Caffeine: Is it dangerous to health? *American Journal of Health Promotion* 2:13–21.

Weissler, J., and A. Mootz. 1990. Pulmonary disease in AIDS patients. *American Journal of Medical Sciences* 300:330–43.

Welder, A., and R. Melchert. 1993. Cardiotoxic effects of cocaine and anabolic-androgenic steroids in the athlete. *Journal of Pharmacological and Toxicological Methods* 29:61–68.

Wexner, S. 1990. Sexually transmitted diseases of the colon, rectum, and anus. The challenge of the nineties. *Diseases of the Colon and Rectum* 33:1048–62.

Wichmann, S., and D. Martin. 1994. Snuffing out smokeless tobacco use. *Physician and Sportsmedicine* 22 (April): 97–110.

Willett, W., and D. Hunter. 1993. Diet and breast cancer. *Contemporary Nutrition* 18 (3,4): 1–4.

Williams, M. 1991. Alcohol, marijuana, and beta blockers. In *Ergogenics: Enhancement of performance in exercise and sport,* ed. D. Lamb and M. Williams. Dubuque, Iowa.: Brown & Benchmark.

Williams, M. 1994. Physical activity, fitness, and substance misuse and abuse. In *Physical activity, fitness, and health,* eds. C. Bouchard, et al. Champaign, Ill.: Human Kinetics.

Wooldridge, W. 1991. Syphilis. A new visit from an old enemy. *Postgraduate Medicine* 89:193–202.

Specific Studies

Abdullah, A., et al. 1993. Treatment of external genital warts comparing cryotherapy (liquid nitrogen) and trichloroacetic acid. *Sexually Transmitted Diseases* 20:344–45.

Bianchi, C., et al. 1993. Alcohol consumption and the risk of acute myocardial infarction in women. *Journal of Epidemiology and Community Health* 47:308–11.

Blum, K., et al. 1990. Allelic association of human dopamine D_2 receptor gene in alcoholism. *Journal of the American Medical Association* 263:2055–60.

Chu, S., et al. 1990. Cigarette smoking and the risk of breast cancer. *American Journal of Epidemiology* 131:244–53.

Coate, D. 1993. Moderate drinking and coronary heart disease mortality: Evidence from NHANES I and the NHANES I follow-up. *American Journal of Public Health* 83:888–90.

Conway, T., and T. Cronan. 1992. Smoking, exercise, and physical fitness. *Preventive Medicine* 21:723–34.

Cos, K., et al. 1993. The combined effects of aerobic exercise and alcohol restriction on blood pressure and serum lipids: A two-way factorial study in sedentary men. *Journal of Hypertension* 11:191–201.

Curry, S., et al. 1990. Intrinsic and extrinsic motivation for smoking cessation. *Journal of Consulting and Clinical Psychology* 58:310–16.

Dyer, A., et al. 1990. Alcohol intake and blood pressure in young adults: The CARDIA study. *Journal of Clinical Epidemiology* 43:1–13.

Ernster, V., et al. 1990. Smokeless tobacco use and health effects among baseball players. *Journal of the American Medical Association* 264:218–24.

Fenton, L., et al. 1993. Prevalence of maternal drug use near time of delivery. *Connecticut Medicine* 57:655–69.

Fiore, M., et al. 1990. Methods used to quit smoking in the United States. Do cessation programs help? *Journal of the American Medical Association* 263:2760–65.

Frankel-Conrat, H., and B. Singer. 1988. Nucleoside adducts are formed by cooperative reactions of acetaldehyde and alcohols: Possible mechanism for the role of alcohol in carcinogenesis. *Proceedings of the National Academy of Sciences* 85:3758–61.

Freund, K., et al. 1993. The health risks of smoking. The Framingham Study: 34 years of follow-up. *Annals of Epidemiology* 3:417–24.

Friedenreich, C., et al. 1993. A cohort study of alcohol consumption and risk of breast cancer. *American Journal of Epidemiology* 137:512–20.

Gaziano, J., et al. 1993. Moderate alcohol intake, increased levels of high-density lipoprotein and its subfractions, and decreased risk of myocardial infarction. *New England Journal of Medicine* 329:1829–34.

Goldberg, R., et al. 1994. A prospective study of the health effects of alcohol consumption in middle-aged and elderly men. The Honolulu Program. *Circulation* 89:651–59.

Grodstein, F., et al. 1993. Relation of female infertility to consumption of caffeinated beverages. *American Journal of Epidemiology* 137:1353–60.

Haglund, B., and S. Cnattingius. 1990. Cigarette smoking as a risk factor for sudden infant death syndrome: A population-based study. *American Journal of Public Health* 80:29–32.

Hartung, G., et al. 1990. Effect of alcohol dose on plasma lipoprotein subfractions and lipolytic enzyme activity in active and inactive men. *Metabolism* 39:81–86.

Humble, C., et al. 1990. Passive smoking and 20-year cardiovascular disease mortality among nonsmoking wives, Evans County, Georgia. *American Journal of Public Health* 80:599–601.

Kawachi, I., et al. 1993. Smoking cessation in relation to total mortality rates in women. A prospective cohort study. *Annals of Internal Medicine* 119:992–1000.

Klatsky, A., et al. 1992. Alcohol and mortality. *Annals of Internal Medicine* 117:646–54.

Kovacs, J., et al. 1995. Increases in CD4 T lymphocytes with intermittent courses of interleukin-12 in patients with human immunodeficiency virus infection. *New England Journal of Medicine* 332:567–75.

Lane, J., et al. 1990. Caffeine effects on cardiovascular and neuroendocrine responses to acute psychosocial stress and their relationship to level of habitual caffeine consumption. *Psychosomatic Medicine* 52:320–26.

LaPerriere, A., et al. 1991. Aerobic exercise training in an AIDS risk group. *International Journal of Sports Medicine* 12:S53–S57.

Leanderson, P., and C. Tagesson. 1994. Cigarette tar promotes neutrophil-induced DNA damage in cultured lung cells. *Environmental Research* 64:103–11.

Linn, S., et al. 1993. High-density lipoprotein cholesterol and alcohol consumption in US white and black adults: Data from NHANES II. *American Journal of Public Health* 83:811–16.

Livingston, G., et al. 1990. Induction of nuclear aberrations by smokeless tobacco in epithelial cells of human oral mucosa. *Environmental and Molecular Mutagenesis* 15:136–44.

Longnecker, M., et al. 1988. A meta-analysis of alcohol consumption in relation to risk of breast cancer. *Journal of the American Medical Association* 260:652–56.

MacArthur, R., et al. 1993. Supervised exercise training improves cardiopulmonary fitness in HIV-infected persons. *Medicine and Science in Sports and Exercise* 25:684–88.

Meilman, P. 1993. Alcohol-induced sexual behavior on campus. *Journal of American College Health* 42:27–31.

Melchior, J., et al. 1993. Resting energy expenditure in human immunodeficiency virus-infected patients: Comparison between patients with and without secondary infections. *American Journal of Clinical Nutrition* 57:614–19.

Melnick, S., et al. 1993. Sexually transmitted diseases among young heterosexual urban adults. *Public Health Reports* 108:673–79.

Meyer, F., and E. White. 1993. Alcohol and nutrients in relation to colon cancer in middle-aged adults. *American Journal of Epidemiology* 138:225–36.

Ockene, J., et al. 1990. The relationship of smoking cessation to coronary heart disease and lung cancer in the Multiple Risk Factor Intervention Trial (MRFIT). *American Journal of Public Health* 80:954–58.

Orcutt, J., and L. Harvey. 1991. The temporal patterning of tension reduction: Stress and alcohol use on weekdays and weekends. *Journal of Studies on Alcohol* 52:415–24.

Perez-Reyes, M., et al. 1988. Interaction between marijuana and ethanol: Effects on psychomotor performance. *Alcoholism* 12:268–76.

Rehm, J., et al. 1993. Effects on mortality of alcohol consumption, smoking, physical activity, and close personal relationships. *Addiction* 88:101–12.

Rigsby, L., et al. 1992. Effects of exercise training on men seropositive for the human immunodeficiency virus-1. *Medicine and Science in Sports and Exercise* 24:6–12.

Robbins, A., et al. 1994. Cigarette smoking and stroke in a cohort of U.S. male physicians. *Annals of Internal Medicine* 120:458–62.

Rosmarin, P., et al. 1990. Coffee consumption and serum lipids: A randomized, crossover clinical trial. *American Journal of Medicine* 88:349–56.

Sandler, D., et al. 1993. Cigarette smoking and risk of acute leukemia: Associations with morphology and cytogenetic abnormalities in bone marrow. *Journal of the National Cancer Institute* 85:1994–2003.

Schmitz, J., et al. 1993. Cognitive and affective responses to successful coping during smoking cessation. *Journal of Substance Abuse* 5:61–72.

Schonwetter, D., et al. 1993. Type A behavior and alcohol consumption: Effects on resting and post-exercise bleeding time, thromboxane and prostacyclin metabolites. *Prostaglandins, Leukotrienes and Fatty Acids* 48:143–48.

Suter, P., et al. 1992. The effect of ethanol on fat storage in healthy subjects. *New England Journal of Medicine* 326:983–87.

Swanson, C., et al. 1993. Moderate alcohol consumption and the risk of endometrial cancer. *Epidemiology* 4:530–36.

Terney, R., and L. McLain. 1990. The use of anabolic steroids in high school students. *American Journal of Diseases in Children* 144:99–103.

Watters, J., et al. 1994. Syringe and needle exchange as HIV/AIDS prevention for injection drug users. *Journal of the American Medical Association* 271:115–20.

Werch, C. 1990. Behavioral self-control strategies for deliberately limiting drinking among college students. *Addictive Behaviors* 15:118–28.

Williamson, D., et al. 1991. Smoking cessation and severity of weight gain in a national cohort. *New England Journal of Medicine* 324:739–45.

Wu, T., et al. 1988. Pulmonary hazards of smoking marijuana as compared with tobacco. *New England Journal of Medicine* 318:347–51.

Wynd, C. 1992. Relaxation imagery used for stress reduction in the prevention of smoking relapse. *Journal of Advanced Nursing* 17:294–302.

10

EXERCISE AND NUTRITION CONCERNS FOR WOMEN

Key Terms

amenorrhea
anorexia athletica
anorexia nervosa
athletic amenorrhea
binge-purge syndrome
bulimia

bulimia nervosa
dysmenorrhea
eating disorders
estrogen
eumenorrhea
female athlete triad

menarche
menopause
menses
menstrual cycle
nulliparity
oligomenorrhea

peak bone mass
premenstrual syndrome (PMS)
secondary amenorrhea
syndrome
teratogens
testosterone

Key Concepts

■ The design of an exercise program for cardiovascular endurance, flexibility, or strength, and of a dietary-exercise program for weight control is the same for both males and females.

■ The effects of exercise and weight control on the menstrual cycle appear to be associated with changes in the levels of estrogen, a hormone involved in the regulation of the menstrual cycle.

■ Excessive concern with controlling body weight through diet and exercise may lead to anorexia nervosa, a serious mental disorder more common in women.

■ The interaction of exercise training with the menstrual cycle is a double-edged sword relative to women's health, some of the effects are beneficial, while other effects, although somewhat rare, may be harmful.

■ Although the cause of secondary amenorrhea in physically active females has not been determined, several associated factors include prior menstrual problems, increased stress, weight loss, low body fat, inadequate dietary fat and protein, and high intensity or increased duration of exercise.

■ Secondary amenorrhea is associated with an increased loss of bone mass that may predispose an individual to osteoporosis.

■ Exercise, diet, and stress management may be useful to help reduce the severity of physical and psychological symptoms associated with the premenstrual syndrome (PMS).

■ Exercise after menopause is important to help prevent or delay bone loss, but hormone replacement or drug therapy and adequate calcium intake also are important therapeutic techniques.

■ All females need to consume foods rich in iron and calcium, but those who are pregnant may need iron and calcium supplements, additional protein, and other vitamins and minerals, such as folic acid and zinc, in the diet.

■ Proper exercise may lead to a healthier pregnancy, but it is important to develop a high level of fitness before conception and to consult your physician about the intensity and duration of exercise during the pregnancy period.

■ Females who run for exercise should be aware of safety precautions to help prevent personal attack.

INTRODUCTION

Differences between males and females have been studied from physiological, psychological, emotional, social, and intellectual viewpoints. With the exception of the obvious sex differences and several other genetic factors, most reviews have reported that males and females are more similar than dissimilar and adherence to or violation of the principles underlying a Positive Health Life-style will affect health status in both genders in a similar fashion.

However, for some unknown reason but probably related to hormonal differences, women live on the average almost 6 years longer than men. Partially because of this, much of the research on preventive medicine in the past has focused on males. However, there are a number of health concerns that are unique to females and women's health has recently become a priority in the United States. The National Institutes of Health (NIH) has created an Office of Research on Women's Health that launched a 14-year research project entitled the Women's Health Initiative Study designed to study a wide variety of factors that may influence women's health, including nutrition, exercise, stress, substance abuse, and hormone activity. Dr. Bernadine Healy, as director of the NIH, stated in regard to women's health the good news is that women live longer, but the bad news is that their quality of life is not what it could be, noting that women experience more disease and debilitating illness than men.

In this regard, adopting a Positive Health Life-style may be especially important for women. The principles and guidelines relative to the development of a Positive Health Life-style are applicable to both males and females. The design of a dietary program for weight control or of exercise programs for the development of cardiovascular fitness, muscular strength, or flexibility is identical for both sexes. In general, women will realize the same physiological and psychological benefits from exercise training and proper nutrition as men (see fig. 10.1). For example, an aerobic exercise program will increase their maximal oxygen uptake and cardiovascular efficiency, improve their serum lipid profile, and help them lose excess body fat. Such benefits may have significant health implications for women, because although occurring later in life than in men, coronary heart disease is the leading cause of mortality among women in the United States. Recent research by Steven Blair and his associates at the Institute for Aerobics Research has shown that higher levels of physical fitness are associated with lower mortality rates in women, a finding previously noted only for men, further enhancing their longevity advantage. Additionally, adoption of a Positive Health Life-style may enhance women's quality of life during their later years by helping prevent debilitating illnesses.

Although the design, implementation, and benefits of a Positive Health Life-style are similar for both men and women, several aspects of exercise and nutrition are of special concern to women. This chapter briefly addresses these concerns.

The Role of Weight Control, Exercise, and Nutrition in the Menstrual Cycle

The onset of puberty represents the time in life when an individual becomes capable of reproduction. In boys, puberty normally occurs between the ages of twelve and sixteen, with an average of approximately fourteen years, while the range for girls is nine to seventeen, with an average of twelve years.

The sex differences after puberty are due to the differential effects of the major hormones secreted by the gonads. Testosterone is secreted by the testes in males, and estrogen is secreted from the ovary in females. Both males and females produce estrogen and testosterone, but the quantities of estrogen and testosterone are greater in the female and male, respectively. The adrenal gland also secretes androgens, hormones similar to testosterone, but these androgens may be converted into a form of estrogen by certain body tissues, particularly fat tissue.

Testosterone stimulates the development of the typical male secondary sex characteristics and is a major anabolic hormone that leads to a rapid increase in the growth rate and formation of muscle tissue typical of adolescent males. **Estrogen** secretion is responsible for the development of the female secondary sex characteristics, including an increase in the amount of body fat and the preparation of the uterus to support pregnancy. The menstrual cycle is functionally related to both of these processes.

Females ovulate approximately once a month. After ovulation, the graafian follicle undergoes some changes, forming a structure known as the corpus luteum. The corpus luteum begins to produce significant amounts of progesterone, a hormone that increases the vascularity, or blood vessels, of the lining of the uterus. If the egg is fertilized by sperm, it will be implanted in the uterine lining. However, if fertilization and implantation do not occur, this vascularity is not needed, and hormonal changes, primarily a decrease in estrogen and progesterone, lead to its dissolution and the onset of menstruation, or **menses.** The sequence of events between menses, involving ovulation and the preparation for pregnancy, is referred to as the menstrual cycle.

Although other secondary sex changes may occur in the female prior to the first onset of menses, or **menarche,** it is usually used as the primary marker for the onset of puberty. Normal menses, known as **eumenorrhea,** continues throughout adulthood and ceases somewhere between the ages of thirty-five and fifty-five. This cessation of menses is known as **menopause.**

Although the role of various hormones in the regulation of the menstrual cycle are fairly well established, the factors that control the onset of menarche, the maintenance of eumenorrhea, and the onset of menopause are not as precisely known. The control of the reproductive cycle involves a complex interaction of hormones released from the hypothalamus, the pituitary gland, the ovaries, the corpus luteum, the adrenal gland, and fat cells. The hypothalamus is the major control center in the brain that regulates the menstrual cycle by carefully monitoring and adjusting blood levels of these hormones. However, as noted in previous chapters, the hypothalamus is also involved in the control of a wide variety of other body functions, including body temperature, hunger, appetite, body weight, and response to stress. Several theories suggest

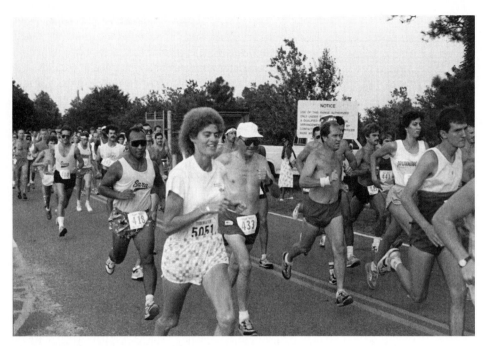

Figure 10.1 *Many women who start running for health and weight control become involved in the competitive aspects of the sport.*

that certain factors, such as a low body weight or excessive stress, interfere with the hypothalamic regulation of the menstrual cycle or estrogen production and may have possible health consequences.

Estrogen is intimately involved in the regulation of the menstrual cycle, but it also impacts significantly upon the development of several major diseases prevalent in the United States. Estrogen is believed to be involved in the production of higher than normals levels of HDL-cholesterol in women, conferring an advantage in the prevention of coronary heart disease. On the other hand, excess levels of estrogen may increase the risk of uterine cancer, while lower levels of estrogen lead to the development of osteoporosis, a loss of bone mass that predisposes women to a higher risk of bone fractures.

Since exercise, nutrition, and weight control are important components of a Positive Health Life-style, let's look at their interactions with the menstrual cycle.

Weight Control and the Menstrual Cycle

As noted in chapter 7, there are some health advantages associated with maintenance of a proper body weight, both in males and females. In the United States, there are powerful societal pressures generated by the fashion and advertising industries for women to be thin, maybe even excessively so. For example, even though the health risks of cigarette smoking are known, some women may continue to smoke because it may help them remain slim. An obsession with having a low body weight may lead to a number of different eating disorders that may have serious health consequences. **Eating disorders** are characterized by gross disturbances in eating behavior, according to the American Psychiatric Association. Low level of self-esteem is one of the major underlying characteristics of individuals with the major eating disorders.

Bulimia, or **bulimia nervosa,** is an eating disorder characterized by a loss of control over the impulse to binge on food; the satiety center of bulimics appears to be less responsive to cues that normally terminate eating, such as a distended stomach. The bulimic repeatedly ingests large quantities of food and then forces himself or herself to vomit in order to avoid weight gain. This practice is referred to as the **binge-purge syndrome.** Purging-type bulimics may also misuse laxatives, diuretics, and enemas. Some bulimics, the nonpurging type, do not engage in self-induced vomiting, but may use other techniques, such as fasting or excessive exercise, to control body weight. Bulimics are generally overconcerned with their body weight, and thus bulimia is more prevalent in females than males. The prevalence of bulimia in the general population is about 2 to 3 percent; however, it may be much higher among college students, possibly as high as 10 percent. College females aged eighteen to twenty-two are one of the most afflicted groups, many of whom use bulimia as a weight-control method to cope with the stress of college life. Bulimia spans the body-weight continuum, and many bulimics have a normal body weight, but body weight may fluctuate frequently due to alternating binges and fasts and the use of diuretics or laxatives. Adverse health effects of bulimia include erosion of tooth enamel, tears in the esophagus, aspiration pneumonia, and heart failure, all of which may be vomiting-induced. The American Psychiatric Association criteria for bulimia nervosa are presented in table 10.1.

Anorexia nervosa is a complex eating disorder that is not completely understood but is thought to be a symptom of mental illness, characterized by a fear of fatness that results in a self-induced starvation. The cause of the obsession is not known but may be related to family or societal pressures to be thin. It appears that the person with the highest probability of

Table 10.1 American Psychiatric Association Diagnostic Criteria for Bulimia Nervosa

1. Recurrent episodes of binge eating. An episode of binge eating is characterized by both of the following:
   a. eating, in a discrete period of time (e.g., within any 2-hour period), an amount of food that is definitely larger than most people would eat during a similar period of time and under similar circumstances
   b. a sense of lack of control over eating during the episode (e.g., a feeling that one cannot stop eating or control what or how much one is eating)
2. Recurrent inappropriate compensatory behavior in order to prevent weight gain, such as self-induced vomiting; misuse of laxatives, diuretics, enemas, or other medications; fasting; or excessive exercise.
3. The binge eating and inappropriate compensatory behaviors both occur, on average, at least twice a week for 3 months.
4. Self-evaluation is unduly influenced by body shape and weight.
5. The disturbance does not occur exclusively during episodes of anorexia nervosa.

Specify Type

Purging Type: during the current episode of bulimia nervosa, the person has regularly engaged in self-induced vomiting or the misuse of laxatives, diuretics, or enemas

Nonpurging Type: during the current episode of bulimia nervosa, the person has used other inappropriate compensatory behaviors, such as fasting or excessive exercise, but has not regularly engaged in self-induced vomiting or the misuse of laxatives, diuretics, or enemas

Source: American Psychiatric Association: Diagnostic and Statistical Manual of Mental Disorders. *Fourth Edition, Revised, Washington, D.C.: American Psychiatric Association, 1994.*

Table 10.2 American Psychiatric Association Diagnostic Criteria for Anorexia Nervosa

1. Refusal to maintain body weight at or above a minimally normal weight for age and height (e.g., weight loss leading to maintenance of body weight less than 85% of that expected; or failure to make expected weight gain during period of growth, leading to body weight less than 85% of that expected).
2. Intense fear of gaining weight or becoming fat, even though underweight.
3. Disturbance in the way in which one's body weight or shape is experienced, undue influence of body weight or shape on self-evaluation, or denial of the seriousness of the current low body weight.
4. In postmenarcheal females, amenorrhea (i.e., the absence of at least three consecutive menstrual cycles). A woman is considered to have amenorrhea if her periods occur only following hormone (e.g., estrogen) administration.

Specify Type

Restricting Type: during the current episode of anorexia nervosa, the person has not regularly engaged in binge-eating or purging behavior (i.e., self-induced vomiting or the misuse of laxatives, diuretics, or enemas)

Binge-Eating/Purging Type: during the current episode of anorexia nervosa, the person has regularly engaged in binge-eating or purging behavior (i.e., self-induced vomiting or the misuse of laxatives, diuretics, or enemas)

Source: American Psychiatric Association: Diagnostic and Statistical Manual of Mental Disorders. *Fourth Edition, Revised, Washington, D.C.: American Psychiatric Association, 1994.*

developing anorexia nervosa is a perfectionistic and self-critical individual who comes from an upper-middle socioeconomic status. The prevalence of anorexia nervosa is relatively low, about 1 percent or less in the general population, but reported to be as high as 2 percent in college students. Although anorexia nervosa does occur in males, approximately 95 percent of those affected with anorexia nervosa are young females. Some anorexics are classified as binge eating/purging types because they engage in these bulimic behaviors, while those who do not binge and/or purge are known as the restrictive type of anorexic. Health consequences of anorexia nervosa can be very serious, including anemia, a decreased heart muscle mass, heart beat arrhythmias attributed to electrolyte imbalances, and even death.

The American Psychiatric Association diagnostic criteria for anorexia nervosa are presented in table 10.2.

Anorexia nervosa is less common than bulimia but is more severe. The basic difference between bulimia and anorexia nervosa is the severe weight loss experienced by anorexics. Although bulimics are at risk because of the dangers associated with vomiting, the fluctuations in body weight are not normally life threatening. The anorexic is more prone to severe acute illnesses due to the excessive weight loss.

Since anorexia nervosa is a serious nervous disorder that may be fatal, professional medical treatment is necessary. The treatment is generally prolonged for several years and involves psychological therapy for both the individual and

his/her family in order to find and eliminate the underlying cause. This is often difficult because the patient is usually self-assured and claims to be in excellent health. The general prognosis is dependent upon the severity of the underlying personality disorder. Some recent investigations have revealed that anorexics may perpetuate their behaviors because starvation may elicit a release of endorphins; thus, they may possibly be addicted to a starvation "high." In severe cases, hospitalization and expert treatment by a physician, possibly involving forced feeding, may be necessary. Additional information may be obtained from the American Anorexia/Bulimia Association, 293 Central Park West, #1R, New York, N.Y. 10024. (212)501–8351.

Although reduction of excess body fat is one of the goals of a Positive Health Life-style, an excessive loss of body weight, as in anorexia nervosa, is not compatible with such a life-style since it may lead to some serious health problems such as osteoporosis. Many females who engage in exercise for health and weight control may become involved in competitive sports (see fig. 10.1), which may continue to confer both physical and psychological health benefits. However, in some sports, such as gymnastics and distance running, excess body weight may hinder performance. In recent years, the term **anorexia athletica** has been applied to athletes or others who exercise excessively and are overly concerned with their weight and who also exhibit some of the diagnostic criteria associated with anorexia nervosa. Studies have revealed that approximately 20 to 40 percent of female athletes exhibit such criteria, particularly in sports emphasizing leanness or a specific body weight. What may begin as a means to control weight for athletic competition on a short-term basis, such as dieting for several months over a competitive season, may develop into a long-term medical problem. Several investigators have suggested that special attention be devoted to young female athletes, particularly those involved in sports such as gymnastics and ballet, for they may meet the age and socioeconomic-status criteria that predispose them to anorexia nervosa. Mimi Johnson, a physician specializing in pediatric and young adult sports medicine, recommends that physicians tailor the preparticipation examination for female athletes to help screen for eating disorders. In general, however, anorexia athletica appears to be limited to the time when an athlete is preparing for competition and fades away when the athletic season is completed and the athlete resumes normal dietary habits.

It is important to note that research conducted over the past 10 years has revealed that even moderate losses of body weight, particularly in those who exercise, may be associated with the cessation of menstruation, or **amenorrhea,** and an increased risk for the development of osteoporosis.

Exercise and the Menstrual Cycle

The American College of Obstetricians and Gynecologists, in its statement on women and exercise, notes that a proper exercise program is an important component of a Positive Health Life-style, conferring health benefits throughout the life cycle for both males and females. Although body fat is distributed differently in males and females, research has supported the role of exercise in a comprehensive weight loss program for everyone. Moreover, for females in particular, some research findings have revealed several interesting implications regarding the potential health effects of exercise during three different time frames of the life cycle—the premenarche stage, the menstrual stage, and the postmenopausal stage.

The Premenarche Stage

Epidemiological research has suggested several possible health effects resulting from habitual physical activity and exercise in young girls prior to the onset of puberty; however, some of these effects will not be evidenced until later in life. One implication is that since exercise helps stimulate the development of bone mass, girls who exercise may develop stronger bones with greater stores of calcium and thus be less prone to osteoporosis as they get older. In general, research findings have revealed that young women who have exercised early in life have greater bone densities, or **peak bone mass** compared to more sedentary girls.

On the other hand, intensive training prior to menarche may be associated with a higher incidence of menstrual irregularities. The age at which menarche occurs may be delayed. Research by Rose Frisch and her associates at Harvard University revealed that girls who exercised extensively prior to menarche did not experience their first menses until an average age of fifteen years, over two years later than more sedentary girls. Moreover, once they began to menstruate, they were more prone to menstrual disturbances. Frisch proposes that these physiological changes in the menstrual cycle are associated with low levels of body fat caused by high levels of exercise. She theorizes that since the body fat stores are very low, there is a decreased capacity to convert circulating androgens into estrogen; the decreased levels of estrogen may contribute to menstrual irregularities such as amenorrhea. Additionally, some preliminary research data suggest that maintenance of a very low body weight during the growth years may retard the growth process, decreasing the potential maximal height of the child.

Although there may be some possible long-term health risks associated with these physiological changes, there may also be some possible long-term health benefits as noted below.

The Menstrual Stage

The monthly **menstrual cycle,** which averages about 28 days, is usually divided into four phases associated with changes in the endometrium, the mucous membrane lining the uterus. Menstruation, the period of uterine bleeding, lasts 4 to 5 days; the follicular phase represents the maturation of the follicle for release of the egg and lasts about 14 days; the luteal phase lasts about 10 to 14 days and involves the development of the corpus luteum and increased production of progesterone; and the premenstrual phase lasts about 1 to 2 days and involves shrinkage of the corpus luteum and other structures designed to support pregnancy.

The interaction of the menstrual cycle and exercise can be viewed from two points. First, what is the effect of the menstrual cycle on physical performance? Second, what effect does exercise have upon the menstrual cycle?

A number of research studies have been conducted about the first question, and probably the best conclusion is that the effects of the different phases of the menstrual cycle on physical performance depend on the individual. Although exercise performance during menstruation is worse in some women, others have no problem and some athletes have even achieved record-breaking performances during the active-flow period. For some women, performance seems to be best during the follicular and early luteal phases, particularly in high-intensity exercise. On the contrary, some evidence suggests that performance in aerobic endurance events may be impaired in the premenstrual phase; this may be related to the increased water retention and body weight at that time.

There appear to be no physical or physiological reasons that a woman cannot exercise during any phase of the menstrual cycle. Each woman should monitor her physical condition during each phase, particularly as it relates to her feelings toward her ability to exercise. In particular, she should evaluate differences between the premenstrual phase and the follicular and luteal phases, the phases where the most marked differences are likely to occur.

Can exercise affect the menstrual cycle? It appears that it can; some of the effects may increase health risks, while other effects may be beneficial.

Increased Health Risks   Some individuals develop a condition labeled as **athletic amenorrhea,** a form of **secondary amenorrhea** in which menstrual flow stops for prolonged periods of time, usually a minimum of three regular cycles. Athletic amenorrhea, observed primarily in runners and ballet dancers, has also been noted in other female athletes as well. **Oligomenorrhea** refers to infrequent bleeding and also appears to occur more frequently among physically active females. Depending upon which of the above definitions is used, secondary amenorrhea or oligomenorrhea, studies have revealed that the percentage of female exercisers who experience these clinical symptoms ranges from less than 5 percent to over 30 percent. The **female athlete triad** (disordered eating, amenorrhea, and osteoporosis) is a recent term coined to depict the sequence of events which may occur in young active females who exercise intensely to lose body weight.

At the present time, the cause of athletic amenorrhea and oligomenorrhea is not known, although it is believed to be due to changes in complex hormonal interactions among the hypothalamus, pituitary gland, and the ovaries. Exercise, per se, is not believed to be the causative factor, and no single mechanism associated with exercise has been identified as the cause of hormonal changes, but exercise appears to interact with a number of other possible factors, including the following:

1. Prior menstrual problems. Individuals with irregular periods before initiating an exercise training program may be more susceptible to athletic amenorrhea and oligomenorrhea.

2. Stress. As noted in chapter 8, stress can create a number of hormonal changes in the body by affecting the hypothalamus. These hormonal changes may disrupt the normal menstrual cycle. For example, the hypothalamus influences the pituitary gland, which secretes several gonadotropic hormones that help regulate the ovaries, which secrete estrogen, so hypothalamic stress may modify estrogen dynamics. Exercise is a physical stressor and may be a psychological stressor in competitive athletics.

3. Weight loss and low body weight or low body fat. Women who lose body weight rapidly or have low levels of body fat appear to be more prone to amenorrhea. Rose Frisch indicates that the loss of 10 to 15 pounds of body fat may trigger amenorrhea. As noted previously, fat cells convert androgens to estrogen, so a decreased amount of body fat may influence levels of this hormone.

4. Distance and intensity of exercise. Runners who log over 30 miles per week or who do high-intensity exercises are more likely to be amenorrheic. The distance and intensity of exercise may be related to increased stress levels in some individuals.

5. Inadequate fat and protein in the diet. The low fat levels may decrease cholesterol production necessary for the formation of estrogen. Low dietary protein may signal the body that there are insufficient stores to support pregnancy, and the menstrual cycle may cease.

6. Increased body temperature during exercise. The increased temperature may disrupt optimal functioning of the hypothalamus and create a hormonal imbalance.

7. Young age and nulliparity. Athletic amenorrhea appears to be more prevalent in the young and in those who never have had children (**nulliparity**). Young girls who undertake strenuous physical training before puberty are also more susceptible.

In general, the amenorrhea experienced by runners and other athletes appears to be reversible once training has stopped. However, as a point of caution, there may be a number of other reasons that a woman becomes amenorrheic, and they may have serious medical implications. If you do develop amenorrhea, consult a gynecologist, preferably one who is sports oriented, for a full medical checkup to determine if there is a medical problem not associated with your exercise program.

If the amenorrhea persists, you may be at increased risk for the development of osteoporosis. Although osteoporosis is prevalent primarily in older women, recent research has suggested that women who develop athletic amenorrhea may experience a premature loss of bone mass due to decreased estrogen levels. Estrogen receptors in the bone may help regulate the activity of calcitonin, a hormone involved in bone-tissue formation. Although exercise is generally advocated as a means to prevent osteoporosis in women, it does not appear to counteract the adverse effects associated with the decreased estrogen levels seen in athletic amenorrhea. Although all findings are not in total agreement, a substantial number of studies have shown that amenorrheic athletes have lower bone-density levels in non-weight-bearing bones, such as the spine, and are more prone to musculo-skeletal injuries, such as stress fractures, than athletes who have normal menstruation.

The suggested medical treatment for this condition may vary, dependent upon the viewpoint of several leading endocrinologists, and may include hormone replacement therapy, usually varying combinations of estrogen or progesterone. Oral contraceptives have been prescribed by some physicians. As noted above, consultation with an appropriate physician is recommended. Osteoporosis is discussed further in chapter 11.

Another problem associated with amenorrhea is anovulation, or the inability to ovulate and thus conceive a child. Women who desire to become pregnant may need to curtail their exercise in order to gain weight and ovulate naturally.

Possible Health Benefits   Research from Frisch and her associates at Harvard has suggested a possible benefit from lower estrogen levels. Although her research is epidemiological and may involve some methodological problems, former college athletes experienced a significantly lower rate of breast cancer and cancer of the reproductive system when compared to nonathletes. Frisch theorized that the athletes, who were leaner than the nonathletes, had lower levels of estrogen, particularly the high-potency type of estrogen believed to be associated with the development of cancer.

Exercise may also be helpful in the treatment or prevention of several physical or psychological problems often associated with various phases of the menstrual cycle, particularly the premenstrual and menstruation phases. These problems are usually grouped under the general terms of the premenstrual syndrome or dysmenorrhea and are discussed later in this chapter.

The Post-Menopausal Stage

Menopause is the final cessation of menstruation, usually between the ages of thirty-five to fifty-five. The age at which menopause occurs appears to be genetically determined and is not influenced to an appreciable extent by environmental factors, although malnutrition and cigarette smoking may cause an earlier onset. There is little evidence to suggest that exercise has any effect upon the age of onset of menopause, but exercise may confer some benefits relative to several of the changes women experience at this time of life.

The production of estrogen decreases dramatically at menopause, and other hormonal changes may occur as well. Rapid hormonal changes may be involved in the etiology of hot flashes, mood changes, depression, irritability, and fatigue often seen with menopause. Although there is little research regarding the effect of exercise upon these unpleasant symptoms, the improved body image and reduction of stress associated with exercise may help minimize some of them.

Decreased estrogen levels at menopause may pose several significant health implications, particularly an increased risk for coronary heart disease (CHD) and osteoporosis, but exercise may help reduce the magnitude of these problems. As noted in chapter 3, aerobic exercise may help reduce some of the risk factors associated with CHD, such as high blood pressure, elevated serum lipid levels, and obesity. Estrogen replacement therapy may help prevent CHD by increasing HDL-cholesterol levels, as will exercise.

Relative to osteoporosis, a number of studies also have shown that weight-bearing exercise alone can help slow down the rate of bone loss that occurs after menopause; walking and jogging will benefit the hip joint, while upper-body exercises, such as weight lifting, will benefit the spine. However, the recommended treatment or prevention program involves the triad of hormone replacement or drug therapy, adequate calcium intake, and weight-bearing exercise. A physician should be consulted for proper advice relative to hormone replacement or newer medical techniques that are evolving to prevent the loss of bone mass.

Nutrition and the Menstrual Cycle

The guidelines presented in chapter 6 should provide adequate nutrition for most females; however, these guidelines may be modified somewhat by changes in the menstrual cycle and exercise habits. A major concern of the average female is obtaining a sufficient amount of iron in the diet. Iron is the major nutrient deficiency in the American diet, especially for women because they need one and a half times as much iron as men. The increased need is due to iron loss through menstrual bleeding. Moreover, women who exercise have an even greater need, for they may lose iron through sweat and by other means. Thus, women should include foods that are high in iron content in their diet, such as lean meats, fish, legumes, iron enriched or fortified cereals, and whole grain products. Other foods high in iron are highlighted in table 6.10 on page 118. Women who are on a low-Calorie diet to lose weight may find it impossible to obtain sufficient iron through dietary sources and may need a dietary supplement, such as a typical one-a-day vitamin pill with 15 milligrams of iron. After menopause the iron requirement of women is comparable to that of men, 10 milligrams per day.

Females of all ages also need adequate calcium in the diet, but most surveys reveal that most adults and many children are currently obtaining less than the RDA of approximately 1,000 milligrams per day. Since inadequate calcium intake may be a predisposing factor for the development of osteoporosis in later years, foods high in calcium should be stressed in the diet during the premenarche and menstrual stage of life. It is especially important to have adequate calcium intake during the growing years to increase peak bone mass, a kind of calcium reservoir for later years when calcium loss from bone accelerates. Adequate calcium intake would appear to be especially important to women who become amenorrheic. A list of foods high in calcium is presented in table 6.10 on page 118. Dairy foods such as skim milk and low-fat cheese are excellent sources. A number of nutritionists recommend that the intake of calcium be increased to 1,200 to 1,500 milligrams following menopause. As with iron, women who are on a low-Calorie diet may find it difficult to obtain adequate calcium through dietary sources and may benefit from a supplement of about 600 milligrams per day.

Exercise, Nutrition, and Stress Management in the Treatment of the Premenstrual Syndrome and Dysmenorrhea

A **syndrome** is defined as a group of signs or symptoms that characterize a particular disease or abnormal condition. A wide variety of unpleasant symptoms are associated with the **premenstrual syndrome (PMS),** including physical symptoms such as abdominal bloating, swelling of the arms and legs, weight gain, tenderness of the breasts, headache, backache, constipation, increased appetite, craving for sweets or salty foods, insomnia, nausea, and vomiting. PMS may also be characterized by psychological symptoms such as low self-esteem, anxiety, irritability, anger, moodiness, tearfulness, lethargy, and depression. These symptoms usually occur in the time between ovulation and menstruation, or the luteal and premenstrual phases, 7 to 10 days just prior to menstruation, and remit with menstruation.

PMS is classified as an abnormal condition, not a disease, because surveys indicate that 70 to 90 percent of all normal adult women may experience one or more of the symptoms at one time or another. Some women appear to be free of PMS symptoms, others experience symptoms on an irregular basis, while others experience one or more of the symptoms on a regular basis. In most women, the symptoms are usually mild; however, they may be moderate to severe in others. PMS has actually been utilized as a legal defense in court trials involving homicide, the women claiming temporary insanity.

The cause of PMS is not known, but it is believed to be due to an imbalance of hormones and brain chemicals during the luteal phase. It may involve complex interactions between the hypothalamus and the production of sex hormones such as estrogen and progesterone; brain neurotransmitters such as endorphins, norepinephrine, and serotonin; and several adrenal gland hormones like epinephrine and aldosterone. Inadequate or excessive amounts of these hormones may contribute to the physical or psychological symptoms observed in PMS. Some of these hormonal changes may be linked to hypoglycemia, or low blood sugar, one of the theories associated with PMS, since the symptoms are similar. Research data linking a lack of serotonin to PMS are impressive, for drugs that increase serotonin levels have been shown to decrease emotional distress and some physical symptoms in women with severe cases.

Many of the symptoms of PMS may occur for other reasons, such as a headache caused by excessive stress. To determine if you suffer from PMS, keep a careful diary of your menstrual cycle and the appearance of any of these physical or psychological symptoms. If one or more symptoms appear on a regular basis during the luteal and premenstrual phases, you may be experiencing hormonal changes associated with PMS. Laboratory Inventory 10.1 may be used as a model to track your symptoms during the menstrual cycle.

Treatment programs for PMS depend upon the symptoms and their severity. Currently there is no cure for PMS, so the objective of therapeutic approaches is to reduce the severity of the symptoms. Research has shown that mild psychological symptoms such as anxiety may be relieved by various stress management procedures, such as the relaxation techniques discussed in chapter 8.

Aerobic exercise may also be helpful. One study found that jogging 30 to 40 minutes four times a week helped reduce the severity of the symptoms associated with PMS. Other researchers have suggested that exercise will help improve the hormonal status, such as an increased production of endorphins and epinephrine, and may alleviate some of the physical and psychological symptoms. Guidelines for developing an aerobic exercise program are presented in chapters 2 and 3. Other types of exercise, such as resistance exercise, may be helpful but not as effective as aerobic exercise.

Modifying the diet may also be helpful. Although research findings are not conclusive, some individuals who experience PMS may benefit from an increased intake of certain vitamins or minerals or from other dietary modifications. Vitamin B_6 helps in the release of various hormones that may help alleviate some of the adverse psychological symptoms associated with PMS. Natural food sources of B_6 include protein foods such as lean meats, fish, and poultry. Some research has shown that B_6 supplements may help relieve the psychological depression associated with PMS. If B_6 supplements are taken, they should not exceed 50 milligrams per day, for some neurological problems have been observed with higher dosages. Vitamin E may also help reduce the severity of PMS symptoms by inhibiting the action of certain natural chemicals in the body known as prostaglandins. Good sources of vitamin E include vegetable oils and whole grain breads and cereals. Supplements of about 400 IU daily have been found to be effective in one study. Minerals such as magnesium, potassium, and zinc may be helpful. For example, lack of magnesium may interfere with the action of serotonin. Magnesium is widely distributed in foods, particularly nuts, seafood, whole grains, legumes, and green, leafy vegetables; potassium is found in a variety of natural foods, including whole grains, nuts, and fruits and vegetables, particularly bananas; zinc is richest in animal protein such as meats, fish, and poultry.

A diet high in complex carbohydrates, low to moderate in protein, and low in fat has been advocated as the Healthy American Diet for the prevention of various chronic diseases, but it may also help relieve some of the symptoms of PMS. Such a diet may prevent hypoglycemia, or low blood sugar, which has been associated with PMS symptoms. Additionally, several investigators have theorized that high-carbohydrate diets may increase the production of brain neurotransmitters such as serotonin to help alleviate some of the PMS psychological symptoms because of their calming action.

Eliminating or reducing caffeine consumption appears to help reduce the occurrence of PMS symptoms, particularly in women who become irritable or anxious. In one study, the prevalence of PMS symptoms was dose dependent, the most symptoms occurring in those college students who drank eight to ten cups of coffee per day. Reducing salt intake may also help reduce water retention in the body, thus reducing some of the bloating and swelling that often occurs.

In general, the guidelines presented in chapter 6 should help you design a healthful diet to provide adequate carbohydrate, vitamin, and mineral nutrition to reduce PMS symptoms.

If you experience mild symptoms of PMS, you may wish to experiment with these safe and healthful stress management, exercise, and diet therapeutic approaches, modifying them if necessary. For example, if you experience excessive swelling and weight gain that makes jogging or running unpleasant, substitute non-weight-bearing exercises such as swimming or bicycling. A broad overview is presented in table 10.3.

For more severe cases of PMS, medical or psychological treatment may be necessary. Although a number of research studies involving the use of drugs to treat PMS have shown placebos to be equally effective, there is substantial clinical

Table 10.3 Positive Health Life-Style Techniques to Help Reduce PMS Symptoms and/or Dysmenorrhea

Stress Management

Practice meditation
Engage in relaxation techniques
Perform aerobic exercise in a relaxing environment

Exercise

Perform aerobic exercise
Do flexibility exercises for the pelvic region
Do strength exercises for the abdominal area

Nutrition

Consume a diet high in complex carbohydrates, low to moderate in protein, and low in fat
Eat foods rich in vitamins B_6 and E
Eat foods rich in magnesium, potassium, and zinc
Reduce the amount of salt and sodium in the diet
Consider a supplement of vitamin B_6 (no greater than 50 milligrams/day) and vitamin E (no greater than 400 IU/day)

Substance Use

Eliminate or reduce caffeine content in the diet
Eliminate or reduce the consumption of alcohol
Stop or decrease the amount of cigarette smoking

evidence to suggest that some medications such as diuretics, antidepressants, and those that raise serotonin levels, such as fluoxetine, are helpful for some individuals. A physician should be consulted for proper medical advice.

Some women periodically experience **dysmenorrhea,** painful cramps associated with menstruation. Aerobic exercise may aggravate the condition in some individuals, so they may wish to exercise less strenuously. Flexibility exercises for the lower back and pelvic area, as discussed in chapter 5 and illustrated in figures 5.8 to 5.11, may help alleviate the symptoms. Women who are more physically fit seem to experience this problem less frequently.

The Role of Nutrition and Exercise in Pregnancy

Most women who are pregnant are under the care of a physician, usually a gynecologist or obstetrician, who will provide guidance to maximize the chances of a safe and healthy pregnancy. Today, many physicians are in tune with the concepts underlying a Positive Health Life-style and recommend such a life-style to their pregnant patients, for although a Positive Health Life-style is important for all of us, it is particularly desirable for the woman who is pregnant, not only for her health but for the health of her child. In this regard, most physicians will recommend abstinence from cigarette smoking and alcohol consumption during pregnancy in order to prevent the possibility of health problems associated with a low birth weight or the fetal alcohol syndrome. Physicians will also counsel against the use of certain drugs and excessive vitamin A supplementation that interfere with normal development of the fetus and cause birth defects. Such drugs are known as **teratogens.**

Physicians will also offer guidance on nutrition, weight control, and exercise during pregnancy. The following discussion is in accord with the recommendations advanced by the American College of Obstetricians and Gynecologists (ACOG).

Nutrition and Pregnancy

Research indicates that women who are underweight or who fail to gain adequate weight during pregnancy have a greater tendency to give birth to children of lower body weight, a condition associated with increased health problems in the newborn child. Thus, physicians may recommend that underweight women who desire to become pregnant attempt to reach an ideal body weight prior to pregnancy. Some guidelines on how to do this were presented in chapter 7.

During pregnancy, the recommended total weight gain is approximately 20 to 30 pounds. The weight gain is necessary not only to sustain the growth and development of the fetus, but also to sustain the growth of supporting structures and to develop a reserve for breast feeding once the child is born. Women who are pregnant need to increase their caloric intake by about 15 percent in order to support this weight gain. The daily increase will be lower during the first trimester (3 months) of pregnancy, approximately 150 additional Calories, compared to the last trimester, about 350 additional Calories per day. For physically active women, additional Calories will be needed to account for those expended through exercise.

Because the requirement for almost every nutrient increases during pregnancy, these additional Calories should be quality Calories, adhering to the principles of nutrient density discussed in chapter 6. In particular, foods rich in high-quality protein, iron, calcium, zinc, and folic acid should be stressed because these requirements increase sharply during pregnancy and lactation. High-protein foods can help supply the additional 10–15 grams of protein recommended, but supplements containing iron, zinc, and folic acid are usually prescribed by physicians, for it may be difficult to obtain the recommended amounts through the diet. Incidentally, for women who may become pregnant, health authorities recommend a folic acid intake of approximately 400 micrograms, which may be obtained by eating more folic acid-rich foods or taking a supplement to complement dietary sources. Folic acid may help prevent neural tube defects—serious diseases of the spinal cord that may cause paralysis in the newborn. Folic acid supplements actually should be taken before pregnancy, if possible. For individuals at risk for neural tube defects, physicians may recommend higher dosages of folic acid. Calcium supplements may also be recommended if dietary intake is inadequate. Prenatal vitamin-mineral supplements are available, but it is important not to take vitamin megadoses during pregnancy, for excesses of some, particularly vitamin A, may be teratogenic.

Following pregnancy, women who breast feed should continue to eat a healthful diet to insure high quality breast milk. Many women may diet and exercise to lose the excess body fat accumulated during pregnancy, but weight loss should be gradual, maybe about 1 pound per week. Although caloric intake may be decreased somewhat, the Calories should consist of nutrient-dense foods, as discussed in chapter 6. A physician may provide appropriate guidelines for dieting postpartum.

Exercise and Pregnancy

Exercise and pregnancy are not mutually exclusive, but whether or not you should exercise during pregnancy and the type of exercise program you should follow may be dependent upon your fitness level or health status at the start of your pregnancy. The fitness boom stimulated considerable research interest into the interaction of exercise and pregnancy, providing us with some general guidelines. In response to inquiries from patients and physicians, the ACOG recently updated their guidelines for exercise during pregnancy and the postpartum period. A summary of these and other guidelines are presented in table 10.4, although ACOG recommends that an exercise prescription during pregnancy should be individualized and include an overall health assessment.

Although several sports gynecologists have criticized these guidelines for being overly conservative for some women (such as the recommendation not to exceed an exercise heart rate of 140 beats per minute) or not being based upon objective research data (such as the recommendation against bouncing type exercises), the ACOG contends that they have made these recommendations for the average woman and, if in error, they prefer to err toward the side of safety. With some modifications, the following discussion is consistent with the ACOG guidelines and the recommendations of other gynecologists.

Physically Fit Women

Mona Shangold, a gynecologist and marathon runner, has noted that the key to fitness during pregnancy is to become fit before pregnancy, for your body will have already adapted to the stress of exercise. Most women who are exercising can continue to exercise through the eighth or ninth month of pregnancy, although their exercise intensity and duration will need to be curtailed. Based upon current research findings, the following appear to be prudent guidelines for women who have been exercising prior to pregnancy.

1. Relative to exercise intensity, research has suggested that physically fit women with uncomplicated pregnancies may exercise at intensity levels adhering to the recommendations of the American College of Sports Medicine for healthy adults noted in chapter 3, and not experience stunted fetal growth or other adverse pregnancy outcomes. Nevertheless, don't overdo it! Stop when fatigued and do not exercise to exhaustion. Women who are fit may continue to exercise to the ACSM guidelines, but their exercise intensity may decrease as they gain weight through the pregnancy (fig. 10.2). Additionally, some investigators suggest the target HR may not be the best approach to use during later stages of pregnancy. Using the ratings of perceived exertion (RPE) or listening to your body during exercise as Shangold suggests may be helpful. As your pregnancy progresses,

Table 10.4 General Guidelines and Recommendations for Exercise during Pregnancy

1. Regular exercise (at least three times per week) is preferable to intermittent activity. Competitive activities should be discouraged.
2. Vigorous exercise should not be performed in hot, humid weather or during a period of febrile illness (fever).
3. Ballistic movements (jerky, bouncy motions) should be avoided. Exercise should be done on a wooden floor or a tightly carpeted surface to reduce shock and provide a sure footing. If running or walking, use well-cushioned, supportive footwear, and exercise on a flat, even surface.
4. Do not overstretch. Deep flexion or extension of joints should be avoided because of connective-tissue laxity. Activities that require jumping, jarring motions or rapid changes in direction should be avoided because of joint instability.
5. Vigorous exercise should be preceded by a warm-up of 5 minutes or longer. Slow walking or stationary cycling at low resistance are good examples.
6. Vigorous exercise should be followed by a warm-down that includes gentle static stretching. Moderate walking is a good example. Again, do not overstretch.
7. Heart rate should be measured at times of peak activity. Target heart rates and limits established in consultation with the physician should not be exceeded. Also use the rating of perceived exertion (RPE) as a guide to your exercise intensity.
8. Gradually reduce the intensity of the exercise during the second and third trimesters. Enjoy your workouts, and do not make them competitive. Breathlessness is an indication that the exercise may be too intense.
9. Care should be taken to gradually rise from the floor to avoid orthostatic hypotension and fainting. Some form of activity involving the legs should be continued for a brief period, such as walking in place.
10. Drink plenty of fluids before and after exercise to prevent dehydration. If necessary, interrupt exercise to replenish body fluids.
11. Women who have had sedentary life-styles should begin with physical activity of very low intensity and increase exercise intensity and duration very gradually.
12. If the mode of exercise, such as running, becomes uncomfortable during the latter stages of pregnancy, switch to other modes of aerobic exercise such as swimming, bicycling, or aerobic dance.
13. No exercise should be performed in the supine (lying on the back) position after the first trimester.
14. Exercises that employ the Valsalva maneuver should be avoided (see page 64).
15. Caloric intake should be adequate to meet not only the extra energy needs of pregnancy, but also of the exercise performed.
16. Activity should be stopped and the physician consulted if any unusual symptoms, such as joint pain, irregular heartbeats, vaginal bleeding, dizziness, or severe fatigue, appear.

Source: American College of Obstetricians and Gynecologists. Exercise during Pregnancy and the Postpartum Period. ACOG Technical Bulletin, *Number 189, February, 1994.*

walking may elicit the same RPE and heart-rate response as running previously did. You may need to adjust your RPE as your pregnancy advances, because they may underestimate your heart rate. The talk-test, or being able to carry on a conversation comfortably, may be a useful guide as well. Modify your exercise as you advance through pregnancy.

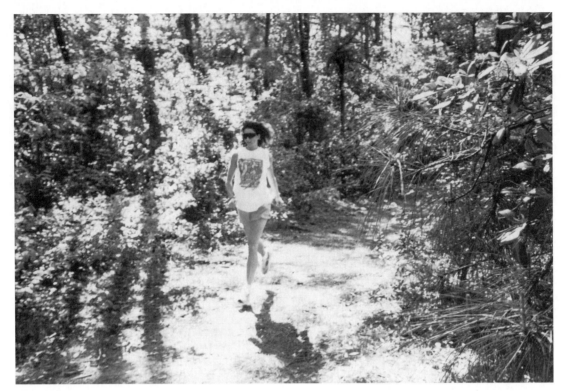

Figure 10.2 *You may perform aerobic exercise into the latter stages of pregnancy if your physician approves.*

2. The duration of the exercise stimulus period should be about 15 to 20 minutes, which is adequate to produce a training effect. The exercise stimulus period should be preceded by a warm-up and followed by a warm-down that includes milder aerobic activities and gentle stretching.

3. Exercise should be done on a regular basis. The ACSM guidelines of 3 to 4 days per week appear adequate; however, exercise may also be done daily.

4. Stretching exercises should not be maximal in nature. During pregnancy, hormones are released that increase the laxity in connective tissues such as ligaments, so it is possible that the joints may be more prone to injury if overly stretched. Strenuous bouncing exercises or other exercises that stress the joints may be contraindicated for the same reason.

5. Exercise should not be performed under environmental conditions that may pose an excessive heat stress. The body temperature should not exceed 101° F. Although little information is available concerning the effect on the fetus of excessive body temperature in humans, research with animals has shown teratogenic effects. Exercising in water has been shown to keep the body temperature cooler than a comparable amount of exercise on land, and the buoyancy effect helps reduce jarring movements and also helps prevent injuries. Drink plenty of fluids to prevent dehydration, which can lead to an increase in body temperature. Exercise may also be contraindicated under other environmental conditions, such as scuba

diving because of increased water pressure at depth, and hiking at high altitudes, because of the decreased oxygen pressure in the atmospheric air.

6. Mona Shangold suggests that resistance training may be good exercise during pregnancy. Increasing the strength of the quadriceps (thigh) muscles will make it easier to arise from a chair in the later months of pregnancy. Another benefit will be greater strength and endurance levels to carry the newborn child. However, exercises that invoke the Valsalva response, as discussed in chapter 4, should be avoided.

7. Be cautious in doing exercises while lying on your back. Some gynecologists suggest that this position may decrease the blood flow to the fetus. Also, some women experience a rapid drop in blood pressure as they get up, which may cause dizziness and fainting. Many of the exercises done on the back are to strengthen the abdominal muscles or to stretch the lower back muscles to help prevent or relieve low back pain, but other exercises, such as a pelvic tilt exercise against a wall and those noted in chapter 5 (figures 5.8 and 5.11), may be substituted.

8. Avoid exercises that may increase the risk of injury, such as loss of balance and falling or any impact trauma to the abdominal area.

9. You should gradually resume your normal exercise program during the postpartum period, for many of the physiological effects of pregnancy last for 4 to 6 weeks postpartum. Take your time getting back to prepregnancy exercise levels.

10. Stop exercising, and see your physician if you feel pain, experience bleeding, or have other unusual symptoms. If you have any questions about your personal exercise program, a knowledgeable physician should be consulted.

Sedentary Women

For those women who have been sedentary prior to pregnancy, but who desire to start an exercise program during pregnancy, caution is in order. It is probably best if the exercise program is individually prescribed by your physician. In general, the exercise intensity should be low, adhering to the ACOG guidelines of less than 140 heartbeats per minute. Exercise duration should be about 15 to 20 minutes three to four times per week. This intensity, duration, and frequency of exercise should provide sufficient stimulus to improve fitness and yet be safe. Walking is a highly recommended exercise but so too are swimming and water exercises, both non-weight-bearing exercises that confer other advantages to pregnant women as mentioned previously.

High-Risk Women

Exercise may be restricted or contraindicated for some women who may be at high risk, either for their own health or the health of the fetus. This includes those who have existing diseases or health conditions such as heart disease, anemia, and high blood pressure, those with ruptured membranes, cervical bleeding, or a weak cervix, and those with histories of premature labor, multiple miscarriages, or low birth weights. Exercise is advisable only if your pregnancy is normal and uncomplicated. Consult your physician for advice.

Fetal Health

A number of studies have revealed that exercise programs that adhere to ACOG or ACSM guidelines have no detrimental effect upon the fetus and the health of the newborn child and may actually be helpful to both the mother and child. Exercise during pregnancy does not appear to affect the mode of delivery, the gestational age at delivery, the fetal birth weight, the duration of labor, or the presence of obstetric complications, but it has been associated with fewer upper respiratory problems in the newborn. The mother may have a more rapid return to normal body weight following birth and may also experience fewer lower back pain problems.

Lactation

There appear to be no significant risks associated with the resumption of exercise postpartum in women who breast feed their baby. Schelkun and Potera both reviewed several studies focusing on this issue, and reported that exercise exerted no adverse effects on the quality of breast milk. Although women may safely lose weight while lactating, adequate energy and fluid intake are necessary to support milk production. A safe weight loss is about one pound per week, but women, especially those who are lean, should consult with their physician.

Running Safety

As noted previously, running, jogging, and walking are highly recommended aerobic activities because of their simplicity and practicality. Guidelines to minimize the chances of health risks or injuries by exercising safely with aerobic exercises were presented in chapter 3, but it appears important to include some additional guidelines for women at this point, because women who run for exercise may be at risk of personal attack. Although there is little evidence regarding the number of women who are attacked running or walking, the national publicity centering on the recent brutal attack and rape of a young woman running in Central Park has heightened this safety concern of women runners. In response to this concern, the Road Runners Club of America (RRCA) has issued some safety tips for female runners. With some modifications, the following highlight the major recommendations of the RRCA.

1. Run with a partner. Running in a group is even safer.
2. Run in familiar areas, avoiding areas that are unpopulated such as deserted streets or isolated trails. Avoid any area or person that you feel may be unsafe.
3. When running on the streets, face traffic in order to observe approaching vehicles.
4. When running at night, wear reflective clothing. Avoid unlit areas. Run clear of parked cars, alleyways, bushes, or other places where someone may hide.
5. Always stay alert to your surroundings. Do not wear a headphone so you may hear clearly.
6. Ignore verbal harassment. Pretend you do not hear it and continue to run, keeping your distance.
7. Do not wear jewelry, because it may be an incentive for robbery and attack.
8. Carry a whistle or other noisemaker, and use it immediately if threatened.
9. Carry an antipersonnel deterrent such as Mace or related chemicals to repress an attack. Learn how to use it rapidly.
10. Inform your family or your friends of your running route. Change your route periodically to avoid a regular pattern.
11. Carry identification with you, including important medical information such as blood type or a diabetic condition.
12. Carry change for a phone call; know the location of telephones and open businesses. Contact the police immediately if something happens to you or someone else.

The RRCA has developed a video and brochure dealing with safety of women runners. Contact the RRCA at 1150 South Washington Street, Suite 250, Alexandria, Va. 22314, (703) 836–0558 for more information if interested.

References

Books

American Psychiatric Association. 1994. *Diagnostic and statistical manual of mental disorders (4th ed. rev.) DSM-IV.* Washington, D.C.: APA.

Artal, R., and R. Wiswell, eds. 1985. *Exercise in pregnancy.* Baltimore: Williams & Wilkins.

Lensky, J. 1994. *Women, sport and physical activity: Selected research themes.* Glouster, Canada: Sport Information Research Center.

Melpomene Institute. 1990. *The bodywise woman: Reliable information on physical activity and health.* Englewood Cliffs, N.J.: Prentice-Hall.

Shangold, M., and G. Mirkin. 1985. *The complete sports medicine book for women.* New York: Simon and Schuster.

Swinney, B. 1993. *Eating expectantly. The essential eating guide and cookbook for pregnancy.* Colorado Springs, Colo. Fall River Press.

Williams, M. 1995. *Nutrition for fitness and sport.* Dubuque: Brown & Benchmark.

Yates, A. 1991. *Compulsive exercise and the eating disorders.* New York: Brunner/Mazel.

Reviews

Albers, M. 1990. Osteoporosis: A health issue for women. *Health Care for Women International* 11:11–19.

American College of Obstetricians and Gynecologists. 1993. Women and exercise. *International Journal of Gynecology and Obstetrics* 42:179–88.

American College of Obstetricians and Gynecologists. 1994. Exercise during pregnancy and the postpartum period. *ACOG Technical Bulletin* 189 (February): 1–5.

Anderson, J., and J. Metz. 1993. Contributions of dietary calcium and physical activity to primary prevention of osteoporosis in females. *Journal of the American College of Nutrition* 12: 378–83.

Aronson, R., et al. 1993. The effect of maternal cigarette smoking on low birth weight and preterm birth in Wisconsin. *Wisconson Medical Journal* 92:613–17.

Artal, R., et al. 1990. Orthopedic problems in pregnancy. *Physician and Sportsmedicine* 18 (September): 93–105.

Blair, S., et al. 1993. Physical activity, physical fitness, and all-cause mortality in women: Do women need to be more active? *Journal of the American College of Nutrition* 12:368–71.

Carbon, R. 1992. Exercise, amenorrhoea and the skeleton. *British Medical Bulletin* 48:546–60.

Carpenter, M. 1994. Physical activity, fitness, and health of the pregnant mother and fetus. In *Physical activity, fitness, and health,* eds. C. Bouchard, et al. Champaign, Ill.: Human Kinetics.

Chuong, C., and E. Dawson. 1992. Critical evaluation of nutritional factors in the patholphysiology and treatment of premenstrual syndrome. *Clinical Obstetrics and Gynecology* 35:679–92.

Clark, N. 1993. How to help the athlete with bulimia: Practical tips and a case study. *International Journal of Sports Nutrition* 3:450–60.

Constantini, N., and M. Warren. 1994. Physical activity, fitness, and reproductive health in women. In *Physical activity, fitness, and health,* eds. C. Bouchard, et al. Champaign, Ill.: Human Kinetics.

Consumers Union. 1993. Premenstrual syndrome: Does anything help? *Consumer Reports on Health* 5:61–63.

Dalsky, G. 1990. Effect of exercise on bone: Permissive influence of estrogen and calcium. *Medicine and Science in Sports and Exercise* 22:281–85.

Dewey, K., and M. McCrory. 1994. Effects of dieting and physical activity on pregnancy and lactation. *American Journal of Clinical Nutrition* 59:446S–452S.

Dustan, H. 1990. Coronary artery disease in women. *Canadian Journal of Cardiology* 6:19B–21B.

Fishbein, E., and M. Phillips. 1990. How safe is exercise during pregnancy? *Journal of Obstetric, Gynecologic, and Neonatal Nursing* 19:45–49.

Frisch, R. 1988. Fatness and fertility. *Scientific American* 258:88–95.

Gambrell, R. 1992. Update on hormone replacement therapy. *American Family Physician* 46:87S–96S.

Gizis, F. 1992. Nutrition in women across the life span. *Nursing Clinics of North America* 27:971–82.

Greene, J. 1993. Exercise-induced menstrual irregularities. *Comprehensive Therapy* 19:116–20.

Hargarten, K. 1994. Menopause: How exercise mitigates symptoms. *Physician and Sportsmedicine* 22 (January): 48–56.

Harris, R. 1991. Anorexia nervosa and bulimia nervosa in female adolescents. *Nutrition Today* 26 (March/April): 30–34.

Haynes, E. 1993. Dietary iron needs in exercising women: A rational plan to follow in evaluating iron status. *Medicine, Exercise, Nutrition, and Health* 2:203–12.

Holloway, M. 1994. Trends in women's health: A global view. *Scientific American* 271:76–83.

Johnson, M. 1992. Tailoring the preparticipation exam to female athletes. *Physician and Sportsmedicine* 20 (July): 61–72.

Lambert, G. 1988. Short review: Exercise and the premenstrual syndrome. *Journal of Applied Sport Science Research* 2:16–19.

Laraia, M., and G. Stuart. 1990. Bulimia. A review of nutritional and health behaviors. *Journal of Child and Adolescent Psychiatric Mental Health Nursing* 3:91–97.

Lebrun, C. 1993. Effect of the different phases of the menstrual cycle and oral contraceptives on athletic performance. *Sports Medicine* 16:400–430.

Liebman, B. 1995. For women only. *Nutrition Action Health Letter* 22 (March): 4–7.

Lokey, E., and Z. Tran. 1989. Effects of exercise training on serum lipid and lipoprotein concentration in women: A meta-analysis. *International Journal of Sports Medicine* 10:424–29.

Loucks, A. 1990. Effects of exercise training on the menstrual cycle: Existence and mechanisms. *Medicine and Science in Sports and Exercise* 22:275–80.

Loucks, A. 1994. Physical activity, fitness, and female reproductive mortality. In *Physical activity, fitness, and health,* eds. C. Bouchard, et al. Champaign, Ill: Human Kinetics.

Lurie, S., and R. Borenstein. 1990. The premenstrual syndrome. *Obstetrical and Gynecological Survey* 45:220–28.

Malina, R. 1983. Menarche in athletes: A synthesis and hypothesis. *Annals of Human Biology* 10:1–24.

Marcus, R., et al. 1992. Osteoporosis and exercise in women. *Medicine and Science in Sports and Exercise* 24:S301.

Marsh, M., and J. Stevenson. 1993. Alternatives to HRT in prevention and treatment. *Baillieres Clinical Rheumatology* 7:549–60.

Matkovic, V., and J. Ilich. 1993. Calcium requirements for growth: Are current recommendations adequate? *Nutrition Reviews* 51:171–80.

McGanity, W., et al. 1994. Nutrition in pregnancy and lactation. In *Modern nutrition in health and disease,* eds. M. Shils, et al. Philadelphia: Lea & Febiger.

McMurray, R., et al. 1993. Recent advances in understanding maternal and fetal responses to exercise. *Medicine and Science in Sports and Exercise* 25:1305–21.

Mortola, J. 1992. Assessment and management of premenstrual syndrome. *Current Opinions in Obstetrics and Gynecology* 4:877–85.

Munnings, F. 1988. Exercise and estrogen in women's health: Getting a clearer picture. *Physician and Sportsmedicine* 16 (May): 152–61.

National Dairy Council. 1993. Focus on nutrition and women's health. *Dairy Council Digest* 64:19–24.

Nattiv, A. 1994. The female athlete triad: Managing an acute risk to long-term health. *Physician and Sportsmedicine* 22 (January): 60–68.

Nattiv, A., and B. Mandelbaum. 1993. Injuries and special concerns in female gymnasts. *Physician and Sportsmedicine* 21 (July): 66–82.

Potera, C. 1994. Exercise is safe for lactating women. *Physician and Sportsmedicine* 22 (August): 13.

Prior, J., et al. 1992. Reproduction for the athletic woman. New understandings of physiology and management. *Sports Medicine* 14:190–99.

Provost, J. 1989. Eating disorders in college students. *Psychiatric Medicine* 7:47–58.

Ravnikar, V. 1993. Diet, exercise, and lifestyle in preparation for menopause. *Obstetrics and Gynocology Clinics of North America* 20:365–78.

Robinson, G., and P. Garfinkel. 1990. Problems in the treatment of premenstrual syndrome. *Canadian Journal of Psychiatry* 35:199–206.

Rock, C., and J. Curran-Celentano. 1994. Nutritional disorder of anorexia nervosa: A review. *International Journal of Eating Disorders* 15:187–203.

Schelkun, P. 1991. Exercise and breast-feeding mothers. *Physician and Sportsmedicine* 19 (April): 109–16.

Seeman, E., et al. 1993. Peak bone mass, a growing problem? *International Journal of Fertility and Menopausal Studies* 38 (Supplement 2): 77–82.

Shangold, M. 1990. Exercise in the menopausal woman. *Obstetrics and Gynecology* 75 (Supplement 4): 53S–58S.

Shroyer, J. 1990. Becoming streetwise: Guidelines for female runners. *Physician and Sportsmedicine* 18 (February): 121–25.

Silverstone, P. 1992. Is chronic self-esteem the cause of eating disorders? *Medical Hypotheses* 39:311–15.

Snyder, J. 1990. Aerobic exercise during pregnancy. *Journal of the American Board of Family Practice* 3:50–53.

Somogyi, A., and H. Beck. 1993. Nurturing and breast-feeding: Exposure to chemicals in breast milk. *Environmental Health Perspectives* 101 (Supplement 2): 45–52.

St. Jeor, S. 1993. The role of weight management in the health of women. *Journal of the American Dietetic Association* 93:1007–12.

Suominen, H. 1993. Bone mineral density and long term exercise. An overview of cross-sectional athlete studies. *Sports Medicine* 16:316–30.

Tucker, J., and R. Whalen. 1991. Premenstrual syndrome. *International Journal of Psychiatry in Medicine* 21:311–41.

Vogel, J., and K. Friedl. 1992. Body fat assessment in women. Special considerations. *Sports Medicine* 13:245–69.

Wichmann, S., and D. Martin. 1992. Heart disease: Not for men only. *Physician and Sportsmedicine* 20 (August): 138–48.

Wichmann, S., and D. Martin. 1993. Eating disorders in athletes. Weighing the risks. *Physician and Sportsmedicine* 21 (May): 126–35.

Williford, H., et al. 1993. Exercise prescription for women. *Sports Medicine* 15:299–311.

Wolfe, L., and M. Mottola. 1993. Aerobic exercise in pregnancy: An update. *Journal of Applied Physiology* 18:119–47.

Wolfe, L., et al. 1994. Maternal exercise, fetal well-being and pregnancy outcome. *Exercise and Sport Sciences Reviews* 22:145–94.

Wurtman, J. 1990. Carbohydrate craving. Relationship between carbohydrate intake and disorders of mood. *Drugs* 39 (Supplement 3): 49–52.

Yeager, K., et al. 1993. The female athlete triad: Disordered eating, amenorrhea, osteoporosis. *Medicine and Science in Sports and Exercise* 25:775–77.

Zeanah, M., and S. Schlosser. 1993. Adherence to ACOG guidelines on exercise during pregnancy: Effect on pregnancy outcome. *Journal of Obstetric, Gynocologic, and Neonatal Nursing* 22:329–35.

Specific Studies

Bachrach, L., et al. 1990. Decreased bone density in adolescent girls with anorexia nervosa. *Pediatrics* 86:440–47.

Ballard, J., et al. 1990. The effect of high level physical activity (8.5 METs or greater) and estrogen replacement therapy upon bone mass in postmenopausal females aged 50–69 years. *International Journal of Sports Medicine* 11:208–14.

Barr, S., et al. 1994. Restrained eating and ovulatory disturbances: Possible implications for bone health. *American Journal of Clinical Nutrition* 59:92–97.

Bernstein, L., et al. 1987. The effects of moderate physical activity on menstrual cycle patterns in adolescence: Implications for breast cancer prevention. *British Journal of Cancer* 55:681–85.

Caplan, G., et al. 1993. The benefits of exercise in postmenopausal women. *Australian Journal of Public Health* 17:23–26.

Clapp, J. 1989. The effects of maternal exercise on early pregnancy outcome. *American Journal of Obstetrics and Gynecology* 161:1453–57.

Cockerill, I., et al. 1992. Mood, mileage and the menstrual cycle. *British Journal of Sports Medicine* 26:145–50.

Cokkinades, V., et al. 1990. Menstrual dysfunction among habitual runners. *Women and Health* 16:59–69.

Davis, C., and J. Fox. 1993. Excessive exercise and weight preoccupation in women. *Addictive Behaviors* 18:201–11.

Devlin, M., et al. 1990. Metabolic abnormalities in bulimia nervosa. *Archives of General Psychiatry* 47:144–48.

Drinkwater, B., et al. 1984. Bone mineral content of amenorrheic and eumenorrheic athletes. *New England Journal of Medicine* 311:277–81.

Drinkwater, B., et al. 1990. Menstrual history as a determinant of current bone density in young athletes. *Journal of the American Medical Association* 263:545–48.

Fast, A., et al. Low-back pain in pregnancy. Abdominal muscles, sit-up performance, and back pain. *Spine* 15:28–30.

Fenley, J., et al. 1990. Untreated anorexia nervosa. A case study of the medical consequences. *General Hospital Psychiatry* 75:264–70.

Frisch, R., et al. 1985. Lower prevalence of breast cancer and cancers of the reproductive system among former college athletes compared to non-athletes. *British Journal of Cancer* 52:885–91.

Goodale, I., et al. 1990. Alleviation of premenstrual syndrome symptoms with the relaxation response. *Obstetrics and Gynecology* 75:549–55.

Gorsky, R., et al. 1994. Relative risks and benefits of long-term estrogen replacement therapy: A decision analysis. *Obstetrics and Gynecology* 83:161–66.

Groer, M., and C. Ohnesorge. 1993. Menstrual-cycle lengthening and reduction in premenstrual distress through guided imagery. *Journal of Holistic Nursing* 11:286–94.

Hatch, M., et al. 1993. Maternal exercise during pregnancy, physical fitness, and fetal growth. *American Journal of Epidemiology* 137:1105–14.

Hetland, M., et al. 1993. Running induces menstrual disturbances but bone mass is unaffected, except in amenorrheic women. *American Journal of Medicine* 95:53–60.

Laesale, R., et al. 1990. Mood changes and physical complaints during the normal menstrual cycle in healthy young women. *Psychoneuroendocrinology* 15:131–38.

Martin, D, and M. Notelovitz. 1993. Effects of aerobic training on bone mineral density of postmenopausal women. *Journal of Bone Mineral Research* 8:931–36.

McMurray, R., et al. 1993. Thermoregulation of pregnant women during aerobic exercise on land and in the water. *American Journal of Perintology* 10:178–82.

Metheny, W., and R. Smith. 1989. The relationship among exercise, stress, and primary dysmenorrhea. *Journal of Behavioral Medicine* 12:569–86.

Mortola, J., et al. 1989. Depressive episodes in premenstrual syndrome. *American Journal of Obstetrics and Gynecology* 161:1682–87.

Mortola, J., et al. 1990. Diagnosis of premenstrual syndrome by a simple, prospective, and reliable instrument: The calendar of premenstrual experience. *Obstetrics and Gynecology* 76:302–7.

Myburgh, K., et al. 1993. Low bone mineral density at axial and appendicular sites in amenorrheic athletes. *Medicine and Science in Sports and Exercise* 25:1197–1202.

O'Neill, M., et al. 1992. Accuracy of Borg's ratings of perceived exertion in the prediction of heart rates during pregnancy. *British Journal of Sports Medicine* 26:121–24.

Patton, G. 1988. Mortality in eating disorders. *Psychological Medicine* 18:947–51.

Pierce, E., et al. 1993. Scores on exercise dependence among dancers. *Perceptual Motor Skills* 76:531–35.

Pivarnik, J., et al. 1993. Effects of maternal aerobic fitness on cardiorespiratory responses to exercise. *Medicine and Science in Sports and Exercise* 25:993–98.

Quadagno, D., et al. 1991. The menstrual cycle: Does it affect athletic performance. *Physician and Sportsmedicine* 19 (March): 121–24.

Reid, I., et al. 1993. Effect of calcium supplementation on bone loss in postmenopausal women. *New England Journal of Medicine* 328:460–64.

Rejeski, W., et al. 1992. Acute exercise: Buffering psychosocial stress responses in women. *Health Psychology* 11:355–62.

Rossignol, A., and H. Bonnlander. 1990. Caffeine-containing beverages, total fluid consumption, and premenstrual syndrome. *American Journal of Public Health* 80:1105–10.

Seeman, E., et al. 1992. Osteoporosis in anorexia nervosa: The influence of peak bone density, bone loss, oral contraceptive use, and exercise. *Journal of Bone Mineral Research* 7:1467–74.

Steege, J., and J. Blumenthal. 1993. The effects of aerobic exercise on premenstrual symptoms in middle-aged women: A preliminary study. *Journal of Psychsomatic Research* 37:127–33.

Sundgot-Borgen, J. 1994. Risk and trigger factors for the development of eating disorders in female elite athletes. *Medicine and Science in Sports and Exercise* 26:414–19.

Telch, C., and W. Agras. 1993. The effects of a very low calorie diet on binge eating. *Behavior Therapy* 24:177–93.

Touyz, S., et al. 1993. Anorexia nervosa in males: A report of 12 cases. *Australia and New Zealand Journal of Psychiatry* 27:512–17.

Wolfe, L., et al. 1994. Effects of pregnancy and chronic exercise on respiratory responses to graded exercise. *Journal of Applied Physiology* 76:1928–36.

Wurtman, J., et al. 1989. Effect of nutrient intake on premenstrual depression. *American Journal of Obstetrics and Gynecology* 161:1228–34.

Yuk, V., et al. 1990. Towards a definition of PMS: A factor analytic evaluation of premenstrual change in non-complaining women. *Journal of Psychosomatic Research* 34:439–46.

11
▼▼▼

HEALTHFUL AGING: REDUCING THE RISK OF CHRONIC HEALTH PROBLEMS

Key Terms

angina
arrhythmia
arteriosclerosis
arthritis
atherosclerosis
blood pressure
cancer
cerebral vascular accident
   (CVA)

chronic disease
claudication
contributory risk factors
coronary artery disease (CAD)
coronary heart disease (CHD)
coronary occlusion
coronary thrombosis
diabetes mellitus
high blood pressure

hypertension
insulin
insulin reaction
ischemia
life expectancy
life span
low back pain syndrome
lumbar lordosis
major risk factors

myocardial infarct
neoplasm
osteoarthritis
peripheral vascular disease
   (PVD)
plaque
rheumatoid arthritis
stroke

Key Concepts

■ Health benefits will be provided no matter in what stage of life the Positive Health Life-style is initiated, but for optimal results, the earlier in life it is started, the better.

■ Although the average life span in the United States should be about eighty-five years, it is actually only about seventy-five years; the average death is ten years premature.

■ Most premature deaths in the United States today are due to chronic diseases (such as coronary heart disease), many of which are preventable to some degree by development of a Positive Health Life-style early in life.

■ Major risk factors associated with the development of coronary heart disease are high blood pressure, high blood lipids, and cigarette smoking. Heredity, obesity, diabetes, stressful life-style, improper diet, and lack of physical activity are some of the contributory risk factors.

■ High blood pressure (hypertension) is a major disease afflicting nearly one out of every five Americans, but because it displays no consistent obvious symptoms, it often remains undetected; blood pressure should be checked regularly.

■ A stroke may be caused by diseased blood vessels in the brain. The condition is associated with the same risk factors as coronary heart disease and high blood pressure.

■ Peripheral vascular disease is arteriosclerosis in blood vessels other than those of the heart or brain.

■ Obesity is one of the major health problems in the United States. Although it is simply defined as an excess storage of Calories, many different factors may cause the caloric imbalance.

■ Diabetes, a major disease in the United States, is a condition in which the body cannot properly metabolize carbohydrates; diet, exercise, and weight control may be useful preventive and treatment methods.

■ Cancer is the second leading cause of death in the United States and is projected to be the leading cause by the year 2000, but a healthy life-style may help prevent its development.

■ The keys to prevent low back problems are to avoid positions or movements that may subject the back to injury, to increase flexibility of the muscles in the low back region, and to increase strength of the abdominal musculature.

■ Osteoporosis (softening of the bone) is usually a disease of older adults, but preventive measures should be initiated in young adulthood.

■ Arthritis is a disease of the cartilage in the joints and, although the cause and cure are not known, the severity of its effects may be lessened by a proper exercise program.

■ A Positive Health Life-style may help prevent and treat many of the major chronic diseases found in the United States today.

INTRODUCTION

As we get older, there are certain ages often used as markers for entrance into a new sphere of life, such as thirteen as a beginning teenager, twenty-one for entrance into adulthood, and forty for the beginning of middle age. As noted in chapter 1, age is a relative term, but, nevertheless, we often think of the growth and development process throughout life in terms of "ages" or certain periods of life defined by our age. For example, one classification system views our development in seven ages: infancy (under two), childhood (two to twelve), adolescence or teen years (thirteen to nineteen), young adulthood (twenty to forty), middle age (forty to sixty), the senior years (sixty to eighty), and the old-age years (over eighty). The principles underlying the development of a Positive Health Life-style are basically the same throughout all seven of these age categories, and benefits of adopting various components of such a life-style may accrue at any age.

Ideally, the development of a Positive Health Life-style should begin as early in life as possible. Unfortunately, this does not appear to be the case in the United States, since many of our young children and adolescents are in poor physical condition. Results of several national surveys, including the National Children and Youth Fitness Study II, have revealed that our children have been getting fatter over the past twenty years, which possibly may be linked to the widespread use of television and other modes of physical inactivity by our youth. Moreover, Dr. Bernard Gutin recently noted that many children, even five- and six-year olds, have several coronary heart-disease risk factors such as low fitness levels, obesity, and elevated blood pressure. On the other hand, proper education programs stressing exercise and nutrition can significantly increase children's levels of physical activity and help them adopt healthier dietary practices. Aerobic exercise programs for children and adolescents should be fun oriented. Hopefully, the emphasis on school-based fitness programs by several national organizations, such as the American Alliance for Health, Physical Education, Recreation, and Dance and the President's Council on Physical Fitness and Sports will help reverse the trend toward poorer fitness and health in our youth.

As a college student, you are most likely at the age of young adulthood, but some of you may be middle aged or older. Hopefully, at this point in the text, you have learned some of the values, both immediate and long-term, of the various components of a Positive Health Life-style and have already incorporated some of them into your life. Immediate benefits, such as an improvement in fitness, a change in physical appearance, a reduction of stress, and an improved psychological well-being may accrue in a short period of time, but to maximize the long-range health benefits you may achieve, such a life-style needs to be lifelong. Now, some of your major concerns for the near future may involve beginning your career, becoming successful in it, and starting a family, all of which will increase your time commitment. Unfortunately, many young physically active individuals often become less active as exercise, which takes time, assumes a lower priority in comparison to work and family, particularly to work. Recent research has indicated that there is an increasing number of individuals who are becoming workaholics, devoting excessive time to work-related responsibilities. They become too busy to exercise. Dietary practices may also change with increased consumption of processed foods, high-Calorie meals on the

run, and greater quantities of alcohol. If you experience such changes, physical inactivity and poor nutrition will reverse the gains you have made and begin to erode your health. Once you have developed a Positive Health Life-style, stay with it. Some guidelines will be presented in chapter 12. A relevant phrase that has been around for years is that nothing is as important as your health. This is a broad statement, of course, but your health status will impact on your job and your family life. The health benefits of a Positive Health Life-style should make you more effective in the other important aspects of your life. There is nothing wrong with devoting considerable energy to becoming successful in your profession, for such success may be a key to enhanced self-esteem and a better life, but not when it impacts negatively on your health. Learn to balance your work, family and social life, and leisure.

Although the health benefits of a Positive Health Life-style are important at all ages, the older you are, the more significant these benefits are to your overall health. Unfortunately, according to C. Carson Conrad, former director of the President's Council on Physical Fitness and Sports, many older Americans are inactive because they have relatively poor knowledge and attitudes about exercise. Moreover, Ausman and Russell indicated that dietary surveys and biochemical tests suggest many of the elderly may have inadequate dietary intakes of some key nutrients, such as calcium and iron. It is important to note that you are never too old to develop a Positive Health Life-style. Research has shown that proper exercise and nutrition programs, even when implemented as late in life as the 60s and 70s, even in the 90s, can elicit physical benefits such as improved cardiovascular functioning, increased muscular strength, decreased blood pressure, and decreased body fat, as well as the psychological benefits of decreased tension, depression, fatigue, and confusion and increased vigor, self-esteem, and independence. A Positive Health Life-style prevents or helps slow the rate of decline of a wide variety of physical and psychological changes that normally occur with aging. This improvement in functional well-being is becoming increasingly important to our country, because nearly one in six Americans will be age sixty-five or over soon after the turn of the century as the "baby boomers" lead to the graying of America.

No matter what your age, a Positive Health Life-style will improve the quality of your life. It may also increase the quantity of your life as well. Some examples have already been presented in earlier chapters, such as smoking cessation to prevent chronic lung diseases, moderation in alcohol consumption to reduce fatal accidents, and safe-sex practices to prevent AIDS. In this chapter, we shall discuss the concept of aging and longevity and focus upon the prevention of chronic diseases, primarily those highlighted in the Public Health Service report *Healthy People 2000: National Health Promotion and Disease Prevention Objectives,* that may decrease the quality and quantity of life .

Aging and Longevity

In chapter 1, we introduced the concept of functional and chronological aging and noted that although we all age chronologically at the same rate, our heredity and life-styles dictate the rate at which we age functionally. It is our functional age that may have significant implications for our

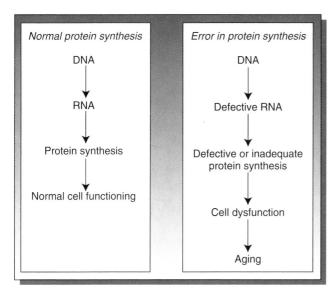

Figure 11.1 *Genetic error theory of aging. The genetic error theory of aging proposes that defective DNA and RNA produce a defective or inadequate amount of protein within a particular cell and thus contribute to the aging of that cell and the related body tissues.*

health, but we still cannot escape some of the gradual changes associated with chronological aging, such as graying hair or lessened visual acuity.

Theories of Aging

Why do we age? Aging is a very complex process that results from the interaction of a wide variety of factors. A number of different theories have been advanced in attempts to explain why we grow older and why aging produces its catabolic effects on the body. The most prominent theories center around genetic control. One genetic theory suggests that aging is an inherited factor—that a genetic clock or tape is present at conception, and cell function ceases when that clock or tape runs out. The second genetic theory (fig. 11.1) is that aging results when the genes that control the synthesis of every cell constituent (primarily proteins) in the body begin to make random errors that eventually disrupt normal cellular functioning. Every cell in the body has a genetic control mechanism designed to make that cell perform its major function—be it to form muscle proteins, produce an enzyme that may be used in energy-producing processes, or manufacture a hormone such as insulin. In simple terms, the genetic material, DNA, activates several types of RNA that control these cellular functions. Thus, the cumulative effect of random errors eventually disrupts this process and may result in cellular dysfunction. Fries and Crapo, in their book on the aging process, *Vitality and Aging,* suggest that the second theory has the most supporting evidence. One possibility is a decreased production of human growth hormone (HGH). Recent research has shown that HGH supplementation to men over age sixty with low levels of HGH reversed some of the effects of aging, effecting a decrease in body fat and an increase in lean body mass and bone mass. Although the primary control of aging in a given individual appears to be genetic, environmental factors such as

nutrition may modify the aging process. For example, excess production of free radicals (highly reactive atoms) in the body cells, possibly due to a vitamin deficiency or excessive alcohol intake, may interfere with normal DNA activity.

Longevity

How long can you expect to live? According to Fries and Crapo, the **life span** (the biological limit to the length of life) of humans has been constant for at least 100,000 years, and no change is anticipated in the near future. Researchers have recently noted that even if we found a cure for major fatal diseases, such as heart disease and cancer, the average life span would be about eighty-five years; that is, the average American could expect to live to be about eighty-five, although some would live fewer or more years. Fries and Crapo see a maximal life span of one hundred, with the possibility of some individuals passing that barrier. However, life span must be differentiated from life expectancy. **Life expectancy** represents the number of years of life expected for a given individual or population. Life expectancy and life span do not necessarily coincide. For example, although the average lifespan may be eighty-five, the average life expectancy in the United States is about seventy-five, being several years lower for men and several years higher for women. Thus, on the average, Americans are not attaining their full potential life span. Why?

Premature Death

Life expectancy has increased tremendously over the course of this century. For example, in the year 1900 the average individual died 38 years prematurely, and only about 50 percent of the population lived to age sixty. In more recent years, the average person dies approximately ten years prematurely, with nearly 85 percent of the population living to age sixty. Most of this increase in life expectancy has not resulted from extension of the natural life span, but rather from the elimination of premature death from such infectious diseases as tuberculosis, diphtheria, influenza, kidney disease, and diseases of early infancy that were epidemic in the first half of the century.

Today the most common cause of premature death or disability is **chronic disease** (diseases that develop over a long period of time), such as atherosclerosis and other arterial diseases, cancer, diabetes, chronic obstructive pulmonary disease, cirrhosis, arthritis, and osteoporosis. These conditions account for over 80 percent of all premature deaths and over 90 percent of all disabilities. Although in more recent years some of the increases in life expectancy may be attributed to the decreased incidence rate of some chronic diseases, such as heart disease, the magnitude of the problem is still rather formidable. Accidental deaths have also increased to the point where they, too, are a major cause of premature death, particularly in teenagers and young adults. Additionally, the number of deaths attributed to AIDS is increasing in the young, and it poses a major risk for the future.

Other than premature deaths in the young, most premature deaths are concentrated in the years over sixty and are due to the chronic diseases noted previously. Although we may

Table 11.1 Developmental Stages of Several Chronic Diseases

Age	Stage	Atherosclerosis	Diabetes	Cirrhosis
20 or younger	Start	Elevated cholesterol	Obesity	Drinker
30	Discernable	Small plaques in arteries	Abnormal glucose tolerance	Fatty liver
40	Subclinical	Larger plaques in arteries	Elevated blood glucose	Enlarged liver
50	Threshold	Leg pain on exercise	Sugar in urine	Bleeding in upper intestines
60	Severe	Pain in chest	Drug requirement	Fluid accumulated in abdomen
70	End	Stroke, heart attack	Blindness, nerve damage	Hepatic coma

Source: From Vitality and Aging, *by J. Fries and L. Crapo. Copyright © 1981 by W. H. Freeman and Company. All rights reserved.*

think of these as diseases of old age, their beginnings may start at age twenty or even as early as ages seven or eight. Table 11.1 represents some possible progressions of several of the chronic diseases prevalent in American society today.

If you want to live to obtain the greatest quantity of life then your greatest opportunity is to reduce the possibility of contracting those chronic diseases that are somewhat preventable. Along with increased quantity of life, we would all like increased quality as well—to be full of vim, vigor, and vitality throughout our lives, including old age, and Perls has reported that many in their eighties, nineties, and older are often healthier and more robust than those 20 years younger. Many of the chronic diseases have their beginnings in the early phases of life. Therefore, preventive measures should be initiated early in order to help counteract the disabling effects or premature death caused by such diseases. The earlier a healthy life-style is developed, the better, but life-style modification may have some positive benefits at almost any age. The remainder of this chapter deals with this concept, the development of a life-style conducive to maximizing both the quantity and quality of life by preventing chronic health problems.

Chronic Health Problems

The average American's life expectancy could be increased appreciably—by more than 10 years—if accidental deaths and several major chronic diseases could be reduced. Moreover, the quality of life could also be improved if we could minimize or eliminate the disabling mental and physical effects of these chronic diseases.

Many of the chronic diseases that limit both the quantity and quality of life begin to develop in our early years and may be associated with various risk factors in our particular life-styles. However, various life-style changes could convey certain health benefits. For example, aerobic exercise may help decrease high blood pressure, a low-fat diet may help reduce atherosclerosis, and smoking cessation will improve the health of your lungs. Although many of these life-style changes exert their beneficial effects independently, the benefits are magnified significantly when multiple Positive Health Life-style changes are adopted. Thus, while aerobic exercise, proper nutrition, and smoking cessation may independently reduce the risk of the major chronic disease—coronary heart disease—their collective effect is even greater.

Table 11.2 Major Health Problems That May Be Prevented or Ameliorated by a Positive Health Life-style

Cardiovascular Diseases
Coronary heart disease
Hypertension—high blood pressure
Stroke
Peripheral vascular disease

Metabolic Disorders
Obesity
Diabetes
Cancer

Musculoskeletal Problems
Low back pain
Osteoporosis
Arthritis

The purpose of the remainder of this chapter is to discuss the etiology, or developmental process, of certain chronic diseases and how identifiable risk factors may contribute to it. The focus will be on the various components of a Positive Health Life-style that, when combined, pose the greatest potential for reducing or eliminating these risk factors. Since many of the chronic diseases are interrelated, such as obesity, diabetes, and coronary heart disease, what may be used to prevent or treat one condition may help in the prevention or treatment of others.

The major chronic diseases with which we are concerned may be grouped under three headings. First, cardiovascular (CV) diseases disrupt normal functioning of the heart and blood vessels. The most prevalent disease is coronary heart disease (CHD). Second, although metabolic disorders are numerous, we are concerned primarily with obesity (an imbalance in energy metabolism), diabetes (a disturbance of carbohydrate metabolism), and cancer (an unregulated, disorganized cell growth). And, third, musculoskeletal problems, such as low back pain or arthritis, although not usually life-threatening, may be a source of constant discomfort, impairing the quality of life. An overview of some of the major health problems that may be prevented or ameliorated by a Positive Health Life-style is presented in table 11.2. The etiology of obesity was presented in some detail in chapter 7, so the discussion is somewhat limited in this chapter. Moreover, chronic obstructive pulmonary disease, such as emphysema, covered in chapter 9, will not be addressed in this chapter.

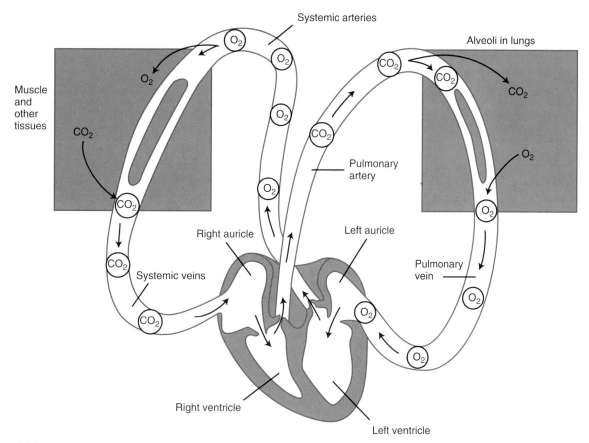

Figure 11.2 *The cardiovascular-respiratory systems. The cardiovascular and respiratory systems function to deliver oxygen (O_2) to all body cells and remove carbon dioxide (CO_2), a metabolic waste product. Oxygen is taken into the lungs from the atmospheric air, and it is diffused into the blood in the alveoli (small air sacs). This oxygenated blood travels to the left side of the heart, where it is eventually pumped to the body tissues (such as muscle tissue) via the arterial blood vessels. The tissues use oxygen for their energy needs, producing carbon dioxide in the process. The carbon dioxide is then returned in the blood to the right side of the heart, where the blood is pumped to the lungs, and the carbon dioxide is expelled from the body.*

Cardiovascular Diseases

Oxygen is the element most vital to life. The most important function of the cardiovascular and respiratory systems is to maintain a constant supply of oxygen to all body tissues according to their needs. Figure 11.2 depicts the interrelationships between the cardiovascular and respiratory systems relative to gaseous exchange of oxygen (O_2) and carbon dioxide (CO_2).

The respiratory system takes in oxygen from the atmospheric air and conveys it to the alveoli (small air sacs in the lungs surrounded by a capillary network). In the alveoli, oxygen is picked up and dissolved in the blood, and carbon dioxide is eliminated from the blood. The bronchi and bronchioli are air pathways that may cause respiratory distress if they become constricted or narrowed for any reason.

The cardiovascular system serves as a plumbing system, functioning to transport the oxygen in the blood throughout the body. The heart serves as a muscular pump to provide the force or pressure for ejecting the blood into the blood vessels, which serve as channels to transport the blood to all living body cells. There are several different types of blood vessels in the body. The major classifications include arteries, capillaries, and veins. The arteries transport blood away from the heart; the capillaries permeate the various tissues and release oxygen and other nutrients to the cells; the veins transport blood back to the heart.

The major health problems associated with the cardiovascular system arise in the blood vessels, primarily the arteries, and, more specifically, the arteries in the heart. The heart is a large muscle with four blood-filled chambers, but the heart itself cannot extract much oxygen directly from the blood in its chambers. Like other organs in the body, it has its own internal network of arteries, capillaries, and veins. The arteries that supply blood to the heart muscle are called coronary arteries—mainly the left coronary, right coronary, and circumflex (fig. 11.3). In order to function efficiently, the coronary arteries and all other arteries throughout the body must maintain a normal interior diameter. When the normal opening of an artery is narrowed or closed, cardiovascular problems develop.

Nearly one out of every two deaths in the United States is due to diseases of the heart and blood vessels. Each year, approximately one million Americans die from some form of cardiovascular disease, including coronary heart disease, stroke, hypertensive disease, rheumatic heart disease, and congenital heart disease.

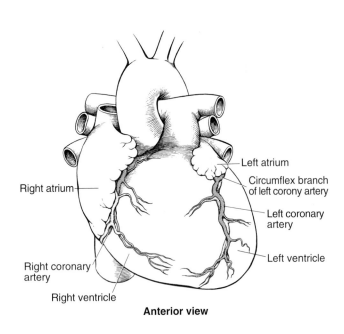

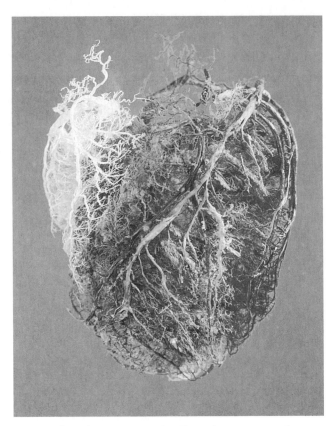

Figure 11.3 *The coronary arteries. The heart muscle itself receives its blood supply from the coronary arteries. The main coronary arteries are the left coronary artery, one of its branches named the* circumflex, *and the right coronary artery. Atherosclerosis of these arteries leads to coronary heart disease.*

Coronary Heart Disease (CHD)

Coronary heart disease is the major disease of the cardiovascular system; of the million deaths noted previously, it is responsible for over half. Although the total percentage of deaths due to coronary heart disease has been declining in recent years, it is still an epidemic and the number one cause of death among Americans, both males and females. Thus, we will look at its etiology and prevention in detail.

Coronary heart disease (CHD) is also known as **coronary artery disease (CAD)** because obstruction of the blood flow in the coronary arteries is responsible for the pathological effects of the disease. The major manifestation of CHD is a heart attack, which results from a sudden stoppage of blood flow to parts of the heart muscle. A decreased blood supply, known as **ischemia,** will deprive the heart of needed oxygen. In some individuals, ischemia results in **angina,** a sharp pain in the chest, jaw, or along the inside of the arm indicative of a mild heart attack. Other terms often associated with a heart attack include **coronary thrombosis,** a blockage of a blood vessel by a clot (thrombus), **coronary occlusion,** which simply means blockage, and **myocardial infarct,** death of heart cells that do not get enough oxygen due to the blocked coronary artery. The major cause of the blocked arteries is atherosclerosis.

Arteriosclerosis

Arteriosclerosis is a term applied to a number of different pathological conditions wherein the arterial walls thicken and lose their elasticity. It is often defined as hardening of the arteries. **Atherosclerosis,** one form of arteriosclerosis, is characterized by deposits of fat, cholesterol (modified or oxidized LDL cholesterol), macrophages (white blood cells that oxidize LDL cholesterol), foam cells (formed from the oxidation of LDL cholesterol), cellular debris, calcium, and fibrin on the inner linings of the arterial wall. These deposits, known as **plaque,** result in a narrowing of the blood channel, making it easier for blood clots to form and eventually resulting in complete blockage of blood flow to vital tissues such as the heart or the brain. Figure 11.4 illustrates the gradual, progressive narrowing of the arterial channel. Figure 11.5 presents a schematic of the content of arterial plaque. Individuals with a genetic predisposition to atherosclerosis may have arteries that form lesions more readily than individuals without such a hereditarial susceptibility.

Atherosclerosis is a slow, progressive disease that begins in childhood and usually manifests itself later in life. Severe coronary atherosclerosis is the cause of almost all heart attacks. Because of its prevalence in industrialized society, scientists throughout the world have been conducting intensive research efforts in attempts to identify the cause or causes of

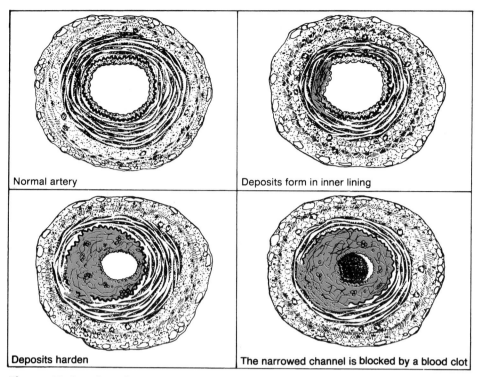

Figure 11.4 *Atherosclerosis. The developmental process of atherosclerosis is illustrated. Deposits of cholesterol, fat, and other debris accumulate in the inner lining of the artery, leading to a decrease or cessation of blood flow to the tissues. Atherosclerosis in the heart is a major cause of coronary heart disease.*

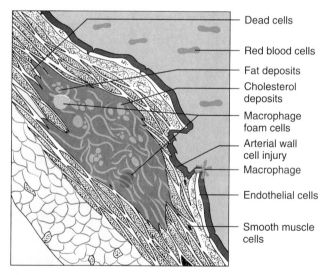

- Dead cells
- Red blood cells
- Fat deposits
- Cholesterol deposits
- Macrophage foam cells
- Arterial wall cell injury
- Macrophage
- Endothelial cells
- Smooth muscle cells

Figure 11.5 *An enlargement of atherosclerotic plaque. Cholesterol, fats, dead cells, and other debris collect within or beneath the inner lining of an artery. There is often an ulceration (opening) in the inner layer of the arterial wall through which the cholesterol and other plaque constituents enter.*

atherosclerosis and CHD. Although the actual cause has not yet been completely identified, considerable evidence has accumulated to help identify those risk factors that may predispose an individual to atherosclerosis and CHD.

Risk Factors

Atherosclerotic coronary heart disease is a complex, multifactorial disease, that is, it has many causes, and research into its etiology has utilized several approaches. One approach involves epidemiological techniques whereby certain populations of people are studied in order to isolate risk factors. For example, a number of epidemiological studies have compared physically active and inactive individuals and found that physical activity may help to prevent the development of CHD. Other research techniques involve experimental studies with both animals and humans and are designed to determine the effect of some factor such as a high-cholesterol diet or jogging on the development of atherosclerosis or the level of blood cholesterol. The results of epidemiological and experimental research have helped document a number of the risk factors associated with CHD. As noted in figure 11.6, this research has also shown that the greater the number and severity of risk factors present, the greater is the predisposition to CHD. Many of these risk factors are presented in Laboratory Inventory 1.1 The Health Life-style Assessment Inventory. You may also complete Laboratory Inventory 11.1, RISKO: A Heart Hazard Appraisal by the American Heart Association.

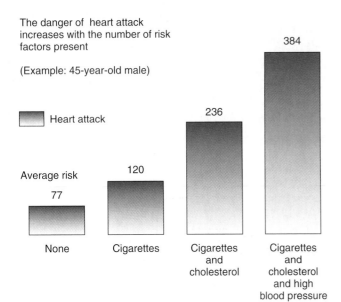

The danger of heart attack increases with the number of risk factors present

(Example: 45-year-old male)

■ Heart attack

Average risk

None — 77
Cigarettes — 120
Cigarettes and cholesterol — 236
Cigarettes and cholesterol and high blood pressure — 384

Figure 11.6 *Risk factors in coronary heart disease. The danger of developing coronary heart disease and experiencing a heart attack increases with the number of risk factors. The three major risk factors are cigarette smoking, high blood serum cholesterol levels, and high blood pressure.*

Table 11.3 Risk Factors Associated with Coronary Heart Disease

Risk Factors	Classification	Positive Health Life-style Modification
*Serum lipid profile Total cholesterol > 240 mg/dL LDL > 160 mg/dL HDL < 35 mg/dL	Major	Proper nutrition; aerobic exercise
*High blood pressure (Hypertension)	Major	Proper nutrition; aerobic exercise
*Smoking	Major	Stop smoking
**ECG abnormalities	Major	Proper nutrition; aerobic exercise
**Obesity	Major	Low-Calorie diet, aerobic exercise
*Diabetes	Major	Proper nutrition; weight loss; aerobic exercise
Stressful life-style	Contributory	Stress management
Dietary intake	Contributory	Proper nutrition
**Sedentary life-style	Contributory	Aerobic exercise
Oral contraceptives	Contributory	Alternative methods of birth control
*Family history	Major	Not modifiable
*Gender; age Male > 45 Female > 55	Major	Not modifiable
Race	Contributory	Not modifiable

*Major risk factors: National Cholesterol Education Program

**May be classified as major risk factor by other professional health organizations

Table 11.3 highlights risk factors that have been identified from epidemiological or experimental studies. **Major risk factors** are those directly related to the development of CHD or atherosclerosis, while **contributory risk factors** may predispose an individual to one of the major risk factors. Differences of opinion exist among health professionals as to the classification of a risk factor as major or contributory. Table 11.3 is based upon a synthesis of reports from various health organizations, including the most recent risk factor classification in the National Cholesterol Education Program. Although several of these risk factors may not be changed, such as family history, gender, and race, many may be modified by adopting a Positive Health Life-style. Let us look briefly at each risk factor and how it is associated with CHD.

Serum Lipid Profile

In atherosclerosis, the plaque that develops in the arterial walls is composed partly of fats and cholesterol. Hence, high levels of blood lipids (triglycerides and cholesterol) are associated with increased levels of plaque formation. As detailed in chapter 6, most triglycerides and cholesterol are carried in the blood as lipoproteins, small capsules of triglycerides, cholesterol, phospholipids (another lipid substance), and protein. The protein acts as a carrier for these lipids, hence the name lipoproteins. Refer back to pages 110–112 and figure 6.7 for a review of lipoprotein composition.

Although high levels of triglycerides are linked to the development of atherosclerosis, the major villain appears to be cholesterol. Some investigators consider hypercholesteremia to be the most important risk factor for development of atherosclerosis. Total cholesterol, expressed in milligrams per 100 milliliters of blood, is important, and as noted in chapter 6, a level below 200 is considered to be desirable, between 200 to 239 is borderline-high, and above 240 is high. However, you should be aware that there is a rather large standard error of measurement involved in some tests of total cholesterol, being on the order of 30 milligrams. What this means is that if your blood cholesterol is reported as 220 (borderline-high), it may be possible that you actually have a cholesterol level of 190 (desirable) or 250 (high) if you vary, respectively, one standard error below or above your actual measurement of 220. For this reason, it may be a good idea to have a second measurement of total cholesterol completed if you are concerned with your total cholesterol level.

The form by which cholesterol is transported in your blood may also be related to the development of atherosclerosis. In general, high levels of low density lipoproteins (LDL) are associated with atherosclerosis. A current theory suggests LDL and other related lipoproteins, such as dense LDL and an abnormal lipoprotein, lipoprotein (a), may be more prone to oxidation by macrophages at an injured site in the arterial epithelium leading to an influx into the cell wall and the formation of plaque. The presence of free oxygen radicals has been suggested to accelerate this process. Levels of LDL less than 130 milligrams per deciliter (100 milliliters) are desirable, whereas levels greater than 160 mg/dL indicate high risk.

Conversely, high levels of high density lipoproteins (HDL), particularly the subfraction HDL_2 and HDL with apoprotein A-I and other apoprotein A subdivisions, appear to be protective against the development of atherosclerosis. Research suggests that HDL interacts with the arterial epithelium, acting as a scavenger by picking up cholesterol from the arterial wall and transporting it to the liver for removal from the body, known as reverse cholesterol transport. HDL may also inhibit LDL oxidation and platelet aggregation, thus helping retard the development of plaque and clots. An HDL level below 35 mg/dL is considered a risk factor, whereas a level greater than 60 mg/dL leads to increased protection. As a matter of fact, the National Cholesterol Education Program indicates you can deduct one risk factor if your HDL level is greater than 60 mg/dL.

Additionally, although triglycerides are not generally recognized as an independent risk factor for CHD, high serum triglyceride levels also increase the risk for arteriosclerosis because they are often associated with increased levels of LDL and decreased levels of HDL. Levels below 200 mg/dL are desirable, while levels above 400 mg/dL represent an increased risk.

If your total blood cholesterol is borderline or high, a determination of the LDL and HDL levels may be desirable for they provide additional information relative to your risk. Based on epidemiological data, several ratios have been developed to assess risk of CHD, with the lower the ratio, the lower the risk.

One common comparison is the ratio of total cholesterol (TC) to the HDL level, or TC/HDL. A ratio of about 4.5:1.0 is associated with an average risk for CHD. For example, an individual with a total cholesterol of 200 and an HDL of 60 would have a ratio of 3.3:1.0 (200/60), or a lower risk, while someone with the same total cholesterol but an HDL of 20 would have a much higher risk with a ratio of 10:1 (200/20).

Another comparison is the ratio of LDL to HDL or LDL/HDL. An LDL to HDL ratio of about 3.5:1.0 is considered to be an average risk for CHD. Thus, a ratio of 140/60, or 2.3:1.0, would be a much lower risk than 140/20, or 7:1.

Other medical laboratory tests are available and may be used to evaluate the causes of a poor lipid profile.

High blood triglyceride and cholesterol levels are often treated with drug therapy, particularly in those with genetic causes, but may also be modified favorably by diet and exercise. In many individuals, diet and exercise may be the first form of medical treatment. Diet may be useful to effectively decrease total cholesterol and LDL, whereas exercise may increase HDL, including A-1 and the HDL_2 subfraction, and decrease serum triglycerides.

It should be noted that there has been some recent concern relative to very low levels of total serum cholesterol, those below 160mg/dL, because they have been associated with increased mortality from digestive diseases and traumatic death, such as suicide, homicide, accidental death, hemorrhagic stroke, and alcohol dependence syndrome. There

may be some cause and effect relationships, because low serum cholesterol may lead to inadequate amounts of serotonin, a neurotransmitter in the brain. Decreased serotonin may lead to depression or aggressive behavior, which may be related to traumatic deaths. Low serum cholesterol may also prolong bleeding time, leading to prolonged hemorrhage. However, several recent reviews by the Consumers Union and Harris questioned a cause and effect relationship, suggesting that low serum cholesterol is the result of illness, not the cause of it. As is well known, alcoholism may affect serum cholesterol levels and is associated with a variety of digestive disorders, suicide, homicide, and accidental death. Harris concluded that low serum cholesterol is not associated with increased mortality in individuals who are classified as healthy. If you are young and healthy, the current advice is not to worry about low serum cholesterol. Although this issue is still being debated, most health professionals suggest it is still beneficial to reduce serum cholesterol to 200 mg/dL or below for health benefits relative to prevention of CHD. For individuals who have a serum cholesterol between 160–199 mg/dL, aggressive techniques to reduce it even further may not be advisable, for the available data do not support an additional protective effect against CHD with levels lower than 160 mg/dL. Additionally, individuals with serum cholesterol levels lower than 160 mg/dL should not attempt to raise it higher, for example by eating high fat diets.

High Blood Pressure

Hypertension, or high blood pressure, is a disease of some magnitude and is discussed in more detail later in this chapter. For now, however, we may note that it is one of the major risk factors associated with CHD and stroke.

Smoking

The degree of CHD risk from cigarette smoking is affected by the number of cigarettes smoked daily (whether or not the smoke is inhaled) and the number of years of smoking. As noted in chapter 9, smoking stresses the cardiovascular system in several ways. Nicotine, a drug present in cigarette smoke, stimulates adrenalin release in the body, which elevates blood pressure by constricting blood vessels and increasing the heart rate. Also, carbon monoxide in the smoke displaces oxygen from hemoglobin and, thus, increases the work load of the heart in delivering oxygen to the tissues. Moreover, certain hydrocarbons in cigarette smoke may act as mutagens (substances that cause a change or transformation) on the cells in the arterial walls, possibly accelerating the atherosclerotic process. However, the American Heart Association has noted that the rate of fatal heart disease in cigarette smokers who stop smoking is nearly as low as for those people who have never smoked.

ECG Abnormalities

The ECG, or electrocardiogram, is a record of the electrical activity generated in the heart. An abnormal pattern or irregular heartbeat (**arrhythmia**) may be indicative of insufficient blood flow and oxygen to part of the heart muscle. In many cases, resting ECGs may not detect these abnormalities, but exercise stress tests, as discussed in chapter 2, usually can detect the presence of CHD. In most cases, an abnormal ECG response is indicative of CHD. Other types of tests may then be conducted to determine the severity of the disease. A prescribed exercise program may help alleviate some ECG abnormalities. Also, although caffeine is generally regarded to be a safe drug, some individuals appear to be susceptible to its effects and experience cardiac arrhythmias, or irregular heartbeats. Such individuals should consult their physicians relative to the use of caffeine in their diet.

Obesity

Excess body fat, particularly when deposited in the abdominal region, predisposes individuals toward high blood pressure and high blood lipid levels, both major risk factors. Obesity is also a factor in the development of adult-onset diabetes, another contributory risk factor. The causes of obesity are complex and have been reviewed in chapter 7, but a low-Calorie diet and aerobic exercise are effective ways to lose excess weight for most individuals.

Diabetes

Individuals with diabetes have an increased risk of CHD and stroke. In essence, the high levels of glucose in the blood of diabetics may damage some of the small blood vessels in the heart or brain. Impaired function of insulin may also interfere with lipid metabolism, leading to hyperlipidemia. Diabetes can be controlled with proper medication, diet, weight reduction, and exercise. An expanded discussion of diabetes is presented later in this chapter.

Stressful Life-Style

Psychological stress is prevalent in today's modern society and may be a factor involved in the development of CHD. As noted in chapter 8, hostility, anger, or constant stress may elicit various hormonal responses in the body, leading to symptoms such as elevated blood pressure or elevated blood lipids, that may predispose an individual to CHD. Stressful situations in life such as job strain should be identified, and actions should be taken to eliminate them whenever possible. The stress-management techniques discussed in chapter 8 may be helpful.

Dietary Intake

A number of different types of foods have been associated with CHD because they increase blood lipid levels or contribute to the development of high blood pressure. Excessive intake of total fat, saturated fat, cholesterol, refined sugars, and alcohol has been associated with high blood lipid levels, whereas excess salt intake may predispose susceptible individuals to high blood pressure. Excessive caloric intake may also contribute to obesity.

Sedentary Life-Style

Steven Blair, a renowned epidemiologist regarding the relationship of exercise to chronic diseases, noted that although some uncertainty remains, it is reasonable to conclude that a low level of physical activity is one of the more important causes of CHD. Carl Casperson, an epidemiologist with the Centers for Disease Control, noted that physical inactivity is as strong a risk factor for CHD as high blood pressure, high blood lipids, and cigarette smoking. In general, people who are physically active experience a lower incidence of heart attacks and clinical symptoms such as chest pain and abnormal ECGs. Also, people who do have heart attacks have a greater survival rate if they have been physically active. The best type of exercise involves aerobic activities that engage the cardiovascular system.

Oral Contraceptives

The use of oral contraceptives may aggravate several of the other risk factors for atherosclerosis, such as an increase in blood pressure, abnormal changes in blood lipids, and the formation of small clots in the arteries or veins, this latter effect being greatly increased in women who also smoke.

Family History

Although there is little evidence to indicate that either CHD or the atherosclerotic process is directly inherited through the genes, there does appear to be a tendency for CHD to run in certain families. This familial tendency may be related to the fact that other risk factors such as high blood lipid levels, high blood pressure, diabetes, and obesity tend to be familial also. If your family has a history of CHD before age sixty, you may be exposed to this risk factor.

Gender

Young females experience fewer heart attacks than males. This protection against CHD may be attributed to estrogen, a female sex hormone that may raise blood levels of HDL-cholesterol. Due to hormonal changes, some of this protection decreases after menopause, and the rate of CHD among women increases sharply. However, the rate of CHD never reaches that of men.

Age

As we get older, our chances of developing CHD increase. Most fatalities from CHD occur after age sixty-five, yet one out of every four deaths does occur under age sixty-five. Increased risks are observed in males after age forty-five and females after age fifty-five.

Race

In the United States, blacks are almost 33 percent more likely to have high blood pressure than are whites. As noted previously, high blood pressure is a major risk factor in CHD. Unfortunately, the cause of this racial tendency toward high blood pressure is not understood at present. Other diseases, such as sickle-cell anemia in blacks, may also be race related.

Positive Health Life-Style

Many of the risk factors associated with CHD may be beneficially affected by the development of a Positive Health Lifestyle. Those that may be modified include high blood pressure, high blood lipid levels, cigarette smoking, obesity, stressful life-style, dietary intake, physical activity, and the use of oral contraceptives.

The risk of CHD decreases when smokers stop their habit. This would appear to be one of the easiest methods to reduce CHD risk. Unfortunately, the smoking habit is so ingrained in some people's life-styles that it is extremely difficult to break. If you don't smoke, don't start! If you do smoke, quit! The guidelines to stop smoking presented in chapter 9 may be helpful. Remembering one thing may help you to quit. Smoking is stupid!

If you use oral contraceptives, it may be wise to have periodic checkups with your physician as to their advisability. If you experience problems, alternative methods of birth control may be used.

Stress-reduction techniques, which have been discussed in detail in chapter 8, provide another mechanism whereby a CHD risk factor may be modified. These techniques may help to counteract some of the adverse effects of a stressful life-style.

Modification of the diet may have a significant impact upon several risk factors. Reduction in the dietary intake of saturated fats, cholesterol, and salt may significantly reduce high blood lipid levels and high blood pressure. A diet low in Calories will help lose excess body fat. An increased intake of complex carbohydrates rich in dietary fiber, both water-soluble and insoluble forms, a balanced, moderate intake of monounsaturated and polyunsaturated fats, and consumption of fish high in omega-3 fish oils may be useful dietary modifications to help prevent atherosclerosis. Niacin supplements may help decrease total and LDL cholesterol while moderate alcohol intake may help increase HDL cholesterol. However, niacin supplements should only be taken under proper medical supervision because of potential liver problems. Individuals who do not drink alcohol should not start for the purpose of reducing the risk of heart disease because of other potential health risks associated with heavy alcohol consumption. The guidelines to healthy eating presented in chapter 6 should be reviewed; diets to prevent obesity are presented in chapter 7.

A properly designed exercise program, primarily aerobic in nature, will remove one risk factor—physical inactivity. William Haskell, an esteemed researcher, and the American Heart Association, in its recent statement on exercise, both noted that regular aerobic physical activity plays a role in both the primary and secondary prevention of CHD. Primary prevention effects of aerobic exercise training include an increased cardiovascular functional capacity and decreased oxygen demand of the heart muscle at any level of physical activity. Aerobic exercise elicits secondary prevention measures as well. Aerobic exercise may help counteract the effects of stress on the body, reduce high blood pressure, help prevent the formation of blood clots, and prevent or reduce obesity and diabetes. Exercise may also beneficially modify the blood lipid profile, decreasing the triglyceride level and increasing the HDL component. When combined with a diet to lose weight, exercise may effectively decrease the LDL component and may help reverse the process of atherosclerosis.

A Positive Health Life-style may not only help to prevent the development of atherosclerosis, but may also lead to regression of coronary artery blockage. In a classic study, Dean Ornish and his colleagues indicated that life-style changes alone helped regress severe coronary atherosclerosis in just one year, and in a recent review, Brown and others noted that the available data support the hypothesis that lowering of serum lipids may lead to regression of atherosclerotic lesions and elicit improved clinical effects.

In summary, there are a variety of life-style changes that may help both men and women in the prevention of atherosclerosis and CHD. The more changes you make, the better your chances.

High Blood Pressure (Hypertension)

Everybody has blood pressure, for without it we would not be able to sustain body metabolism. Simply speaking, **blood pressure** is the force that the blood exerts against the blood vessel walls. Although pressure is present in all types of blood vessels, the arterial blood pressure is the one most commonly measured and most important to our health. Blood pressure is usually measured by a sphygmomanometer, which records the pressure in millimeters of mercury (mmHg). Blood pressure readings are given in two numbers, for example 120/80 mmHg. Systolic blood pressure (the higher number) represents that phase during which the heart is pumping blood through the arterial system when the pressure is greatest against the arterial wall. Increases in the amount of blood being pumped from the heart can increase the systolic blood pressure. The diastolic blood pressure represents that phase when the heart is resting (between beats) and blood is flowing back into it. Two important determinants of blood pressure are the volume of blood in the circulation and the resistance to blood flow, known as peripheral vascular resistance.

High blood pressure, also known as **hypertension** (hyper = high; tension = pressure), is known as a silent disease. The American Heart Association indicates that nearly 60 million Americans have high blood pressure. However, millions do not know they have it because it has no outstanding symptoms. Some general symptoms include headaches, dizziness, and fatigue, but since they can be caused by a multitude of other factors, they may not be recognized as symptoms of high blood pressure. Although a great deal of research has been and is being conducted about the cause of high blood pressure, the exact cause is unknown in about 90 percent of all cases. In these cases, the condition is known as essential hypertension, which cannot be cured, although life-style changes or medications can lower the pressure by reducing the blood volume or decreasing the peripheral vascular resistance. The goal of *Healthy People 2000* is to increase to 90 percent the proportion of people with high blood pressure that are taking actions to reduce it.

The National Research Council has noted that any definition of high blood pressure is arbitrary. Traditionally, physicians have used elevations in diastolic blood pressure as the basis for their diagnosis, but the Joint National Committee on Detection, Evaluation and Treatment of High Blood Pressure (JNCDET) recently released its classification of blood pressure for adults age 18 years and older. It

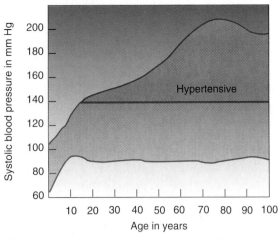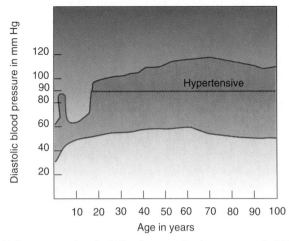

Figure 11.7 *Ranges of systolic and diastolic blood pressures from birth to age one hundred. Blood pressure levels vary among individuals as noted by the wide ranges, particularly as one ages. Systolic hypertension occurs at a pressure of 140 mmHg; diastolic hypertension is rated at 90 mmHg. Note that advancing age increases the probability of hypertension, but even young adults may have high blood pressure.*

Table 11.4	Classification of Blood Pressure for Adults Age 18 Years and Older	
Category	**Systolic (mmHg)**	**Diastolic (mmHg)**
Normal	<130	<85
High Normal	130–139	85–89
Hypertension		
Stage 1 (mild)	140–159	90–99
Stage 2 (moderate)	160–179	100–109
Stage 3 (severe)	180–209	110–119
Stage 4 (very severe)	≥210	≥120

The Fifth Report of the Joint National Committee on Detection, Evaluation, and Treatment of High Blood Pressure, *National Institutes of Health—National Heart, Lung, and Blood Institute*

includes both systolic and diastolic pressures, and rates the severity of high blood pressure from mild to very severe. The classification system is presented in table 11.4.

A number of factors influence the normal range of blood pressure, including age, body position (such as sitting or standing), time of day, recency of exercise, and intake of drugs (such as caffeine, alcohol, or nicotine). As noted in figure 11.7, there is a rather wide range in blood pressure levels, both systolic and diastolic, from one individual to another. For example, at age twenty, the range is about 90 to 145 for systolic and 50 to 95 for diastolic. A level of 140 for systolic and 90 for diastolic is considered to be stage 1 hypertension in the JNCDET classification. Thus, some twenty-year-olds have high blood pressure. You may also note from this figure that as age increases, the upper ranges of both systolic and diastolic pressures also increase, and a greater percentage of individuals become hypertensive. A persistent resting blood pressure of over 140 systolic and/or 90 diastolic is considered high, and medical attention should be sought.

The risk factors that appear to predispose individuals to high blood pressure are similar to those for CHD and atherosclerosis. Hereditarial factors include family history, gender (males being more susceptible), and race (about 33 percent more prevalent in black Americans than in whites). Other risk factors are obesity, a sedentary life-style, use of oral contraceptives, excessive alcohol consumption, low potassium intake, and excessive sodium consumption, particularly in individuals who have increased sodium sensitivity.

High blood pressure is dangerous for several reasons. First, it drastically increases the work load of the heart in pumping the extra blood volume or overcoming the peripheral vascular resistance. This normally leads to an enlarged heart, but over time the increase in heart size becomes excessive, and the efficiency of the heart actually decreases, making it more prone to a heart attack. Second, high blood pressure may directly damage the arterial walls due to constant pressure and thus be a major contributing factor to the development of atherosclerosis and a predisposing factor to CHD and stroke. High blood pressure is a disease unto itself, but it is also a risk factor in the etiology of other diseases. It is one of the most common and important risk factors for CHD.

Positive Health Life-Style

Since high blood pressure is such a potentially dangerous disease, it is important that it be controlled. In many cases, this means the utilization of drug therapy (antihypertension drugs) under a physician's direction. Commonly prescribed drugs include: calcium channel blockers, which may relax both the heart and blood vessels; angiotensin converting enzyme (ACE) inhibitors, which may block the formation of angiotensin, a potent chemical that increases blood pressure; diuretics, which reduce body water levels, and hence blood volume, and thus reduce blood pressure; and, beta-blockers, which block the pressure-raising effect of epinephrine and norepinephrine upon the blood vessels and heart. Unfortunately, drugs may exert other adverse effects or actually increase health risks that may decrease the quality of life, so a nonpharmacologic approach is often a first choice of treatment in cases of mild to moderate hypertension.

Two rather universally accepted Positive Health Life-style changes that reduce blood pressure are a decreased dietary intake of salt and a decrease of body fat. Excessive amounts of salt in the body hold more water, thereby increasing the blood volume, which then increases the blood pressure. Reduction of salt intake is particularly effective in salt-sensitive individuals, those whose blood pressure increases with increased dietary intake of salt and vice versa. Techniques to decrease salt intake are presented in chapter 6 on pages 129–130. The JNCDET also recommended an increase in dietary potassium. Wholesome foods in their natural state, such as fruits and vegetables, are low in sodium and high in potassium as compared to processed foods. Excessive body fat places extra demands on the heart to pump blood through more blood vessels, again increasing the blood pressure. Weight loss programs are detailed in chapter 7.

Stress reduction techniques have been advocated as a means to reduce blood pressure, but results are not as conclusive as with salt restriction and weight loss. Behavioral techniques involving the relaxation response (see chapter 8) have successfully reduced blood pressure in some highly motivated subjects, but the general success of this technique in lowering high blood pressure is still considered to be questionable.

Regular aerobic exercise has also been recommended as a modality to reduce high blood pressure. Since exercise may be an effective means to lose excess body fat, it may exert a beneficial effect through this avenue. However, the exact role or mechanism of exercise as an independent factor in lowering blood pressure has not been totally resolved. Although a number of studies have shown that exercise training by itself helps decrease resting systolic blood pressure in those who are hypertensive and may even elicit a slight decrease in those with normal blood pressure, not all studies are in agreement. In a similar vein, many investigators who have reviewed the relevant research conclude that aerobic exercise is an effective mechanism to reduce high blood pressure, but others suggest that more research is needed to support this viewpoint. Not all individuals will experience a decrease in blood pressure from an exercise program; they may be exercise insensitive, somewhat opposite to individuals who are salt sensitive. Nevertheless, most investigators in this area suggest that the present information appears to be favorable and is sufficient to justify an aerobic exercise program as a useful adjunct for the treatment of high blood pressure. It normally takes months to observe an effect, but average decreases in systolic and diastolic blood pressure approximate 10 mmHg. The interested student is referred to the excellent reviews by James Hagberg and Charles Tipton and the recent position stand of the American College of Sports Medicine relative to physical activity, physical fitness, and hypertension. In general, the ACSM recommends aerobic exercise with large muscle groups at an intensity of 50–85 percent of maximal oxygen uptake or lower (40–70 percent), 20 to 60 minutes in duration, and a frequency of three to five times per week.

Individuals who have high blood pressure should consult with their physicians relative to mode and intensity of exercise. Those with blood pressures above 160/95 mmHg may need to use drugs to lower blood pressure prior to initiating an exercise program. Walking at moderate intensity may be an effective exercise mode. Although aerobic exercise may help to reduce blood pressure at rest and may evoke a lessened blood pressure rise during exercise, a protective effect, other exercises may be

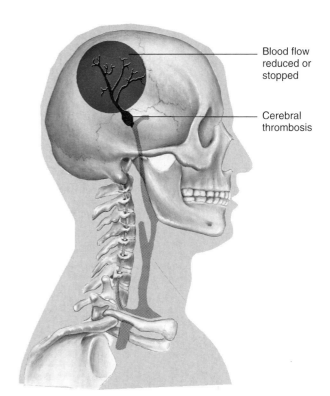

Figure 11.8 *Stroke. A stroke, or apoplexy, is caused by inadequate blood flow to parts of the brain. Ischemic stroke (lack of blood flow) may be caused by atherosclerosis or a cerebral thrombosis, or clot, which decreases blood flow, and hence oxygen, with resultant damage to brain function. Hemorrhagic, or bleeding stroke, may also occur, but is not depicted here. The observable effects depend upon the area of the brain and the amount of tissue damaged.*

harmful. For example, high-intensity aerobic exercise and activities that require intense straining, lifting, or hanging, such as isometric exercises, weight lifting, or pull-ups, should be avoided. The use of hand-held weights in aerobic exercises may also be a concern when used vigorously. These activities create a physiological response that rapidly raises the blood pressure to rather high levels. This increase may be hazardous to someone whose resting blood pressure is already at an elevated level. Nevertheless, although resistance training is not recommended as the only type of exercise a hypertensive individual should do, it is recommended as part of an overall exercise training program. Working at lower intensities may still increase muscular strength and endurance, and may reduce the blood pressure responses when one uses strength during daily activities, such as lifting and carrying grocery bags.

Stroke

Stroke, also known as apoplexy or a **cerebral vascular accident (CVA),** annually afflicts almost 500,000 Americans and is responsible for nearly 153,000 deaths. It is the third leading cause of death in the United States. There are two major types of stroke. An ischemic, or clotting, stroke occurs when the blood supply to the brain is inadequate, usually due to a blocking of the cranial arteries in the brain by atherosclerosis or by a clot traveling from elsewhere in the body (see fig. 11.8). A hemorrhagic, or bleeding, stroke occurs when a cerebral blood vessel ruptures, usually due to high blood pressure.

Other causes may include tumors, which block blood flow to the brain. The severity of the stroke may vary from slight to severe, depending on the location and extent of the brain damage. Many people suffer minor strokes, which may involve a brief loss of memory, dizziness or unsteadiness, speaking difficulty, disturbed vision, or temporary weakness, numbness, or paralysis in the face or extremities. They may recover totally or have some residual effects, such as garbled speech or slight paralysis. Severe strokes lead to major paralysis or death but they are more commonly disabling rather than fatal. Although there is currently no treatment to limit the brain damage in a stroke victim, some promising therapies, such as clot-dissolving drugs, are being studied.

An individual with atherosclerosis and/or high blood pressure is more likely to have a stroke. Thus, the risk factors associated with the development of both of these diseases may contribute to CVA.

Positive Health Life-Style

A Positive Health Life-style that reduces the severity of the risk factors associated with coronary heart disease and high blood pressure is also an effective preventive measure against stroke, particularly abstinence from smoking, appropriate stress management techniques, and proper diet and exercise programs as discussed previously relative to the prevention of atherosclerosis and hypertension. Relative to exercise, recent epidemiological research by Shinton and Sagar found that a history of vigorous exercise early in life, between the ages of 15 to 25, appeared to protect against stroke in later life, but maintaining a lifetime of exercise provided an increasing protection.

Peripheral Vascular Disease (Claudication)

Peripheral vascular disease (PVD) is similar to coronary heart disease (CHD); however, in PVD, the arteriosclerosis is found in blood vessels other than those in the heart. Individuals with PVD experience pain during physical activity, particularly in the calf muscles when walking, referred to as intermittent **claudication,** due to the inability of the vessels to deliver enough blood to the active muscles. The risk factors for CHD and PVD are similar, but diabetes is the most prominent risk factor. PVD reduces life-expectancy by 10 years, primarily because patients commonly have coronary and cerebral atherosclerosis as well.

Positive Health Life-Style

Adoption of the Positive Health Life-style recommended for the prevention of CHD is also prudent behavior to help prevent PVD. Moreover, such a life-style may also help alleviate the symptoms of PVD once the condition has developed. In one of the first studies, researchers at the Longevity Research Institute have shown that exercise and dietary modification have a beneficial effect upon the symptoms of PVD. They found that exercise training, in conjunction with a normal American diet, was effective in prolonging walking endurance without symptoms of pain. However, their dietary program (10 percent fat, 10 percent protein, 80 percent complex carbohydrates, and no cholesterol), in conjunction with exercise training, was even more effective.

Although the results of this study have been contested by other investigators, Radack and Wyderski conducted a meta-analysis (a detailed statistical review) of all studies involving the effect of exercise training on PVD symptoms and concluded that dynamic aerobic exercise training increased pain-free walking distance, which appears to be related to the increased blood flow to the calf muscles noted in other research. In a major review, Barnard supported these conclusions, but indicated the effects of exercise training may be individualized; although many may benefit, some may not, and some may even be worse off. Some data also suggest that vitamin E supplementation may help alleviate the pain in walking associated with PVD. Smoking cessation has also been found to be helpful.

Metabolic Disorders

Metabolism represents the sum total of all the physical and chemical processes in the human body concerned with the energy transformations essential to life. Although general metabolism includes all processes involved in the utilization of ingested nutrients, there are also special types such as carbohydrate metabolism, fat metabolism, and protein metabolism. There are a vast number of different metabolic disorders that are harmful to health, but three of the most prevalent in American society are obesity (unbalanced Calorie metabolism), diabetes (a disorder of carbohydrate metabolism), and cancer (unregulated and disorganized cell growth).

Obesity

Obesity is a metabolic disorder characterized by a disturbance in energy balance that results in a condition marked by excessive deposition and storage of fat throughout the body. Since clinical definitions and the etiology of obesity were covered in chapter 7, we shall simply recap some of the major health-related aspects at this point.

In ancient time Hippocrates, the Greek physician acknowledged to be the father of medicine, noted that death occurs earlier in the obese, and recent research indicates thinner men in midlife have lower death rates. Obesity is a major health problem in the United States, one of epidemic nature. Obesity affects both children and adults, and recent estimates suggest that about 25 to 30 percent of the American population are too fat for optimal health. The Public Health Service has stated in *Healthy People 2000* that one of the major health objectives of the year 2000 is to decrease the proportion of adults and children who are significantly overweight, or obese.

Being obese is associated with a host of health problems—both physical and socioemotional. Reports from the National Institute of Health conclude that being overweight contributes to serious health consequences and have labeled obesity as a killer disease. One report noted that obesity accounts for 15 to

20 percent of the mortality rate and is associated with twenty-six known health conditions, including CHD, high blood pressure, diabetes, kidney disease, cirrhosis of the liver, arthritis, and cancer of the colon and rectum. At particular risk are those with android-type obesity, body fat patterning in which fat is stored primarily in the abdominal region. Android type obesity elicits a series of physiological responses, such as insulin resistance, hyperinsulinemia, lipid abnormalities, impaired clotting processes, and high blood pressure, collectively known as the metabolic syndrome and all of which increase the risk for CHD and diabetes. Additionally, obesity may impair the immune system or modify hormone levels, such as estrogen, which may increase the risk of various cancers, particularly prostrate cancer in men and breast or endometrial cancer in women. Although mild to moderate levels of obesity increase one's health risks, individuals with morbid obesity, defined as being at least 100 pounds over the ideal weight or having a body mass index (BMI) greater than 40, are particularly susceptible to these health problems.

Obesity may also contribute to the development of psychological disturbances, particularly in adolescents and young adults who are conscious of their body images. Body image is a term used to describe the feelings an individual has toward his or her body; a poor body image developed because of obesity can retard proper socioemotional development and impair the quality of life. Being overweight is viewed by many as a handicap to both personal and professional fulfillment, and the term "fattism" has been coined to reflect society's prejudice toward the obese.

Positive Health Life-Style

Morbid obesity merits medical supervision and may involve a combination of many techniques such as surgery, drugs, starvation-type diets, and exercise. An individualized, medically supervised weight-control program is very important for the morbidly obese because there may be a number of associated health risks. Unfortunately, morbid obesity is very resistant to treatment and the vast majority, 95 to 99 percent, of these individuals who lose weight regain it within a year. However, weight-control programs have greater chances for success in individuals who have accumulated excess body fat through environmental conditions such as increased food intake or a sedentary life-style and who do not have a strong genetic predisposition towards obesity.

Basically, there are two general means to treat or prevent obesity. You must either decrease your energy intake or increase your energy output. In essence, you must initiate a low-Calorie diet or an exercise program or both. Just as adding 150 Calories to the daily diet will increase body fat by 15 pounds in one year, so too will decreasing 150 Calories from the daily diet result in an annual loss of 15 pounds. Increasing your exercise by jogging a mile and a half per day will also accomplish basically the same result, a loss of 15 pounds in a year.

A Positive Health Life-style centered around a low-Calorie, nutritious diet, and an aerobic exercise program can

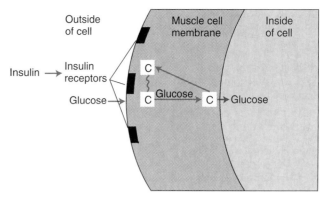

Figure 11.9 *Role of insulin. Insulin binds to insulin receptors in the cell membrane and then activates a carrier system (C). The carrier system transports glucose through the cell membrane to the interior where it is released for further use. One cause of diabetes is a deficiency of insulin receptors in the body. Another cause is insufficient insulin production by the pancreas.*

be a sound means to prevent or treat obesity. Research has indicated that a combination of a nutritious diet and an aerobic exercise program, combined with proper behavior management techniques, is the best approach to weight control. Chapter 7 provides you with such a program. Prevention is more effective than treatment, so the earlier in life that proper weight control is initiated, the better, preferably by the adolescent years. Although youngsters do not normally die of CHD, epidemiological research has recently shown that obese adolescents are at greater risk for chronic disease in adulthood and all-cause mortality compared to their non-obese peers.

Diabetes

There are approximately 6 million known diabetics in the United States, but this may represent only half the actual number of cases because an estimated 50 percent have not been diagnosed. There are about 500,000 new cases diagnosed annually, and it is nearly 1.5 times more prevalent in women than in men. It is a major leading cause of death, claiming 300,000 lives annually, due to both the disease itself and its complications, such as heart attack and stroke. Diabetes affects almost all body tissues. Millions of diabetics suffer consequences such as blindness, high blood pressure, and chronic infections.

Diabetes is a condition in which excessive amounts of urine are excreted from the body daily. It may be caused by such problems as a malfunctioning adrenal or pituitary gland. However, its most common form is **diabetes mellitus,** a disorder in which the body cannot metabolize carbohydrates properly. The main effect is a high level of glucose in the blood. The major problem is associated with **insulin,** a hormone secreted by the pancreas. Insulin is necessary for blood glucose to enter the body cells (fig. 11.9). Diabetics may have a decreased or absent pancreatic production of insulin or a deficiency of insulin receptors in the liver, muscle, and fat tissues so that the insulin, even if it is present in normal amounts or even in excess amounts, may have no effect on the tissues. In essence, diabetics have impaired carbohydrate, or glucose, metabolism. High blood glucose levels exert adverse effects on small blood vessels in the eyes, kidneys, and nerves, leading to blindness, kidney disease, infection, and gangrene; the latter occurs primarily in the feet which may necessitate amputation. As the body turns to fat for its major energy sources, the rise in serum lipids becomes a contributing factor for other diseases, such as atherosclerosis and CHD.

Diabetes may develop in one of two general ways. Juvenile-onset diabetes (type I) usually occurs in children and may be caused by a virus or other toxic agent that appears to trigger an autoimmune response that impairs or destroys the ability of the beta cells in the pancreas to produce insulin. This is the most severe type of diabetes. Heredity does not appear to play a major role in its development. Maturity-onset diabetes (type II) usually develops later in life. Its onset is more gradual, and the disease is usually milder than the juvenile-onset type. Most, but not all, maturity-onset diabetics are overweight, and android-type obesity is a strong risk factor. Nearly 85 percent of these diabetics have a diabetic parent. The two appropriate terms used to describe diabetic patients are insulin-dependent and noninsulin-dependent. All juvenile-onset diabetics and some maturity-onset diabetics have insulin-dependent diabetes mellitus (IDDM), for they must take insulin in order to control the disease. Noninsulin-dependent diabetics (NIDDM) who constitute about 90 percent of all diabetics, may be able to control their blood sugar by proper nutrition, exercise, or prescribed drugs.

Positive Health Life-Style

As with the other diseases discussed previously in this chapter, a Positive Health Life-style can be viewed as both treatment and possible prevention for diabetes. The primary goal of treatment programs is to maintain a normal blood glucose level to prevent damage to blood vessels. Additional goals include favorable changes in the blood lipid profile to prevent atherosclerosis and maintenance of proper body weight to increase insulin sensitivity and blood glucose control. Medical treatment of diabetes usually centers around four aspects—insulin or other drugs, diet, weight control, and exercise. Of these four factors, the latter three are important components of a Positive Health Life-style. IDDM diabetics need medical supervision in order to determine how much insulin they need and how often they should take it. The dosage must be tailored to the life-style of the individual. NIDDM diabetics may need oral drugs to help control their blood glucose by either stimulating insulin secretion or decreasing insulin resistance in the tissues. However, many may attain adequate control with diet, exercise, and weight control.

Both types of diabetics must control their diet. A National Institute of Health conference focusing upon the diet and exercise needs of the diabetic recommended a diet consisting of

50 to 60 percent of Calories from complex carbohydrates
12 to 20 percent of Calories from protein
20 to 30 percent or less of Calories from fat

The carbohydrates should be of the complex type, such as vegetables, beans, whole-grain products, and fruits. An increased fiber content, found naturally in these products, may also be helpful because it may slow down the absorption of carbohydrates in the intestine, thus minimizing the increase in blood glucose. Water-soluble fibers appear to be especially important in this regard. Simple sugars or other carbohydrates that lead to a rapid rise in blood glucose should be avoided. Total and saturated fat content should be low, focusing upon a balance of monounsaturated and polyunsaturated fats. These dietary adjustments will help normalize both blood glucose and serum lipids.

The diet should also be balanced in Calories to maintain the recommended body weight. One of the contributing factors to NIDDM is excessive body fat, particularly abdominal fat. Excessive body fat decreases the number of active insulin receptors in body cells or their sensitivity, and thus, insulin will not function properly. Decreasing caloric intake and the resultant losses of body fat help reactivate these receptors, improving glucose tolerance (the ability of the tissues to metabolize glucose), thus minimizing or eliminating the need for oral drugs by NIDDM diabetics.

Properly prescribed exercise may be an effective adjunct to insulin and diet for the diabetic patient. Aerobic exercise programs are recommended, and the ACSM guidelines regarding intensity, duration, and frequency, as discussed in chapter 3, are deemed appropriate. Exercise facilitates the utilization of glucose by muscle cells, helping lower blood glucose levels. In essence, exercise itself has an insulin-type effect. In addition, exercise increases energy expenditure and helps the individual to lose weight. Furthermore, research also suggests that aerobic exercise may help to improve glucose tolerance and increase insulin sensitivity so that less insulin needs to be secreted by the pancreas. The beneficial effects of exercise on blood glucose regulation are more predominant in NIDDM, although exercise is also highly recommended for those with IDDM. Exercise also lowers blood lipid levels associated with diabetes, for muscle cells also use these lipids for energy. Such an effect may help in the prevention of atherosclerosis, which is often observed in both types of diabetics.

Although the report from the National Institute of Health conference on diet, exercise, and diabetes noted that exercise is a useful adjunct in the treatment of diabetes, it is best used in combination with dietary control. The role of exercise in weight control, particularly the ability to decrease abdominal fat deposits, appears to be its most significant contribution.

Resistance training exercise is also recommended for diabetics, for the increase in muscle mass and possible decrease in body fat will improve insulin sensitivity and blood glucose control. However, resistance exercise training should not replace aerobic exercise, but should be added to it. Both IDDM and NIDDM diabetics may do almost any type of exercise, even Ironman-type triathlons. Some world-class and Olympic athletes are diabetic. However, exercise may be harmful to the diabetic if is not carefully prescribed. Although the blood glucose response to exercise may vary in the diabetic, the major problem is hypoglycemia, or low blood sugar. In particular, this may be a problem in the IDDM diabetic, for exercise stimulates blood flow and, thus, can increase the blood levels of insulin by mobilizing the insulin from its injection site. This increased insulin and the insulin-effect of exercise itself will increase the transport of glucose into the muscle and possibly create hypoglycemia, particularly if exercise is undertaken at the peak of insulin action. This effect, referred to as an **insulin reaction,** may result in loss of consciousness due to inadequate glucose for brain function or acidosis, which can lead to coma. The exercising diabetic should always carry something sweet to eat in case of a hypoglycemic episode and should also make sure that others know that he or she is a diabetic and what an insulin reaction is. Diabetics should not exercise late at night because there may be a delayed effect of exercise to potentiate insulin, possibly leading to hypoglycemia while sleeping.

It is important that diabetics discuss a proper exercise program with their physicians. The use of simple home tests for blood glucose will enable the diabetic to monitor his or her blood glucose daily and observe the effects of exercise. Additionally, some forms of exercise may be contraindicated or modified for diabetics if complications exist. For example, individuals with damage to the blood vessels in the retina of the eye should avoid straining-type exercise, such as intense resistance training, while those prone to foot infections should be careful to protect the feet with appropriate footwear for the activity.

Although these general guidelines relative to diet, exercise, and weight control have been developed for the individual who has diabetes, they may also be very important in its prevention for those who are nondiabetic. Such guidelines may be particularly important to those who may be at increased risk, such as those with diabetic parents. Relative to diet, excessive intake of simple sugars stimulates the pancreas to release insulin in greater quantities. Prolonged consumption of simple sugars may possibly impair the ability of the pancreas to produce insulin. Aerobic exercise is an excellent means to help maintain a normal body weight, which may be one of the reasons that endurance exercise appears to improve glucose tolerance and insulin sensitivity, both of which normally decrease with the aging process. In a recent study, exercise helped prevent adult-onset diabetes in men who were at high risk. Those who exercised somewhat vigorously, engaging in tennis, swimming laps, and jogging, were less likely to develop diabetes than those who were sedentary or who exercised less vigorously, for instance bowling. Again, the more Positive Health Life-style changes you adopt, the greater the health benefits.

Cancer

Cancer, one of the most feared diseases in the United States, involves an unregulated, disorganized growth of cells in the body. The result is the formation of a malignant tumor, technically known as a **neoplasm,** or new cell material. The neoplasm serves no useful function but simply grows at the expense of other healthy cells in the body. The word *cancer* is derived from the Latin for *crab,* or creeping ulcer, for a malignant cancer can spread throughout the entire body.

Cancer may develop in almost any tissue, common sites being the skin, oral cavity, lung, stomach, colon, kidney, liver, prostate, bone, blood, breast, and uterus. One in every three Americans will eventually get cancer. It is the second leading cause of death in the United States, resulting in approximately 500,000 deaths per year. There is an increasing number of cancer cases, not linked solely to the aging process, but also to environmental carcinogenic hazards in addition to smoking, and it is projected that by the year 2000, cancer will surpass coronary heart disease as the number one cause of death in the United States. Skin cancer is the most common form of cancer, but it is not often fatal. Lung cancer is the most prevalent fatal form.

Cancer may go undetected for years, for it may grow slowly and elicit no symptoms. However, there are a number of warning signs and symptoms that may be indicative of cancer. Many of these symptoms are usually minor, but if you experience any of them, consult your physician without delay.

1. Rapid loss of weight without any apparent cause, such as 10 pounds in 10 weeks.
2. A change in bowel habits, such as frequent diarrhea or constipation. Bowel movements that look black or tarry. Rectal bleeding.
3. A change in bladder habits, such as discomfort while urinating or an unusual color, such as pink or red, or unusual appearances, such as cloudy or smoky, of the urine.
4. A sore that does not heal in normal time, about 3 weeks or less.
5. An obvious change in a wart or mole, such as bleeding, itching, or a change in size, shape, or color.
6. A thickening or lump in the breast, testicles, or other body parts.
7. Indigestion or difficulty in swallowing.
8. A persistent cough or hoarseness that lasts for more than a week without apparent reason.
9. Any unusual bleeding or discharge from the mouth (coughed-up phlegm or sputum), the penis, or the vagina.
10. Unexplained pain, such as headaches or abdominal pain.

The cause of cancer is unknown, but a number of epidemiological studies with humans and experimental studies with animals have revealed a variety of substances or agents, known as carcinogens, that may initiate (initiators) or promote (promoters) the cancer process. Other substances have been identified as antipromotors. To briefly recap information presented in chapter 6, an initiator is necessary to trigger the growth of cancer cells, but promoters are necessary for the growth to continue. If the growth progresses, it may reach the metastasis stage in which the cancer spreads to other tissues in the body. Antipromoters may block the supportive effect of the promoter and arrest growth to help prevent progression and metastasis.

The war against cancer is far from over, but some victories have been won. Early detection methods have decreased cancer of the cervix and uterus by nearly 70 percent, while removal of possible carcinogens from processed meats has been associated with a significant decrease in stomach cancer. Although scientists are working on a cure for the various forms of cancers, the current objective is prevention.

Positive Health Life-Style

Although much of the research relative to the effectiveness of a Positive Health Life-style to prevent the development of cancer is epidemiological in nature and thus does not support a cause-and-effect relationship, the following dozen guidelines are prudent suggestions. Some of these suggestions have substantial research support, such as smoking cessation, while others are supported by preliminary data and need further research, such as the role of exercise. Nevertheless, based upon the data available, these recommendations are not likely to do any harm and may do some good in the prevention of cancer. As will be obvious as you review them, they are similar to the prevention of other diseases.

1. Have a regular medical checkup. The earlier cancer is detected, the better is the prognosis for treatment and recovery. The American Cancer Society recommends that women should do a breast self-exam every month, (see figure 11.10) and a Pap smear every year. Between the ages of twenty to forty, women should have a breast physical exam and pelvic examination every three years, and yearly once they are over the age of forty. A baseline mammography examination should be done between the ages of thirty-five and thirty-nine and then every 1 to 2 years as recommended by the physician. Males and females should have a digital rectal exam yearly after the age of forty and other tests, such as blood tests, stool blood tests, and colon examinations, after the age of fifty for detection of rectal, colon, or prostrate (males only) cancer; however, these latter tests may be conducted earlier if there is a family history of rectal cancer. Males should perform self-examination of the testicles monthly (see figure 11.11).

2. Do not smoke. Smoking poses one of the greatest risks for cancer; over 140,000 deaths are attributed to tobacco. As noted in chapter 9, a number of substances found in cigarette smoke and smokeless tobacco are carcinogenic. There are a number of good reasons not to smoke. Prevention of cancer is one of the most important ones. One cancer researcher noted that if you smoke, there is nothing we can do for you; your fate has been sealed.

3. Restrict your intake of alcohol. As noted in chapter 9, alcohol in moderation appears to be safe. However,

excessive amounts lead to increased risk for a variety of cancers, primarily of the digestive tract. Also, in chapter 9, we discussed the relationship between alcohol intake and breast cancer in women. The greater the alcohol intake, the greater the breast cancer risk. Therefore, abstinence or moderation is recommended. Heavy alcohol consumption is also associated with increased risk of cancer of the mouth, throat, and liver. Review chapter 9 for guidelines relative to safe and moderate drinking.

4. Control your body weight. Epidemiological evidence from humans and experimental evidence from animals supports a clear link between obesity and a variety of cancers, particularly cancer of the colon, prostate, breast, endometrium, and pancreas. The diet and exercise guidelines presented in chapter 7 provide the basis for maintaining an optimal body weight.

5. Eat less fat. Increased dietary fat, particularly high levels of saturated and polyunsaturated fats, has been associated with cancer of the colon, rectum, prostate gland, and breast. The epidemiological data linking dietary fat is strongest for colon cancer, but weaker for the other forms of cancer. One hypothesis suggests that the bile salts secreted into the intestine to help digest the fats go through a series of changes caused by intestinal bacteria and eventually form promoters. However, epidemiological evidence suggests that some forms of dietary fat, such as olive oil and fish oils, may not pose a problem. The guidelines presented in chapter 6 may be helpful in reducing the intake of dietary fat.

6. Avoid additives in food. Certain additives are suspected of contributing to cancer, such as nitrates and nitrites used to preserve meats. These compounds may be converted in the intestinal tract into carcinogenic compounds. Read food labels and limit your intake or avoid nitrite-cured meats or those that are smoked or salt-cured. As noted in chapter 6, your diet should consist primarily of natural, wholesome foods with minimal processing.

7. Eat more dietary fiber. Both water-soluble and water-insoluble fiber appear to be beneficial, especially the former. Fiber may function in a variety of ways to minimize the contact of possible carcinogens with the mucosa of the intestinal walls. Insoluble fiber attracts water and dilutes the concentration of carcinogens; it also speeds the transit of materials through the intestine, decreasing the amount of time carcinogens are in the intestine, and insoluble fiber is the major type associated with reduced risk of colon cancer. The soluble fibers may bind with some of the bile salts, leading to an increased excretion in the feces. Foods rich in dietary fiber include the complex carbohydrates such as whole-grain breads, beans, and vegetables.

8. Eat more cruciferous vegetables. These vegetables, also known as the cabbage family, contain certain phytochemicals that may serve as antipromoters in the intestinal tract. As noted in chapter 6, such vegetables include broccoli, cauliflower, brussel sprouts, kale, and all cabbages.

9. Eat more foods rich in beta carotene, vitamin C, and calcium. Epidemiological research suggests that foods high in beta-carotene, which is converted into vitamin A in the body, and vitamin C may serve as antipromoters. Both may function as antioxidants, preventing free radical damage to cells. Vitamin C also has been shown to block the formation of carcinogens from nitrites. Remember the slogan by the American Cancer Society to eat five a day, meaning a *minimum* of five servings of fruits and vegetables daily. Fruits and vegetables are high in these vitamins, particularly the yellow-orange varieties for beta-carotene and citrus fruits for vitamin C. Calcium is believed to function somewhat like soluble fiber, forming insoluble complexes with bile salts or free fatty acids and helping to excrete them in the feces, thereby reducing their potential carcinogenic effect on the walls of the colon. Chapter 6 provides additional information on dietary sources of beta-carotene, vitamin C, and calcium.

10. Avoid excessive exposure to the sun and other possible environmental carcinogens. Ultraviolet rays may trigger cancer in the skin, particularly in light-skinned individuals. Those of Irish descent with red hair are especially vulnerable as are blondes and those with a freckling tendency. If you desire a tanned look, gradual tanning with the use of appropriate sunblock protection (at least #15) is recommended. Safe sunglasses and a broad-brimmed hat are also essential for sunbathing. The sun is especially harmful during the hours of 11 A.M. to 3 P.M.

    Contact with other environmental hazards, such as asbestos, pesticides, solvents, and cleaning fluids should be avoided or minimized as much as possible.

11. Avoid medications that may predispose to cancer such as excessive estrogen or anabolic steroids. Consult with your physician relative to estrogen use.

12. Do aerobic exercise. In a recent interview, Lee indicated that physical activity is emerging as a potential means to reduce the risk of developing cancer. A number of epidemiological studies have suggested that exercise may help in the prevention of several types of cancer. Research by Rose Frisch and her associates at Harvard relative to the beneficial role that exercise may play in the prevention of cancer of the breast and reproductive organs in females was discussed in chapter 10. Research by Ralph Paffenbarger, an internationally renowned epidemiologist, has revealed that men who exercise at a level equivalent to approximately 2,000 Calories per week are less likely to develop cancer. Other recent studies have shown a decreased likelihood of colon cancer in those who exercise on a regular basis, even when other risk factors for colon cancer were controlled. The epidemiological data supportive of a beneficial linkage between exercise and cancer is strongest for prevention of colon cancer.

Although few experimental data are available to support these epidemiological data, some hypotheses have been advanced regarding the mechanisms by which exercise could help to prevent cancer. First, some investigators suggest that exercise may lead to other life-style changes, such as improved diet habits and smoking cessation, that may decrease the chances of developing cancer. Second, exercise may help to prevent obesity, which, as mentioned previously, is associated with a variety of cancers. Third, exercise may enhance immune function and the production of other natural anticancer agents in the body. For example, by increasing the body temperature and the secretion of epinephrine, exercise has been shown to increase white blood cell production of two small natural proteins in the body, interferon and interleukin-2. Both of these chemicals have been used as antipromoters in the treatment of cancer. In a related manner, exercise may also increase the production of some prostaglandins that promote anticancer activity. Animal studies also have shown that exercise may alter the activity of monocytes and macrophages, both white blood cells, to enhance antitumor effects. In some animal studies, exercise activity has been shown to suppress the development of chemically and virally induced cancers, providing some experimental support for the anticancer effects of exercise. These general effects could help prevent a variety of cancers. However, as noted previously, excessive exercise or overtraining may actually suppress immune function, although no data appear to be available to suggest this would increase the risk for developing cancer.

Relative to specific cancers, research has shown that exercise may increase bowel motility which, comparable to the effects of dietary fiber, will speed intestinal transit time and decrease contact time for possible carcinogens and the colon cell wall, one hypothesis regarding the prevention of colon cancer. Exercise, particularly if it leads to low body fat levels, may depress estrogen formation and reduce the risk of breast cancer in women, a hypothesis advanced by Frisch and discussed in chapter 10. Also, exercise may decrease testosterone levels in males, which may lead to a decreased risk of prostate cancer because it is associated with high levels of testosterone in the body.

Although the data are limited regarding the cancer preventive effect of exercise, they do provide the basis for cautious optimism. Guidelines for an appropriate aerobic exercise program may be found in chapter 3.

Overall, the Positive Health Life-style is associated with an enhanced immune system and other factors that may prevent cancer.

Breast Self-Examination

Breast self-examination (BSE) is a method a woman employs to detect suspicious lumps in her breasts. Such lumps, though not uncommon, can be early indicators of cancer.

Eighty to ninety percent of all breast lumps are *benign* (noncancerous). Such lumps tend to disappear or fluctuate in size during the monthly cycle, being more common during the first few days of the period or around ovulation. Thus, it is best to conduct a BSE about a week after menstruation. If the periods are irregular, BSE should occur at a regular 1-month interval. Women past menopause should perform the exam at the same time each month, such as on the first of the month. Consistent, regular exams will help a woman become familiar with the shapes, colors, texture, and consistency of her own breasts.

In the Shower

Examine your breasts during your bath or shower since hands glide more easily over wet skin. Fingers flat, move them with firm pressure over every part of each breast. Use the right hand to examine the left breast and the left hand for the right breast. Check for any lump, hard knot, or thickening (fig. 11.10, part a).

Before a Mirror

Inspect your breasts with arms at your sides, facing the mirror (fig. 11.10, part b). Next, raise your arms high overhead. Look for any changes in the contour of each breast: a swelling, dimpling of skin, or changes in the nipple.

Next, rest your palms on your hips and press down firmly to flex your chest muscles. Left and right breast will not exactly match—few women's breasts do. Again, look for changes and irregularities. Regular inspection shows what is normal for you and will give you confidence in your examination.

Lying Down

To examine your right breast, while lying down put a pillow or folded towel under your right shoulder. Place your right hand behind your head—this distributes breast tissue more evenly on the chest. With your left hand, fingers flat, press firmly in small circular motions around an imaginary clock face. Begin at outermost top of your right breast for twelve o'clock, then move to one o'clock, and so on around the circle back to twelve. (A ridge of firm tissue in the lower curve of each breast is normal.) Then move one inch inward, toward the nipple, and keep circling to examine every part of your breast, including the nipple. This requires at least three more circles. Now slowly repeat the procedure on your left breast with a pillow under your left shoulder and left hand behind your head. Notice how your beast structure feels.

Finally, squeeze the nipple of each breast gently between the thumb and index finger. Any discharge, clear or bloody, should be reported to your doctor immediately (fig. 11.10, part c).

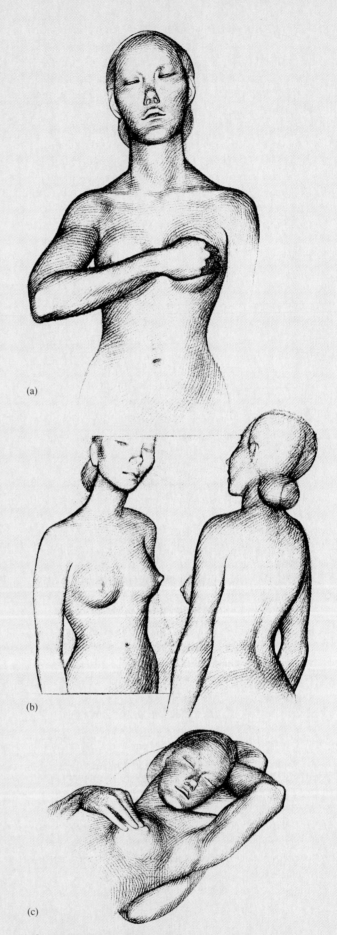

(a)

(b)

(c)

Figure 11.10 *Steps in self-examination of the breasts.*

Self-Examination of the Testicles

Testicular cancer is the most common malignancy in men between twenty-nine and thirty-five years of age.

Early detection of testicular cancer is critical for successful treatment. However, the most common symptom of this cancer is a scrotal lump that progressively increases in size, and in most cases, this lump produces no pain or other symptoms.

While breast self-examination has received wide publicity, many men do not know of the importance of testicular self-examination (TSE). Young men, in particular, should learn and practice the routine monthly. It is recommended that the man examine himself when the skin of the scrotum is relaxed, as after a warm shower or bath. A normal testis is smooth, egg shaped, and firm, with the epididymis perceived as a raised area at the rear of the testis (fig. 11.11, part a). Using the thumb and fingertips, the man should feel the entire surface of the testis for any lump, hardening, or enlargement. Any suspicious areas should be reported to a physician immediately (fig. 11.11, part b).

Cases of testicular cancer are increasing in number. TSE is one important way a male can perhaps avoid the dire consequences of the disease and take responsibility for his own health.

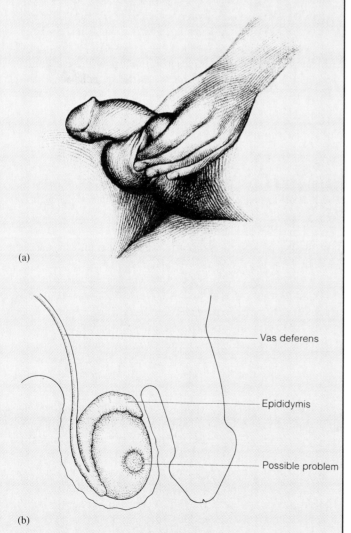

(a)

(b)

Figure 11.11 *Testicular self-examination.*

Musculoskeletal Disorders

As the name suggests, musculoskeletal disorders afflict either the muscular system, the skeletal system, or both. Although there are a wide variety of these disorders, three types of musculoskeletal disorders that may be influenced by a Positive Health Life-style are of special interest. These disorders, or diseases, are low back pain, osteoporosis, and arthritis.

Low Back Pain

The skeletal spine is a remarkable structure designed to support a good portion of the body's weight, to transmit this weight to the lower part of the body, to protect the delicate spinal cord of the nervous system, to serve as a shock absorber, and to provide movement in all directions. Figure 11.12 is a lateral view of the spine and shows the various curves and muscle groups that have an impact upon spine movement and stability, two different types of joints, and the sciatic nerve. The discs of cartilage between each vertebra serve as shock absorbers and are also part of one of the two types of joints in the spine where all movement can occur. The curves in the spine develop naturally and are necessary for the spine to perform its major functions. The stability of the spine involves an interaction between the natural curves, the discs, ligaments, and the extensive musculature.

Unfortunately, the lower part of the back, particularly the lumbar-sacral area, may be subjected to excessive stresses that may lead to the **low back pain syndrome,** characterized by dull, aching pain in the lumbar region and occasional bursts of sharp pain when certain movements of the low back area are performed. Low back pain is one of the most common chronic health problems in the United States. It accounts for over 25 percent of all injuries and nearly 40 percent of all workmen's compensation claims, costing American industry billions of dollars yearly in compensation and medical expenses. Research has also revealed that nearly 25 percent of physically fit college students have experienced low back pain. One of the goals of *Healthy People 2000* is to reduce disability from chronic disabling diseases, such as low back pain, by exercising to increase muscular strength and endurance and flexibility.

There are a number of causes of low back pain, including structural deformities and direct trauma to the spinal column. However, the usual cause of low back injury is mechanical trauma due to improper lifting techniques, lifting too heavy a load, or improper posture. Recent research suggests that most back problems are due to seemingly insignificant activities like bending over to pick up a pencil or some light object. Such movements may place excessive stresses upon the spinal column, leading to a tear in soft tissues such as the muscles or ligaments or damage to one of the joints. The most common damage appears to be to the capsule in the joint between several of the processes, or facets, of the vertebra (joint B in fig. 11.12) known as the facet syndrome. With very heavy loads and in older individuals, the cartilage disc may be damaged. In this latter situation, the outer surface of the disc ruptures and exerts pressure on nerves in the

Labels on figure (b): Vas deferens, Epididymis, Possible problem

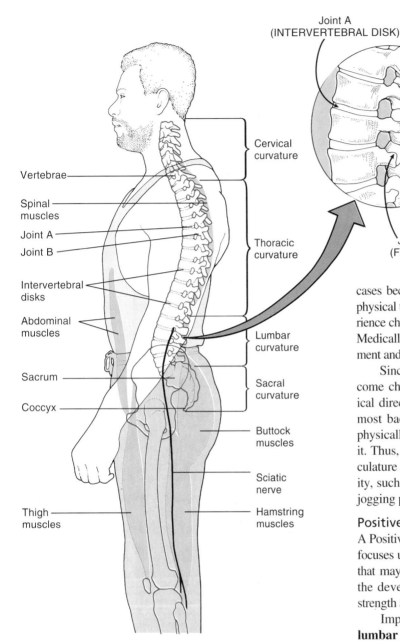

Joint A
(INTERVERTEBRAL DISK)

Cervical
curvature

Vertebrae

Spinal
muscles

Joint A

Joint B

Intervertebral
disks

Abdominal
muscles

Thoracic
curvature

Sacrum

Coccyx

Lumbar
curvature

Sacral
curvature

Buttock
muscles

Sciatic
nerve

Thigh
muscles

Hamstring
muscles

Spinal vertebrae

Joint B
(FACETS)

Figure 11.12 *Lateral view of the spine. Among the five segments of the spine, the cervical region curves forward in the neck area, the thoracic backward in the upper back, and the lumbar forward in the low back region. A disc of fibrocartilage, the intervertebral disc, is located between each of the vertebrae in the spinal column.*

vicinity, usually the sciatic nerve, a condition referred to as sciatica, pain radiating anywhere from the lower back through the buttocks to the calf.

You're not as young as you used to be when your back goes out more than you do; there is greater likelihood of experiencing low back pain as one gets older. After the age of thirty, the vertebral discs begin to lose some of their elasticity and become more prone to injury. It is a fact that over 80 percent of the population will experience low back pain at some time in their lives. Fortunately, in most cases, especially in the young, a few days of rest may relieve the pain completely. Most cases of back pain resolve in 1 to 2 weeks by themselves. However, other

cases become chronic and require medical services, including physical therapy and analgesic drugs for pain relief. If you experience chronic low back pain, a medical examination is in order. Medically oriented back clinics provide comprehensive treatment and prevention programs.

Since low back injury can be quite disabling and may become chronic, preventive techniques are important. A medical director of a back injury research project suggested that most back problems occur because the back has not been physically conditioned for the amount of work people put on it. Thus, a sedentary life-style may predispose the back musculature and ligaments to weakness so that any physical activity, such as lifting objects, chopping wood, or even starting a jogging program, may result in the low back pain syndrome.

Positive Health Life-Style

A Positive Health Life-style to help prevent low back problems focuses upon two areas. The first is the avoidance of behaviors that may increase the risk of back injury, while the second is the development of physical fitness, particularly muscular strength and endurance, flexibility, and proper weight control.

Improper posture may contribute to the development of **lumbar lordosis,** a condition, described as hollow back, in which there is an increased forward curvature, or hyperextension, in the lower back region. Although the body does have a natural forward curve in the lumbar region, it may become excessive and predispose one to low back pain or injury. You may recall in chapter 5 that muscles and ligaments are elastic, and if stretched or shortened consistently, they may become either longer or shorter, respectively. Thus, constant backward slumping while sitting, slouching while standing for long periods of time, or sleeping on the stomach may stretch the abdominal muscles and tighten the lower back muscles, resulting in an increase in the lumbar curve. Be conscious of your posture. Sit properly with good support for the lower back, occasionally stretching as illustrated in figure 11.13. Shift your weight occasionally while standing, contracting your abdominal muscles (tucking your tummy) to help flatten out your lower back. Sleep on your side with your knees curled up, somewhat like a tuck position. These actions may help prevent lumbar lordosis.

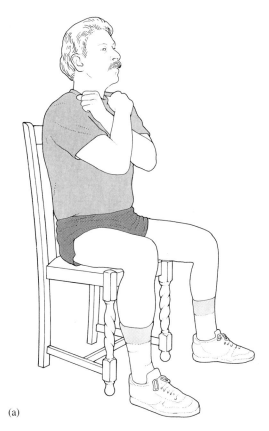

(a)

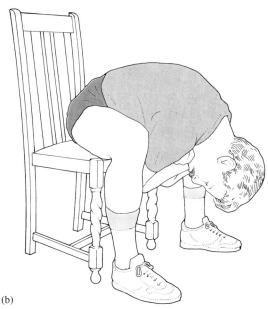

(b)

Figure 11.13 *A sitting exercise to stretch the muscles in the lower back region. (a) Fold your arms across your chest and (b) slowly lower the elbows down between the knees. Hold for 15–60 seconds. Come back up slowly.*

Avoiding various movements and using proper lifting techniques are also recommended behaviors to prevent low back pain. Clinical research supports the following suggestions.

1. Avoid rapid hyperextension movements that will suddenly increase lumbar lordosis, such as that depicted in figure 11.14.

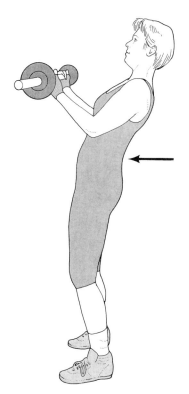

Figure 11.14 *Lumbar lordosis. Lumbar lordosis, or hollow back, is a position in which the normal curve in the lower portion of the back increases toward the front of the body. Any type of movement that causes increased curvature in the lumbar spine region (arrow) may be a causative factor of low back pain.*

2. Do not bend over quickly to touch your toes or to pick up an object while your knees are straight. This action may create tremendous pressure in the lumbar region, primarily when stopping rapidly as you touch your toes and when you begin to straighten up.

3. Keep your back relatively straight, or with a slight lumbar curve, when lifting objects. Tuck your chin, pull your shoulders back slightly, push your chest out a little, and tighten your abdominal muscles. These actions will help lock your lower back. Do not bend at the waist. Grasp the object firmly. Use your leg muscles to lift. It is not necessary to go to a full squat position, but you should avoid the stoop position as much as possible. Use a modified squat style as shown in figure 11.15.

4. When lifting objects, keep them as close to the body as possible. The farther the object is in front of you, the greater the stress on the lower back when lifting. See figure 11.16 for the rationale.

5. Do not attempt to lift or carry objects that are too heavy for you. A sudden shift of the weight may place an excessive stress on the lower back area. You may wish to wear a protective custom-fitted lumbar support or weight belt if you do a lot of lifting.

Although there is no absolute proof that a certain amount of strength is needed to prevent low back pain, or that exercise training will help you recover faster, a proper exercise program is theorized to be sound preventive medicine because it may

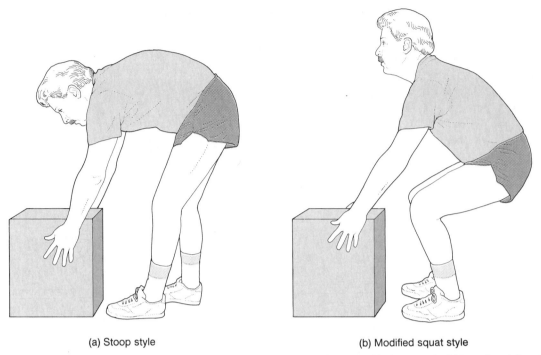

(a) Stoop style   (b) Modified squat style

Figure 11.15 *Methods of lifting. The stoop style (a) should be avoided. A modified squat style (b) is preferred, keeping the back as straight as possible or with a slight lumbar curve.*

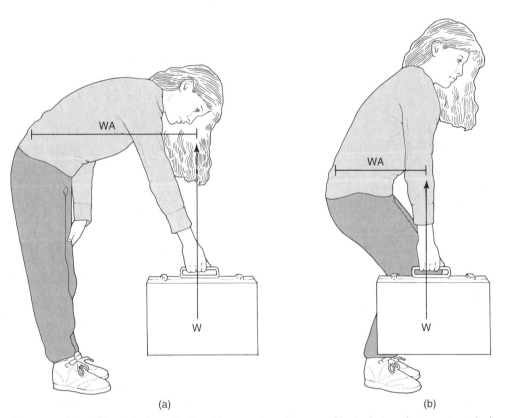

(a)   (b)

Figure 11.16 *Lifting techniques. Position (a) represents an improper lifting technique that may stress the ligaments and muscles of the back, putting excessive stress on the lower lumbar region. The total resistance is equal to the product of the weight (W) times the weight area (WA), which is the perpendicular distance from the weight to the lower lumbar joints. Position (b) minimizes the weight arm and thus decreases the total resistance that needs to be overcome.*

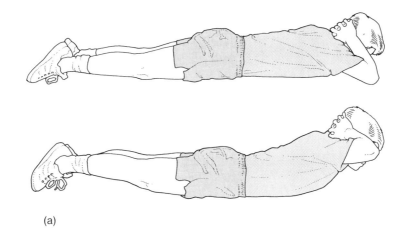

(a)

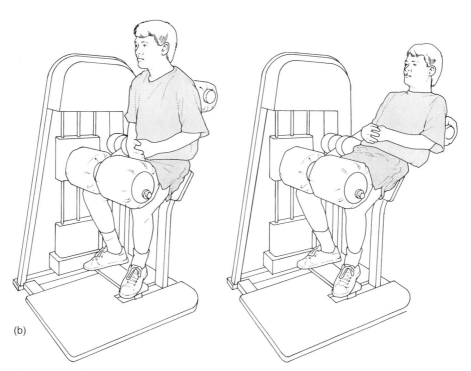

(b)

Figure 11.17 *Exercises to strengthen extensor muscles of the lower back. (a) Lie on a mat or padded surface. Keep your pelvis on the floor and hyperextend your back slowly. Hold the up position for 2 to 3 seconds. Repeat eight to twelve times. (b) Start in the up position and extend the back against the padded resistance. Set the resistance on the machine so that you may do eight to twelve repetitions. Follow the principles of resistance training discussed in chapter 4.*

help prevent an initial injury or recurrences. Some studies have indicated that exercise training may decrease back complaints and the intensity of back pain. Four specific components appear to be especially important.

1. The abdominal muscles must be strengthened. As noted in chapter 4, these muscles help pull up on the pelvic bone, thus rotating it backward and helping to flatten out the lower back. A strong set of abdominals will help prevent sagging of the lower back. Exercises to increase the strength and endurance of these muscles were presented in chapter 4. Use Laboratory Inventory 4.3 to evaluate the fitness of your abdominal muscles.

2. The flexibility of the lower back muscles and hamstrings should be increased. Tightened musculature and ligaments in these areas may contribute to the development of low back problems. A variety of exercises to increase the flexibility of the soft tissues in this region were presented in chapter 5. Laboratory Inventory 5.1 provides you with an assessment of lower back and hamstring flexibility.

3. The back extensor muscles must be strengthened. Figure 11.17 illustrates two exercises to increase the strength of the extensors in the lumbar region of the back. Because these exercises involve extension or

hyperextension of the lower back, do them slowly and avoid the sensation of pain. For the mat exercise, keep your pelvis on the floor and hyperextend your back slowly, holding the up position for 2 to 3 seconds. Repeat eight to twelve times. You may set the resistance on the machine so that you may do eight to twelve repetitions, following the principles of resistance training discussed in chapter 4.

4. Excess body fat will also place a stress on the lower back since much of the fat is normally deposited in the abdominal region, contributing to the development of lumbar lordosis. Proper weight control through diet and exercise, as covered in chapter 7, is an important consideration in the prevention of low back pain.

Osteoporosis

Osteoporosis is a disorder characterized by increased thinness and fragility of the bone structure resulting from a decreased bone density, mainly because calcium is lost from the bones faster than it is replaced. It usually occurs in older individuals, particularly women, and is associated with an increased susceptibility to bone fractures. Recent estimates suggest osteoporosis (see figure 11.18) is responsible for over 1.5 million fractures per year, including more than a half million spine fractures and a quarter million hip fractures. Such events seriously impair the quality of life in otherwise healthy people.

The major cause of osteoporosis appears to be a deficiency of estrogen, for an inescapable conclusion supported by research is that decreases in estrogen levels lead to bone loss. Bone loss may occur in women of all ages due to low estrogen levels. For example, young female athletes who become amenorrheic may experience premature bone loss; the role of estrogen relative to bone formation under such circumstances was discussed on page 227 in chapter 10. Surgical removal of the ovaries at a young age may also lead to an estrogen deficiency.

However, osteoporosis is a major health problem primarily for older women, particularly those over the age of fifty, the average age of menopause. More than 60 percent of women between ages fifty-five to sixty-four have osteoporosis, and the percentage is even higher in older age groups. Although age, gender, and low levels of estrogen are three primary risk factors, others include a family history of osteoporosis, race (white or oriental), leanness, and early menopause. Secondary, or contributing, risk factors include calcium deficiency, a sedentary life-style, smoking, excessive alcohol intake, and certain medications.

Positive Health Life-Style

Even though osteoporosis is a problem associated with age, those who have a lower bone mass to begin with will be at greater risk at menopause. Indeed, the most important factor determining the risk of osteoporosis is the peak bone mass at menopause. Thus, the key to treatment of osteoporosis is prevention. Young women need to develop peak bone mass, the optimal amount within genetic limitations, prior to age twenty-five, and attempt to keep the bone mass high in the

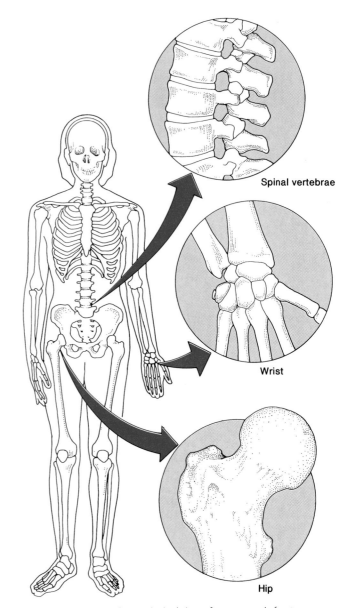

Figure 11.18 *Three principal sites of osteoporosis fractures.*

advancing years. Thus, it would appear prudent for young women to develop a lifetime exercise program and obtain the RDA for calcium in the diet. The earlier the better.

Calcium intake should be adequate, averaging about 1,200 milligrams per day in childhood through age twenty-five, 1,000 milligrams or higher per day during adulthood, and possibly 1,200–1,500 milligrams for postmenopausal women. Dairy products represent the major source of calcium in the American diet; one glass of milk or its equivalent contains about 300 milligrams. Other foods rich in calcium are the dark-green, leafy vegetables. Additional information on calcium intake may be found in chapter 6. Women who do not consume dairy products may need calcium supplements.

Calcium supplements come in a variety of forms, such as calcium carbonate, calcium lactate, and calcium gluconate, and are found in certain antacids, such as Tums. The bioavailability may vary considerably according to the brand, and there is speculation that antacids may actually interfere with calcium absorption. Be sure to check the label for the calcium content per tablet, which may range from 50–600 milligrams depending on the brand. For those who desire to take a calcium supplement, it may be wise to take a tablet with about 200 milligrams at meals three times a day, rather than one tablet with 600 milligrams, for it appears that more calcium is absorbed when the intake is spread throughout the day. Moreover, when the supplement is combined with meals, gastric acidity and slower transit time in the gut promote calcium absorption. Daily supplementation of 600 milligrams calcium, combined with a dietary intake of 500–600 milligrams, should provide adequate calcium nutrition for most individuals. However, the point should be stressed that careful selection of foods will provide the calcium you need from the daily diet, thus eliminating the need for supplements.

Although supplements up to 600 milligrams per day do not appear to pose much danger, excessive amounts may contribute to abnormal heart contractions, constipation, and the development of kidney stones in susceptible individuals, particularly those with a family history of kidney problems. Moreover, excessive dietary calcium may interfere with the absorption of other key minerals, notably iron and zinc. The National Research Council recommends against supplementation to a total much above the RDA.

Exercise, particularly weight-bearing exercise such as jogging, aerobic walking, or aerobic dancing, may not only help to maintain normal bone mass, but may actually increase the bone-mineral content in body segments that are exercised, such as the spine and hip region. In its recent position stand on osteoporosis and exercise, the American College of Sports Medicine concluded that weight-bearing physical activity is essential for the normal development and maintenance of a healthy skeleton. Exercises that are not weight bearing, such as swimming and bicycling, may not be as effective. Resistance training is also highly recommended. Epidemiological research has shown that female bodybuilders have greater bone mass compared to endurance athletes, and some experimental research has shown gains in bone mass following a weight-training program. However, with any exercise program, adequate calcium intake appears to help maximize gains in bone mass during the years of bone growth to optimize peak bone mass. Following menopause, exercise may help to maintain bone mass, but does not appear to reverse bone loss. Exercise training may also help the elderly maintain balance and experience fewer falls, the major cause of bone fractures in the aged.

It is important to reiterate that excessive exercise and other behaviors associated with eating disorders, as discussed in chapter 10, may actually lead to loss of bone mass and contribute to the premature development of osteoporosis.

As noted in chapter 10, the use of hormone replacement therapy, usually estrogen, or other pharmaceuticals that help prevent bone loss is very important in the prevention of osteoporosis and can effectively interact with adequate calcium intake and exercise to help maintain bone integrity, particularly during prolonged amenorrhea or after menopause. For women who are estrogen deficient and want to prevent osteoporosis, estrogen therapy is a must. Although exercise and diet may complement hormone replacement therapy, they are not substitutes for it. The need for such therapy should be determined in consultation with an appropriate physician since there may be some medical problems associated with excess estrogen.

Cigarette smoking and excess alcohol intake may interfere with estrogen and calcium metabolism, so cessation of smoking and the use of alcohol in moderation will eliminate two risk factors for osteoporosis. Helpful guidelines have been presented in chapter 9.

It is important to realize that these preventive measures associated with a Positive Health Life-style need to begin early and be continued throughout life for optimal bone development. However, even if they are not implemented until later in life (even at age sixty to seventy), they may still help to maintain bone density or at least help to decrease the rate of bone loss.

Arthritis

A *joint* is located wherever two bones come together in the body. There are a number of different types of joints, but most are of the diarthrodial (moving) type. A typical joint (fig. 11.19) is surrounded by a synovial membrane that secretes a lubricant (synovial fluid) to help reduce friction in the joint. The ends of the bones are covered with cartilage, which serves to provide a smoother surface and, as a result, creates less friction.

Arthritis, translated literally, means inflammation of the joint, but the term is used to cover a number of different conditions (over one-hundred) that cause pain in the joints. Over thirty million Americans experience some form of arthritis serious enough to necessitate medical care. An extensive discussion of the various forms of arthritis is beyond the scope of this book, but the two major types are highlighted in relation to the Positive Health Life-style.

Rheumatoid arthritis is the most serious form and may cause crippling. It may occur at any age (even in children) and may affect almost all body tissues. It affects more women than men. The disease causes inflammation in the synovial lining surrounding the joint. The inflammation may eventually invade and destroy the cartilage, increasing friction within the joint and causing pain. The cause of rheumatoid arthritis is still a mystery, but infection and a malfunctioning immune system in the body are two current theories. There is no known cure, although certain medications may help control the disease. For individuals who develop rheumatoid arthritis, proper exercise is recommended therapy. Most of the damage to the joint from rheumatoid arthritis occurs in the first year or two, so many physicians are using new drugs, such as Rheumatrex, that may arrest rheumatic fever before significant damage is done.

Osteoarthritis, the most common form of arthritis, usually occurs later in life. Nearly forty million people have osteoarthritis. There are basically two forms. *Primary osteoarthritis* occurs without any apparent cause, usually appears in women, and

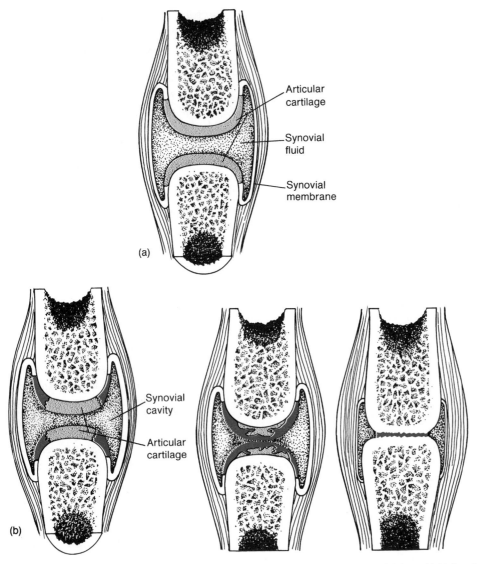

Figure 11.19 *Structure of a joint. (a) A simplified schematic of a typical diarthrodial (movable) joint. (b) The onset of arthritis and the progressive destruction of the articular cartilage.*

affects the smaller joints. *Secondary osteoarthritis* may result from excessive wear and tear, or mechanical stress, of a joint. It usually affects the weight-bearing joints such as the knee and hip. The cartilage in the joint simply wears out, creating increased friction and pain. No cure for osteoarthritis exists and damage done cannot be undone, but the disease process may be controlled with medication, such as anti-inflammatory agents, and a rest-exercise rehabilitation program.

Positive Health Life-Style

Exercise appears to be the one component of the Positive Health Life-style that may be helpful to the individual with arthritis. In most cases, exercises are prescribed by a physician and may be done either with the help of a physical therapist or by the individual alone. Although exercise training may confer some benefits to patients with either rheumatoid arthritis or osteoarthritis, research indicates not all will benefit. Exercise programs need to be individualized. The major purpose of the

exercise program is to maintain or increase the current range-of-motion or flexibility of the joint without increased pain levels. The exercises are specific to the joint that is affected.

Resistance training is important to increase the strength of the muscles around the joints. Isometric, isotonic, and isokinetic training programs may be used, as described in chapter 4. Figure 11.20 depicts an isometric exercise for the muscles that extend the knee, and similar isometric exercises may be done to strengthen specific muscle groups any time of the day.

Aerobic exercise programs adhering to the American College of Sports Medicine standards are appropriate for arthritic patients. Walking is an appropriate exercise for most individuals if not painful, but smooth, low-impact, non-weight bearing activities, such as cycling, skating, cross-country skiing, and rowing may also be enjoyable and effective. Exercise in water is excellent therapy, for the buoyancy effect reduces the stress on the joints to help make exercising almost painless. Warm water also helps to relax the muscles.

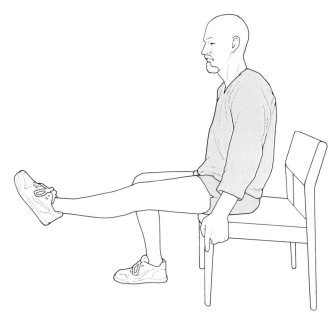

Figure 11.20 *Isometric exercise to increase strength of the muscles affecting the knee joint. Isometric exercises may be used almost any time of the day to increase the strength of nearly any muscle group in the body. Isometrics may be particularly helpful to arthritics because limited movement of the joint occurs. In this case, the muscles should be contracted isometrically for 5 to 10 seconds, and repeated eight to twelve times. This exercise, as well as others, may be done several times per day.*

Some, but not all, research has revealed that rheumatoid arthritic patients may exercise aerobically more intensely than previously believed. They may increase their cardiovascular fitness while decreasing their perceived pain level, with no increase in joint inflammation. Moreover, other research has revealed that exercise training may decrease the progression of destructive changes within the joints of individuals with rheumatoid arthritis. For arthritic individuals, a properly designed exercise program may or may not alleviate stiffness, pain, or swollen joints, but it will improve aerobic capacity, strength, muscle function and, just as important, psychological well-being.

A question is often raised concerning the possibility that habitual exercise programs may contribute to the development of osteoarthritis because of an increased rate of wear and tear. There is clear evidence that athletes or others involved in physical work may develop arthritis specific to a joint that is stressed repeatedly in their sports or work, particularly so if it is injured at one time or another. Baseball pitchers may have problems with their elbows; football players may have problems with their knees; ballet dancers may have problems with their ankles; and carpenters may have problems with their wrists and hands.

However, several studies have indicated that osteoarthritis is not an inevitable consequence of long-term training, either resistance training or aerobic endurance training such as running, if exercise is conducted comfortably within a normal range of motion. A radiological (X-ray) study of the upper and lower limbs of experienced weight lifters revealed significant degenerative changes in 20 percent of those investigated, but the percentage was no different from that found in the general population for that age group. This suggests that habitual resistance training neither increases nor decreases the possibility of developing osteoarthritis.

In a recent detailed review of studies involving exercise and osteoarthritis, Panush concluded that runners without underlying biomechanical problems of the lower extremities do not develop osteoarthritis at a rate any different from nonrunners. Furthermore, a study of Finnish runners also revealed that primary osteoarthritis of the hip joint was slightly less in the runners as compared to a control group. These investigators noted that the physical strain to which runners' hips are exposed does not contribute to the development of osteoarthritis. They suggested that rhythmical compression and release of the joint cavity by the running motion stimulates the flow of synovial fluid and benefits the nutrition of the joint cartilage.

Based upon recent reviews of the available evidence, it would appear that normal, habitual exercise does not accelerate the development of osteoarthritis. However, joints that are excessively stressed and injured may be more prone to become arthritic. Whether the legion of individuals who are physically active now will be more likely to develop arthritis later in life remains to be seen, since we have very little data at this point. Given some conflicting data from radiographic studies, Panush indicates that long-term, high-intensity, high-mileage running perhaps should not be entirely dismissed as a potential risk factor for premature osteoarthritis. It seems, however, that the increased risk is minimal compared with the other benefits of habitual exercise, and exercise may actually improve joint health.

Summary

Leroy (Satchel) Paige, the venerable major league baseball player who seemed to pitch forever, was once asked by a reporter how old he was, and he replied with a question: "How old would you be if you didn't know how old you was?" Chronologically, we get older every day; it is unavoidable. If we smoke, live a sedentary life-style, do not eat properly, drink alcohol in excess, and experience high levels of stress, we will also age faster physiologically every day, becoming not only old, but fat, weak, and ill as well. We may have a chronological age of thirty, but a functional age of sixty. To paraphrase Satchel, we will be older than we really are.

Although we can do nothing about our chronological age, we may be able to maintain a younger functional age by adopting a Positive Health Life-style. The information in this and preceding chapters has presented you with the essential knowledge concerning the design and implementation of programs that constitute a Positive Health Life-style and the health benefits that result from such programs to enhance the quality and quantity of your life. To reap the maximal benefits, a Positive Health Life-style needs to be lifelong. Although you may have already implemented some healthy changes in your life, such as starting to exercise, the hardest part is to maintain these changes over your lifetime. Adherence to a Positive Health Life-style is the focus of the next chapter.

References

Books

American Alliance for Health, Physical Education, Recreation and Dance. 1988. *Physical best.* Reston, Va.:AAHPERD.

Arthritis Foundation. 1981. *Arthritis. The basic facts.* Atlanta: The Arthritis Foundation.

Bouchard, C., et al., eds. 1994. *Physical activity, fitness, and health.* Champaign, Ill.: Human Kinetics.

Cooper, K. 1988. *Controlling cholesterol.* New York: Bantam Books.

Fries, J., and L. Crapo. 1981. *Vitality and aging.* San Francisco: W. H. Freeman.

Hochschuler, S. 1991. *Back in shape.* Boston: Houghton Mifflin.

Mackinnon, L. 1992. *Exercise and immunology.* Champaign, Ill.: Human Kinetics.

National Institute of Health. National Heart, Lung, and Blood Institute. 1993. *The fifth report of the Joint National Committee on Detection, Evaluation, and Treatment of High Blood Pressure.* Bethesda, Md.: National Institutes of Health, Number 93-1008.

National Research Council. 1989. *Diet and health: Implications for reducing chronic disease risk.* Washington, D.C.: National Academy Press.

Nuland, S. 1995. *How we die.* New York: Vintage Books.

Rowland, T. 1990. *Exercise and children's health.* Champaign, Ill.: Human Kinetics.

Schatz, M. 1992. *Back care basics: A doctor's gentle yoga program for back and neck pain relief.* Berkeley, Calif.: Rodale Press.

United States Department of Health and Human Services. Public Health Service. 1991. *Healthy people 2000: National health promotion and disease prevention objectives.* Washington D.C.: U.S. Government Printing Office.

Reviews

Allegrante, J., et al. 1993. Walking education program for patients with osteoarthritis of the knee: Theory and intervention strategies. *Health Education Quarterly* 20:63–81.

Allen, S. 1993. Primary osteoporosis. Methods to combat bone loss that accompanies aging. *Postgraduate Medicine* 93:43–50.

American College of Sports Medicine. 1993. American College of Sports Medicine. Position Stand. Physical activity, physical fitness, and hypertension. *Medicine and Science in Sports and Exercise* 25 (10): i–x.

American College of Sports Medicine. 1994. American College of Sports Medicine. Position Stand. Exercise for patients with coronary artery disease. *Medicine and Science in Sports and Exercise* 26 (3): i–v.

American College of Sports Medicine. 1995. ACSM position stand on osteoporosis and exercise. *Medicine and Science in Sport and Exercise.* 27: in press.

Anderson, J., and J. Metz. 1993. Contributions of dietary calcium and physical activity to primary prevention of osteoporosis in females. *Journal of the American College of Nutrition* 12: 378–83.

Arakawa, K. 1993. Hypertension and exercise. *Clinical and Experimental Hypertension* 15:1171–79.

Assmann, G., et al. 1993. High density lipoproteins, reverse transport of cholesterol, and coronary artery disease. *Circulation* 87:III-34.

Atkinson, M., and N. Maclaren. 1990. What causes diabetes? *Scientific American* 263:62–71.

Ausman, L., and B. Russell. 1994. Nutrition in the elderly. In *Modern nutrition in health and disease,* eds. M. Shils, et al. Philadelphia: Lea & Febiger.

Badimon, J., et al. 1993. Coronary atherosclerosis. A multifactorial disease. *Circulation* 87 (Supplement II):II-3–II-16.

Barnard, R. J. Physical activity and claudication. In *Physical activity, fitness, and health,* eds. C. Bouchard, et al. Champaign, Ill.: Human Kinetics.

Berg, A., et al. 1994. Physical activity and lipoprotein lipid disorders. *Sports Medicine* 17:6–21.

Biering-Sorenson, F., et al. 1994. Physical activity, fitness, and back pain. In *Physical activity, fitness, and health,* eds. C. Bouchard, et al. Champaign, Ill.: Human Kinetics.

Birge, S. 1993. Osteoporosis and hip fracture. *Clinics in Geriatric Medicine* 9:69–86.

Bjorntorp, P. 1992. Abdominal obesity and the metabolic syndrome. *Annals of Medicine* 24:465–68.

Blair, S. 1993. 1993 C. H. McCloy Research Lecture: Physical activity, physical fitness, and health. *Research Quarterly for Exercise and Sport* 64:365–76.

Boulware, D., and S. Byrd. 1993. Optimizing exercise programs for arthritis patients. *Physician and Sportsmedicine* 21 (April):104–18.

Brown, B., et al., 1993. Lipid lowering and plaque regression. New insights into prevention of plaque disruption and clinical events in coronary disease. *Circulation* 87:1781–89.

Brown, W. 1994. Lipoprotein disorders in diabetes mellitus. *Medical Clinics of North America* 78:143–61.

Cartee, G. 1994. Aging skeletal muscle: Response to exercise. *Exercise and Sport Sciences Review* 22:91–120.

Caspersen, C. 1987. Physical inactivity and coronary heart disease. *Physician and Sportsmedicine* 15 (November): 43–44.

Cavenee, W., and R. White. 1995. The genetic basis of cancer. *Scientific American* 272 (March): 72–79.

Chestnut, C. 1989. Is osteoporosis a pediatric disease? Peak bone mass attainment in the adolescent female. *Public Health Reports* 104 (Supplement): 50–54.

Cohen, L. 1987. Diet and cancer. *Scientific American* 257 (November): 42–48.

Consumers Union. 1992. Is reducing your cholesterol harmful? *Consumer Reports on Health* 4:81–93.

Consumers Union. 1993. Does exercise fight cancer? *Consumer Reports on Health* 5:12–13.

Consumers Union. 1994. Detecting breast cancer early: Still the best hope. *Consumer Reports on Health* 6:61–63.

Consumers Union. 1994. Does exercise prevent heart attacks—or cause them? *Consumer Reports on Health* 6:133–35.

Consumers Union. 1995. Cutting cholesterol: More vital than ever. *Consumer Reports on Health* 7:3–15.

Crastes de Paulet, A. 1990. Free radicals and aging. *Annales de Biologie Clinique* 48:323–30.

Curb, J., et al. 1990. Effective aging. *Journal of the American Geriatrics Society* 38:827–28.

Curfman, G. 1993. The health benefits of exercise. *New England Journal of Medicine* 328:574–76.

Daley, M., and B. Berman. 1993. Rehabilitation of the elderly patient with arthritis. *Clinics in Geriatric Medicine* 9:783–801.

DeMarco, T., and K. Sidney. 1989. Enhancing children's participation in physical activity. *Journal of School Health* 59:337–40.

Drinkwater, B. 1994. Physical activity, fitness, and osteoporosis. In *Physical activity, fitness, and health,* eds. C. Bouchard, et al. Champaign, Ill.: Human Kinetics.

Durstine, J. L., and W. Haskell. 1994. Effects of exercise training on plasma lipids and lipoproteins. *Exercise and Sport Sciences Reviews* 22:477–521.

Egg Nutrition Center. 1994. Apo A-IV-2 gene protective against high cholesterol diet. *Nutrition Close-Up* 11 (3):1–2.

Eichner, E. 1987. Exercise, lymphokines, calories, and cancer. *Physician and Sportsmedicine* 15 (June): 109–18.

Eisman, J., et al. 1993. Peak bone mass and osteoporosis prevention. *Osteoporosis International* 3:56–60.

Ekdahl, C. 1990. Muscle function in rheumatoid arthritis. Assessment and training. *Scandinavian Journal of Rheumatology Supplement* 86:9–61.

Epstein, F. 1993. Strategies for primary coronary heart disease prevention. *Cor et Vasa* 35:16–19.

Ershow, A., and S. Skarlatos. 1993. Diet and risk factors for coronary heart disease: An update. *Contemporary Nutrition* 18 (1):1–2.

Evans, W. 1992. Exercise, nutrition, and aging. *Journal of Nutrition* 122 (3 Supplement): 796–801.

Fagard, R., and C. Tipton. 1994. Physical activity, fitness, and hypertension. In *Physical activity, fitness, and health* eds. C. Bouchard, et al. Champaign, Ill.: Human Kinetics.

Fentem, P. 1992. Exercise in prevention of disease. *British Medical Bulletin* 48: 630–50.

Fitzgerald, B., and G. McLatchie. 1980. Degenerative joint disease in weightlifters. Fact or fiction. *British Journal of Sports Medicine* 14: 97–101.

Fletcher, G., et al. 1992. Statement on exercise. Benefits and recommendations for physical activity programs for all Americans. *Circulation* 86:340–44.

Freudenheim, J., and S. Graham. 1989. Toward a dietary prevention of cancer. *Epidemiologic Reviews* 11:229–35.

Friedman, R. (Ed.) 1988. Caffeine update: The news is mostly good. *University of California, Berkeley Wellness Letter* 4 (July): 4–5.

Gilmer, H., et al. 1993. Lumbar disk disease: Pathophysiology, management and prevention. *American Family Physician* 47: 1141–52.

Grieve, D. 1977. The dynamics of lifting. *Exercise and Sports Science Review* 5: 157–79.

Gudat, U., et al. 1994. Physical activity, fitness and non-insulin-dependent (Type II) diabetes mellitus. In *Physical activity, fitness, and health,* eds. C. Bouchard, et al. Champaign, Ill.: Human Kinetics.

Hagberg, J. 1994. Physical activity, fitness, health, and aging. In *Physical activity, fitness, and health,* eds. C. Bouchard, et al. Champaign, Ill.: Human Kinetics.

Haskell, W. 1994. Health consequences of physical activity: Understanding and challenges regarding dose-response. *Medicine and Science in Sports and Exercise* 26:649–60.

Haskell, W. 1995. Physical activity in the prevention and management of coronary heart disease. *Physical Activity and Fitness Research Digest* 2(1):1–8.

Hoffman, D. 1993. Arthritis and exercise. *Primary Care* 20: 895–910.

Hoffman-Goetz, L. 1994. Exercise, natural immunity, and tumor metastasis. *Medicine and Science in Sports and Exercise* 26:157–63.

Horton, E. 1991. Exercise and decreased risk of NIDDM. *New England Journal of Medicine* 325:196–98.

Houston, M. 1992. Exercise and hypertension. Maximizing the benefits in patients receiving drug therapy. *Postgraduate Medicine* 92:139–44, 150.

Ike, R., et al. 1989. Arthritis and aerobic exercise: A review. *Physician and Sportsmedicine* 17:128–39.

Jacobs, D., et al. 1992. Report of the conference on low blood cholesterol: Mortality associations. *Circulation* 86: 1046–60.

Kahn, C. 1991. Age-reversing drugs. *Longevity* 3 (January): 39–52.

Kriska, A., et al. 1994. The potential role of physical activity in the prevention of non-insulin-dependent diabetes mellitus: The epidemiological evidence. *Exercise and Sport Sciences Reviews* 22:121–43.

Kritchevsky, D. 1990. Nutrition and breast cancer. *Cancer* 66:1321–25.

Kushner, R. 1993. Body weight and mortality. *Nutrition Reviews* 51: 127–36.

LaRosa, J. 1990. At what levels of total low- or high-density lipoprotein cholesterol should diet/drug therapy be initiated? United States guidelines. *American Journal of Cardiology* 65: 7F–10F.

Leaf, D. 1990. Overweight: Assessment and management issues. *American Family Physician* 42:653–60.

Lee, I-M. 1994. Physical activity, fitness, and cancer. In *Physical activity, fitness, and health,* eds. C. Bouchard, et al. Champaign, Ill.: Human Kinetics.

Lee, I-M. 1995. Physical activity and cancer. *Physical Activity and Fitness Research Digest* 2(2):1–8

Levine, D., et al. 1993. Behavior changes and the prevention of high blood pressure. Workshop II. *Circulation* 88: 1387–90.

Liebman, B. 1995. Dodging cancer with diet. *Nutrition Action Health Letter* 22 (January/February): 4–7.

Massie, M. 1992. To combat hypertension, increase activity. *Physician and Sportsmedicine* 20 (May): 88–111.

Mazzeo, R. 1994. The influence of exercise and aging on immune function. *Medicine and Science in Sports and Exercise* 26:586–92.

Mera, S. 1993. Atherosclerosis and coronary heart disease. *British Journal of Biomedical Sciences* 50:235–48.

Micheli, L. 1993. How I manage low-back pain in athletes. *Physician and Sportsmedicine* 21 (March): 183–94.

Miller, N. 1990. Raising high density lipoprotein cholesterol: The biochemical pharmacology of reverse cholesterol transport. *Biochemical Pharmacology* 40:403–10.

Montgomery, A. 1988. Cholesterol tests: How accurate are they? *Nutrition Action Health Letter* 15 (May): 4–7.

Moore, S. 1994. Physical activity, fitness, and atherosclerosis. In *Physical activity, fitness, and health,* eds. C. Bouchard, et al. Champaign, Ill.: Human Kinetics.

Morris, C., and V. Froelicher. 1993. Cardiovascular benefits of improved exercise capacity. *Sports Medicine* 16: 225–36.

Morris, J. 1994. Exercise in the prevention of coronary heart disease: Today's best buy in public health. *Medicine and Science in Sports and Exercise* 26: 807–14.

Munnings, F. 1993. Strength training. Not only for the young. *Physician and Sportsmedicine* 21 (April): 133–40.

Newsholme, E., and M. Parry-Billings. 1994. Effects of exercise on the immune system. In *Physical activity, fitness, and health,* eds. C. Bouchard, et al. Champaign, Ill.: Human Kinetics.

Niewoehner, C. 1993. Osteoporosis in men. Is it more common than we think? *Postgraduate Medicine* 93:59–70.

Olshansky, S., et al. 1990. In search of Methuselah: Estimating the upper limits to human longevity. *Science* 250:634–40.

Paffenbarger, R. 1994. 40 years of progress: Physical activity, health and fitness. In *American College of Sports Medicine—40th Anniversary Lectures* Indianapolis, Ind.: ACSM.

Panush, R. 1994. Physical activity, fitness, and osteoarthritis. In *Physical activity, fitness, and health,* eds. C. Bouchard, et al. Champaign, Ill.: Human Kinetics.

Pascale, M., and W. Grana. 1989. Does running cause osteoarthritis? *Physician and Sportsmedicine* 17 (March): 157–66.

Patterson, J., and K. Adams, Jr. 1993. Pathophysiology of heart failure. *Pharmacotherapy* 13:73S–81S.

Perls, T. 1995. The oldest old. *Scientific American* 272 (January): 70–76.

Plowman, S. 1992. Physical activity, physical fitness, and low back pain. *Exercise and Sport Sciences Reviews* 20:221–42.

Plowman, S. 1993. Physical fitness and healthy low back function. *Physical Activity and Fitness Research Digest* 1(3):1–8.

Poehlman, E., et al. 1994. Endurance exercise in aging humans: Effects on energy metabolism. *Exercise and Sport Sciences Reviews* 22:251–54.

Pope, M. 1989. Risk indicators in low back pain. *Annals of Medicine* 21:387–92.

Potter, J. 1993. Colon cancer—do the nutritional epidemiology, the gut physiology and the molecular biology tell the same story? *Journal of Nutrition* 123:418–23.

Public Health Service. 1987. Summary of findings from National Children and Youth Fitness Study II. *Journal of Physical Education, Recreation, and Dance* 58 (November–December): 49–96.

Public Health Service. 1993. Public health focus: Physical activity and the prevention of coronary heart disease. *Morbidity and Mortality Weekly Report* 42:669–72.

Quinn, S. 1993. Diabetes and diet. We are still learning. *Medical Clinics of North America* 77:773–82.

Radack, K., and R. Wyderski. 1990. Conservative management of intermittent claudication. *Annals of Internal Medicine* 113:135–46.

Ravussin, E., et al. 1993. Risk factors for the development of obesity. *Annals of the New York Academy of Sciences* 683:141–50.

Riggs, B. 1990. A new option for treating osteoporosis. *New England Journal of Medicine* 323:124–25.

Rimmer, J. 1990. Flexibility and strength exercises for persons with arthritis. *Clinical Kinesiology* 44:90–96.

Robison, J., et al. 1993. Obesity, weight loss, and health. *Journal of the American Dietetic Association* 93:445–49.

Rooney, E. 1993. Exercise for older patients: Why it's worth your effort. *Geriatrics* 48 (November): 68–77.

Rosenson, R. 1993. Low levels of high-density lipoprotein cholesterol (hypoalphalipoproteinemia). An approach to management. *Archives of Internal Medicine* 153:1528–38.

Rothenberg, R., and J. Koplan. 1990. Chronic disease in the 1990s. *Annual Review of Public Health* 11:267–96.

Safer, M. 1990. Aging and its effects on the cardiovascular system. *Drugs* 39 (Supplement 1): 1–8.

Samples, P. 1990. Exercise encouraged for people with arthritis. *Physician and Sportsmedicine* 18 (January): 123–27.

Sasco, A. 1992. Tobacco and cancer: How to react to the evidence. *European Journal of Cancer Prevention* 1:367–73.

Schwartz, C., et al. 1993. A modern view of atherogenesis. *American Journal of Cardiology* 71:9B–14B.

Sharkey, B. 1987. Functional vs chronologic age. *Medicine and Science in Sports and Exercise* 19:174–78.

Shephard, R. 1993. Exercise and aging: Extending independence in older adults. *Geriatrics* 48:61–64.

Shephard, R. 1993. Exercise in the prevention and treatment of cancer. An update. *Sports Medicine* 15:258–80.

Sherman, C. 1994. Reversing heart disease. Are lifestyle changes enough? *Physician and Sportsmedicine* 22 (January): 91–95.

Simons-Morton, B., et al. 1987. Children and fitness; a public health perspective. *Research Quarterly for Exercise and Sport* 58:295–303.

Simopoulos, A. 1990. The relationship between diet and hypertension. *Comprehensive Therapy* 16:25–30.

Soukup, J., and J. Kovaleski. 1993. A review of the effects of resistance training for individuals with diabetes mellitus. *Diabetes Education* 19:307–12.

Stallone, D. 1994. The influence of obesity and its treatment on the immune system. *Nutrition Reviews* 52:37–50.

Sternfeld, B. 1992. Cancer and the protective effect of physical activity: The epidemiological evidence. *Medicine and Science in Sports and Exercise* 24:1195–1209.

Stevenson, J. 1990. Pathogenesis, prevention, and treatment of osteoporosis. *Obstetrics and Gynecology* 75 (Supplement 4): 36S–41S.

St Jeor, S. 1993. The role of weight management in the health of women. *Journal of the American Dietetic Association* 93:1007–12.

Stokes, J. 1990. Cardiovascular risk factors. *Cardiovascular Clinics* 20:3–20.

Tal, A. 1993. Oral hypoglycemic agents in the treatment of type II diabetes. *American Family Physician* 48:1089–95.

Tanji, J. 1990. Hypertension Part 1: How exercise helps. *Physician and Sportsmedicine* 18 (July): 77–82.

Tanji, J. 1990. Hypertension Part 2: The role of medication. *Physician and Sportsmedicine* 18 (August): 87–91.

Tate, C., et al. 1994. Mechanisms for the responses of cardiac muscle to physical activity in old age. *Medicine and Science in Sports and Exercise* 26: 561–67.

Tipton, C. 1991. Exercise, training, and hypertension: An update. *Exercise and Sport Sciences Reviews* 19:447–505.

Trachtenbarg, D. 1990. Treatment of osteoporosis. What is the role of calcium? *Postgraduate Medicine* 87: 263–66.

Van Itallie, T., and A. Simopoulos. 1993. Summary of the national obesity and weight control symposium. *Nutrition Today* 28 (July/August): 33–35.

Weinerman, S., and R. Bockman. 1990. Medical therapy of osteoporosis. *Orthopedic Clinics of North America* 21:109–24.

Woods, J., and J. M. Davis. 1994. Exercise, monocyte/macrophage function, and cancer. *Medicine and Science in Sports and Exercise* 26:147–57.

Wood, P. 1994. Physical activity, diet and health: Independent and interactive effects. *Medicine and Science in Sports and Exercise* 26:838–43.

World Hypertension League. 1993. Nonpharmacological interventions as an adjunct to the pharmacological treatment of hypertension: A statement by WHL. *Journal of Human Hypertension* 7:159–64.

Yeater, R., and I. Ullrich. 1992. Hypertension and exercise. Where do we stand? *Postgraduate Medicine* 91: 429–36.

Young, J. 1995. Exercise prescription for individuals with metabolic disorders. *Sports Medicine* 19:43–54.

Young, J., and N. Ruderman. 1993. Exercise and metabolic disorders. In *Principles of exercise biochemistry,* ed. J. Poortmans. Basel, Switzerland: Karger.

Zierath, J., and H. Wallberg-Henriksson. 1992. Exercise training in obese diabetic patients. *Sports Medicine* 14: 171–89.

Zivin, J., and D. Choi. 1991. Stroke therapy. *Scientific American* 265: 56–63.

Specific Studies

Aoyagi, Y., and S. Katsuta. 1990. Relationship between the starting age of training and physical fitness in old age. *Canadian Journal of Sport Sciences* 15:65–71.

Ballard-Barbash, R., et al. 1990. Physical activity and risk of large bowel cancer in the Framingham Study. *Cancer Research* 50:3610–13.

Cohen, L., et al. 1992. Voluntary exercise and experimental mammary cancer. *Advances in Experimental Medicine and Biology* 322:41–59.

Dalsky, G., et al. 1988. Weight-bearing exercise training and lumbar bone mineral content in postmenopausal women. *Annals of Internal Medicine* 108:824–28.

Davis, D., et al. 1994. Decreasing cardiovascular disease and increasing cancer among whites in the United States from 1973 through 1987. Good news and bad news. *Journal of the American Medical Association* 271:431–37.

Faas, A., et al. 1993. A randomized, placebo-controlled trial of exercise therapy in patients with acute low back pain. *Spine* 18:1388–95.

Fiatarone, M., et al, 1990. High-intensity strength training in nonagenarians: Effects on skeletal muscle. *Journal of the American Medical Association* 263:3029–34.

Folsom, A., et al. 1993. Body fat distribution and 5-year risk of death in older women. *Journal of the American Medical Association* 269:483–87.

Frisch, R., et al. 1987. Lower lifetime occurrence of breast cancer and cancers of the reproductive system among former college athletes. *International Journal of Fertility* 32:217–25.

Gemmell, H., and B. Jacobson. 1990. Incidence of sacroiliac joint dysfunction and low back pain in fit college students. *Journal of Manipulative and Physiological Therapeutics* 13:63–67.

Gleeson, P., et al. 1990. Effects of weight lifting on bone mineral density in premenopausal women. *Journal of Bone and Mineral Research* 5:153–58.

Granhed, H., et al. 1987. The loads on the lumber spine during extreme weight lifting. *Spine* 12:146–49.

Graves, J., et al. 1994. Pelvic stabilization during resistance training: Its effect on the development of lumbar extension strength. *Archives of Physical and Medical Rehabilitation* 75:210–15.

Grove, K., and B. Londeree. 1992. Bone density in postmenopausal women: High impact vs low impact exercise. *Medicine and Science in Sports and Exercise* 24:1190–94.

Gundewall, B., et al. 1993. Primary prevention of back symptoms and absence from work. A prospective randomized study among hospital employees. *Spine* 18:587–94.

Gutin, B., et al. 1990. Blood pressure, fitness, and fatness in 5- and 6-year-old children. *Journal of the American Medical Association* 264:1123–27.

Hagberg, J. 1987. Effect of training on the decline of VO_{2MAX} with aging. *Federation Proceedings* 46:1830–33.

Hansen, T., et al. 1993. Long term physical training in rheumatoid arthritis. A randomized trial with different training programs and blinded observers. *Scandinavian Journal of Rheumatology* 22:107–12.

Harris, T., et al. 1992. The low cholesterol-mortality association in a national cohort. *Journal of Clinical Epidemiology* 45:595–601.

Hart, D., et al. 1987. Effect of lumbar posture on lifting. *Spine* 12:138–45.

Hebert, L., and G. Miller. 1987. Newer heavy load lifting methods help firms reduce back injuries. *Occupational Health and Safety* 56:57–60.

Heinrich, C., et al. 1990. Bone mineral content of cyclically menstruating female resistance and endurance trained athletes. *Medicine and Science in Sports and Exercise* 22:558–63.

Helmrich, S., et al. 1991. Physical activity and reduced occurrence of non-insulin-dependent diabetes mellitus. *New England Journal of Medicine* 325:147–52.

Hiatt, W., et al. 1990. Benefit of exercise conditioning for patients with peripheral arterial disease. *Circulation* 81:602–9.

Hull, S., et al. 1994. Exercise training confers anticipatory protection from sudden death during acute myocardial ischemia. *Circulation* 89:548–52.

Hunt, S., et al. 1990. Health related behavior in hypertension. *Journal of Human Hypertension* 4:49–52.

Jarvikoski, A., et al. 1993. Outcome of two multimodal back treatment programs with and without intensive physical training. *Journal of Spinal Disorders* 6:93–98.

Kasch, F., et al. 1988. A longitudinal study of cardiovascular stability in active men aged 45 to 65 years. *Physician and Sportsmedicine* 16 (January): 117–25.

Kasch, F., et al. 1993. Effect of exercise on cardiovascular ageing. *Age and Ageing* 22:5–10.

Kavanagh, T., and R. Shephard. 1990. Can regular sports participation slow the aging process? Data on Masters athletes. *Physician and Sportsmedicine* 18 (June): 94–104.

Kusaka, Y., et al. 1992. Healthy lifestyles are associated with higher natural killer cell activity. *Preventive Medicine* 21:602–15.

LaCroix, A., et al. 1993. Maintaining mobility in late life. II. Smoking, alcohol consumption, physical activity, and body mass index. *American Journal of Epidemiology* 137:858–69.

Lane, N., et al. 1990. Running, osteoarthritis, and bone density: Initial 2-year longitudinal study. *American Journal of Medicine* 88:452–59.

Lee, I-M., et al. 1993. Body weight and mortality. A 27-year follow-up of middle-aged men. *Journal of the American Medical Association* 270:2823–28.

Minor, M., et al. 1989. Efficacy of physical conditioning exercise in patients with rheumatoid arthritis and osteoarthritis. *Arthritis and Rheumatism* 32:1396–1405.

Moy, C., et al. 1993. Insulin-dependent diabetes mellitus, physical activity, and death. *American Journal of Epidemiology* 137:74–81.

Nieman, D., et al. 1993. Physical activity and immune function in elderly women. *Medicine and Science in Sports and Exercise* 25:823–31.

Oberman, A., et al. 1990. Pharmacologic and nutritional treatment of mild hypertension: Changes in cardiovascular risk status. *Annals of Internal Medicine* 112:89–95.

Ornish, D., et al. 1990. Can lifestyle changes reverse coronary heart disease? The Lifestyle Heart Trial. *Lancet* 336:129–33.

Paffenbarger, R., et al. 1986. Physical activity, all-cause mortality, and longevity of college alumni. *New England Journal of Medicine* 314:605–13.

Prasad, K., and J. Kalra. 1993. Oxygen free radicals and hypercholesterolemic atherosclerosis: Effect of vitamin E. *American Heart Journal* 125:958–73.

Pukkala, E., et al. 1993. Life-long physical activity and cancer risk among Finnish female teachers. *European Journal of Cancer Prevention* 2:369–76.

Richter, E., et al. 1992. Metabolic responses to exercise. Effects of endurance training and implications for diabetes. *Diabetes Care* 15:1767–76.

Roberston, G., et al. 1993. Effects of exercise on total and segmental colon transit. *Journal of Clinical Gastroenterology* 16:300–303.

Rudman, D., et al. 1990. Effects of human growth hormone in men over 60 years old. *New England Journal of Medicine* 323:1–5.

Sale, D., et al. 1994. Effect of training on the blood pressure response to weight lifting. *Canadian Journal of Applied Physiology* 19:60–74.

Sarna, S., et al. 1993. Increased life expectancy of world class male athletes. *Medicine and Science in Sports and Exercise* 25:237–44.

Sellers, T., et al. 1993. Association of body fat distribution and family histories of breast and ovarian cancer with risk of postmenopausal breast cancer. *American Journal of Epidemiology* 138:799–803.

Shinton, R., and G. Sagar. 1993. Lifelong exercise and stroke. *British Medical Journal* 307:231–34.

Snow-Harter, C., et al. 1990. Muscle strength as a predictor of bone mineral density in young women. *Journal of Bone and Mineral Research* 5:589–95.

Somers, V., et al. 1991. Effects of endurance training on baroreflex sensitivity and blood pressure in borderline hypertension. *Lancet* 337:1363–68.

Tilyard, M., et al. 1992. Treatment of postmenopausal osteoporosis with calcitriol or calcium. *New England Journal of Medicine* 326:357–62.

Wynd, C. 1992. Relaxation imagery used for stress reduction in the prevention of smoking relapse. *Journal of Advanced Nursing* 17:294–302.

Young, D., et al. 1993. Associations between changes in physical activity and risk factors for coronary heart disease in a community based sample of men and women: The Stanford Five-City Project. *American Journal of Epidemiology* 138:205–16.

12

STAYING WITH THE POSITIVE HEALTH LIFE-STYLE

Key Terms

adherence
positive addiction
relapse

Key Concepts

- Health behaviors that constitute a Positive Health Life-style should be practiced for a lifetime to provide you with maximum benefits.

- Adherence is the ability to stick with your positive health behavior changes, not just for several months in a college course, but for a lifetime.

- One of the most important factors in adherence to the Positive Health Life-style is your attitude; you should try to develop a positive addiction to various health behaviors.

- Setting reasonably difficult goals and objectives and successfully attaining them through a planned program will help enhance your self-esteem and improve your chances of adherence.

- If you do suffer a relapse, such as reverting to a sedentary life-style because of an injury, review the principles in the appropriate chapter and establish new goals and objectives to help restore your Positive Health Life-style to normal.

- Although you may successfully implement healthful behavioral changes on your own, social support from family, friends, and the community help to foster adherence to such behavior changes.

- Commercial health/fitness clubs and weight loss centers may help some individuals initiate and continue with exercise or weight loss programs, but the quality of such programs may vary. Be sure to investigate the qualifications and suitability of the staff, facilities, equipment, and management of such commercial programs before joining.

INTRODUCTION

At the beginning of this course, you completed The Health Life-style Assessment Inventory (Laboratory Inventory 1.1) in order to evaluate your health behaviors in a variety of areas that may impact upon your health, such as exercise, nutrition, and smoking status. One purpose for taking this inventory was to identify those behaviors that may exert a positive impact upon your health. A concomitant purpose was to alert you to possible negative health behaviors that increase your risk of experiencing various health problems now and in the future. The purpose of your college course, then, was to help reaffirm the value of your positive health behaviors, such as not smoking, and to provide you with appropriate knowledge and skills to help you implement more positive health behaviors, such as eating a healthful diet.

In conjunction with your college course, the focus of this text has been on the development of a set of health behaviors supported by medical science that may enhance the quality, and possibly the quantity, of your life. You may not have covered all of the preceding chapters in this text because of time constraints, but if you have, you should possess the knowledge and skills to implement positive health behaviors such as the following:

1. Exercise properly for development of aerobic fitness, muscular strength and endurance, and flexibility
2. Eat healthful foods
3. Maintain a healthful body weight
4. Manage stress through recommended stress-reduction techniques
5. Abstain from cigarette smoking
6. Abstain from or use moderation in alcohol consumption
7. Avoid use of illegal drugs
8. Practice healthful sex behaviors

At this point it might be of interest to you to retake The Health Life-style Assessment Inventory and compare the findings with your initial inventory in order to see what changes you have made as a result of taking this college course. If not part of your course requirements, you may also wish to repeat several of the laboratory inventories, such as The Rockport Fitness Walking Test (Inventory 3.5), in order to assess fitness changes following several months of aerobic exercise training. By retaking some of the laboratory inventories, you will probably find that you have made several positive health behavior changes and also have improved your health or fitness status.

In chapter 1 we talked about behavioral change; proper knowledge may change your attitude about a certain behavior, which may then lead to behavioral changes. Subsequent chapters then provided information to help you initiate behavioral changes consistent with the Positive Health Life-style. Although the focus of this book has been on behavioral changes to enhance wellness, it is important to note that wellness is not simply a collection of behaviors, but a life-style, an internalized feeling that you will do all you possibly can to optimize your health status. In order to maximize the health benefits of the Positive Health Life-style, it must be lifelong.

In general, initiating a positive health behavior change is not difficult, and this college course may have helped you initiate several such behavioral changes. However, maintaining behavioral changes may be difficult for some individuals, who may slip back to previous unhealthy behaviors. For example, many individuals have made resolutions at one time or another to start exercising to improve their fitness level or to lose some excess body fat. In the beginning, they may have implemented an exercise program with great enthusiasm and expectations. Unfortunately, for a number of reasons such as lack of time, they may lose this initial enthusiasm and resume a sedentary life-style. More than 50 percent of the people who start to exercise quit within 6 months, and even a greater proportion of individuals do not maintain weight loss or smoking cessation within 6 months of beginning such programs.

The purpose of this brief chapter is to discuss recommendations that will help you maximize your chances to adhere to the Positive Health Life-style. The major focus will be on exercise adherence, primarily because exercise may be the key positive health behavior, as it may have a positive impact on other health behaviors such as weight control and stress management ∎

Adherence

In relation to the Positive Health Life-style, **adherence** is the ability to stick with your positive health behavior changes, not just for several months in a college course, but for a lifetime. Although adherence to a behavioral change may depend on the particular behavior (e.g., different factors may influence adherence to an exercise program versus staying cigarette free), several general factors will maximize your chances to adhere to behaviors consistent with a Positive Health Life-style.

Because exercise is so important, researchers have looked at reasons that people stop exercising. The most-cited reasons include lack of time and facilities, inconvenience, boredom, injury, and lack of results. Smoking cessation is also a very important behavior change, and research has found that individuals resume smoking for several reasons, including adverse effects associated with nicotine withdrawal, stress, and weight gain. Similar reasons may exist relative to the discontinuance of other positive health behaviors. These reasons are not insurmountable obstacles and do not have to occur. For example, those who desire to stop smoking may use nicotine patches to alleviate the effects of nicotine withdrawal, relaxation techniques to help reduce stress, and an appropriate diet and exercise program to counteract weight gain.

Researchers have also looked at factors that help enhance adherence to a Positive Health Life-style, particularly exercise. The following points may help you stick with the various behaviors of the Positive Health Life-style by helping you get through the hard times. Although most of these points are directed at exercise, they may be applied to other life-style changes, such as dieting, smoking cessation, and weight control.

Attitude

One of the most important factors in adherence to the Positive Health Life-style is your attitude. Although most of you should now possess the information to know why a Positive Health Life-style is good for you, you need to develop a personal health ethic and a related set of positive health behaviors that will maximize the health of your mind and body, and you need to practice these behaviors daily until you develop a deeply ingrained attitude and commitment to such a life-style.

Think of it as a **positive addiction,** the formation of a habit that has positive, not negative, effects on your health. Develop a positive addiction to exercise, to healthful eating, to reduction of stress, and to other health behaviors that minimize risks to your physical and mental well-being. However, as noted in chapters 8 and 10, beware of becoming overzealous, because health behaviors that generally are regarded to be beneficial, such as exercise and losing excess body fat, may actually lead to impaired health if they lead to a negative addiction, such as exercising excessively or developing an obsession for thinness and an associated eating disorder.

One of the key determinants of your attitude is your degree of self-motivation, often referred to as your will power or self-control. Laboratory Inventory 12.1 enables you to obtain a brief assessment of your self-motivation level. Possibly the initial motivation for you to start exercising was this college course. Your motivation may possibly have been extrinsic; that is, your instructor may have motivated you to exercise in order to obtain a desirable grade. Although extrinsic motivation may be useful to help us initiate and continue with an exercise program for a short time, the motivation needs to be internalized in order to enhance the possibility of maintaining an exercise program for a lifetime. For some, exercising to lose body fat helps provide a personal sense of purpose to exercise, and may improve adherence if they feel exercise is an important behavior to maintain their desirable body appearance. They have developed a sense of intrinsic motivation. You need to develop an intrinsic sense of motivation that the Positive Health Life-style is one of the most important principles underlying your everyday activities. Your adherence to exercise and other positive life-style behaviors will be reinforced if you experience the perceived benefits, such as increased energy levels, improved mood, less stress, improved body image, better sleep, and possibly even an enhanced sexuality, all benefits that can enhance the quality of your life and help you develop a sense of intrinsic motivation.

A positive addiction will help you persevere through the hard times. The "no pain, no gain" theory of exercise may have some application to training for sports competition, but it is not applicable to health-related fitness training. Exercise does not have to hurt or be painful to give you health benefits. However, although ease and enjoyment of your exercise choice is important, there are times when exercise may encroach upon your time, be inconvenient, or seem like hard work. During these times, it is important to use your positive addiction to overcome barriers to exercise. By working through the hard times, you are laying the groundwork for a lifetime program.

Self-Efficacy and Self-Esteem

As discussed in chapter 1, one very important determinant of behavior change is self-efficacy, or self-confidence, your belief that you can accomplish the goals and objectives that you establish for yourself. The Self-Efficacy Potential for Health Behavior Change (Laboratory Inventory 1.2) taken at the beginning of the course provided you with an opportunity to assess your potential for making positive health behavior changes and may be a useful tool to evaluate yourself periodically.

A feeling of high self-esteem has been associated with high levels of adherence. One of the important determinants of enhanced self-esteem is success, and as you continue with the Positive Health Life-style you will observe various changes, such as a favorable change in body composition, that will enhance your body image and self-esteem. But in order to achieve success through attainment of your goals and objectives, they must be reasonable and attainable.

Planning Goals and Objectives

Remember, nothing breeds success like success. To be successful in achieving some goals, such as losing 50 pounds of body fat, may take considerable time, so you need to plan intermediate objectives which may serve as markers for success as you move towards your ultimate goal. Also remember, no initial objective is too small and no subsequent increase in objectives is too small in pursuit of your final goal. In making health behavior changes, you may receive advice and consultation from others, such as your course instructor, but it is important that you set your own goals and objectives. As part of this college course you may have established certain goals and objectives for yourself. Your ultimate goal may have been to jog 3 miles nonstop, but you may have established a number of smaller, more achievable short-term objectives, such as jogging 1 mile, in pursuit of your long-range goal.

You should establish daily, weekly, or monthly goals relative to the various components of your Positive Health Life-style. In some cases, you may establish daily objectives, such as eating a vegetarian diet for one day. In other cases, you may wish to set weekly goals, such as jogging 20 miles in one week, or monthly goals, such as losing 4 pounds. If you like competition, compete with yourself to achieve your objectives or goals. Whatever the case, you need to develop reasonably difficult objectives that are attainable and that provide you with the opportunity for success. Chapters 3 to 9 should have provided you with the necessary information to make an informed decision on establishment of reasonable objectives and goals in each of the major health promotion areas.

Part of your planning for exercise should also include a definite time and place. Set aside a definite time and place to exercise. Use time-management procedures, establishing a routine for exercise just as you do with other facets of your life. Try to foresee barriers to exercise. If you find that a change in your daily schedule may disrupt your planned exercise time or location, develop alternate plans. Your positive addiction towards exercise may help here, possibly motivating you to rise an hour earlier to give you the time, or finding three 10-minute periods during the day for brisk walks. Do exercise along with other daily activities. For example, walk briskly with your dog or watch the evening news while pedalling your stationary bicycle in the den. Be creative! Make exercise one of the most important parts of your daily schedule.

Record Keeping

Write a contract specifying your goals and objectives. You may sign it yourself or have a family member or colleague sign it with you. Keep a record of your daily activities and progress. Keeping a log of your daily workout may be useful for a variety of reasons. For one, it will help you evaluate your progress. Also, it may be a clue to the onset of an injury. For example, you may note that a rapid increase in your weekly running mileage is associated with sore, tender calf muscles. Information was presented in earlier chapters to help you establish a proper exercise program to meet your objectives while helping you avoid common injuries.

You should also periodically evaluate your progress toward or maintenance of various health behavior objectives and goals, because such evaluations may be used to see if you have achieved your objectives and to modify them accordingly. Retake the appropriate tests, such as The Rockport Fitness Walking Test (Laboratory Inventory 3.5), step test to monitor your heart rate as discussed in Laboratory Inventory 3.4, chapter 3, or the Daily State Anxiety Inventory discussed in Laboratory Inventory 8.1, chapter 8, to help you maintain a Positive Health Life-style.

Reward System

Another factor that will help you achieve your goals and objectives is a reward system. Set up a reward system for yourself to help reinforce your positive health behaviors. For example, treat yourself to a banana split or some other delicacy after you have completed one of your objectives for the week. Even though you may be on a diet to lose weight, a Positive Health Life-style does not mean total abstinence from all of life's pleasures. Although certain nutritional practices are important in weight-loss programs, occasional deviations are not harmful. For someone who is exercising and dieting to lose weight, a favorite food may be an appropriate reward. You may devise your own reward system for various health behavior changes you undertake.

Relapse Prevention

When undergoing most health behavior changes, there are often occasional lapses, or slips, such as significantly exceeding your caloric intake or missing exercise for several days. Such lapses may be caused by a variety of events, including changes in your daily schedule. For example, you may have a hectic business trip with numerous luncheon and dinner meetings and little chance to exercise. Lapses are generally temporary, but it is important to prevent a lapse in your program towards your health goal from becoming a **relapse**, i.e., slipping back to previous unhealthy behaviors such as a sedentary life-style or obesity. Relapses may be caused by a variety of factors, but the chances of relapse may be lessened by careful planning. For example, let's look at your choice of exercise. You may choose from a wide variety of exercises that will enhance your aerobic fitness or help you lose excess body fat. You should choose those that are fun or that bring you joy or a sense of satisfaction. You should also select a variety of exercises, so if for one reason or another you are unable to perform your desired exercise, such as swimming, you may be able to substitute another, such as running.

Relapses often occur during periods when you may feel depressed. Using an appropriate stress-management technique presented in chapter 8 may be a sound preventive approach.

If you suffer a simple relapse, such as eating a whole pack of cookies while on a diet, put the episode behind you and get back on your daily program. No one is perfect, and we all make mistakes or lose self-control occasionally. If you suffer a more prolonged relapse, simply reset your goals. Use the guidelines in the specific chapter to help you get back on the program and restore your Positive Health Life-style to normal.

Social Environment

With appropriate knowledge, you may initiate many of the health behavior changes discussed in this book, such as exercise, weight loss, smoking cessation, and stress management, by yourself without assistance from others. However, one of the key elements for adherence to any health behavior change is appropriate social support, such as that offered by your family, friends, and professionals in the community.

For many individuals, exercise is usually more enjoyable if done with others. Finding a partner to exercise with may help you both commit to a daily exercise program, while joining a running, cycling, or health club will help you develop friendships with others who have similar exercise and health interests. Involve other members of your family in exercise; it will help give you some quality family time. For some individuals in programs such as weight control, smoking cessation, and substance abuse, professional social support may be essential to guarantee adherence and provide formal relapse prevention training.

Most communities have a variety of public and private organizations that may provide appropriate support for various health behavior changes or for individuals with specific health problems. Your local telephone book, both the white and yellow pages, may provide you with local contacts. In the white pages, simply look under health agencies for your local city government listing, or for a specific agency, such as the American Cancer Society or American Heart Association for a listing of local affiliates. In the yellow pages look under health/fitness facilities for local health clubs; look under social service organizations for a variety of health-related programs.

Health/Fitness Clubs and Commercial Weight-Loss Centers

Some individuals need the social atmosphere and/or facilities and equipment of an exercise spa or aerobic dance class to motivate them to exercise or lose weight. Since the fitness boom began, hundreds of new companies have developed, both nationally and locally, in attempts to capitalize financially on America's increased interest in physical fitness. Today, we have centers specializing in aerobics to music, such as aerobic dancing or Jazzercise®, which advertise improved aerobic fitness through fun exercise; we have weight-training programs with highly sophisticated and expensive equipment, which advertise the development of strength and cardiovascular endurance; we have numerous weight-reduction spas, or salons, which advertise quick and easy weight loss; and we even have the no-exercise exercise spas, which advertise that motorized tables will do our exercises for us while we simply lie there.

The American College of Sports Medicine has estimated that 10 million individuals now exercise at health/fitness facilities, that another 50 million may join during the 1990s, and the weight loss industry is a billion dollar business. These health/fitness clubs and commercial weight control centers may provide a social atmosphere or social support, but they may vary greatly in cost and quality.

If you desire to join a health/fitness club, the American College of Sports Medicine has developed a brochure to provide you with information to help you make an informed decision. You may request a copy of the *ACSM Health Fitness Facility Consumer Selection Guide* by writing to the ACSM National Center at P.O. Box 1440, Indianapolis, Ind., 46206–1440. The following are some of the key points.

1. The staff should have an appropriate educational background and certification from a nationally recognized professional organization, such as the American College of Sports Medicine or the Aerobic and Fitness Association of America. They should check your medical status, be able to evaluate your current fitness level, help you plan an appropriate exercise program, establish goals and objectives, and evaluate your progress.

2. The facility should have enough space, adequate and safe equipment, and specific programs to meet your exercise needs, and should be open at times convenient to your daily schedule. The facility should also be a member of a nationally recognized professional organization, such as the Association for Fitness in Business.

3. Hopefully, you should be able to obtain a trial membership or guest pass in order to evaluate the facility and its staff before joining. Check the facility for crowding at your normal exercise time. You should also have access to written materials describing the programs and associated costs of joining. Be wary of long-term contracts and high pressure sale techniques.

4. You should contact the local Better Business Bureau or similar organization for information to determine the reputation of the company and its management.

You should also investigate the quality of commercial weight loss programs before enrolling in one. The weight loss industry is a billion dollar business, and such programs may be very costly to join, in some cases running into thousands of dollars. Unfortunately, there is little governmental control over many of these programs, but many of the national programs have recently been cited by the Federal Trade Commission for false advertising claims. Although some programs may be well-designed, others may not provide appropriate programs for safe and effective long-term weight loss.

If you want to enroll in a commercial weight loss program, what do authorities recommend you should receive for your money? Some of the considerations are similar to those for evaluating health/fitness facilities. The following points are summarized from the report of a task force to establish weight loss guidelines for the state of Michigan. Free copies of the full report, Toward Safe Weight Loss, may be obtained from The Center for Health Promotion, Michigan Department of Public Health, P.O. Box 30195, Lansing, Mich., 48909.

1. The staff should be well-trained in their specialty, preferably having appropriate educational backgrounds, such as a physician, nurse, dietician, or exercise physiologist.

2. You should receive a medical screening, verifying you have no medical or psychological condition that might be exacerbated by weight loss through dieting or exercise. All risks of the program should be identified, and you should sign an informed consent form.

3. A reasonable weight goal should be established given your weight history and the rate of weight loss, after the first two weeks, should not exceed two pounds per week. You should receive an individualized treatment plan based on your weight loss goal, and the program should include a nutrition education program that stresses permanent life-style changes in your eating habits, an appropriate diet and exercise program, and behavior modification techniques.

4. The diet should be one that:
   a. Contains no less than 1,000 Calories per day
   b. Is between 10–30 percent fat Calories
   c. Has at least 100 grams of carbohydrate per day
   d. Should provide at least 100 percent of the RDA; supplements, if used, should not exceed 100 percent of the RDA
   e. If under medical supervision, 600 Calories and 50 grams of carbohydrate per day are minimal levels

5. Aerobic exercise should follow appropriate standards relative to mode, intensity, duration, and frequency, and should be an exercise program you can live with for a lifetime.

6. There should be a weight maintenance phase in the program once you have achieved your weight loss goal. This should be a high priority to help you maintain your healthy body weight.

Summary

A Positive Health Life-style does not have to be boring and ascetic. If it did, most people would not want to adhere to it for a lifetime. You do not have to abstain completely from premium ice cream, prime rib, alcohol, or a variety of other pleasures you enjoy, because a Positive Health Life-style is compatible with most of the pleasures of life in proper moderation.

In order for the health behaviors that constitute a Positive Health Life-style to be effective and to serve as personal preventive medicine, they must be lifelong. An old

Chinese proverb notes that a journey of 1,000 miles begins with a single step. So too, a Positive Health Life-style may begin with that first jogging or aerobic walking step. Make such a personal choice and commitment now. Your body and mind will thank you for years to come. Hopefully, you will become an ambassador for such a life-style and spread the word to your family and friends, and in particular to the youth of the world. To quote John Locke, "A sound mind in a sound body is a short but full description of a happy state in the world."

References

Books

American College of Sports Medicine. 1992. *ASCM's Health/fitness standards and guidelines.* Champaign, Ill.: Human Kinetics.

Blair, S. 1991. *Living with exercise.* Dallas: American Health Publishing Company.

Bouchard, C., et al. eds. 1994. *Physical activity, fitness, and health.* Champaign, Ill.: Human Kinetics.

Dishman, R. 1988. *Exercise adherence: Its impact on public health.* Champaign, Ill.: Human Kinetics.

Dishman, R. 1994. *Advances in exercise adherence.* Champaign Ill.: Human Kinetics.

United States Department of Health and Human Services. 1986. *Clinical opportunities for smoking intervention.* Washington, D.C.: U.S. Government Printing Office.

Reviews

Carmody, T. 1992. Preventing relapse in the treatment of nicotine addiction: Current issues and future directions. *Journal of Psychoactive Drugs* 24:131–58.

Consumers Union. 1993. How to start an exercise habit you can stick with. *Consumer Reports on Health* 5:69–71.

Dishman, R. 1994. Advances in exercise adherence. Champaign, Ill.: Human Kinetics.

Dishman, R. 1994. Prescribing exercise intensity for healthy adults using perceived exertion. *Medicine and Science in Sports and Exercise* 26:1087–94.

Dishman, R., and J. Sallis. 1994. Determinants and interventions for physical activity and exercise. In *Physical Activity, fitness, and health,* eds. C. Bouchard, et al. Champaign, Ill.: Human Kinetics.

Foreyt, J., and G. Goodrick. 1991. Factors common to successful therapy for the obese patient. *Medicine and Science in Sports and Exercise* 23:292–97.

Hall, S., et al. 1991. Relapse prevention. *NIDA Research Monograph* 106:279–92.

King, A. 1994. Community and public health approaches to the promotion of physical activity. *Medicine and Science in Sports and Exercise* 26:1405–12.

Levin, S. 1993. Does exercise enhance sexuality? *Physician and Sportsmedicine* 21 (March): 199–203.

Mayer, J., Ed. 1991. Pointers for sticking with it. *Tufts University Diet & Nutrition Letter* 9 (September): 6.

Perri, M., et al. 1993. Strategies for improving maintenance of weight loss. Toward a continuous care model of obesity management. *Diabetes Care* 16:200–209.

Sallis, J. 1994. Influences on physical activity of children, adolescents, and adults or determinants of active living. *Physical Activity and Fitness Research Digest* 1 (August): 1–8.

Stamford, B. 1993. Getting off the couch—and staying off. *Physician and Sportsmedicine* 21 (November): 101–2.

Westover, S., and R. Lanyon. 1990. The maintenance of weight loss after behavioral treatment. A review. *Behavior Modification* 14:123–27.

Whitehead, J. 1993. Physical activity and intrinsic motivation. *Physical Activity and Fitness Research Digest* 1 (May): 1–8.

Wichmann, S., and D. Martin. 1992. Exercise excess. Treating patients addicted to fitness. *Physician and Sportsmedicine* 20 (May): 193–200.

Specific Studies

Cohen, S., and E. Lichtenstein. 1990. Perceived stress, quitting smoking, and smoking relapse. *Health Psychology* 9:466–78.

DeBusk, R., et al. 1990. Training effects of long versus short bouts of exercise in healthy subjects. *American Journal of Cardiology* 65:1010–13.

Duncan, T., and E. McAuley. 1993. Social support and efficacy cognitions in exercise adherence: A latent growth curve analysis. *Journal of Behavioral Medicine* 16:199–218.

Gauvin, L. 1990. An experiential perspective on the motivational features of exercise and lifestyle. *Canadian Journal of Sport Sciences* 15:51–58.

Hofstetter, C., et al. 1991. Illness, injury, and correlates of aerobic exercise and walking: A community study. *Research Quarterly for Exercise and Sport* 62:1–9.

Lavery, M., and J. Loewy. 1993. Identifying predictive variables for long-term weight change after participation in a weight loss program. *Journal of the American Dietetic Association* 93:1017–24.

Lynch, D., et al. 1992. Adherence to exercise interventions in the treatment of hypercholesterolemia. *Journal of Behavioral Medicine* 15:365–77.

Marcus, B., et al. 1992. Self-efficacy and the stages of exercise behavior change. *Research Quarterly for Exercise and Sport* 63:60–66.

Marcus, B., and A. Stanton. 1993. Evaluation of relapse prevention and reinforcement interventions to promote exercise adherence in sedentary females. *Research Quarterly for Exercise and Sport* 64:447–52.

McAuley, E. 1993. Self-efficacy and the maintenance of exercise participation in older adults. *Journal of Behavioral Medicine* 16:103–13.

Montgomery, S., and G. Dunbar. 1993. Paroxetine is better than placebo in relapse prevention and the prophylaxis of recurrent depression. *International Clinical Psychopharmacology* 8:189–95.

Pargman, D., and L. Green. 1990. The type A behavior pattern and adherence to a regular running program by adult males ages 25 to 39 years. *Perceptual and Motor Skills* 70:1040–42.

Robison, J., et al. 1992. Effects of a 6-month incentive-based exercise program on adherence and work capacity. *Medicine and Science in Sports and Exercise* 24:85–93.

Spielman, A., et al. 1992. The cost of losing: An analysis of commercial weight-loss programs in a metropolitan area. *Journal of American College of Nutrition* 11:36–41.

Stoffelmayr, B., et al. 1992. A program model to enhance adherence in work-site-based fitness programs. *Journal of Occupational Medicine* 34:156–61.

Wynd, C. 1992. Relaxation imagery used for stress reduction in the prevention of smoking relapse. *Journal of Advanced Nursing* 17:294–302.

1.1
▼▼▼

The Health Life-Style Assessment Inventory

Introduction

The purpose of this inventory of life-styles is to increase your level of awareness of the areas in your life over which you have some control and that have a direct impact on your health.

Awareness does not cause change, but it is a necessary first step. This life-style assessment survey will help you identify behaviors that may affect your health, some positively and some negatively. Use the insights you gain to plan life-style changes that may improve your health.

THIS LABORATORY IS FOR YOUR OWN PERSONAL USE AND EVALUATION. IT NEED NOT BE SUBMITTED TO THE INSTRUCTOR.

Following completion of this laboratory inventory, completion of Laboratory Inventory 1.2 will help you identify those negative health factors that you may have the greatest potential to change.

Directions

Put a check beside each statement that applies to you, unless otherwise noted.

1. Physical Activity/Physical Fitness

_____ I do some form of vigorous exercise for at least 20–30 minutes three times a week or more.

_____ I do exercises that enhance my muscle tone, strength, and endurance two times a week or more.

_____ I use part of my leisure time participating in individual, family, or team physical activities such as gardening, walking, bowling, golf, and baseball at least 30 minutes per day most days of the week.

_____ I don't get fatigued easily while doing physical work.

_____ I would say that my level of physical fitness is higher than that of most of the people in my age group.

2. Eating Habits

_____ In general, I can identify foods that are low in total fat, saturated fat, cholesterol, and sugar, and high in starch and fiber.

_____ I eat a variety of foods each day, such as fruits and vegetables, whole-grain breads and cereals, lean meats, dairy products, dry peas and beans, and nuts and seeds.

_____ I limit the amount of fat, saturated fat, and cholesterol I eat (including fat in meats, eggs, butter, margarine, cream, whole milk, and organ meats such as liver).

_____ I limit the amount of salt I eat by cooking with only small amounts, not adding salt at the table, and avoiding salty snacks and other highly processed foods.

_____ I avoid eating too much sugar, especially frequent snacks of sticky candy or soft drinks.

3. Weight/Body Fat

_____ According to height and weight charts, I am in the average range.

_____ I have not been on a weight-reduction diet in the past year.

_____ There is no place on my body that I can pinch an inch of fat.

_____ I am satisfied with the way my body looks.

_____ None of my family, friends, or health-care professionals has ever urged me to lose weight.

4. Blood Pressure

_____ I have had my blood pressure checked within the last 6 months.

_____ I have never had high blood pressure.

_____ I do not currently have high blood pressure.

_____ I make a conscious effort to avoid salt in my diet.

_____ There is no history of high blood pressure in my family.

With permission of John Cavendish, Ed.D.; and in part, the Public Health Service.

5. Cholesterol Levels

_____ I know my blood cholesterol level.

_____ My total blood cholesterol is less than 200 milligrams.

_____ My LDL cholesterol is less than 130 milligrams.

_____ My total cholesterol:HDL cholesterol level is less than 4:5.

_____ I know how to favorably modify blood cholesterol levels by diet and exercise, or I am aware that my blood cholesterol level is high, and I am undertaking life-style changes to lower it.

6. Stress Control/Personal Relationships

_____ I find it easy to relax and express my feelings freely.

_____ I recognize events or situations likely to be stressful for me and use appropriate stress-reduction techniques.

_____ I have close friends, relatives, or others whom I can talk to about personal matters and call on for help when needed.

_____ I rarely feel tense or nervous.

_____ I participate in group activities, such as church and community organizations, or hobbies that I enjoy.

7. Rest/Sleep

_____ I almost always get between 7 and 9 hours of sleep a night.

_____ I do *not* have trouble falling asleep or waking up.

_____ I wake up few, if any, times during the night.

_____ I feel rested and ready to go when I get up in the morning.

_____ Most days, I have a lot of energy.

8. Car Safety

_____ I always use seat belts when I drive.

_____ I always use seat belts when I am a passenger.

_____ I have not had an automobile accident in the past 3 years.

_____ I have not had a speeding ticket or other moving violation for the past 3 years.

_____ I never ride with a driver who has had more than two drinks.

9. Alcohol Use

_____ I avoid drinking alcoholic beverages (particularly if pregnant), or I drink fewer than two drinks a day.

_____ In the past year, I have not driven an automobile after having more than two drinks.

_____ When I'm under stress, I do not drink more.

_____ I do not do things when I'm drinking that I later regret.

_____ I have not experienced any problem because of my drinking in the past.

10. Tobacco Use

_____ I have never smoked cigarettes. (Score 5 and move to Risky Behaviors below.)

_____ I haven't smoked cigarettes in the past year.

_____ I do not use any other form of tobacco (pipes, cigars, chewing tobacco).

_____ I smoke only low-tar and low-nicotine cigarettes.

_____ I smoke less than one pack of cigarettes a day.

11. Risky Behaviors

_____ I do not abuse prescription drugs.

_____ I do not smoke or use marijuana.

_____ I do not use cocaine or similar drugs.

_____ I do not use anabolic steroids.

_____ I practice safe sex habits.

12. Life Satisfaction

_____ If I had my life to live over, I wouldn't make all that many changes.

_____ I've accomplished most of the things that I've set out to do in my life.

_____ I can't think of an area in my life that really disappoints me.

_____ I am a happy person.

_____ Compared to the people with whom I grew up, I feel I've done as well or better than most of them with my life.

Scoring:

Record the number of checks (from 0 to 5) for each of the twelve areas. Then add up the numbers to determine your total score.

Area	Subscore
Physical Activity/Physical Fitness	1
Eating Habits	2
Weight/Body Fat	0
Blood Pressure	4
Cholesterol Levels	0
Stress Control/Personal Relationships	1
Rest/Sleep	3
Car Safety	3
Alcohol Use	5
Tobacco Use	3
Risky Behaviors	5
Life Satisfaction	2

Total Score = _____ 29 _____

Interpreting Your Score

A score of 48–60	Healthier than average life-style
A score of 30–47	Average life-style
A score of 0–29	Below average: need for improvement ✓
*Scores of less than 3 in any one of the twelve areas	Need for improvement in that area

*Scores of less than 3 in any area may be listed as a negative health factor for Laboratory Inventory 1.2, which will help you identify negative health behaviors that you believe you may be able to change. Also, even though you may have a score of 3 or 4 in an area, one health behavior in that area may be classified as a negative health factor. For example, under the area of Risky Behaviors you may not use any of the drugs listed, but you may not practice safe sex habits which will put you at risk for sexually-transmitted diseases.

1.2 ✓ due monday

▼▼▼

Self-Efficacy Potential for Health Behavior Change

Laboratory Inventory 1.1 is designed to provide you with an awareness of your health-related life-style behaviors. If you rated high (positive health factors) in some of the twelve areas, you may possess a Positive Health Life-style related to those factors and may need to undertake little, if any, action to change. On the other hand, those areas in which you scored low (negative health factors), if modified favorably, may benefit your health. The purpose of this laboratory is to help you identify those negative health behaviors that you may have the greatest potential to change. This laboratory will take some time and critical self-assessment on your part.

First, after completing Laboratory Inventory 1.1, list those areas you feel are positive health factors in your life in the Positive Health Factors column, and those that are negative health factors in the Negative Health Factors column. You may list either an entire category, such as Eating Habits, or just parts of a category, such as consuming too much sugar.

Positive Health Factors	Negative Health Factors	Total SEPCS Score	Priority Ranking
Physical activity/Fitness,	Cholesterol levels	33	3
I limit the amount of fat I eat	eat more fruit veg,	36	2
I am in avg. range for height/	area in my	40	1
Blood Pressure weight	life that dis-		
Stress Control/Personal rel.	appoints me		
Sleep			
I always use seat belts			
Alcohol Use			
Tobacco Use			
I am a happy person			

For each of the Negative Health Factors that you list above, try to determine your potential for change by using the Self-Efficacy Potential for Change Scale (SEPCS) for each negative factor. Respond to each of the ten items in the SEPCS with a numerical value of 0–5 according to how strongly you feel about that item, using the following numerical scale:

Extremely Strong = 5
Very Strong = 4
Strong = 3
Weak = 2
Very Weak = 1
Extremely Weak = 0

Your total score for each Negative Health Factor will range from 0–50. You should calculate the score on a separate sheet of paper for each Negative Health Factor, put that score under the column SEPCS, and then prioritize the scores from high to low. If you have six Negative Health Factors, the one with the highest SEPCS will be the first priority, and the one with the lowest will be the sixth. This priority list will assist you in selecting health behavior changes that you may have the greatest likelihood of implementing successfully, although you may not necessarily select the first priority.

Self-Efficacy Potential for Change Scale
Score (0–5)

_____ Your awareness of a problem in this area.
_____ Your belief that this health behavior is impairing your health.
_____ Your belief that a positive change will make you a healthier, happier person.
_____ Your desire to change to a healthier behavior.
_____ Your knowledge of skills to initiate healthful changes.
_____ Your belief in yourself that you can initiate changes.
_____ Your support from your friends and family to help you change.
_____ Your community or other resources to help you change, such as exercise facilities, educational self-help programs, etc.
_____ Your belief in yourself that you can overcome personal barriers to change, such as lack of time, equipment, facilities, or finances.
_____ Your belief in yourself that you can sustain this behavior change for a lifetime.

(handwritten: for pg.281 questions)

Example:

Positive Health Factors	Negative Health Factors	SEPCS Score	Priority
Blood pressure	Physical activity (very little exercise)	22	5
Rest/sleep	Eating habits (too much dietary fat)	40	2
Car safety	Weight/body fat (too much body fat)	42	1
Alcohol use	Stress/personal relationships	38	3
Tobacco use	Cholesterol	34	4
Risky behaviors			
Life satisfaction			

In this case, seven positive health factor areas and five negative health factor areas have been identified. Based on the SEPCS, this individual recognizes that excess body fat is a problem and believes strongly that this negative health factor may be changed. It is the first priority for change, and an appropriate plan should be developed. Eating habits, the second priority, also has a strong potential to be changed, and such a change may impact upon body weight, as would a positive change in physical activity. Interestingly, loss of body fat could have positive influences on the negative factors of stress/personal relationships and cholesterol, reflecting the mind/body concept of the Positive Health Life-style.

(handwritten table)

	chol.	eating	Disappointments	SEPCS
1	2	2	3	
2	2	2	3	
3	2	3	4	
4	2	3	4	
5	4	5	4	
6	5	5	4	
7	4	4	4	
8	4	4	4	
9	4	4	4	
10	4	4	5	
	33	36	40	total

2.1 *due monday*

Exercise Program Implementation

This laboratory is a modification of Project PACE*, the Physician-based Assessment and Counseling for Exercise program developed in conjunction with the Centers for Disease Control and Prevention. Completion of Part A will help you determine your current physical activity level and status. If you are a precontemplator, completion of Part B may help you to get moving. If you are a contemplator, completion of Part C will provide you with some helpful hints for beginning your exercise program. If you are an active, completion of Part D may be helpful to keep you active.

Important: Complete Laboratory Inventory 2.2 if you have any questions regarding health risks associated with starting or increasing the intensity of an exercise program, please check with your physician to see if you need an exercise tolerance (stress) test before you begin.

PART A

Physical Activity Levels Identified in the Self-Assessment Phase of Project PACE**

Precontemplator

1. I do not exercise or walk regularly now, and I do not intend to start in the near future.

Contemplator

2. I do not exercise or walk regularly, but I have been thinking of starting.
3. I am trying to start to exercise or walk. *(or)* During the last month I have started to exercise or walk on occasion or on weekends only.
4. I have exercised or walked infrequently (or on weekends only) for more than 1 month.

Active

5. I am doing vigorous or moderate exercise less than three times a week (or moderate exercise less than 2 hours a week).
6. I have been doing moderate exercise three or more times a week (or more than 2 hours a week) for the last 1 to 6 months.
7. I have been doing moderate exercise three or more times a week (or more than 2 hours a week) for 7 months or more.
8. I have been doing vigorous exercise three to five times a week for 1 to 6 months.
9. I have been doing vigorous exercise three to five times a week for 7 to 12 months.
10. I have been doing vigorous exercise three to five times a week for more than 12 months.
11. I do vigorous exercise six or more times a week.

***Source:** Adapted from Project PACE. Courtesy of Barbara Long, MD. Student Health Services. San Diego State University, San Diego, CA 92182–4701.*

***Select one statement that best describes your activity pattern.*

Getting Out of Your Chair

On your PACE Assessment you said that you are not very interested in physical activity. Have you thought very much about what *you* can get out of being active?

- *Physical Activity can help you feel better*
- *Physical Activity can help you look better*
- *Physical Activity can help you be healthier*

What would be the two most important benefits of physical activity *for you?* Be specific.

1. _____

2. _____

Do you know you can get most of the benefits of physical activity just by *walking* on a regular basis? You do not have to jog or go to aerobics classes to be an exerciser.

Many things can interfere with physical activity. Here are some of the reasons people give for not being physically active. Check the ones that apply most to you.

_____	Exercise is hard work	_____	I do not enjoy exercise
_____	I am usually too tired for exercise	_____	I hate to fail, so I will not start
_____	I do not have anyone to exercise with me	_____	I do not have a safe place to exercise
_____	The weather is too bad	_____	Exercise is boring
_____	There is no convenient place	_____	I do not have the time
_____	I am too overweight	_____	I am too old

What are the two main things that keep you from wanting to be physically active?

1. _____

2. _____

The good news is you can do something about the reasons you are not physically active. If you think of them as *roadblocks* between you and physical activity, you can figure out how to get around them. You can change the roadblock itself *(I will get up earlier in the morning to make time for physical activity)*. You can also change your attitude about the roadblock *(I really can find some time to exercise)*.

How can you get around your two main roadblocks? Look at the ideas on the next page.

1. _____

2. _____

The First Step in Being Physically Active is Getting out of Your Chair.

How to Get Past Roadblocks

Roadblock	How to Get Past It
_____ Exercise is hard work	Pick an activity that you enjoy and that is easy for you. "No pain, no gain" is a myth.
_____ I do not have time	We're only talking about three 30 minute sessions each week. Can you do without three TV shows each week?
_____ I do not enjoy exercise	Do not "exercise." Start a hobby or way of playing that gets you moving.
_____ I am usually too tired to exercise	Tell yourself, "This activity will give me more energy." See if it doesn't happen.
_____ I do not have a safe place to exercise	If your neighborhood is not safe, you can walk at work, walk in a group, or walk in the morning.
_____ I do not have anyone to exercise with me	Maybe you have not asked. A neighbor, family member, or co-worker may be a willing partner. Or you can choose an activity that you enjoy doing by yourself.
_____ There is no convenient place	Pick an activity you can do near your home or work. Walk around your neighborhood or do aerobics with a TV show at home.
_____ I am afraid of being injured	Walking is very safe, and it is an excellent activity to improve your health.
_____ The weather is too bad	There are many activities you can do in your home, in any weather.
_____ Exercise is boring	Listening to music during your activity keeps your mind occupied. Walking, biking, or running can take you past lots of interesting scenery.
_____ I am too overweight	You can benefit from physical activity regardless of your weight. Pick an activity that you are comfortable with, like walking.
_____ I am too old	It's never too late to start. If you are ill, it is important to talk to your doctor about physical activity.

PART C

Planning the First Step

Congratulations. On your PACE Assessment you said that you are ready to make physical activity a regular part of your life. You are taking a big step toward improving your physical and mental health. This form should be able to help you start an activity program you can stick with.

What are the two main benefits you hope to get from being active? Write them down here and think of them often.

1. _____   2. _____

PHYSICAL ACTIVITY MUST BE REGULAR. Plan to do an activity of your choice, 3–5 times per week.

What Activities Are You Going to Do?

Some activities enjoyed by many people are listed on the back. In choosing *your* activity, consider these questions:

- **Do you enjoy it?**   Can you afford the supplies, equipment, facilities, or classes? Are there family or friends to do this activity with you? Can you do it year-round or do you need more than one activity?
  Type(s) of Activity: _____

- **Where will you do your activity?**   Can you do this activity at home or in your neighborhood? Do you have to go to a gym, a park, or a health club? Is this place convenient for you?
  Place(s) for Activity: _____

- **What is the most realistic time for you to do this activity 3 to 5 times per week?**   Will you have to reschedule other activities?
  Days and Times for Activity: _____

- **How long do you plan to do your activity each time?**   Build up time gradually over several weeks. Start with a 5–10 minute workout and build up to 30–60 minutes of moderate activity or 20–40 minutes of vigorous activity.
  Length of Activity: _____

- **Who can support you or help with your new activity program?**   It is ideal for someone to be active with you. You may want to ask someone to encourage you or help you to be active.
  Who will help you, and how: _____

Activities

Moderate	*Vigorous*
Walking (at home, to work, on lunch break)	Jogging
Gardening (must be regular)	Aerobic dance
Hiking	Basketball
Slow cycling	Fast cycling
Folk, square, or popular dancing	Cross-country skiing
Ice and roller skating	Swimming laps
Doubles tennis	Singles tennis and racquet sports
Taking the stairs	Soccer

How to Get Past Roadblocks

Roadblock	*How to Get Past It*
_____ I do not have the time	We're only talking about three 30-minute sessions each week. Can you do without three TV shows each week?
_____ I do not enjoy exercise	Do not "exercise." Start a hobby or an enjoyable activity that gets you moving.
_____ I am usually too tired to exercise	Regular activity will *improve* your energy level. Try it and see for yourself!
_____ The weather is too bad	There are many activities you can do in your own home, in any weather.
_____ Exercise is boring	Listening to music during your activity keeps your mind occupied. Walking, biking, or running can take you past lots of interesting scenery.
_____ I get sore when I exercise	Slight muscle soreness after physical activity is common when you are just starting. It should go away in 2–3 days. You can avoid this by building up gradually and stretching after the activity.

Activity Log

Use this Activity Log to keep track of your physical activity. Write down how long you do your activity as well as positive feelings and experiences. Note any roadblocks that discourage you from doing your activity and do something about them. When this log is full, make one of your own.

Date	Activity	Minutes	Feelings/Comments

Good Luck and Keep Moving!

PART D

Keeping the Pace

Congratulations. You are doing regular physical activity. You have a right to feel proud that you are doing something very positive for yourself. Sometimes you may lose sight of the physical and mental health benefits you are getting from physical activity. What motivates you to stay active?

1. _makes me feel good_ 2. _gives me energy_ 3. _I enjoy exercising mentally & physically_

Review Your Program

By reviewing the activities you are doing now, you can see if any changes need to be made in your plan. The goal is to improve your chances of *staying* active.

What *type(s)* of activity do you usually do? _walking, weight lifting, hiking, stepper_
How many *times a week?* _4_
How long each time? _weight lifting (1hr) , walking (30 min.)_
Who *helps* you or does the activity with you? _boyfriend / friends_
Have you had any *injuries?* _no_
What parts of your activity plan are you *most satisfied* with? _results_
What parts of your activity plan are you *least satisfied* with? _time it takes_
What *changes* might you make in your activity plan to make it more enjoyable, convenient, or safe? _walking different places or at different times_

Getting Back on Track

Most people who are regularly active have stopped at one time or another in the past. Sometimes they stop for a few weeks. Sometimes it is years before they start being active again. Planning ahead by answering these questions now can help you get past roadblocks later.

- If you have stopped regular activity in the past, what caused you to stop? _working full time_

- What could you have done differently that would have helped you stay active or what helped you to get back on track quickly? _Self - motivation_

Keeping the Pace

How confident are you that you can continue to do regular physical activity for the next 3 months?

| *(Please circle)* | NO CONFIDENCE | LOW CONFIDENCE | MEDIUM CONFIDENCE | HIGH CONFIDENCE |

What is reducing your confidence and what can you do to improve it? _____

Look Ahead for Your Roadblocks

What situation or thing is most likely to make you stop being active? _getting acquainted with working full time._

What can you do about this roadblock to prevent it or prepare for it? _workout later or earlier in the day._

What is the best way for you to get back on track if you stop? _energy level declines. Have someone to workout with._

How to Get Back on Track

- Remind yourself it is okay to have a pause in your activity once in a while. Don't be hard on yourself. Feeling guilty will make it more difficult to get back on track.

- You may need some extra help to get going again. Ask family and friends to help and encourage you.

- Ask someone to exercise with you.

- It may be helpful to tell everybody you know that you are restarting your activity plan.

- Use an Activity Log to keep track of your activity again.

- Give yourself small rewards each time you do your physical activity. Make a chart for your refrigerator. Use stickers or gold stars to keep track of your activity. Put change in a jar as a reward. Praising yourself is an effective reward (*"I did it and I'm proud of myself!"*).

- For variety, try new activities.

- Do whatever worked for you in the past to restart physical activity.

2.2
▼▼▼

Revised Physical Activity Readiness Questionnaire (rPAR-Q)*

rPAR-Q & You

rPAR-Q is designed to help you help yourself. Many health benefits are associated with regular exercise, and the completion of rPAR-Q is a sensible first step to take if you are planning to increase the amount of physical activity in your life.

For most people, physical activity should not pose any problem or hazard. rPAR-Q has been designed to identify the small number of adults for whom physical activity might be inappropriate or those who should have medical advice concerning the type of activity most suitable for them.

Common sense is your best guide in answering these few questions. Please read them carefully and check (√) the ☐ YES or ☐ NO opposite the question if it applies to you.

YES   NO

☐   ☑   1. Has a doctor said that you have a heart condition and recommended only medically supervised activity?

☐   ☑   2. Do you have chest pain brought on by physical activity?

☐   ☑   3. Have you developed chest pain in the past month?

☐   ☑   4. Do you tend to lose consciousness or fall over as a result of dizziness?

☐   ☑   5. Do you have a bone or joint disease that could be aggravated by the proposed physical activity?

☐   ☑   6. Has a doctor ever recommended medication for your blood pressure or a heart condition?

☐   ☑   7. Are you aware through your own experience, or a doctor's advice, of any other physical reason against your exercising without medical supervision?

*From Shepard, R. J., S. Thomas, and I. Weller. (1991). "The Canadian Home Fitness Test: 1991 Update." Sports Medicine 1:359, 1991. Used with permission, Adis Press Limited.

If You Answered YES to One or More Questions

If you have not recently done so, consult with your personal physician by telephone or in person BEFORE increasing your physical activity and/or taking a fitness appraisal. Tell your physician what questions you answered YES to on rPAR-Q or present your rPAR-Q copy.

Programs

After medical evaluation, seek advice from your physician as to your suitability for:

- unrestricted physical activity starting off easily and progressing gradually;
- restricted or supervised activity to meet your specific needs, at least on an initial basis. Check in your community for special programs or services.

If You Answered NO to All Questions

If you answered rPAR-Q accurately, you have reasonable assurance of your present suitability for:

- a graduated exercise program—a gradual increase in proper exercise promotes good fitness development while minimizing or eliminating discomfort;
- a fitness appraisal—the Canadian Standardized Test of Fitness (CSTF).

Postpone

If you have a temporary minor illness, such as a common cold.

3.1

Heart Rate Palpation

Practice taking the heart rate (HR) via the technique described on page 36 and as shown in figure 3.12 on page 37. Practice finding the pulse as rapidly as possible so that it may be found readily when needed. Practice taking the HR in pairs, you (the subject) taking your own radial pulse while your partner takes your carotid pulse.

Take the HR under the following situations:

1. After lying down 3 minutes
2. After sitting 3 minutes
3. After standing 3 minutes
4. After doing vigorous jumping jacks for 1 minute (same number each time), record the heart rate during:
    a. a 10-second period from 5 to 15 seconds after the cessation of exercise
    b. a 30-second period after 1 minute of recovery (1 to 1½ minutes after exercise)
    c. a 30-second period after 2 minutes of recovery (2 to 2½ minutes after exercise)

Record your heart rate results below:

	Date _____	Date _____	Date _____	Date _____	Date _____
Lying down	_____	_____	_____	_____	_____
Sitting	_____	_____	_____	_____	_____
Standing	_____	_____	_____	_____	_____
5 to 15 seconds after exercise	_____	_____	_____	_____	_____
1 to 1½ minutes after exercise	_____	_____	_____	_____	_____
2 to 2½ minutes after exercise	_____	_____	_____	_____	_____

3.2

Determination of Target HR and RPE

The following procedure is based upon a walk-jog-run mode of exercise, but it may be adapted to other modes such as bicycling, swimming, rope jumping, aerobic dancing, stair climbing, and others. Simply increase the intensity of the exercise in a consistent fashion and observe the effect on the heart rate.

1. Determine your resting heart rate (RHR) in a relaxed state, preferably just before getting up in the morning. The RHR should be taken several times a day, after you have been resting for an hour or so.

2. Based upon your RHR and your age, consult table 3.3 on page 38 to determine your target HR range.

3. Mark a ½-mile course. Two laps on a ¼-mile course is ideal. If you do not have an accurately measured track area available, design one yourself. There are measuring wheels available, but the following is a simple technique.

   a. Find a measured distance, such as a 100-yard football field.

   b. Walk the distance at your normal pace and count the number of steps you take. Do it several times to ensure accuracy.

   c. Calculate the average number of yards you cover per step. For example, if you take 120 steps to walk 100 yards, your average distance per step is .833 yards (100 yards/120 steps).

   d. Using sidewalks, fields, or other areas by your home, mark off a circular or elliptical course that measures ½ mile (880 yards). You may wish to place markers at 220-yard (⅛ mile) intervals to facilitate recording your pace. A steady pace is reflected by nearly equal times for each of the four 220-yard segments in the ½ mile.

4. Measure your RHR again before you begin to exercise.

5. Walk until you have settled into an even pace and then time yourself for the ½ mile. Immediately measure your heart rate for 6 seconds at the conclusion of the exercise. It is important to measure your recovery heart rate immediately so that it very closely represents your exercise heart rate. Also, during your walk or run, mentally record your RPE, as explained on page 38.

6. Record your heart rate and RPE in the chart and plot them on the graph on page 295. Try to relate the RPE to your heart rate.

7. If you do not reach your target heart rate, rest until your RHR returns to nearly normal (within 5 to 10 beats) and then repeat the ½-mile test at a faster pace. Again, record your heart rate and RPE.

8. Repeat this procedure until you have reached your target heart rate and RPE. You should be exercising at least to the 50 percent level. You may also use this technique to get to the 85 percent level.

9. You may use this technique to determine your true HR max. Keep increasing your speed for the ½ mile until you can go no faster. This procedure should be done only when you are fairly well conditioned.

Record your results below:

	Date ____	Date ____	Date ____	Date ____	Date ____
Target HR for training effect*					
Resting HR	____	____	____	____	____
Predicted HR max (220 – age)	____	____	____	____	____
50% of HR reserve	____	____	____	____	____
85% of HR reserve	____	____	____	____	____
½-mile test					
Trial 1					
Time	____	____	____	____	____
Minutes/mile	____	____	____	____	____
HR	____	____	____	____	____
RPE	____	____	____	____	____
Trial 2					
Time	____	____	____	____	____
Minutes/mile	____	____	____	____	____
HR	____	____	____	____	____
RPE	____	____	____	____	____
Trial 3					
Time	____	____	____	____	____
Minutes/mile	____	____	____	____	____
MR	____	____	____	____	____
RPE	____	____	____	____	____
Trial 4					
Time	____	____	____	____	____
Minutes/mile	____	____	____	____	____
HR	____	____	____	____	____
RPE	____	____	____	____	____

To calculate minutes/mile, simply double your ½-mile time. For example, a ½-mile time of 5:40 is an 11:20 mile.

*Example: Individual 20 years old. RHR = 70. THR = X% (HR max – RHR) + RHR

50% Target HR = .50 (200 – 70) + 70 = 135

85% Target HR = .85 (200 – 70) + 70 = 180

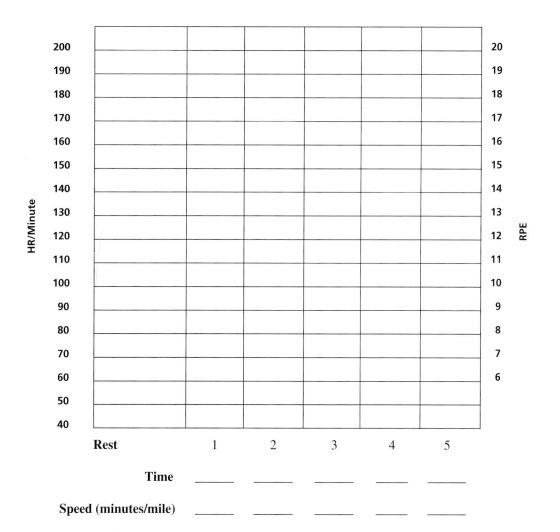

Record resting HR and RPE at rest; then plot HR and RPE at different speeds. See figure 3.16 on page 42 for an example.

3.3

▼▼▼

Cooper's Distance Tests

Administer one of the following tests:

a. 3-mile walking test (no running)

b. 1½-mile running test

The person taking the test should have medical clearance and should have been exercising for 6 to 8 weeks prior to the test. Some other guidelines for taking these tests are presented on pages 33–34. Since the test requires a nearly exhaustive effort, it is helpful if the person is instructed to keep an even pace throughout the test rather than going out too fast or too slow in the early stages.

Other helpful suggestions include the following:

1. Rest both the day before and the day of the test
2. Practice at the actual distance several times before the test day
3. Refrain from eating and smoking for at least 2 to 3 hours prior to the test
4. Warm up adequately
5. Have someone keep you aware of your pace time
6. Warm down after the test by walking or reducing the intensity of the activity

Tables B.1 and B.2 in Appendix B represent the fitness categories for two of the tests developed by Cooper. Table B.3 is a version developed by Draper and Jones for use by college students aged seventeen through twenty-five who are moderately fit. On the appropriate table for your test, find your age category across the top row, locate your sex in the second column, then find the entry that corresponds to your time. For example, an eighteen-year-old female who walked 3 miles in 34 minutes is in the *excellent* fitness category. If a nineteen-year-old male ran the 1½-mile test in 11:22, in what fitness category would he be? The answer is *fair* or *moderate*.

Once you have determined the fitness category, consult table B.4 to predict the $\dot{V}O_{2\,MAX}$ in ml O_2/kg/minute. For the eighteen-year-old female, you would predict 39.0–41.9 ml O_2/kg/minute. The nineteen-year-old male would be 38.4–45.1 ml O_2/kg/minute.

Test Taken:

___ 3-mile walk (no running)

___ 1½-mile running

	Date _____	Date _____	Date _____	Date _____	Date _____
Time	_____	_____	_____	_____	_____
Fitness level	_____	_____	_____	_____	_____
Predicted $\dot{V}O_{2\,MAX}$ (ml O_2/kg/min)	_____	_____	_____	_____	_____

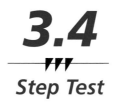

3.4

Step Test

Step tests have been developed for two purposes—to predict aerobic fitness and to help evaluate the effects of training. Keep in mind the limitations of step tests as a means to predict aerobic fitness, as discussed in chapter 3. The 3-minute step test does have a fitness prediction scale, but it is best utilized to evaluate a training effect. You may wish to design your own test for this purpose by using available equipment such as bleacher steps, chairs, locker room benches, etc. Simply establish a rate of stepping such as 18, 24, 30, or 36 4-count steps per minute, and an appropriate test length (3 to 5 minutes).

When administering any step test it is important that the individual maintain the cadence of the stepping. This is critical, as it determines the work rate. A metronome or tape recording may be used to expedite maintenance of cadence. One step involves four beats on the metronome: left up, right up, left down, right down. The individual should completely straighten the knees when coming to the standing position on the bench. It may be advisable to alternate stepping legs so that one leg does not do all the work and develop soreness.

Three-Minute Step Test

The three-minute step test has been developed by Mead and Hartwig for men and women ages eighteen to twenty-six.

Bench height:	12 inches
Stepping cadence:	24 steps/minute
Duration:	3 minutes
Heart rate:	Sit down immediately and record heart rate for exactly 1 minute.

Fitness Index	Males	Females
Superior	68	73
Excellent	69–75	74–82
Good	76–83	83–90
Average	84–92	91–100
Fair	93–99	101–107
Poor	100–106	108–114
Very poor	>107	>115

Figures represent heart rate response as measured for one minute immediately after the step test.

Source: From "A Comparison of the Exercise Tolerance of Post-Rheumatic and Normal Boys," by Frederick Kasch, in Journal of the Association of Physical and Mental Rehabilitation *15:35, 1961. © 1961 American Corrective Therapy Association. Reprinted by permission.*

Record your step test results:

	Date _____	Date _____	Date _____	Date _____	Date _____
Resting HR*	_____	_____	_____	_____	_____
Recovery HR (1 minute)	_____	_____	_____	_____	_____
Fitness index	_____	_____	_____	_____	_____

*Resting heart rate is not necessary but may be of interest to the student from test to test.

For your own individual step test, use the following form to tabulate your data.

	Date _____	Date _____	Date _____	Date _____	Date _____
Individual Step Test					
Step height	_____	_____	_____	_____	_____
Cadence	_____	_____	_____	_____	_____
Duration	_____	_____	_____	_____	_____
Resting HR	_____	_____	_____	_____	_____
Recovery HR (1 minute)	_____	_____	_____	_____	_____

3.5

The Rockport Fitness Walking Test

1. You need to find a measured mile; high school or college tracks are usually about four laps to the mile. You may wish to measure your own mile as explained in Laboratory Inventory 3.2.

2. Stretch and limber up for about 5–10 minutes. Be sure to wear a comfortable pair of walking shoes.

3. Walk as fast as you can for one mile. Your pace should be brisk and steady, yet comfortable.

4. Record your time for one mile.

5. Stop and record your heart rate immediately for 15 seconds. The fitness data for the Rockport Fitness Walking Test are based upon a 15-second heart rate count. Multiply the obtained value by four to get your heart rate per minute.

6. Compare your heart rate to the appropriate chart presented for your age on the next page. For example, if you are a twenty-one-year-old female who completed the test in 16 minutes with a heart rate of 170 beats per minute, you would be classified in the average fitness category. However, it should be noted that the Rockport Fitness Walking Test was developed using a population aged 30–69, and recent research has suggested that the fitness categories may be overestimated for college students aged 20–29. Therefore, if you are in this age range keep this point in mind, although this test is still very useful to evaluate progress for those who use aerobic walking in their fitness program.

7. Repeat the test periodically throughout your training program in order to evaluate changes in fitness. In general, as you become more fit, your time to walk 1 mile should decrease or, if you maintain the same pace, your heart rate for the 1 minute recovery period should also decrease.

Date _____ _____ _____ _____

Time _____ _____ _____ _____

Heart Rate _____ _____ _____ _____

Relative
Fitness Level _____ _____ _____ _____

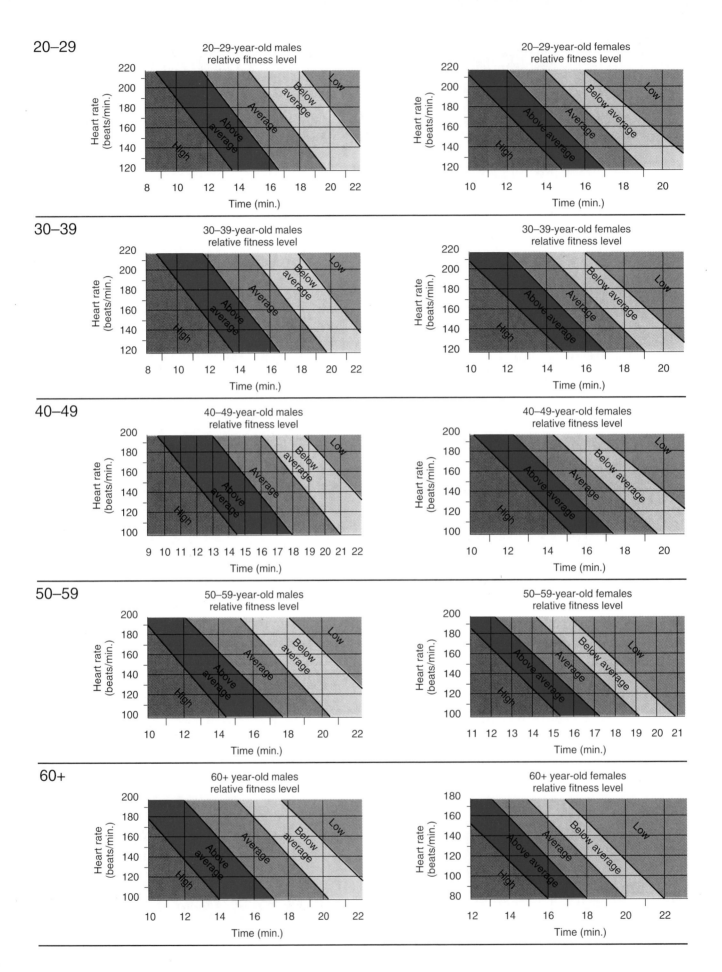

3.6

Exercise Prescription and Contract

Name _____ Age _____

Inclusive dates _____ to _____

Training Heart Rate

Resting HR (RHR) _____

HR max

   Predicted _____

   Actual _____

Target HR Levels

Target HR = X% (HR max – RHR) + RHR

50% _____

60% _____

70% _____

80% _____

85% _____

Fitness goals:

   Short-term   _____

                  _____

   Long-term   _____

                  _____

Exercise prescription:

   Mode   _____

   Warm-up   _____

   Warm-down   _____

Stimulus period	*Date* ____	*Date* ____	*Date* ____	*Date* ____	*Date* ____
Intensity	____	____	____	____	____
Duration	____	____	____	____	____
Frequency	____	____	____	____	____

    By my signature below, I do hereby commit myself to this exercise prescription and will do everything in my power to complete this prescription and attain my short-term and/or long-term fitness goals. I know that the successful completion of this exercise prescription will help me become a regular exerciser and may lead to a lifetime commitment to health through improved physical fitness.

_____ _____

Name (signed)   Date

_____

Witness

4.1

Tests of Upper Body Strength and Endurance

There are numerous tests of muscular strength and endurance, actually one for every resistance-training exercise that you do. As you progress through your resistance-training program, you may actually test your strength periodically for any exercise simply by doing the one repetition maximum test (1RM Test). You may also test your endurance by selecting a set weight to lift and executing as many repetitions as possible.

The test selected for upper body strength and endurance is the bench press, a popular resistance-training exercise that uses the large muscles of the chest and upper arm. Some data is available to provide you with a rough evaluation of your strength and endurance levels in comparison to those of others of your age. These levels may be useful in helping you establish goals in your resistance-training program.

The bench press may be done with free weights (barbell) or with a machine such as the Universal Gym®. The grip should be greater than shoulder width, the feet should be flat on the floor, and the back should be straight. See page 70 for a description.

Strength Ratios for the Bench Press

Upper-body strength (men)*
1 Repetition maximum bench press
Bench press weight ratio = weight pushed ÷ body weight

%	<20	20-29	30-39	40-49	50-59	60+	
99	>1.76	>1.63	>1.35	>1.20	>1.05	>.94	
95	1.76	1.63	1.35	1.20	1.05	.94	S
90	1.46	1.48	1.24	1.10	.97	.89	
85	1.38	1.37	1.17	1.04	.93	.84	
80	1.34	1.32	1.12	1.00	.90	.82	E
75	1.29	1.26	1.08	.96	.87	.79	
70	1.24	1.22	1.04	.93	.84	.77	
65	1.23	1.18	1.01	.90	.81	.74	
60	1.19	1.14	.98	.88	.79	.72	G
55	1.16	1.10	.96	.86	.77	.70	
50	1.13	1.06	.93	.84	.75	.68	
45	1.10	1.03	.90	.82	.73	.67	
40	1.06	.99	.88	.80	.71	.66	F
35	1.01	.96	.86	.78	.70	.65	
30	.96	.93	.83	.76	.68	.63	
25	.93	.90	.81	.74	.66	.60	
20	.89	.88	.78	.72	.63	.57	P
15	.86	.84	.75	.69	.60	.56	
10	.81	.80	.71	.65	.57	.53	
5	.76	.72	.65	.59	.53	.49	VP
1	<.76	<.72	<.65	<.59	<.53	<.49	
N =	60	425	1909	2090	1279	343	

S, superior; E, excellent; G, good; F, fair; P, poor; VP, very poor.
* Data provided by the Institute for Aerobics Research, Dallas, TX (1994).

Upper-body strength (women)*
1 Repetition maximum bench press
Bench press weight ratio = weight pushed ÷ body weight

%	<20	20-29	30-39	40-49	50-59	60+	
99	>.88	>1.01	>.82	>.77	>.68	>.72	
95	.88	1.01	.82	.77	.68	.72	S
90	.83	.90	.76	.71	.61	.64	
85	.81	.83	.72	.66	.57	.59	
80	.77	.80	.70	.62	.55	.54	E
75	.76	.77	.65	.60	.53	.53	
70	.74	.74	.63	.57	.52	.51	
65	.70	.72	.62	.55	.50	.48	
60	.65	.70	.54	.54	.58	.47	G
55	.64	.68	.58	.53	.47	.46	
50	.63	.65	.57	.52	.46	.45	
45	.60	.63	.55	.51	.45	.44	
40	.58	.59	.53	.50	.44	.43	F
35	.57	.58	.52	.48	.43	.41	
30	.56	.56	.51	.47	.42	.40	
25	.55	.53	.49	.45	.41	.39	
20	.53	.51	.47	.43	.39	.38	P
15	.52	.50	.45	.42	.38	.36	
10	.50	.480	.42	.38	.37	.33	
5	.41	.436	.39	.35	.305	.26	VP
1	<.41	<.436	<.39	<.35	<.305	<.26	
N =	20	191	379	333	189	42	

S, superior; E, excellent; G, good; F, fair; P, poor; VP, very poor.
* Data provided by the Institute for Aerobics Research, Dallas, TX (1994).

Strength

After a warm-up, use a trial-and-error approach to test your 1RM. The weight selected for your first lift should be slightly lower than what you know you can lift. Following your first lift, rest for a few minutes, and add additional weights based upon your perception of the effort needed. You should need only about two to four attempts to reach your 1RM. Rest several minutes between each attempt.

The following scale may be used to rate your performance. The ratios are multiplied by your body weight to determine the actual amount of weight you need to lift to be in that category. For example, if you are age twenty and a 150-pound male, you will need to bench press at least 189 pounds in order to be in the 75th percentile and excellent category ($1.26 \times 150 = 189$). If you are a 120-pound female of age twenty, you will need to lift at least 92 pounds to be in the 75th percentile and excellent category ($0.77 \times 120 = 92$).

Endurance

In the bench press test for endurance, males should select a weight that is $\frac{2}{3}$ of their body weight, while females should select a weight that is $\frac{1}{2}$ of their body weight. For example, a 150-pound male would exercise with 100 pounds ($\frac{2}{3} \times 150 = 100$), while a 120-pound female would use 60 pounds ($\frac{1}{2} \times 120 = 60$). Once you have selected the resistance based upon your body weight, do as many repetitions as possible until you are fatigued. You may compare your performance with the following rating scale, appropriate for both males and females of college age.

Rating Scale for Bench Press Repetitions*

Excellent	>14
Above Average	12–13
Average	10–11
Below Average	8–9
Poor	<7

Based on data from Heyward, V. Design for Fitness. Minneapolis: Burgess, 1984.

Date	_____	_____	_____	_____
Bench Press Weight	_____	_____	_____	_____
Body Weight	_____	_____	_____	_____
Bench Press: Body Weight Ratio	_____	_____	_____	_____
Percentile	_____	_____	_____	_____
Fitness Category	_____	_____	_____	_____

4.2

▼▼▼

Test of Lower Body Strength

Strength ratios are also available for a test of lower body strength, but you must have a Universal Gym® with the leg press station in order to conduct this test. The upper leg press is used, with the seat in the middle position. Follow the guidelines for the conduct of the 1RM bench press test in Laboratory Inventory 4.1. To obtain your strength ratio, divide the amount of weight you pressed by your body weight, e.g., 300-pound leg press divided by 150 pounds body weight equals a strength ratio of 2.00. The following ratio scale may be used to indicate your percentile ranking and rating from superior to very poor.

Strength Ratios for the Upper Leg Press (Universal Gym)®

Leg Strength (men)*
1 Repetition maximum leg press
Leg press weight ratio = weight pushed ÷ body weight
Age

%	<20	20-29	30-39	40-49	50-59	60+	
99	>2.82	>2.40	>2.20	>2.02	>1.90	>1.80	
95	2.82	2.40	2.20	2.02	1.90	1.80	S
90	2.53	2.27	2.07	1.92	1.80	1.73	
85	2.40	2.18	1.99	1.86	1.75	1.68	
80	2.28	2.13	1.93	1.82	1.71	1.62	E
75	2.18	2.09	1.89	1.78	1.68	1.58	
70	2.15	2.05	1.85	1.74	1.64	1.56	
65	2.10	2.01	1.81	1.71	1.61	1.52	
60	2.04	1.97	1.77	1.68	1.58	1.49	G
55	2.01	1.94	1.74	1.65	1.55	1.46	
50	1.95	1.91	1.71	1.62	1.52	1.43	
45	1.93	1.87	1.68	1.59	1.59	1.40	
40	1.90	1.83	1.65	1.57	1.46	1.38	F
35	1.89	1.78	1.62	1.54	1.42	1.34	
30	1.82	1.74	1.59	1.51	1.39	1.30	
25	1.80	1.68	1.56	1.48	1.36	1.27	
20	1.70	1.63	1.52	1.44	1.32	1.25	P
15	1.61	1.58	1.48	1.40	1.28	1.21	
10	1.57	1.51	1.43	1.35	1.22	1.16	
5	1.46	1.42	1.34	1.27	1.15	1.08	VP
1	<1.46	<1.42	<1.34	<1.27	<1.15	<1.08	
N =	60	424	1909	2089	1286	347	

S, superior; E, excellent; G, good; F, fair; P, poor; VP, very poor.
* Data provided by the Institute for Aerobics Research, Dallas, TX (1994).

Leg Strength (women)*
1 Repetition maximum leg press
Leg press weight ratio = weight pushed ÷ body weight
Age

%	<20	20-29	30-39	40-49	50-59	60+	
99	>1.88	>1.98	>1.68	>1.57	>1.43	>1.43	
95	1.88	1.98	1.68	1.57	1.43	1.43	S
90	1.85	1.82	1.61	1.48	1.37	1.32	
85	1.81	1.76	1.52	1.40	1.31	1.32	
80	1.71	1.68	1.47	1.37	1.25	1.18	E
75	1.69	1.65	1.42	1.33	1.20	1.16	
70	1.65	1.58	1.39	1.29	1.17	1.13	
65	1.62	1.63	1.33	1.27	1.12	1.08	
60	1.59	1.50	1.33	1.23	1.10	1.04	G
55	1.51	1.47	1.31	1.20	1.08	1.01	
50	1.45	1.44	1.27	1.18	1.05	.99	
45	1.42	1.40	1.24	1.15	1.08	.97	
40	1.38	1.37	1.21	1.13	.99	.93	F
35	1.33	1.32	1.18	1.11	.97	.90	
30	1.29	1.27	1.15	1.08	.95	.88	
25	1.25	1.26	1.12	1.06	.92	.86	
20	1.22	1.22	1.09	1.02	.88	.85	P
15	1.19	1.18	1.05	.97	.84	.80	
10	1.09	1.14	1.00	.94	.78	.72	
5	1.06	.99	.96	.85	.72	.63	VP
1	<1.06	<.99	<.96	<.85	<.72	<.63	
N =	20	192	281	337	192	44	

S, superior; E, excellent; G, good; F, fair; P, poor; VP, very poor.
* Data provided by the Institute for Aerobics Research, Dallas, TX (1994).

Date	_____	_____	_____	_____
Leg Press Weight	_____	_____	_____	_____
Body Weight	_____	_____	_____	_____
Leg Press: **Body Weight Ratio**	_____	_____	_____	_____
Percentile	_____	_____	_____	_____
Fitness Category	_____	_____	_____	_____

4.3
Test for Abdominal Muscle Endurance

Although you may test yourself for abdominal muscular strength by the 1RM technique, such tests are not usually conducted, for they may expose the low back to injury. Thus, most abdominal muscle tests focus upon endurance.

The most prevalent test for abdominal muscle endurance is the curl-up. The knees are bent, feet are flat on the floor, arms are crossed over your chest, and the chin is tucked to the chest. See figure 4.24d on page 82 for an illustration. The feet may be held down lightly for testing purposes. On the up-phase, touch your elbows to your thighs; on the down-phase, go back until your shoulder blades touch the floor. Keep your chin tucked to your chest throughout the exercise. Record the total number of curl-ups that you do in 1 minute. Use the following scale to evaluate your performance:

Standard Values for 1-minute Sit-up Endurance

	Age (yr)				
Rating	20–29	30–39	40–49	50–59	60+
Men					
Excellent	>48	>40	>35	>30	>25
Good	43–47	35–39	30–34	25–29	20–24
Average	37–42	29–34	24–29	19–24	14–19
Fair	33–36	25–28	20–23	15–18	10–13
Poor	<32	<24	<19	<14	<9
Women					
Excellent	>44	>36	>31	>26	>21
Good	39–43	31–35	26–30	21–25	16–20
Average	33–38	25–30	19–25	15–20	10–15
Fair	29–32	21–24	16–18	11–14	6–9
Poor	<28	<20	<15	<10	<5

Date _____ _____ _____ _____

Number of Sit-Ups _____ _____ _____ _____

Fitness Rating _____ _____ _____ _____

4.4

Weekly Resistance-Training Record

Weekly Resistance-Training Record, Basic Eight Exercises

	Chest (Bench Press)		Back (Lats Exercise)		Thigh (Half Squat)		Shoulder (Lateral Raise)		Calf (Heel Raise)		Front Arm (Curls)		Back Arm (Seated Press)		Abdominal Area (Curl-ups)	
Date _____	Wt	Reps	Wt	Reps	Wt	Reps	Wt	Reps	Wt	Reps	Wt	Reps	Wt	Reps	Wt	Reps
Set 1																
Set 2																
Set 3																
Set 4																
Set 5																
Date _____ Set 1																
Set 2																
Set 3																
Set 4																
Set 5																
Date _____ Set 1																
Set 2																
Set 3																
Set 4																
Set 5																
Date _____ Set 1																
Set 2																
Set 3																
Set 4																
Set 5																

The sequence of exercises should be

1. Bench press—chest muscles
2. Lat machine pull down or bent-arm pullover—back muscles
3. Half squat—thigh muscles
4. Standing lateral raise—shoulder muscles
5. Heel raise—calf muscles
6. Standing curl—front upper arm muscles
7. Seated overhead press—back upper arm muscles
8. Curl-up—abdominal muscles

A weekly record form, similar to this one, should be used to keep track of your progress.

5.1

▼▼▼

Sit-and-Reach Test for Lower Back and Hamstring Flexibility

Assume a position as in the following figure. Feet, preferably bare or stockinged, should be flat against the surface. Knees should be kept flat on the floor, preferably by a partner who holds them down. Place one hand on top of the other, and bend forward as far as you can with fingertips on the ruler. The ruler should extend 9 inches (23 centimeters) in front of the support. Measure the reach to the nearest centimeter or half inch. See the flexibility rating scale for interpretation of the results.

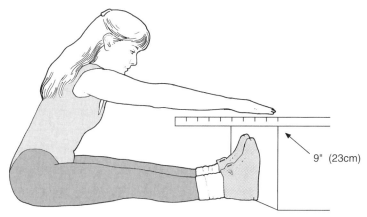

9" (23cm)

Position for the sit-and-reach test of flexibility in the low back and hamstring area.

Standard Values for Trunk Flexion in Inches (centimeters)

Rating	Age (yr)				
	20–29	30–39	40–49	50–59	60+
Men					
Excellent	>22 (56)	>21 (53)	>20 (51)	>19 (48)	>18 (46)
Good	19–21 (48–53)	18–20 (46–51)	17–19 (43–48)	16–18 (41–46)	15–17 (38–43)
Average	13–18 (33–46)	12–17 (30–43)	11–16 (28–41)	10–15 (25–38)	9–14 (23–36)
Fair	10–12 (25–30)	9–11 (23–28)	8–10 (20–25)	7–9 (18–23)	6–8 (15–20)
Poor	<9 (23)	<8 (20)	<7 (18)	<6 (15)	<5 (13)
Women					
Excellent	>24 (61)	>23 (58)	>22 (56)	>21 (53)	>20 (51)
Good	22–23 (56–58)	21–22 (53–56)	20–21 (51–53)	19–20 (48–51)	18–19 (46–48)
Average	16–21 (41–53)	15–20 (38–51)	14–19 (36–48)	13–18 (33–46)	12–17 (30–43)
Fair	13–15 (33–38)	12–14 (30–36)	11–13 (28–33)	10–12 (25–30)	9–11 (23–28)
Poor	<12 (30)	<11 (28)	<10 (25)	<9 (23)	<8 (20)

Reprinted from Y's Way to Physical Fitness (1982); Golding L., Myers, C., and Sinning, W., with permission of the YMCA of the USA, 101 N. Wacker Drive, Chicago, IL 60606.

Date				
Trunk Flexion (inches)				
Fitness Rating				

5.2

Shoulder Rotation Test for Shoulder Joint Flexibility

This test is a general measure of your overall shoulder flexibility. You will need a rope about 60 inches long and a ruler. First, measure the shoulder width from the tip of each deltoid muscle. Next, with your hands in front of your body, grasp one end of the rope with your left hand and a few inches away with your right hand. Now keep your arms straight, and move them straight forward, upward, and then backward and downward as you attempt to rotate the rope behind your head and to your lower back. As you meet resistance in rotating your shoulders, let the rope slide through your right hand so your hands become just far enough apart to let them rotate behind your back. Try to keep this distance to a minimum. After you have completed the maneuver, measure the rope distance between your hands. Subtract your shoulder width from the rope measurement and compare your results with the rating scale on the next page. The rating scale is somewhat arbitrary but may be useful if you are concerned with your shoulder flexibility. Use this test periodically to measure your progress as you pursue a flexibility exercise program for your shoulder, chest, and upper back areas.

Date _____   _____   _____   _____

Shoulder Rotation (inches) _____   _____   _____   _____

Performance Level _____   _____   _____   _____

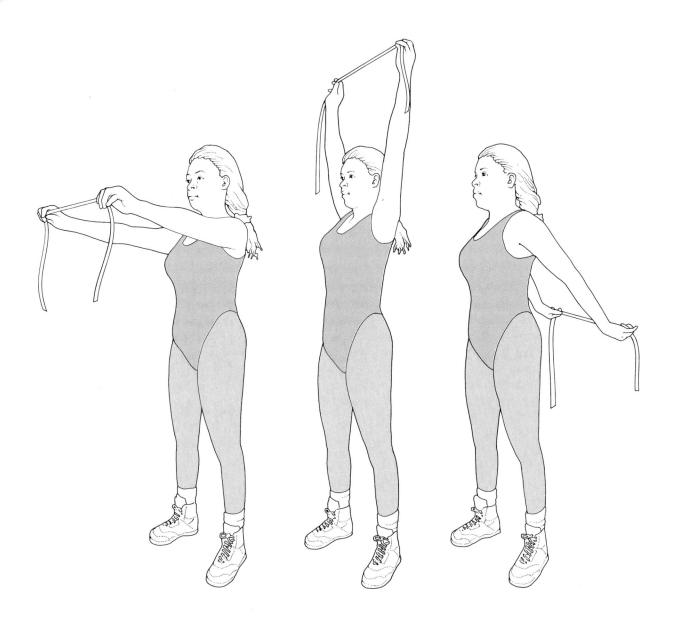

Norms in Inches for Shoulder Rotation Test, College Students

Performance Level	Men	Women
Advanced	7–Less	5–Less
Advanced intermediate	11½–7¼	9¾–5¼
Intermediate	14½–11¾	13–10
Advanced beginner	19¾–14¾	17¾–13¼
Beginner	20 and above	18 and above

Reprinted by permission from Barry L. Johnson and Jack K. Nelson, Practical Measurements for Evaluation in Physical Education. *© 1986 by Macmillan Publishing Company.*

5.3

▼▼▼

Ankle Flexion Test for Ankle Flexibility

This test is a general measure of ankle flexibility, with particular focus on the calf muscles and the Achilles tendon. Stand facing a wall, and lean into it so that your hands, chin, and chest are against the wall; keep your knees and body straight, and keep your heels flat on the floor (see the figure below). Your goal is to get as much distance between the wall and your feet while still keeping the heels flat on the floor and your hands, chin and chest in contact with the wall. Have a partner measure two distances: (1) the distance between your toes and the wall and (2) the distance from the floor to your chin while you are standing straight, not leaning against the wall. Subtract your lean distance from the standing chin height, and compare the results with the table below. The rating scale is somewhat arbitrary but may be useful if you are concerned with your ankle joint flexibility. Use this test periodically to measure your progress as you pursue a flexibility exercise program for your calf and Achilles tendon area.

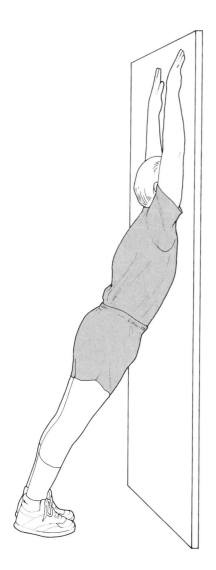

Norms in Inches for Ankle Flexion Test, College Students		
Performance Level	Men	Women
Advanced	26½ and below	24¼ and below
Advanced intermediate	29½–26¾	26½–24½
Intermediate	32½–29¾	30¼–26¾
Advanced beginner	35¼–32¾	31¾–30½
Beginner	35½ and above	32 and above

Reprinted by permission from Barry L. Johnson and Jack K. Nelson, Practical Measurements for Evaluation in Physical Education. © 1986 by Macmillan Publishing Company.

Date _____ _____ _____ _____

Ankle Flexion (inches) _____ _____ _____ _____

Performance Level _____ _____ _____ _____

6.1

▼▼▼

Classification of Daily Food Intake into the Six Exchange Lists and Determination of Caloric, Carbohydrate, Fat, and Protein Intake

This Laboratory Inventory may take considerable time and effort if you do it by hand, but the results may provide you with some useful information concerning your dietary intake. It may also be a good means to become familiar with the Food Exchanges System so that when you select a food to eat, you may know what its general content is in the form of Calories, carbohydrate, protein, and fat. However, computer software is available that will facilitate this process and provide you with a more detailed analysis of your diet, including dietary fiber, vitamins, minerals, and other nutrients. Whichever method you use, try to become familiar with the nutrient content of the foods you eat.

To do this laboratory, keep a record of everything you eat and drink for one day, including the specific amounts. Carry a notepad with you to record what you eat immediately. Be sure to note the ingredients of combination foods such as casseroles, pizza, and sandwiches. Use the form below to record the type of food, the Exchange List it is on, and the amount. If you are uncertain as to which exchange it is in, consult Appendix A.

Appendix A should also be used to determine the number of exchanges in the amount you have consumed. Use the following information to give you the Calories and the grams of carbohydrate, fat, and protein in each exchange. Multiplying the number of exchanges times these values will give you the total Calories, carbohydrate, fat, and protein in the food. Another good idea is to use the nutrition information on the foods' labels to record Calories, carbohydrate, fat, and protein intake.

Exchange	Calories	Carbohydrate (Grams)	Fat (Grams)	Protein (Grams)
Milk				
Skim, very low fat	90	12	0	8
Low fat	120	12	5	8
Whole	150	12	8	8
Meat				
Lean	55	0	3	7
Medium-fat	75	0	5	7
High-fat	100	0	8	7
Starch/bread	80	15	0	3
Fruit	60	15	0	0
Vegetable	25	5	0	2
Fat	45	0	5	0

Daily Food Intake

(1) Food	(2) Exchange List	(3) Amount	(4) Number of Exchanges	(5) Calories per Exchange	(6) Total Calories (4)×(5)
					Total _____

When you have completed recording the data on the form, perform the following calculations.

1.

Exchange	Total Number	Multiplied by	Calories per Exchange	Calories
Milk				
Skim, very low fat	_____	×	90	_____
Low fat	_____	×	120	_____
Whole	_____	×	150	_____
Meat				
Lean	_____	×	55	_____
Medium-fat	_____	×	75	_____
High-fat	_____	×	100	_____
Starch/bread	_____	×	80	_____
Fruit	_____	×	60	_____
Vegetable	_____	×	25	_____
Fat	_____	×	45	_____

2. Total Calories: _____ (column 6)

3. Total grams of carbohydrate: _____ grams (column 8)

4. Percent of carbohydrate in diet:

grams of carbohydrate _____ × 4 Calories = _____ carbohydrate Calories

carbohydrate Calories ÷ total Calories × 100 = _____ %

(7) Grams of Carbohydrate per Exchange	(8) Total Grams of Carbohydrate (4)×(7)	(9) Grams of Fat per Exchange	(10) Total Grams of Fat (4)×(9)	(11) Grams of Protein per Exchange	(12) Total Grams of Protein (4)×(11)
	Total _____		Total _____		Total _____

5. Total grams of fat: _____ grams (column 10)
6. Percent of fat in diet:

   grams of fat _____ × 9 Calories = _____ fat Calories

   fat Calories ÷ total Calories × 100 = _____ %

7. Total grams of protein: _____ grams (column 12)
8. Percent of protein in diet:

   grams of protein _____ × 4 Calories = _____ protein Calories

   protein Calories ÷ total Calories × 100 = _____ %

After completing this Laboratory Inventory, ask yourself the following questions. Did I get *at least* two to three milk exchanges, five to six meat, four starch/bread, one to two fruit, three to four vegetable, and one to two fat? Did I get about 60 percent of my Calories from carbohydrate? Analyze the content for simple and complex carbohydrates if you have that information available. Is the percentage of fat Calories less than 30 percent? Do I have about 10 to 12 percent or more of my Calories as protein? The answers to these questions may give you some insight into any needed dietary changes.

Doing this Laboratory Inventory is also good preparation for chapter 7. You may relate this information to Laboratory Inventories 7.4, 7.5, and 7.6 relative to weight control.

The day of the week that you select should be typical of your average diet. A more representative account is a three-day analysis. For a college student, this might be a Monday, Thursday, and Saturday, representing two different class schedule days and one weekend day. Calculate each day separately to see if you are balancing the diet over a week's time.

If computer software is available for an analysis of your dietary nutrients, this process will be facilitated.

6.2

▼▼▼

Center for Science in the Public Interest
How's Your Diet

The 40 questions below will help you focus on the key features of your diet. The (+) or (–) numbers under each set of answers instantly pat you on the back for good habits or alert you to problems you may not even realize you have.

The Grand Total rates your overall diet, on a scale from "Great" to "Arghh!"

The quiz focuses on fat, cholesterol, sodium, sugar, fiber, and vitamins A and C. It doesn't attempt to cover everything in your diet. Also, it doesn't try to measure precisely how much of these key nutrients you eat. (Computer dietary-analysis software programs are available for this purpose.)

What the quiz will do is give you a rough sketch of your current eating habits and, implicitly, suggest what you can do to improve them.

Finally, please don't despair over a less-than-perfect score. A healthy diet isn't built overnight.

Instructions

- Under each answer is a number with a + or – sign in front of it. Circle the number that is directly beneath the answer you choose. That's your score for the question. (If you use a pencil, you can erase your answers and give the quiz to someone else.)
- Circle only one number for each question, unless the instructions tell you to "average two or more scores if necessary."
- How to average. In answering question 18, for example, if you drink club soda (+3) and coffee (–1) on a typical day, add the two scores (which gives you +2) and then divide by 2. That gives you a score of +1 for the question. If averaging gives you a fraction, round it to the nearest whole number.
- If a question doesn't apply to you, skip it.
- Pay attention to serving sizes. For example, a serving of vegetables is ½ cup. If you usually eat one cup of vegetables at a time, count it as two servings.
- Add up all your + scores and your – scores.
- Subtract your – scores from your + scores. That's your GRAND TOTAL.

Quiz

1. How many times per week do you eat unprocessed red meat (steak, roast beef, lamb or pork chops, burgers, etc.)?
   (a) never   (b) 1 or less   (c) 2–3   (d) 4–5   (e) 6 or more
     +3   +2   0   –1   –3

2. After cooking, how large is the serving of red meat you usually eat? (To convert from raw to cooked, reduce by 25 percent. For example, 4 oz. of raw meat shrinks to 3 oz. after cooking. There are 16 oz. in a pound.)
   (a) 8 oz. or more   (b) 6–7 oz.   (c) 4–5 oz.   (d) 3 oz. or less   (e) don't eat red meat
       –3   –2   –1   0   +3

3. Do you trim the visible fat when you cook or eat red meat?
   (a) yes   (b) no   (c) don't eat red meat
     +1   –3   0

4. How many times per week do you eat processed meats (hot dogs, bacon, sausage, bologna, luncheon meats, etc.)? (OMIT products that contain one gram of fat or less per serving.)
   (a) none   (b) less than 1   (c) 1–2   (d) 3–4   (e) 5 or more
     +3   +2   0   –1   –3

5. What kind of ground meat or pountry do you usually eat?
   (a) regular ground beef   (b) lean ground beef   (c) ground round   (d) ground turkey   (e) Healthy Choice
           −3   −2   0   +1   +2
   (f) don't eat ground meat
        +3

6. What type of bread do you usually eat?
   (a) whole wheat or other whole grain   (b) rye   (c) pumpernickel   (d) white, "wheat," French, or Italian
              +3   +2   +2   −2

7. How many times per week do you eat deep-fried foods (fish, chicken, vegetables, potatoes, etc.)?
   (a) none   (b) 1–2   (c) 3–4   (d) 5 or more
    +3   0   −1   −3

8. How many servings of non-fried vegetables do you usually eat per day? (One serving = ½ cup. INCLUDE potatoes.)
   (a) none   (b) 1   (c) 2   (d) 3   (e) 4 or more
    −3   0   +1   +2   +3

9. How many servings of cruciferous vegetables do you usually eat per week? (ONLY count kale, broccoli, cauliflower, cabbage, Brussels sprouts, greens, bok choy, kohlrabi, turnip, and rutabaga. One serving = ½ cup.)
   (a) none   (b) 1–3   (c) 4–6   (d) 7 or more
    −3   +1   +2   +3

10. How many servings of vitamin-A-rich fruits or vegetables do you usually eat per week? (ONLY count carrots, pumpkin, sweet potatoes, cantaloupe, spinach, winter squash, greens, and apricots. One serving = ½ cup.)
    (a) none   (b) 1–3   (c) 4–6   (d) 7 or more
     −3   +1   +2   +3

11. How many times per week do you eat at a fast-food restaurant? (INCLUDE burgers, fried fish or chicken, croissant or biscuit sandwiches, topped potatoes, and other main dishes. OMIT meals of just plain baked potato, broiled chicken, or salad.)
    (a) never   (b) less than 1   (c) 1   (d) 2   (e) 3   (f) 4 or more
     +3   +1   0   − 1   −2   −3

12. How many servings of grains rich in complex carbohydrates do you eat per day? (One serving = 1 slice of bread, 1 large pancake, 1 cup whole grain cold cereal, or ½ cup cooked cereal, rice, pasta, bulgur, wheat berries, kasha, or millet. OMIT heavily-sweetened cold cereals.)
    (a) none   (b) 1–3   (c) 4–5   (d) 6–8   (e) 9 or more
     −3   0   +1   +2   +3

13. How many times per week do you eat fish or shellfish? (OMIT deep-fried items, tuna packed in oil, shrimp, squid, and mayonnaise-laden tuna salad—a little mayo is okay.)
    (a) never   (b) 1–2   (c) 3–4   (d) 5 or more
     −2   +1   +2   +3

14. How many times per week do you eat cheese? (INCLUDE pizza, cheeseburgers, veal or eggplant parmigiana, cream cheese, etc. OMIT low-fat or fat-free cheeses.)
    (a) 1 or less   (b) 2–3   (c) 4–5   (d) 6 or more
      +3   +2   −1   −3

15. How many servings of fresh fruit do you eat per day?
    (a) none   (b) 1   (c) 2   (d) 3   (e) 4 or more
     −3   0   +1   +2   +3

16. Do you remove the skin before eating poultry?
    (a) yes   (b) no   (c) don't eat poultry
     +3   −3   0

17. What do you usually put on your bread or toast? (AVERAGE two or more scores if necessary.)
    (a) butter or cream cheese   (b) margarine or peanut butter   (c) diet margarine   (d) jam or honey   (e) fruit butter
           −3   −2   −1   0   +1
    (f) nothing
       +3

18. Which of these beverages do you drink on a typical day? (AVERAGE two or more scores if necessary.)
    (a) water or club soda   (b) fruit juice   (c) diet soda   (d) coffee or tea   (e) soda, fruit "drink," or fruit "ade"
         +3   +1   −1   −1   −3

19. Which flavorings do you most frequently add to your foods? (AVERAGE two or more scores if necessary.)
    (a) garlic or lemon juice   (b) herbs or spices   (c) salt or soy sauce   (d) margarine   (e) butter   (f) nothing
             +3   +3   −2   −2   −3   +3

20. What do you eat most frequently as a snack? (AVERAGE two or more scores if necessary.)
    (a) fruits or vegetables   (b) sweetened yogurt   (c) nuts   (d) cookies or fried chips   (e) granola bar
             +3   +2   −1   −2   −2
    (f) candy bar or pastry   (g) nothing
             −3   0

21. What is your most typical breakfast? (SUBTRACT an extra 3 points if you also eat bacon or sausage.)
    (a) croissant, danish, or doughnut   (b) eggs   (c) pancakes or waffles   (d) cereal or toast
             −3   −3   −2   +3
    (e) low-fat yogurt or cottage cheese   (f) don't eat breakfast
             +3   0

22. What do you usually eat for dessert?
    (a) pie, pastry, or cake   (b) ice cream   (c) fat-free cookies or cakes   (d) frozen yogurt or ice milk
             −3   −3   −1   +1
    (e) non-fat ice cream or sorbet   (f) fruit   (g) don't eat dessert
             +1   +3   +3

23. How many times per week do you eat beans, split peas, or lentils?
    (a) none   (b) 1   (c) 2   (d) 3 or more
        −2   +1   +2   +3

24. What kind of milk do you drink?
    (a) whole   (b) 2% low-fat   (c) 1% low-fat   (d) ½% or skim   (e) none
        −3   −1   +2   +3   0

25. What dressings or toppings do you usually add to your salads? (ADD two or more scores if neccessary.)
    (a) nothing, lemon, or vinegar   (b) fat-free dressing   (c) low- or reduced-calorie dressing   (d) regular dressing
             +3   +2   +1   −1
    (e) croutons or bacon bits   (f) cole slaw, pasta salad, or potato salad
             −1   −1

26. What sandwich fillings do you eat most frequently? (AVERAGE two or more scores if necessary.)
    (a) luncheon meat   (b) cheese or roast beef   (c) peanut butter   (d) low-fat luncheon meat
             −3   −1   0   +1
    (e) tuna, salmon, chicken, or turkey   (f) don't eat sandwiches
             +3   0

27. What do you usually spread on your sandwiches? (AVERAGE two or more scores if necessary.)
    (a) mayonnaise   (b) light mayonnaise   (c) catsup, mustard, or fat-free mayonnaise   (d) nothing
             −2   −1   0   +2

28. How many egg yolks do you eat per week? (ADD 1 yolk for every slice of quiche you eat.)
    (a) 2 or less   (b) 3–4   (c) 5–6   (d) 7 or more
             +3   0   −1   −3

29. How many times per week do you eat canned or dried soups? (OMIT low-sodium, low-fat soups.)
    (a) none   (b) 1–2   (c) 3–4   (d) 5 or more
        +3   0   −2   −3

30. How many servings of a rich source of calcium do you eat per day? (One serving = ⅔ cup milk or yogurt, 1 oz. cheese, 1½ oz. sardines, 3½ oz. salmon, 5 oz. tofu made with calcium sulfate, 1 cup greens or broccoli, or 200 mg. of a calcium supplement.)
    (a) none   (b) 1   (c) 2   (d) 3 or more
        −3   +1   +2   +3

31. What do you usually order on your pizza? (Vegetable toppings include green pepper, mushrooms, onions, and other vegetables. SUBTRACT 1 point from your score if you order extra cheese.)
    (a) no cheese with vegetables   (b) cheese with vegetables   (c) cheese   (d) cheese with meat toppings   (e) don't eat pizza
             +3   +1   0   −3   +2

32. What kind of cookies do you usually eat?
    (a) graham crackers or ginger snaps   (b) oatmeal   (c) sandwich cookies (like Oreos)
                        +1   −1   −2
    (d) chocolate coated, chocolate chip, or peanut butter   (e) don't eat cookies
                        −3   +3

33. What kind of frozen dessert do you usually eat? (SUBTRACT 1 point from your score for each topping you use—whipped cream, hot fudge, nuts, etc.)
    (a) gourmet ice cream   (b) regular ice cream   (c) sorbet, sherbet, or ices   (d) frozen yogurt, fat-free ice cream, or ice milk
            −3   −1   +1   +1
    (e) don't eat frozen desserts
            +3

34. What kind of cake or pastry do you usually eat?
    (a) cheesecake, pie, or any microwave cake   (b) cake with frosting or filling   (c) cake without frosting
                    −3   −2   −1
    (d) unfrosted muffin, banana bread, or carrot cake   (e) angelfood or fat-free cake   (f) don't eat cakes or pastries
                    0   +1   +3

35. How many times per week does your dinner contain grains, vegetables, or beans, but little or no animal protein (meat, poultry, fish, eggs, milk, or cheese)?
    (a) none   (b) 1–2   (c) 3–4   (d) 5 or more
        −1   +1   +2   +3

36. Which of the following salty snacks do you typically eat? (AVERAGE two or more scores if necessary.)
    (a) potato chips, corn chips, or packaged popcorn   (b) reduced-fat potato or tortilla chips   (c) salted pretzels
                    −3   −2   −1
    (d) unsalted pretzels or baked corn or tortilla chips   (e) homemade air-popped popcorn   (f) don't eat salty snacks
                    +1   +3   +3

37. What do you usually use to saute vegetables or other foods? (Vegetable oil includes safflower, corn, canola, olive, sunflower, and soybean.)
    (a) butter or lard   (b) more than one tablespoon of margarine or vegetable oil
            −3   −1
    (c) no more than one tablespoon of margarine or vegetable oil   (d) no more than one tablespoon of olive oil   (e) water or broth
                    0   +1   +2

38. What kind of cereal do you usually eat?
    (a) whole grain (like oatmeal or Shredded Wheat)   (b) low-fiber (like Cream of Wheat or Corn Flakes)
                    +3   0
    (c) sugary low-fiber (like Frosted Flakes)   (d) granola
                    −1   −2

39. With what do you make tuna salad, pasta salad, chicken salad, etc?
    (a) mayonnaise   (b) light mayonnaise   (c) non-fat mayonnaise   (d) low-fat yogurt   (e) non-fat yogurt
            −2   −1   0   +2   +3

40. What do you typically put on your pasta? (ADD one point if you also add sauteed vegetables. (AVERAGE two or more scores if necessary.)
    (a) tomato sauce   (b) tomato sauce with a little parmesan   (c) white clam sauce   (d) meat sauce or meat balls
            +3   +3   +1   −2
    (e) Alfredo, pesto, or other creamy sauce
            −3

Your Grand Total

+59 to +116	GREAT!	You're a nutrition superstar. Give yourself a big (non-butter) pat on the back.
0 to +58	GOOD	Pin your Quiz on the nearest wall.
−58 to −1	FAIR	Hang in there. Tape CSPI's Nutrition Scoreboard poster to your refrigerator for a little friendly help.
−117 to −59	ARGHH!	Stop lining the cat box with *Nutrition Action Healthletter*. Empty your refrigerator and cupboard. It's time to start over.

7.1

Prediction of Body Fat Percentage

A. Skinfold Caliper Technique

In order to make accurate measurements, it is best to use skinfold calipers that have pressure built into the instrument itself. However, some of the less expensive plastic models may also be effective.

1. Take a full fold of fat between the thumb and index finger, being sure to separate the fat from the underlying muscle. Measurements must include only the skinfold, not clothing such as leotards, shirts, etc.

2. Hold the skin firmly and place the contact surface of the calipers at the base of the fold about ½ inch below your fingers.

3. Release the grip on the calipers slowly so that full pressure is exerted at the base of the fold. Continue to hold the skin.

4. Take recordings to the nearest ½ millimeter after the needle comes to a full stop. Duplicate the measurements until two consecutive measurements agree within ½ millimeter.

B. Skinfold Sites (See appropriate figures.)

Females	Males
Triceps	Chest
Thigh	Thigh
Suprailium	Abdomen

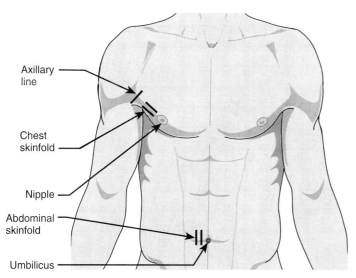

The chest and abdomen skinfold. Chest—A diagonal fold is taken between the axillary fold and the nipple. Abdomen—A vertical fold is taken about 2.5 centimeters (1 inch) to the side of the umbilicus.

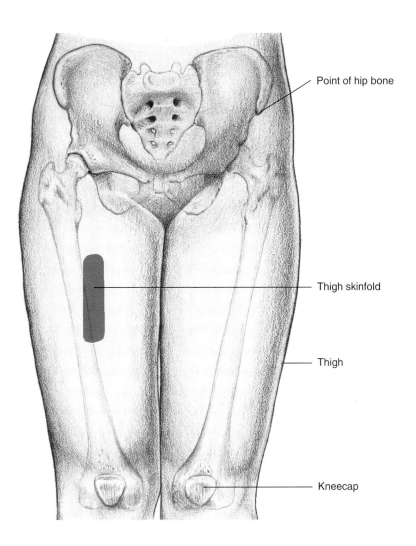

Point of hip bone

Thigh skinfold

Thigh

Kneecap

The thigh skinfold. A vertical fold is taken on the front of the thigh midway between the anterior iliac spine and the patella.

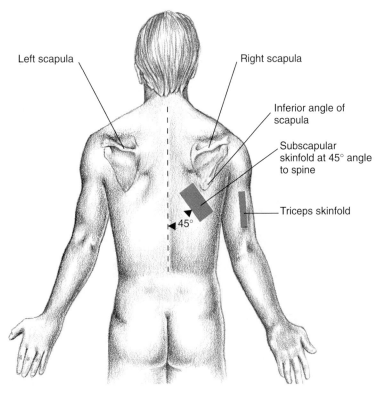

Left scapula

Right scapula

Inferior angle of scapula

Subscapular skinfold at 45° angle to spine

Triceps skinfold

45°

The triceps and subscapular skinfolds. In triceps skinfold, a vertical fold is taken over the triceps muscle one-half the distance from the acromion process to the olecranon process at the elbow. The subscapular skinfold is taken just below the lower angle of the scapula at about a 45° angle to the spinal column.

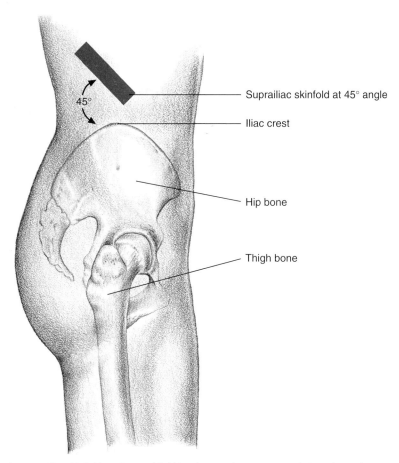

Suprailiac skinfold at 45° angle

Iliac crest

Hip bone

Thigh bone

The suprailiac skinfold. A diagonal fold is taken at about a 45° angle just above the crest of the ilium.

C. Calculation of percent body fat

Use the appropriate formula for your gender or enter the sum of the three skinfold sites in the table on the following pages for your age and gender.

D. Calculation of pounds of body fat

Your body weight in pounds × your percent body fat

Generalized Equations for Predicting Body Fat

Women*

$BD = 1.0994921 - 0.0009929\,(X_1) + 0.0000023\,(X_1)^2 - 0.0001392\,(X_2)$
BD = Body density
X_1 = Sum of triceps, thigh, and suprailium skinfolds
X_2 = Age

Men**

$BD = 1.10938 - 0.0008267\,(X_1) + .0000016\,(X_1)^2 - 0.0002574\,(X_2)$
BD = Body density
X_1 = Sum of chest, abdomen, and thigh skinfolds
X_2 = Age

To calculate percent body fat, plug into Siri's equation $\left(\dfrac{4.95}{BD} - 4.5\right) \times 100$

---

*From Jackson, A.; Pollock, M.; and Ward, A. 1980. Generalized equations for predicting body density of women. Medicine and Science in Sports and Exercise, 12:175–82. Reprinted by permission of Physician and Sportsmedicine, a McGraw-Hill publication.

**Jackson, A., and Pollock, M. 1978. Generalized equations for predicting body density of men. British Journal of Nutrition. 40:497–504. Reprinted by permission of Physician and Sportsmedicine, a McGraw-Hill publication.

Percent Fat Estimate for Men: Sum of Chest, Abdomen, and Thigh Skinfolds

Sum of Skinfolds (mm)	Under 22	23–27	28–32	33–37	38–42	43–47	48–52	53–57	Over 57
				Age to Last Year					
8–10	1.3	1.8	2.3	2.9	3.4	3.9	4.5	5.0	5.5
11–13	2.2	2.8	3.3	3.9	4.4	4.9	5.5	6.0	6.5
14–16	3.2	3.8	4.3	4.8	5.4	5.9	6.4	7.0	7.5
17–19	4.2	4.7	5.3	5.8	6.3	6.9	7.4	8.0	8.5
20–22	5.1	5.7	6.2	6.8	7.3	7.9	8.4	8.9	9.5
23–25	6.1	6.6	7.2	7.7	8.3	8.8	9.4	9.9	10.5
26–28	7.0	7.6	8.1	8.7	9.2	9.8	10.3	10.9	11.4
29–31	8.0	8.5	9.1	9.6	10.2	10.7	11.3	11.8	12.4
32–34	8.9	9.4	10.0	10.5	11.1	11.6	12.2	12.8	13.3
35–37	9.8	10.4	10.9	11.5	12.0	12.6	13.1	13.7	14.3
38–40	10.7	11.3	11.8	12.4	12.9	13.5	14.1	14.6	15.2
41–43	11.6	12.2	12.7	13.3	13.8	14.4	15.0	15.5	16.1
44–46	12.5	13.1	13.6	14.2	14.7	15.3	15.9	16.4	17.0
47–49	13.4	13.9	14.5	15.1	15.6	16.2	16.8	17.3	17.9
50–52	14.3	14.8	15.4	15.9	16.5	17.1	17.6	18.2	18.8
53–55	15.1	15.7	16.2	16.8	17.4	17.9	18.5	19.1	19.7
56–58	16.0	16.5	17.1	17.7	18.2	18.8	19.4	20.0	20.5
59–61	16.9	17.4	17.9	18.5	19.1	19.7	20.2	20.8	21.4
62–64	17.6	18.2	18.8	19.4	19.9	20.5	21.1	21.7	22.2
65–67	18.5	19.0	19.6	20.2	20.8	21.3	21.9	22.5	23.1
68–70	19.3	19.9	20.4	21.0	21.6	22.2	22.7	23.3	23.9
71–73	20.1	20.7	21.2	21.8	22.4	23.0	23.6	24.1	24.7
74–76	20.9	21.5	22.0	22.6	23.2	23.8	24.4	25.0	25.5
77–79	21.7	22.2	22.8	23.4	24.0	24.6	25.2	25.8	26.3
80–82	22.4	23.0	23.6	24.2	24.8	25.4	25.9	26.5	27.1
83–85	23.2	23.8	24.4	25.0	25.5	26.1	26.7	27.3	27.9
86–88	24.0	24.5	25.1	25.7	26.3	26.9	27.5	28.1	28.7
89–91	24.7	25.3	25.9	26.5	27.1	27.6	28.2	28.8	29.4
92–94	25.4	26.0	26.6	27.2	27.8	28.4	29.0	29.6	30.2
95–97	26.1	26.7	27.3	27.9	28.5	29.1	29.7	30.3	30.9
98–100	26.9	27.4	28.0	28.6	29.2	29.8	30.4	31.0	31.6
101–103	27.5	28.1	28.7	29.3	29.9	30.5	31.1	31.7	32.3
104–106	28.2	28.8	29.4	30.0	30.6	31.2	31.8	32.4	33.0
107–109	28.9	29.5	30.1	30.7	31.3	31.9	32.5	33.1	33.7
110–112	29.6	30.2	30.8	31.4	32.0	32.6	33.2	33.8	34.4
113–115	30.2	30.8	31.4	32.0	32.6	33.2	33.8	34.5	35.1
116–118	30.9	31.5	32.1	32.7	33.3	33.9	34.5	35.1	35.7
119–121	31.5	32.1	32.7	33.3	33.9	34.5	35.1	35.7	36.4
122–124	32.1	32.7	33.3	33.9	34.5	35.1	35.8	36.4	37.0
125–127	32.7	33.3	33.9	34.5	35.1	35.8	36.4	37.0	37.6

Reprinted by permission of Physician and Sportsmedicine, *a McGraw-Hill publication.*

Percent Fat Estimate for Women: Sum of Triceps, Suprailium, and Thigh Skinfolds

Sum of Skinfolds (mm)	Under 22	23–27	28–32	33–37	38–42	43–47	48–52	53–57	Over 57
				Age to Last Year					
23–25	9.7	9.9	10.2	10.4	10.7	10.9	11.2	11.4	11.7
26–28	11.0	11.2	11.5	11.7	12.0	12.3	12.5	12.7	13.0
29–31	12.3	12.5	12.8	13.0	13.3	13.5	13.8	14.0	14.3
32–34	13.6	13.8	14.0	14.3	14.5	14.8	15.0	15.3	15.5
35–37	14.8	15.0	15.3	15.5	15.8	16.0	16.3	16.5	16.8
38–40	16.0	16.3	16.5	16.7	17.0	17.2	17.5	17.7	18.0
41–43	17.2	17.4	17.7	17.9	18.2	18.4	18.7	18.9	19.2
44–46	18.3	18.6	18.8	19.1	19.3	19.6	19.8	20.1	20.3
47–49	19.5	19.7	20.0	20.2	20.5	20.7	21.0	21.2	21.5
50–52	20.6	20.8	21.1	21.3	21.6	21.8	22.1	22.3	22.6
53–55	21.7	21.9	22.1	22.4	22.6	22.9	23.1	23.4	23.6
56–58	22.7	23.0	23.2	23.4	23.7	23.9	24.2	24.4	24.7
59–61	23.7	24.0	24.2	24.5	24.7	25.0	25.2	25.5	25.7
62–64	24.7	25.0	25.2	25.5	25.7	26.0	26.2	26.4	26.7
65–67	25.7	25.9	26.2	26.4	26.7	26.9	27.2	27.4	27.7
68–70	26.6	26.9	27.1	27.4	27.6	27.9	28.1	28.4	28.6
71–73	27.5	27.8	28.0	28.3	28.5	28.8	29.0	29.3	29.5
74–76	28.4	28.7	28.9	29.2	29.4	29.7	29.9	30.2	30.4
77–79	29.3	29.5	29.8	30.0	30.3	30.5	30.8	31.0	31.3
80–82	30.1	30.4	30.6	30.9	31.1	31.4	31.6	31.9	32.1
83–85	30.9	31.2	31.4	31.7	31.9	32.2	32.4	32.7	32.9
86–88	31.7	32.0	32.2	32.5	32.7	32.9	33.2	33.4	33.7
89–91	32.5	32.7	33.0	33.2	33.5	33.7	33.9	34.2	34.4
92–94	33.2	33.4	33.7	33.9	34.2	34.4	34.7	34.9	35.2
95–97	33.9	34.1	34.4	34.6	34.9	35.1	35.4	35.6	35.9
98–100	34.6	34.8	35.1	35.3	35.5	35.8	36.0	36.3	36.5
101–103	35.3	35.4	35.7	35.9	36.2	36.4	36.7	36.9	37.2
104–106	35.8	36.1	36.3	36.6	36.8	37.1	37.3	37.5	37.8
107–109	36.4	36.7	36.9	37.1	37.4	37.6	37.9	38.1	38.4
110–112	37.0	37.2	37.5	37.7	38.0	38.2	38.5	38.7	38.9
113–115	37.5	37.8	38.0	38.2	38.5	38.7	39.0	39.2	39.5
116–118	38.0	38.3	38.5	38.8	39.0	39.3	39.5	39.7	40.0
119–121	38.5	38.7	39.0	39.2	39.5	39.7	40.0	40.2	40.5
122–124	39.0	39.2	39.4	39.7	39.9	40.2	40.4	40.7	40.9
125–127	39.4	39.6	39.9	40.1	40.4	40.6	40.9	41.1	41.4
128–130	39.8	40.0	40.3	40.5	40.8	41.0	41.3	41.5	41.8

Reprinted by permission of Physician and Sportsmedicine, *a McGraw-Hill publication.*

7.2

▼▼▼

Determination of Desirable Body Weight

There are a number of different techniques utilized to determine a desirable body weight. The following three methods offer you an estimate of an appropriate body weight. Method A is based upon height-weight charts. Method B is based on the Body Mass Index (BMI). Method C is based upon body fat percentage. Method D does not determine a desirable body weight but provides an assessment of desirable body fat distribution.

Method A

1. Measure your height.
2. Measure your elbow width and determine your frame size from table A on the next page.
   _____ Elbow width   _____ Frame size
3. Consult table B or C below to determine your desirable weight range. The midpoint is halfway into the range.
   _____ Height
   _____ Frame size
   _____ Desirable weight range
   _____ Midpoint of range
4. Obtain your current weight (as close to nude weight as feasible).
   _____ Current body weight
5. Determination of desirable weight. You should attempt to reach the midpoint or lower end of the range.

   Current body weight – Desirable weight = Pounds of fat to lose

   Your data:

   Current body weight – Midpoint of range = Pounds of fat to lose

   _____ – _____ = _____

   Current body weight – Low end of range = Pounds of fat to lose

   _____ – _____ = _____

Table A Approximation of Body Frame Size

Extend your arm and bend the forearm upward at a 90 degree angle. Keep fingers straight and turn the inside of your wrist toward your body. If you have a caliper, measure the space between the two prominent bones on either side of your elbow. Without a caliper, place thumb and index finger of your other hand on these two bones. Measure the space between your fingers against a ruler or tape measure. Compare it with the accompanying tables that list elbow measurements for medium-framed men and women. Measurements lower than those listed indicate that you have a small frame. Higher measurements indicate a larger frame.

Height (ft./in.)	Elbow Breadth (in.)
Men (1″ Heels)	
5′2″–5′3″	2½″–2⅞″
5′4″–5′7″	2⅝″–2⅞″
5′8″–5′11″	2¾″–3″
6′0″–6′3″	2¾″–3⅛″
6′4″	2⅞″–3¼″
Women (1″ Heels)	
4′10″–4′11″	2¼″–2½″
5′0″–5′3″	2¼″–2½″
5′4″–5′7″	2⅜″–2⅝″
5′8″–5′11″	2⅜″–2⅝″
6′0″	2½″–2¾″

Source: Used with permission of the Metropolitan Life Insurance Company.

Table B Desirable Weights for Males Aged Twenty-Five and Over

Height		Small Frame		Medium Frame		Large Frame	
(ft./in.)	(cm.)	(lb.)	(kg.)	(lb.)	(kg.)	(lb.)	(kg.)
6'3"	190.5	157–168	71.2–76.2	165–183	74.9–83.0	175–197	79.4–89.3
6'2"	188.0	153–164	69.4–74.4	160–178	72.6–80.8	171–192	77.6–87.1
6'1"	185.4	149–160	67.6–72.6	155–173	70.3–78.5	166–187	75.3–84.8
6'0"	182.9	145–155	65.8–70.3	151–168	68.5–76.2	161–182	73.0–82.6
5'11"	180.3	141–151	64.0–68.5	147–163	66.7–74.0	157–177	71.2–80.3
5'10"	177.8	137–147	62.1–66.7	143–158	64.9–71.7	152–172	69.0–78.0
5'9"	175.3	133–143	60.3–64.9	139–153	63.1–69.4	148–167	67.1–75.3
5'8"	172.7	129–138	58.5–62.6	135–149	61.2–67.6	144–163	65.3–74.0
5'7"	170.2	125–134	56.7–60.8	131–145	59.4–65.8	140–159	63.5–72.1
5'6"	167.6	121–130	54.9–59.0	127–140	57.6–63.5	135–154	61.2–69.9
5'5"	165.1	117–126	53.1–57.2	123–136	55.8–61.7	131–149	59.4–67.6
5'4"	162.6	114–122	51.7–55.3	120–132	54.4–59.9	128–145	58.1–65.8
5'3"	160.0	111–119	50.3–54.0	117–129	53.1–58.5	125–141	56.7–64.0
5'2"	157.5	108–116	49.0–52.6	114–126	51.7–57.2	122–137	55.3–62.1
5'1"	154.9	105–113	47.6–51.3	111–122	50.3–55.3	119–134	54.0–60.8

Height measured without shoes.
Source: Used with permission of the Metropolitan Life Insurance Company.

Table C Desirable Weights for Females Aged Twenty-Five and Over

Height		Small Frame		Medium Frame		Large Frame	
(ft./in.)	(cm.)	(lb.)	(kg.)	(lb.)	(kg.)	(lb.)	(kg.)
5'10"	177.8	134–144	60.8–65.3	140–155	63.5–70.3	149–169	67.6–76.6
5'9"	175.3	130–140	59.0–63.5	136–151	61.7–68.5	145–164	65.8–74.4
5'8"	172.7	126–136	57.2–61.7	132–147	59.9–66.7	141–159	64.0–72.1
5'7"	170.2	122–131	55.3–59.4	128–143	58.1–64.9	137–154	62.1–69.9
5'6"	167.6	118–127	53.5–57.6	124–139	56.2–63.1	133–150	60.3–68.1
5'5"	165.1	114–123	51.7–55.8	120–135	54.4–61.2	129–146	58.5–66.2
5'4"	162.6	110–119	49.9–54.0	116–131	52.6–59.4	125–142	56.7–64.4
5'3"	160.0	107–115	48.5–52.2	112–126	50.8–57.2	121–138	54.9–62.6
5'2"	157.5	104–112	47.2–50.8	109–122	49.4–55.3	117–134	53.1–60.8
5'1"	154.9	101–109	45.8–49.4	106–118	48.1–53.5	114–130	51.7–59.0
5'0"	152.4	98–106	44.4–48.1	103–115	46.7–52.2	111–127	50.3–57.6
4'11"	149.8	95–103	43.1–46.7	100–112	45.4–50.8	108–124	49.0–56.2
4'10"	147.3	92–100	41.7–45.4	97–109	44.0–49.4	105–121	47.6–54.9
4'9"	144.7	90–97	40.8–44.0	94–106	42.6–48.1	102–118	46.3–53.5

For women between eighteen and twenty-five, subtract one pound for each year under twenty-five. Height measured without shoes.
Source: Used with permission of the Metropolitan Life Insurance Company.

Method B

The BMI uses the metric system, so you need to determine your weight in kilograms and your height in meters. The formula is:

$$\frac{\text{Body weight in kilograms}}{(\text{Height in meters})^2}$$

Dividing your body weight in pounds by 2.2 will give you your weight in kilograms. Multiplying your height in inches by 0.0254 will give you your height in meters.

Your weight in kilograms = $\dfrac{(\text{Your weight in pounds})}{2.2}$ = _____

Your height in meters = (Your height in inches) × 0.0254 = _____

BMI = $\dfrac{\text{Body weight in kilograms}}{(\text{Height in meters})^2}$ = _____

A BMI range of 20 to 25 is considered to be normal, but a suggested desirable range for females is 21.3 to 22.1 and for males is 21.9 to 22.4. BMI values above 27.8 for men and 27.3 for women have been associated with increased incidence rates for several health problems, including high blood pressure and diabetes. The American Dietetic Association, in their position statement on nutrition and physical fitness, notes that a BMI greater than 30 is classified as obese.

If you want to lower your body weight to a more desirable BMI, such as 22, use the following formula to determine what that weight should be; the weight is expressed in kilograms, so multiplying it by 2.2 will give you the desired weight in pounds.

Kilograms body weight = Desired BMI × (Height in meters)^2

Here's a brief example for a woman who weighs 187 pounds and is 5′9″ tall; her BMI calculates to be 27.7, so her weight poses a health risk. If she wants to achieve a BMI of 23, she will need to reduce her weight to 155 pounds.

Kilograms body weight = 23 × (1.753)^2 = 70.6

70.6 kg × 2.2 = 155 pounds

Kilograms body weight = (Your desired BMI) × (Your height in meters)^2

Kilograms body weight = _____ × _____ = _____

_____ kg × 2.2 = _____ pounds

Method C

For this method, you will need to know your body fat percentage as determined by Laboratory Inventory 7.1 or another appropriate technique. You will also need to determine the body fat percentage you desire to be. You may use table 7.3 on page 145 as a guideline.

You will need to do the following calculations for the formula:

1. Determine your current lean body weight (LBW). Multiply your current body weight in pounds by your current percent body fat expressed as a decimal (20 percent would be .20) to obtain your pounds of body fat. Subtract your pounds of body fat from your current weight to give you your lean body weight (LBW).
2. Determine your desired body fat percentage and express it as a decimal.

Desired body weight = $\dfrac{\text{LBM}}{1.00 - \text{Desired \% body fat}}$

As an example, suppose we have a 200-pound male who is currently at 25 percent body fat but desires to get down to 20 percent as his first goal. Multiplying his current weight by his current percent body fat yields 50 pounds of body fat (200 × .25 = 50); subtracting this from his current weight yields a LBM of 150 (200 – 50). If we plug his desired percent of 20 into the formula, he will need to reach a body weight of 187.5 to achieve this first goal.

Desired body weight = $\dfrac{150}{1.00 - .20}$ = $\dfrac{150}{.8}$ = 187.5

Your current body weight _____
Your current percent body fat _____
Your pounds of body fat _____
Your LBW _____
Your desired percent body fat _____

Desired body weight = $\dfrac{\text{LBW}}{1.00 - ?}$ = _____ = _____

Method D

The waist:hip ratio (WHR) is a measure of regional fat distribution. Using a flexible, preferably metal, tape, measure the narrowest section of the bare waist as seen from the front while standing. Measure the hip girth at the largest circumference, which could be the hips, buttocks, or thighs, while standing. Wear tight clothing. Do not compress skin and fat with pressure from the tape. The measurement may be in either the English or metric system.

Waist girth _____

Hip girth _____

Determine the ratio by dividing the waist girth by the hip girth.

$$\frac{\text{Waist girth}}{\text{Hip girth}} = \text{_____}$$

Compare your result to the rating scale for health risk, based on data from Van Itallie, T. B. Topography of body fat: Relationship to risk of cardiovascular and other diseases. In *Anthropometric standardization reference manual,* ed. T. G. Lohman, et al. Champaign, Ill.: Human Kinetics.

Waist:Hip Ratio Health Risk Rating Scale

	Men	Women
Higher risk	>.95	>.85
Moderately high risk	.90–.95	.80–.85
Lower risk	<.90	<.80

7.3

---▼▼▼---

Calculation of Daily Energy Expenditure Based on the Physical Activity Factor Classification System

This laboratory provides a means to calculate your daily energy expenditure based on a physical activity classification system developed by the National Research Council. For the next laboratory (Laboratory Inventory 7.4), which deals with energy deficits for weight loss, you may use the figure calculated in this Laboratory Inventory instead of assuming a given number of Calories per pound body weight. You may also use computer programs to calculate your daily energy expenditure if available.

In this laboratory, you will need to determine your daily resting energy expenditure (REE), keep a record of your daily activities over a typical 24-hour period, calculate your overall average daily multiple of the REE, and then calculate your total daily energy expenditure. An abbreviated example is provided on page 341.

Step 1: Calculate your daily REE. For your sex and age, use the table below, and multiply the appropriate number of Calories by your body weight in kilograms, and add the appropriate number. You may also calculate a 10 percent range of daily caloric expenditure. An example is provided in the table for both a male and female.

(Body weight in kg) × (number of Calories) + (   ) = _____

(   ) × (   ) + (   ) = _____

Range:

(.10 × RMR) = _____   RMR + 10% = _____

                           RMR − 10% = _____

Estimation of the Daily Resting Energy Expenditure (based on age, gender, and body weight in kilograms)

Age (years)	Equation
Males	
3–9	(22.7 × body weight) + 495
10–17	(17.5 × body weight) + 651
18–29	(15.3 × body weight) + 679
30–60	(11.6 × body weight) + 879
>60	(13.5 × body weight) + 487
Example	
154-lb male, age 20	10% range
154 lbs/2.2 = 70 kg	.10 × 1750 = 175
(15.3 ×70) + 679 = 1750	± 10% = 1575–1925
Females	
3–9	(22.5 × body weight) + 499
10–17	(12.2 × body weight) + 746
18–29	(14.7 × body weight) + 496
30–60	(8.7 × body weight) + 829
>60	(10.5 × body weight) + 596
Example	
121-lb female, age 20	10% range
121 lbs/2.2 = 55 kg	.10 × 1304 = 130
(14.7 × 55) + 496 = 1304	± 10% = 1174–1434

Reprinted with permission from Recommended Dietary Allowances, *10th edition,* © 1989 by the National Academy of Sciences. Published by National Academy Press, Washington, DC.

Step 2. Determine your average daily physical activity factor. Keep a daily log of your physical activities, including sleeping, sitting, standing, leisure activities, exercise, etc. You will be asked to classify these activities as resting, very light, light, moderate, or heavy, so you may wish to peruse the table below relative to the physical activity factor classification system. Do not modify your daily behaviors; do what you normally do on a typical day.

Actual Time	*Total Hours or Portion of an Hour*	*Activity*	*Multiple of REE*
12:00– _____	_____	_____	_____
_____	_____	_____	_____
_____	_____	_____	_____
_____	_____	_____	_____
_____	_____	_____	_____
_____	_____	_____	_____
_____	_____	_____	_____
_____	_____	_____	_____
_____	_____	_____	_____
_____	_____	_____	_____
_____	_____	_____	_____
_____	_____	_____	_____
_____	_____	_____	_____
_____	_____	_____	_____
_____	_____	_____	_____
_____	_____	_____	_____
_____	_____	_____	_____
_____	_____	_____	_____
_____	_____	_____	_____
_____	_____	_____	_____
_____	_____	_____	_____
_____	_____	_____	_____
_____	_____	_____	_____
_____ -12:00	_____	_____	_____

Physical Activity Factor Classification System

Activity	Multiple of REE
1. **Resting:** Sleeping, reclining while watching TV	1.0
2. **Very light:** Sitting and standing activities, such as driving, playing cards, typing	1.5
3. **Light:** Activities comparable to walking at a leisurely pace, light housework, sports such as golf, bowling, archery	2.5
4. **Moderate:** Walking at a pace of 3.5–4.0 mph, active gardening, sports such as cycling, tennis, dancing	5.0
5. **Heavy:** Faster walking, stair and hill climbing, more active sports such as basketball, soccer	7.0

Reprinted with permission from Recommended Dietary Allowances, *by the National Academy of Sciences. Published by National Academy Press, Washington, DC. © 1989.*

Step 3. Calculate overall daily average physical activity factor. First, summarize your activity in the five different areas. Then, multiply the total number of hours for each activity times the multiple of the REE. Divide this total number by 24, the number of hours in a day.

Summary

Activity	Total Number of Hours	Multiple of REE	Total Number of Hours × Multiple of REE
Resting	_____	1.0	_____
Very Light	_____	1.5	_____
Light Activity	_____	2.5	_____
Moderate Activity	_____	5.0	_____
Heavy Activity	_____	7.0	_____
Total	24		_____

Calculate overall daily average physical activity factor:

Total number of hours × multiple of REE/24

(   )/24 = _____

Step 4. Calculate the total daily energy expenditure by multiplying the overall daily average physical activity factor (Step 3) by the REE calculated in Step 1.

Calculate Daily Energy Expenditure:

(Overall daily average of the physical activity factor) × (REE)
(   ) × (   ) = _____

You may also use the upper and lower ranges calculated in step 1 to provide you with other estimates of your daily caloric needs. For a weight-loss program, you may desire to use the lower estimate.

(Overall daily average of the physical activity factor) × (upper level REE)
(   ) × (   ) = _____

(Overall daily average of the physical activity factor) × (lower level REE)
(   ) × (   ) = _____

You may use this answer in Laboratory Inventory 7.4 as the basis for your estimated daily caloric expenditure to maintain your current body weight, provided you have been maintaining that weight and this represents your typical daily activities.

Example:

A twenty-year-old female who weighs 132 pounds, or 60 kilograms, is very physically active. Her calculated daily resting energy expenditure is 1378 Calories ($14.7 \times 60 = 882 + 496 = 1378$). Her upper estimate is 1516 ($1378 + 138$), while her lower estimate is 1240 ($1378 - 138$). Let us assume her daily activity levels were: rest, 8 hours; very light activity, 8 hours; light activity, 4 hours; moderate activity, 2 hours; and heavy activity, 2 hours.

Activity	Total Number of Hours	Multiple of REE	Total Number of Hours × Multiple of REE
Resting	8	1.0	8.00
Very Light	8	1.5	12.00
Light Activity	4	2.5	10.00
Moderate Activity	2	5.0	10.00
Heavy Activity	2	7.0	14.00
Total	24		54.00

Average daily physical activity factor = 54/24 = 2.25

Total daily energy expenditure = 2.25 × 1378 = 3,100 Calories

7.4
▼▼▼

Calculation of Daily Caloric Deficit Needed to Lose Two Pounds of Body Fat per Week

Note: May be adjusted to lose less weight per week. A 3,500 Calorie deficit per week is the equivalent of 1 pound of body weight. See table 7.13 on page 162 for daily caloric deficits and number of days to lose a given amount of weight. Also, if you use the caloric value calculated in Step 4 of Laboratory Inventory 7.3, which already accounts for daily physical activity, you need only complete Steps 2 and 5 of this laboratory inventory. If the caloric value calculated in Laboratory Inventory 7.3 is keeping you at your current weight, simply put that value in Step 2 and then subtract 1,000.

1. Calculate the number of daily Calories needed to maintain current body weight. Since you will calculate exercise calories in number 3, use the sedentary level of 14 Calories per pound body weight and calculate the following:

(Calories per pound body weight)	×	(Body weight in pounds)	=	Number of daily Calories to maintain body weight
___14___	×	_____	=	_____

2. Since 2 pounds of body fat equals 7,000 Calories, and there are 7 days in the week, you must achieve a daily dietary caloric deficit of 1,000 Calories (7,000 ÷ 7).

Number of daily Calories to maintain body weight	−	Daily dietary deficit	=	Number of daily Calories to lose 2 pounds per week
_____	−	___1,000___	=	_____

3. Calculate average number of daily exercise Calories for 1 week in your planned aerobic program. See Appendix C for appropriate exercise Calories. Divide the total exercise Calories expended by 7 to get your daily average.

Day	Exercise	Calories Expended
Monday	_____	_____
Tuesday	_____	_____
Wednesday	_____	_____
Thursday	_____	_____
Friday	_____	_____
Saturday	_____	_____
Sunday	_____	_____
Total Calories expended		_____
Daily average number of exercise Calories expended		_____

4. Add the average daily exercise Calories to the daily dietary Calories without exercise to calculate the total number of Calories you may consume and still lose 2 pounds of body fat per week.

Number of daily Calories to lose 2 pounds per week	+	Average daily exercise Calories	=	Total number of daily dietary Calories you may consume
_____	+	_____	=	_____

5. Plot your weight losses on the accompanying graph. Keep in mind that actual weight losses may not parallel caloric deficits due to reasons noted in chapter 7. You may duplicate this chart to plot your weight loss over several months.

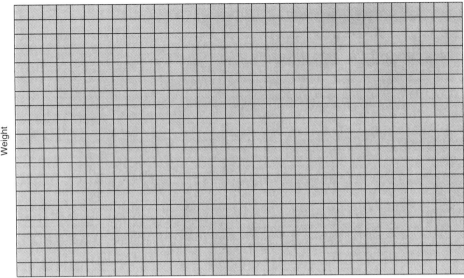

Weight

Dates

7.5

▼▼▼

Developing Your Personal Diet

1. Calculate the number of Calories you need per day. See Laboratory Inventory 7.3 or 7.4 for guidelines.
2. Use table 7.8 on page 154 to determine how many servings you need from each Food Exchange. If the exact number of Calories you need is not listed, simply add or subtract Food Exchanges as needed. For example, if you needed 3,000 Calories, add 500 Calories to the 2,500-Calorie diet plan by including an additional two lean meat exchanges (110 Calories), three starch/bread exchanges (240 Calories), one fruit exchange (60 Calories) and one skim milk exchange (90 Calories).
3. If you make adjustments to the diet plan in table 7.8 on page 154, multiply the number of servings by the Calories per serving as a check on your total Calories.
4. Select appropriate foods from the Exchange Lists in Appendix A.

Personal Diet: Calories _____	Number of Servings	Calories Per Serving	Total Calories	Foods Selected
Breakfast				
Milk, skim		90		
Meat, lean		55		
Fruit		60		
Vegetable		25		
Starch/bread		80		
Fat		45		
Beverage		0		
Lunch				
Milk, skim		90		
Meat, lean		55		
Fruit		60		
Vegetable		25		
Starch/bread		80		
Fat		45		
Beverage		0		
Dinner				
Milk, skim		90		
Meat, lean		55		
Fruit		60		
Vegetable		25		
Starch/bread		80		
Fat		45		
Beverage		0		
Snacks				
Milk, skim		90		
Meat, lean		55		
Fruit		60		
Vegetable		25		
Starch/bread		80		
Fat		45		
Beverage		0		
Total Calories			_____	

7.6

A Guide to Weight Gaining

The keys to gaining weight, primarily muscle mass, are to create a positive caloric balance through increased caloric intake and to use a resistance-training program for most of the major muscle groups in the body. Use the following as a guide to increasing your caloric intake while assuring that the weight gain is muscle tissue and not body fat.

1. From Laboratory Inventory 7.3 or table 7.5 on page 150, determine how many Calories you need daily simply to maintain body weight. If you use Laboratory Inventory 7.3 to calculate your daily average energy expenditure, which already accounts for your daily physical activity, including exercise, you need only simply add 400 to 500 Calories to the daily average. Because you are trying to gain weight, you might add these Calories to the upper range.

2. Plan to expend about 300 Calories per day exercising. Three or four days per week should involve a weight-training program as described in chapter 7. Each session will take about an hour. Four days per week should involve aerobic activities lasting approximately 20 to 30 minutes. Each of these types of activities will expend a total of approximately 300 Calories daily when based on a 7-day week.

3. Consume an additional 400 to 500 Calories per day to add 1 pound per week.

4. Total the Calories from steps 1 to 3 to determine your recommended daily caloric intake. Then refer to table 7.8 on page 154 to design your own diet plan as suggested in Laboratory Inventory 7.5.

5. Use a good cloth or steel tape to take body measurements. Be sure you take them at the same points about once a week. Those body parts measured should include the neck, upper arm, chest, abdomen, thigh, and calf. This is to insure that body weight gains are proportionately distributed. You should look for good gains in the chest and limbs; the abdominal girth increase should be kept low because that is where the fat will increase the most. If you have skinfold calipers, then various skinfold measures can also be used to check on body fat levels. See Laboratory Inventory 7.1 for the skinfold technique.

Personal data:

1. Number of Calories to maintain body weight   _____
2. Daily exercise Calories   _____ +300 _____
3. Add 400 to 500 Calories for 1 pound gain per week   _____ +400 _____
4. Recommended daily caloric intake (Total steps 1 to 3)   _____

5. Body measurements

	Date _____	Date _____	Date _____	Date _____	Date _____
Girths:					
Neck	_____	_____	_____	_____	_____
Upper arm	_____	_____	_____	_____	_____
Chest	_____	_____	_____	_____	_____
Abdomen	_____	_____	_____	_____	_____
Thigh	_____	_____	_____	_____	_____
Calf	_____	_____	_____	_____	_____
Skinfolds:					
Triceps	_____	_____	_____	_____	_____
Abdominal	_____	_____	_____	_____	_____
Thigh	_____	_____	_____	_____	_____
Chest	_____	_____	_____	_____	_____
Suprailium	_____	_____	_____	_____	_____

8.1

Daily State Anxiety

This laboratory provides you with a quick method to assess your level of state anxiety on a daily basis. It utilizes several pairs of adjectives that may describe your mood for any given day, focusing basically upon your feelings of tension, depression, anger, confusion, and time urgency. The adjectives are placed on a continuum. For example, low levels of tension are reflected by the terms *relaxed* and *calm,* whereas high levels of tension are represented by the adjectives *tense* and *tight.*

First, look at the terms on each end of the continuum and decide how you feel today, e.g., relaxed and calm or tense and tight. Then, use the following as a guide to the magnitude of your feelings on each of the five pairs of terms. For example, if you feel extremely relaxed and calm, place a check in the 0 column for relaxed, calm. However, if you are mildly or slightly tense or tight, place a check under the 3 column towards that side of the continuum. The scale below will focus upon the first set of adjectives, so simply substitute the other terms as you evaluate your feelings.

0 = Very (extremely) calm, relaxed
1 = Moderately (quite) calm, relaxed
2 = Mildly (slightly) calm, relaxed
3 = Mildly (slightly) tight, tense
4 = Moderately (quite) tight, tense
5 = Very (extremely) tight, tense

	0	1	2	3	4	5	
Relaxed, calm	___	___	___	___	___	___	Tense, tight
Joyful, happy	___	___	___	___	___	___	Depressed, unhappy
Pleasant, friendly	___	___	___	___	___	___	Hostile, unfriendly
Sharp, attentive	___	___	___	___	___	___	Foggy, confused
Leisurely, unhurried	___	___	___	___	___	___	Rushed, hurried

To score, simply sum the total of your check marks for the five sets of adjectives. Use the following scale as a guide to your general level of state anxiety.

0–7 = Low stress or anxiety level
8–16 = Moderate stress or anxiety level
17–25 = High stress or anxiety level

If you recognize that you are at a higher level of stress than normal, use one or more of the stress-reduction techniques discussed in chapter 8 to help you cope better throughout the day.

8.2

▼▼▼

Stress and You

This is a four-part test. The first three parts are designed to measure your vulnerability to certain types of stress and to increase your awareness of stress and how it affects you. The fourth part gives you some idea of how well you cope with stressful situations.

These tests were developed by Dr. Daniel Girdano and Dr. George Everly at The University of Maryland and may be found in their text *Controlling Stress and Tension.*

If you have any concerns or questions about your answers to this assessment, you may want to discuss them with a qualified counselor, your family physician, or other medical professionals. For additional information on stress, write or call the National Institute of Mental Health, Public Inquiries Section, 5600 Fishers Lane, Rockville, MD 20857, (301) 443–4513 or the National Mental Health Association, Information Center, 1021 Prince Street, Alexandria, VA 22314–2971, (800) 969–6642.

Stress Test Part One

Read and choose the most appropriate answer for each of the ten questions.

1. When I can't do something "my way," I simply adjust to do it the easiest way.
   a) Almost always true b) Usually true c) Usually false d) Almost always false
2. I get "upset" when someone in front of me drives slowly.
   a) Almost always true b) Usually true c) Usually false d) Almost always false   3
3. It bothers me when my plans are dependent upon others.
   a) Almost always true b) Usually true c) Usually false d) Almost always false   3
4. Whenever possible, I tend to avoid large crowds.
   a) Almost always true b) Usually true c) Usually false d) Almost always false   3
5. I am uncomfortable when I have to stand in long lines.
   a) Almost always true b) Usually true c) Usually false d) Almost always false   3
6. Arguments upset me.
   a) Almost always true b) Usually true c) Usually false d) Almost always false   4
7. When my plans don't "flow smoothly," I become anxious.
   a) Almost always true b) Usually true c) Usually false d) Almost always false   3
8. I require a lot of room (space) in which to live and work.
   a) Almost always true b) Usually true c) Usually false d) Almost always false   3
9. When I am busy at some task, I hate to be disturbed.
   a) Almost always true b) Usually true c) Usually false d) Almost always false   2
10. I believe that "All good things are worth waiting for."
    a) Almost always true b) Usually true c) Usually false d) Almost always false

Score ___26___

Scoring Part One

To score: 1 and 10: a = 1 pt, b = 2 pts, c = 3 pts, d = 4 pts

            2 through 9: a = 4 pts, b = 3 pts, c = 2 pts, d = 1 pt

This test measures your vulnerability to the stress of being "frustrated," i.e., inhibited. Scores in excess of 25 seem to suggest some vulnerability to this source of stress.

Stress Test Part Two

Circle the letter of the response option that best answers the following ten questions.

How often do you

1. find yourself with insufficient time to complete your work?
   a) Almost always b) Very often c) Seldom d) Never
2. find yourself becoming confused and unable to think clearly because too many things are happening at once?
   a) Almost always b) Very often c) Seldom d) Never
3. wish you had help to get everything done?
   a) Almost always b) Very often c) Seldom d) Never
4. feel your boss/professor simply expects too much from you?
   a) Almost always b) Very often c) Seldom d) Never
5. feel your family/friends expect too much from you?
   a) Almost always b) Very often c) Seldom d) Never
6. find your work infringing upon your leisure hours?
   a) Almost always b) Very often c) Seldom d) Never
7. find yourself doing extra work to set an example for those around you?
   a) Almost always b) Very often c) Seldom d) Never
8. find yourself doing extra work to impress your superiors?
   a) Almost always b) Very often c) Seldom d) Never
9. have to skip a meal so that you can get work completed?
   a) Almost always b) Very often c) Seldom d) Never
10. feel that you have too much responsibility?
    a) Almost always b) Very often c) Seldom d) Never

Score 20

Scoring Part Two

To score: a = 4 pts, b = 3 pts, c = 2 pts, d = 1 pt

Total up your score for this exercise.

This text measures your vulnerability to "overload" (having too much to do). Scores in excess of 25 seem to indicate vulnerability to this source of stress.

Stress Test Part Three

Answer all questions as is generally true for you.

1. I hate to wait in lines.
    a) Almost always true b) Usually true c) Seldom true d) Never true

2. I often find myself "racing" against the clock to save time.
    a) Almost always true b) Usually true c) Seldom true d) Never true

3. I become upset if I think something is taking too long.
    a) Almost always true b) Usually true c) Seldom true d) Never true

4. When under pressure, I tend to lose my temper.
    a) Almost always true b) Usually true c) Seldom true d) Never true

5. My friends tell me that I tend to get irritated easily.
    a) Almost always true b) Usually true c) Seldom true d) Never true

6. I seldom like to do anything unless I can make it competitive.
    a) Almost always true b) Usually true c) Seldom true d) Never true

7. When something needs to be done, I'm the first to begin even though the details may still need to be worked out.
    a) Almost always true b) Usually true c) Seldom true d) Never true

8. When I make a mistake, it is usually because I've rushed into something without giving it enough thought and planning.
    a) Almost always true b) Usually true c) Seldom true d) Never true

9. Whenever possible, I try to do two things at once, like eating while working, or planning while driving or bathing.
    a) Almost always true b) Usually true c) Seldom true d) Never true

10. When I go on a vacation, I usually take some work along just in case I get a chance to do it.
    a) Almost always true b) Usually true c) Seldom true d) Never true

Score _____

Scoring Part Three

To score: a = 4 pts, b = 3 pts, c = 2 pts, d = 1 pt

This test measures the presence of compulsive, time-urgent, and excessively aggressive behavioral traits. Scores in excess of 25 suggest the presence of one or more of these traits.

Stress Test Part Four

How do you cope with the stress in your life? There are numerous ways, some more effective than others. Some coping strategies may actually be as harmful as the stress they are used to alleviate. This scale was created largely on the basis of results compiled by clinicians and researchers who sought to identify how individuals effectively cope with stress. This scale is an educational tool, not a clinical instrument. Therefore, its purpose is to inform you, the reader, of ways by which you can effectively and healthfully cope with the stress in your life. At the same time, a point system gives you some indication of the relative desirability of the coping strategies you are currently using. Simply follow the instructions given for each of the fourteen items listed. When you have completed all of the items, total your points and consult the scoring procedure.

_____ 1. Give yourself 10 points if you feel that you have a supportive family around you.

_____ 2. Give yourself 10 points if you actively pursue a hobby.

_____ 3. Give yourself 10 points if you belong to some social or activity group (other than your family) that meets at least once a month.

_____ 4. Give yourself 15 points if you are within 5 pounds of your "ideal" body weight, considering your height and bone structure.

_____ 5. Give yourself 15 points if you practice some form of "deep relaxation" at least 3 times a week. Deep relaxation exercises include meditation, imagery, yoga, etc.

_____ 6. Give yourself 5 points for each time you exercise for 30 minutes or longer during the course of an average week (15 points maximum).

_____ 7. Give yourself 5 points for each nutritionally balanced and wholesome meal you consume during the course of an average day (15 points maximum).

_____ 8. Give yourself 5 points if you do something that you really enjoy and that is "just for you" during the course of an average week.

_____ 9. Give yourself 10 points if you have some place in your home that you can go in order to relax and/or be by yourself.

_____ 10. Give yourself 10 points if you practice time management techniques in your daily life.

_____ 11. Subtract 10 points for each pack of cigarettes you smoke during the course of an average day.

_____ 12. Subtract 5 points for each evening during the course of an average week that you take any form of medication or chemical substance (including alcohol) to help you sleep.

_____ 13. Subtract 10 points for each day during the course of an average week that you consume any form of medication or chemical substance (including alcohol) to reduce your anxiety or just calm you down.

_____ 14. Subtract 5 points for each evening during the course of an average week that you bring work home—work that was meant to be done at your place of employment.

Score _____

Scoring Part Four

Calculate your total score. A "perfect" score is 115 points. If you scored in the 50–60 range, you probably have an adequate collection of coping strategies for most common sources of stress. However, you should keep in mind that the higher your score, the greater your ability to cope with stress in an effective and healthful manner.

9.1

Do You Have a Problem with Substance Abuse?

The following questions are based on the diagnostic criteria for psychoactive substance dependence listed by the American Psychiatric Association in their publication, *Diagnostic and Statistical Manual of Mental Disorders*.

These criteria pertain to various psychoactive substances, including alcohol, marijuana, amphetamines, cocaine, narcotics, and various prescription drugs, such as antidepressants. If you respond positively to at least three of the following questions, you should consult a health professional.

1. Do you often take more of a psychoactive substance than you originally intended?
2. Have you tried unsuccessfully a number of times to cut down or control substance use?
3. Do you spend a great deal of your time using the substance, or in ways to obtain the substance or to recover from using it?
4. Does the use of the substance interfere with the accomplishment of other responsibilities, such as work, school, family, and community obligations or the personal safety of yourself and others?
5. Have you decreased or given up participation in important social, recreational, or occupational activities because of substance use?
6. Do you continue to use the substance even though you experience a social, psychological, or physical problem associated with its use?
7. Have you found that you need increased amounts of the substance in order to develop the psychoactive effects you once experienced with lower doses, or do you have decreased psychoactive effects with doses that used to elicit the desired effects?
8. Do you experience specific withdrawal symptoms, such as anxiety or shakiness, when you do not take the substance on your regular schedule?
9. If you do experience withdrawal symptoms, do you take the substance to relieve them?

9.2

Self-Test on Drinking Habits and Alcoholism

Here is a self-test to help you review the role alcohol plays in your life. These questions incorporate some of the common symptoms of alcoholism. This test is intended to help you determine if you or someone you know needs to find out more about alcoholism; it is not intended to be used to establish the diagnosis of alcoholism.

	Yes	No
1. Do you drink heavily when you are disappointed, under pressure, or have had a quarrel with someone?	____	____
2. Have you ever been unable to remember part of the previous evening, even though your friends say you didn't pass out?	____	____
3. When drinking with other people, do you try to have a few extra drinks when others won't know about it?	____	____
4. Are you in more of a hurry to get your first drink of the day than you used to be?	____	____
5. Do you sometimes feel a little guilty about your drinking?	____	____
6. When you're sober, do you sometimes regret things you did or said while drinking?	____	____
7. Have you tried switching brands or drinks, or following different plans to control your drinking?	____	____
8. Have you sometimes failed to keep promises you made to yourself about controlling or cutting down on your drinking?	____	____
9. Have you ever had a DWI (driving while intoxicated) or DUI (driving under the influence of alcohol) violation, or any other legal problem related to your drinking?	____	____
10. Do you try to avoid family or close friends while you are drinking?	____	____

Any "yes" answer indicates you may be at greater risk for alcoholism. More than one "yes" answer may indicate the presence of an alcohol-related problem or alcoholism, and the need for consultation with an alcoholism professional. To find out more, contact the National Council on Alcoholism and Drug Dependence in your area.

Reprinted courtesy of the National Council on Alcoholism and Drug Dependence. For a brochure that contains these and other questions, please contact NCADD, 12 West 21st Street, New York, NY, 10010.

9.3

Why Do You Smoke?

Here are some statements made by people to describe what they get out of smoking cigarettes. How often do you feel this way when smoking them? Circle one number for each statement. **Important: Answer every question.**

		Always	Frequently	Occasionally	Seldom	Never
A.	I smoke cigarettes in order to keep myself from slowing down.	5	4	3	2	1
B.	Handling a cigarette is part of the enjoyment of smoking it.	5	4	3	2	1
C.	Smoking cigarettes is pleasant and relaxing.	5	4	3	2	1
D.	I light up a cigarette when I feel angry about something.	5	4	3	2	1
E.	When I run out of cigarettes, I find it almost unbearable until I can get them.	5	4	3	2	1
F.	I smoke cigarettes automatically, without even being aware of it.	5	4	3	2	1
G.	I smoke cigarettes to stimulate me, to perk myself up.	5	4	3	2	1
H.	Part of the enjoyment of smoking a cigarette comes from the steps I take to light up.	5	4	3	2	1
I.	I find cigarettes pleasurable.	5	4	3	2	1
J.	When I feel uncomfortable or upset about something, I light up a cigarette.	5	4	3	2	1
K.	I am very much aware of when I'm not smoking a cigarette.	5	4	3	2	1
L.	I light up a cigarette without realizing I still have one burning in the ashtray.	5	4	3	2	1

Source: *U.S. Department of Health, Education and Welfare.* The Smoker's Self-Test. *DHEW Publication No. (CDC) 75–8716. Washington, D.C.: U.S. Government Printing Office.*

M. I smoke cigarettes to give me a lift.	5	4	3	2	1
N. When I smoke a cigarette, part of the enjoyment is watching the smoke as I exhale it.	5	4	3	2	1
O. I want a cigarette most when I'm comfortable and relaxed.	5	4	3	2	1
P. When I feel blue or want to take my mind off cares and worries, I smoke cigarettes.	5	4	3	2	1
Q. I get a real gnawing hunger for a cigarette when I haven't smoked for a while.	5	4	3	2	1
R. I've found a cigarette in my mouth and didn't remember putting it there.	5	4	3	2	1

1. Enter the number you have circled for each question in the spaces below, putting the number you have circled to question A over line A, to question B over line B, etc.
2. Add the three scores on each line to get your totals. For example, the sum of your scores over lines A, G, and M gives you your score on Stimulation; lines B, H, and N give the score on Handling, etc.

Totals

_____ +	_____ +	_____ =	_____	
A	G	M		Stimulation
_____ +	_____ +	_____ =	_____	
B	H	N		Handling
_____ +	_____ +	_____ =	_____	
C	I	O		Pleasurable Relaxation
_____ +	_____ +	_____ =	_____	
D	J	P		Crutch: Tension Reduction
_____ +	_____ +	_____ =	_____	
E	K	Q		Craving: Psychological Addiction
_____ +	_____ +	_____ =	_____	
F	L	R		Habit

Scores can vary from 3 to 15. Any score 11 and above is high; any score 7 and below is low.

The six factors measured by this test describe ways of experiencing or managing certain kinds of feelings. Three of these feeling-states represent the positive feelings people get from smoking: (1) a sense of increased energy or *stimulation*, (2) the satisfaction of *handling* or manipulating things, and (3) the enhancing of *pleasurable feelings* accompanying a state of well-being. The fourth is the *decreasing of negative feelings* by reducing a state of tension or feelings of anxiety, anger, shame, etc. The fifth is a complex pattern of increasing and decreasing "craving" for a cigarette, a *psychological addiction* to cigarettes. The sixth is *habit* smoking, which takes place in an absence of feeling—purely automatic smoking.

A score of 11 or above on any factor indicates that this factor is an important source of satisfaction for you. The higher your score (15 is the highest), the more important a particular factor is in your smoking and the more useful the discussion of that factor can be in your attempt to quit.

A few words of warning. If you give up smoking, you may have to get along without the satisfactions that smoking gives you. Either that, or you will have to find some more acceptable way of getting this satisfaction. In either case, you need to know just what it is you get out of smoking before you can decide whether to forego the satisfactions it gives you.

1. Stimulation. If you score high or fairly high on this factor, it means that you are one of those smokers who is stimulated by the cigarette—you feel that it helps wake you up, organize your energies, and keep you going. If you try to give up smoking, you may want a safe substitute—a brisk walk or moderate exercise—whenever you feel the urge to smoke.

2. Handling. Handling things can be satisfying, but there are many ways to keep your hands busy without lighting up or playing with a cigarette. Why not toy with a pen or pencil? Or try doodling. Or play with a coin, a piece of jewelry, or some other harmless object. There are plastic cigarettes to play with; you might even use a real cigarette if you can trust yourself not to light it.

3. Accentuation of pleasure—pleasurable relaxation. It is not always easy to find out whether you use the cigarette to feel good, that is, get real, honest pleasure out of smoking (factor 3) or to keep from feeling bad (factor 4). About two-thirds of smokers score high or fairly high on accentuation of pleasure, and about half of those also score as high or higher on reduction of negative feelings.

   Those who do get real pleasure out of smoking often find that an honest consideration of the harmful effects of their habit is enough to help them quit. They substitute eating, social activities, and physical activities—within reasonable bounds—and find they do not seriously miss their cigarettes.

4. Reduction of negative feelings, or "crutch." Many smokers use the cigarette as a kind of crutch in moments of stress or discomfort, and on occasion it may work; the cigarette is sometimes used as a tranquilizer. But the heavy smoker, the person who tries to handle severe personal problems by smoking many times a day, is apt to discover that cigarettes do not help him deal with his problems effectively.

   When it comes to quitting, this kind of smoker may find it easy to stop when everything is going well, but he/she may be tempted to start again in a time of crisis. Again, physical exertion, eating, or social activity—in moderation—may serve as useful substitutes for cigarettes, even in times of tension. The choice of a substitute depends on what will achieve the same effect without having any appreciable risk.

5. "Craving" or psychological addiction. Quitting smoking is difficult for the person who scores high on this factor. For him/her, the craving for the next cigarette begins to build up the moment he/she puts one out, so tapering off is not likely to work. He/she must go "cold turkey."

   It may be helpful for him/her to smoke more than usual for a day or two, so that the taste for cigarettes is spoiled, and then isolate himself/herself completely from cigarettes until the craving is gone. Giving up cigarettes may be so difficult and cause so much discomfort that once he/she does quit, he/she will find it easy to resist the temptation to go back to smoking because he/she knows that some day he/she will have to go through the same agony again.

6. Habit. This kind of smoker is no longer getting much satisfaction from cigarettes. He/she just lights them frequently without even realizing he/she is doing so. He/she may find it easy to quit and stay off if he/she can break the habit patterns he/she has built up. Cutting down gradually may be quite effective if there is a change in the way the cigarettes are smoked and the conditions under which they are smoked. The key to success is becoming aware of each cigarette smoked. This can be done by asking, "Do I really want this cigarette?" You may be surprised at how many you do not want.

Summary

If you do not score high on any of the six factors, chances are that you do not smoke very much or have not been smoking for very many years. If so, giving up smoking and staying off should be easy.

If you score high on several categories, you apparently get several kinds of satisfaction from smoking and will have to find several solutions. Certain combinations of scores may indicate that giving up smoking will be especially difficult. Those who score high on both factor 4 and factor 5, reduction of negative feelings and craving, may have a particularly hard time in going off smoking and in staying off. However, there are ways of doing it; many smokers represented by this combination have been able to quit.

Others who score high on factors 4 and 5 may find it useful to change their patterns of smoking and cut down at the same time. They can try to smoke fewer cigarettes, smoke them only half-way down, use low-tar-and-nicotine cigarettes, and inhale less often and less deeply. Nicotine patches are available to help wean the smoker from the addictive effects of nicotine. After several months of this temporary solution, they may find it easier to stop completely.

You must make two important decisions: (1) whether to try to do without the satisfactions you get from smoking or find an appropriate, less hazardous substitute, and (2) whether to try to cut out cigarettes all at once or taper off.

Your scores should guide you in making both of these decisions.

9.4

Do You Really Want to Quit Smoking?

Answer each question, circling the number that most accurately indicates how you feel.

	Completely Agree	Somewhat Agree	Somewhat Disagree	Completely Disagree
A. Cigarette smoking might give me a serious illness.	4	3	2	1
B. My cigarette smoking sets a bad example for others.	4	3	2	1
C. I find cigarette smoking to be a messy kind of habit.	4	3	2	1
D. Controlling my cigarette smoking is a challenge to me.	4	3	2	1
E. Smoking causes shortness of breath.	4	3	2	1
F. If I quit smoking cigarettes, it might influence others to stop.	4	3	2	1
G. Cigarettes cause damage to clothing and other personal property.	4	3	2	1
H. Quitting smoking would show that I have willpower.	4	3	2	1
I. My cigarette smoking will have a harmful effect on my health.	4	3	2	1
J. My cigarette smoking influences others close to me to take up or continue smoking.	4	3	2	1
K. If I quit smoking, my sense of taste or smell would improve.	4	3	2	1
L. I do not like the idea of feeling dependent on smoking.	4	3	2	1

Enter the numbers you have circled to each test question in the appropriate space below, entering the number you circled to answer question A over line A, to question B over line B, and so on.

```
____ + ____ + ____  =  _____
  A      E      I          Health

____ + ____ + ____  =  _____
  B      F      J          Example

____ + ____ + ____  =  _____
  C      G      K          Esthetics

____ + ____ + ____  =  _____
  D      H      L          Mastery
```

Total the three scores across on each line to get your totals. For example, the sum of your scores over line A, E, and I gives your score on Health; lines B, F, and J give your score on Example, and so on.

Scores can vary from three to twelve. Any score nine and above is high; any score six and below is low. A *high* score on any of the following indicates that you are motivated by the factor to help you quit smoking.

Health—You believe smoking is potentially hazardous to your health.

Example—You believe you are an example to others and may influence their smoking behavior. By not smoking, your younger brother or sister may follow your example.

Esthetics—You believe that smoking is a bad habit that may be aesthetically damaging. It smells and creates a mess.

Mastery—You want to be able to control your behavior and not be dependent upon smoking.

Source: *U.S. Department of Health, Education and Welfare.* The Smoker's Self-Test. *Public Health Service Publication No. 2013. Washington, D.C.: U.S. Government Printing Office, 1969.*

10.1

Monthly Record of Physical and Psychological Symptoms During My Menstrual Cycle

This laboratory will help you plot the occurrence of symptoms associated with the premenstrual syndrome (PMS) over a menstrual cycle. You may duplicate this page to track your symptoms over several cycles. Listed below are some common physical and psychological (emotional) symptoms that may occur throughout your cycle, particularly during the days prior to menstruation. Try to visualize the small block for each day on a scale ranging from 0 to 10 in a degree of severity of the symptom, with 0 being the complete absence of the symptom, 1 to 3 being degrees of mild symptoms, 4 to 7 being degrees of moderate symptoms, and 8 to 10 being degrees of severe symptoms. Fill in the proportion of the block accordingly, e.g., empty for completed absence of the symptom, about one-third full for a mild symptom, about half to two-thirds full for moderate symptoms, and nearly full or full for severe symptoms. At the end of the month, your graphical display should highlight those symptoms that appear most frequently, and plotting this graph over several months will show you how regular such symptoms might occur. Mild to moderate symptoms may be alleviated by some of the life-style changes discussed in chapter 10, while more severe symptoms may need the attention of a physician.

Month _____ Year _____	1	2	3	4	5	6	7	8	9	10	11	12	13	14	15	16	17	18	19	20	21	22	23	24	25	26	27	28	29	30	31
Psychological symptoms																															
Anxiety; tension																															
Confusion; forgetfulness																															
Depression; sadness																															
Disinterest																															
Irritability; anger																															
Lethargy; fatigue																															
Low self-esteem																															
Moodiness																															
Tearfulness																															
Others:																															
Physical symptoms																															
Breast tenderness																															
Bloating; weight gain																															
Constipation; diarrhea																															
Cramps																															
Food cravings; increased appetite																															
Headache; backache																															
Hot flashes																															
Insomnia; disturbed sleep																															
Nausea; vomiting																															
Others:																															

11.1

Cardiovascular Disease Risk Factor Inventory
RISKO: A Heart Hazard Appraisal

Men

Find the column for your age group. Everyone starts with a score of 10 points. Work down the page *adding* points to your score or *subtracting* points from your score.

			54 OR YOUNGER		55 OR OLDER	
1. **WEIGHT**	☐	weight category A	STARTING		STARTING	
Locate your weight category in the table for men, on p. 369. If you are in. . .	☐	weight category B	SCORE	10	SCORE	10
	☐	weight category C	SUBTRACT 2		SUBTRACT 2	
	☐	weight category D	SUBTRACT 1		ADD 0	
			ADD 1		ADD 1	
			ADD 2		ADD 3	
			EQUALS		**EQUALS**	
2. **SYSTOLIC BLOOD PRESSURE**	A	119 or less	SUBTRACT 1		SUBTRACT 5	
Use the "first" or "higher" number from your most recent blood pressure measurement. If you do not know your blood pressure, estimate it by using the letter for your weight category. If your blood pressure is. . .	B	between 120 and 139	ADD 0		SUBTRACT 2	
	C	between 140 and 159	ADD 0		ADD 1	
	D	160 or greater	ADD 1		ADD 4	
			EQUALS		**EQUALS**	
3. **BLOOD CHOLESTEROL LEVEL**	A	199 or less	SUBTRACT 2		SUBTRACT 1	
Use the number from your most recent blood cholesterol test. If you do not know your blood cholesterol, estimate it by using the letter for your weight category. If your blood cholesterol is. . .	B	between 200 and 224	SUBTRACT 1		SUBTRACT 1	
	C	between 225 and 249	ADD 0		ADD 0	
	D	250 or higher	ADD 1		ADD 0	
			EQUALS		**EQUALS**	
4. **CIGARETTE SMOKING**	☐	do not smoke	SUBTRACT 1		SUBTRACT 2	
If you. . .	☐	smoke less than a pack a day	ADD 0		SUBTRACT 1	
(If you smoke a pipe, but not cigarettes, use the same score adjustment as those cigarette smokers who smoke less than a pack a day.)	☐	smoke a pack a day	ADD 1		ADD 0	
	☐	smoke more than a pack a day	ADD 2		ADD 3	
			FINAL SCORE EQUALS		**FINAL SCORE EQUALS**	

Women

Find the column for your age group. Everyone starts with a score of 10 points. Work down the page *adding* points to your score or *subtracting* points from your score.

		54 OR YOUNGER		**55 OR OLDER**	
1. WEIGHT *Locate your weight category in the table for women on p. 369. If you are in. . .*	□ weight category A □ weight category B □ weight category C □ weight category D	STARTING SCORE SUBTRACT 2 SUBTRACT 1 ADD 1 ADD 2 **EQUALS**	10	STARTING SCORE SUBTRACT 2 SUBTRACT 1 ADD 1 ADD 1 **EQUALS**	10
2. SYSTOLIC BLOOD PRESSURE *Use the "first" or "higher" number from your most recent blood pressure measurement. If you do not know your blood pressure, estimate it by using the letter for your weight category. If your blood pressure is. . .*	A 119 or less B between 120 and 139 C between 140 and 159 D 160 or greater	SUBTRACT 2 SUBTRACT 1 ADD 0 ADD 1 **EQUALS**		SUBTRACT 3 ADD 0 ADD 3 ADD 6 **EQUALS**	
3. BLOOD CHOLESTEROL LEVEL *Use the number from your most recent blood cholesterol test. If you do not know your blood cholesterol, estimate it by using the letter for your weight category. If your blood cholesterol is. . .*	A 199 or less B between 200 and 224 C between 225 and 249 D 250 or higher	SUBTRACT 1 ADD 0 ADD 0 ADD 1 **EQUALS**		SUBTRACT 3 SUBTRACT 1 ADD 1 ADD 3 **EQUALS**	
4. CIGARETTE SMOKING *If you. . .*	□ do not smoke □ smoke less than a pack a day □ smoke a pack a day □ smoke more than a pack a day	SUBTRACT 1 ADD 0 ADD 1 ADD 2 **FINAL SCORE EQUALS**		SUBTRACT 2 SUBTRACT 1 ADD 1 ADD 4 **FINAL SCORE EQUALS**	

Weight Table for Men

Look for your height (without shoes) in the far left column and then read across to find the category into which your weight (in indoor clothing) would fall. Because both blood pressure and blood cholesterol are related to weight, an estimate of these risk factors for each weight category is printed at the bottom ot the table.

YOUR HEIGHT		WEIGHT CATEGORY (lbs.)			
FT	IN	A	B	C	D
5	1	up to 123	124–148	149–173	174 plus
5	2	up to 126	127–152	153–178	179 plus
5	3	up to 129	130–156	157–182	183 plus
5	4	up to 132	133–160	161–186	187 plus
5	5	up to 135	136–163	164–190	191 plus
5	6	up to 139	140–168	169–196	197 plus
5	7	up to 144	145–174	175–203	204 plus
5	8	up to 148	149–179	180–209	210 plus
5	9	up to 152	153–184	185–214	215 plus
5	10	up to 157	158–190	191–221	222 plus
5	11	up to 161	162–194	195–227	228 plus
6	0	up to 165	166–199	200–232	233 plus
6	1	up to 170	171–205	206–239	240 plus
6	2	up to 175	176–211	212–246	247 plus
6	3	up to 180	181–217	218–253	254 plus
6	4	up to 185	186–223	224–260	261 plus
6	5	up to 190	191–229	230–267	268 plus
6	6	up to 195	196–235	236–274	275 plus
ESTIMATE OF SYSTOLIC BLOOD PRESSURE		119 or less	120 to 139	140 to 159	160 or more
ESTIMATE OF BLOOD CHOLESTEROL		199 or less	200 to 224	225 to 249	250 or more

Weight Table for Women

Look for your height (without shoes) in the far left column and then read across to find the category into which your weight (in indoor clothing) would fall. Because both blood pressure and blood cholesterol are related to weight, an estimate of these risk factors for each weight category is printed at the bottom of the table.

YOUR HEIGHT		WEIGHT CATEGORY (lbs.)			
FT	IN	A	B	C	D
4	8	up to 101	102–122	123–143	144 plus
4	9	up to 103	104–125	126–146	147 plus
4	10	up to 106	107–128	129–150	151 plus
4	11	up to 109	110–132	133–154	155 plus
5	0	up to 112	113–136	137–158	159 plus
5	1	up to 115	116–139	140–162	163 plus
5	2	up to 119	120–144	145–168	169 plus
5	3	up to 122	123–148	149–172	173 plus
5	4	up to 127	128–154	155–179	180 plus
5	5	up to 131	132–158	159–185	186 plus
5	6	up to 135	136–163	164–190	191 plus
5	7	up to 139	140–168	169–196	197 plus
5	8	up to 143	144–173	174–202	203 plus
5	9	up to 147	148–178	179–207	208 plus
5	10	up to 151	152–182	183–213	214 plus
5	11	up to 155	156–187	188–218	219 plus
6	0	up to 159	160–191	192–224	225 plus
6	1	up to 163	164–196	197–229	230 plus
ESTIMATE OF SYSTOLIC BLOOD PRESSURE		119 or less	120 to 139	140 to 159	160 or more
ESTIMATE OF BLOOD CHOLESTEROL		199 or less	200 to 224	225 to 249	250 or more

Understanding Heart Disease

In the United States it is estimated that close to 550,000 people die each year from coronary heart disease. Coronary artery disease is the most common type of heart disease and the leading cause of death in the United States and many other countries.

Coronary heart disease is the result of coronary atherosclerosis. Coronary atherosclerosis is the name of the process by which an accumulation of fatty deposits leads to a thickening and narrowing of the inner walls of the arteries that carry oxygenated blood and nutrients to the heart muscle. The effect is similar to that of a water pipe clogged by deposits.

The resulting restriction of the blood supply to the heart muscle can cause injury to the muscle as well as angina (chest pain). If the restriction of the blood supply is severe or if it continues over a period of time, the heart muscle cells fed by the restricted artery suffer irreversible injury and die. This is known as a myocardial infarction or heart attack.

Scientists have identified a number of factors which are linked with an increased likelihood or risk of developing coronary heart disease. Some of these risk factors, like aging, being male, or having a family history of heart disease, are unavoidable. However, many other significant risk factors, including all of the factors used to determine your RISKO score, can be changed to reduce the likelihood of developing heart disease.

Appraising Your Risk

- The RISKO heart hazard appraisal is an indicator of risk for adults who do not currently show evidence of heart disease. However, if you already have heart disease, it is very important that you work with your doctor in reducing your risk.
- The original concept of RISKO was developed by the Michigan Heart Association.
- It has been further developed by the American Heart Association with the assistance of Drs. John and Sonja McKinlay in Boston. It is based on the Framingham, Stanford, and Chicago heart disease studies. The format of RISKO was tested and refined by Dr. Robert M. Chamberlain and Dr. Armin Weinberg of the National Heart Center at the Baylor College of Medicine in Houston.
- RISKO scores are based upon four of the most important modifiable factors which contribute to the development of heart disease. These factors include your weight, blood pressure, blood cholesterol level, and use of tobacco.
- The RISKO score you obtain measures your risk of developing heart disease in the next several years, provided that you currently show no evidence of such disease.
- THE RISKO heart hazard appraisal is not a substitute for a thorough physical examination and assessment by your physician. Rather, it will help you learn more about your risk of developing heart disease and will indicate ways in which you can reduce this risk.

Reproduced with permission. RISKO, 1985. Copyright American Heart Association.

What Your Score Means

0-4	You have one of the lowest risks of heart disease for your age and sex.
5-9	You have a low to moderate risk of heart disease for your age and sex but there is some room for improvement.
10-14	You have a moderate to high risk of heart disease for your age and sex, with considerable room for improvement on some factors.
15-19	You have a high risk of developing heart disease for your age and sex with a great deal of room for improvement on all factors.
20 & Over	You have a very high risk of developing heart disease for your age and sex and should take immediate action on all risk factors.

Warning

- If you have diabetes, gout, or a family history of heart disease, your actual risk will be greater than indicated by this appraisal.
- If you do not know your current blood pressure or blood cholesterol level, you should visit your physician or health center to have them measured. Then figure your score again for a more accurate determination of your risk.
- If you are overweight, have high blood pressure or high blood cholesterol, or smoke cigarettes, your long-term risk of heart disease is increased even if your risk in the next several years is low.

How to Reduce Your Risk

- Try to quit smoking permanently. There are many programs available.
- Have your blood pressure checked regularly, preferably every twelve months after age 40. If your blood pressure is high, see your physician. Remember blood pressure medicine is only effective if taken regularly.
- Consider your daily exercise (or lack of it). A half hour of brisk walking, swimming or other enjoyable activity should not be difficult to fit into your day.
- Give some serious thought to your diet. If you are overweight, or eat a lot of foods high in saturated fat or cholesterol (whole milk, cheese, eggs, butter, fatty foods, fried foods) then changes should be made in your diet. Look for the *American Heart Association Cookbook* at your local bookstore.
- Visit or write your local Heart Association for further information and copies of free pamphlets on many related subjects including:
  - Reducing your risk of heart attack.
  - Controlling high blood pressure.
  - Eating to keep your heart healthy.
  - How to stop smoking.
  - Exercising for good health.

Some Words of Caution

- If you have diabetes, gout, or a family history of heart disease, your real risk of developing heart disease will be greater than indicated by your RISKO score. If your score is high and you have one or more of these additional problems, you should give particular attention to reducing your risk.
- If you are a woman under 45 years or a man under 35 years of age, your RISKO score represents an upper limit on your real risk of developing heart disease. In this case, your real risk is probably lower than indicated by your score.
- Using your weight category to estimate your systolic blood pressure or your blood cholesterol level makes your RISKO score less accurate.
- Your score will tend to overestimate your risk if your actual values on these two important factors are average for someone of your height and weight.
- Your score will underestimate your risk if your actual blood pressure or cholesterol level is above average for someone of your height or weight.

12.1

Self-Motivation Assessment

Read the following statements and circle the *number beneath the letter* that corresponds to how characteristic that behavior is of you. Answer every item and be as honest as possible. Keep your responses to yourself.

A. extremely uncharacteristic of me
B. somewhat uncharacteristic of me
C. neither characteristic nor uncharacteristic of me
D. somewhat characteristic of me
E. extremely characteristic of me

Self-Motivation Assessment Scale

A	B	C	D	E	
(5)	4	3	2	1	1. I get discouraged easily.
5	(4)	3	2	1	2. I don't work any harder than I have to.
1	(2)	3	4	5	3. I seldom, if ever, let myself down.
(5)	4	3	2	1	4. I'm just not the goal-setting type.
(1)	2	3	4	5	5. I'm good at keeping promises, especially the ones I make to myself.
5	(4)	3	2	1	6. I don't impose much structure on my activities.
1	2	(3)	4	5	7. I have a very hard-driving, aggressive personality.

Scoring: Simply add the total of your seven scores. If the total is 24 or less, you are more subject to dropping out. The lower the score, the greater the possibility that you will drop out.

total 24

Source: *Rod K. Dishman, Ph.D., University of Georgia; William Ickes, Ph.D., University of Texas.*

A

Food Exchange Lists

The reason for dividing food into six different groups is that foods vary in their carbohydrate, protein, fat, and Calorie content. Each exchange list contains foods that are alike—each choice contains about the same amount of carbohydrate, protein, fat, and Calories.

The following chart shows the amount of these nutrients in one serving from each exchange list. As you read the exchange lists, you will notice that one choice often is a larger amount of food than another choice from the same list. Because foods are so different, each food is measured or weighed so the amount of carbohydrate, protein, fat, and Calories is the same in each choice.

You will notice symbols on some foods in the exchange groups. Foods that are high in fiber (3 grams or more per normal serving) have a ⚶ symbol. High-fiber foods are good for you. It is important to eat more of these foods.

Foods that are high in sodium (400 milligrams or more of sodium per normal serving) have a ⬛ symbol. It's a good idea to limit your intake of high-salt foods, especially if you have high blood pressure.

If you have a favorite food that is not included in any of these groups, ask your dietitian about it. That food can probably be worked into your meal plan, at least now and then.

Exchange List	Carbohydrate (grams)	Protein (grams)	Fat (grams)	Calories
Starch/bread	15	3	trace	80
Meat				
Lean	—	7	3	55
Medium-fat	—	7	5	75
High-fat	—	7	8	100
Vegetable	5	2	—	25
Fruit	15	—	—	60
Milk				
Skim	12	8	trace	90
Lowfat	12	8	5	120
Whole	12	8	8	150
Fat	—	—	5	45

Starch/Bread List

Each item in this list contains approximately 15 grams of carbohydrate, 3 grams of protein, a trace of fat, and 80 Calories. Whole-grain products average about 2 grams of fiber per serving. Some foods are higher in fiber. Those foods that contain 3 or more grams of fiber per serving are identified with the fiber symbol ⚶ .

You can choose your starch exchanges from any of the items on this list. If you want to eat a starch food not on this list, the general rule is

- ½ cup of cereal, grain, or pasta is one serving
- 1 ounce of a bread product is one serving

Your dietitian can help you be more exact.

Cereals/Grains/Pasta

⚶ Bran cereals, concentrated (such as Bran Buds®, All Bran®)	⅓ cup
⚶ Bran cereals, flaked	½ cup
Bulgur (cooked)	½ cup
Cooked cereals	½ cup
Cornmeal (dry)	2½ tbsp.
Grapenuts	3 tbsp.
Grits (cooked)	½ cup
Other ready-to-eat unsweetened cereals	¾ cup
Pasta (cooked)	½ cup
Puffed cereal	1½ cup
Rice, white or brown (cooked)	⅓ cup
Shredded wheat	½ cup
⚶ Wheat germ	3 tbsp.

Dried Beans/Peas/Lentils

⚶ Beans and peas (cooked) (such as kidney, white, split, blackeye)	⅓ cup
⚶ Lentils (cooked)	⅓ cup
⚶ Baked beans	¼ cup

Starchy Vegetables

⚜ Corn	½ cup
⚜ Corn on cob, 6 in. long	1
⚜ Lima beans	½ cup
⚜ Peas, green (canned or frozen)	½ cup
⚜ Plantain	½ cup
Potato, baked	1 small (3 oz.)
Potato, mashed	½ cup
Squash, winter (acorn, butternut)	¾ cup
Yam, sweet potato, plain	⅓ cup

Bread

Bagel	½ (1 oz.)
Bread sticks, crisp, 4 in. long × ½ in.	2 (⅔ oz.)
Croutons, low fat	1 cup
English muffin	½
Frankfurter or hamburger bun	½ (1 oz.)
Pita, 6 in. across	½
Plain roll, small	1 (1 oz.)
Raisin, unfrosted	1 slice (1 oz.)
⚜ Rye, pumpernickel	1 slice (1 oz.)
Tortilla, 6 in. across	1
White (including French, Italian)	1 slice (1 oz.)
Whole wheat	1 slice (1 oz.)

Crackers/Snacks

Animal crackers	8
Graham crackers, square 2½ in.	3
Matzoth	¾ oz.
Melba toast	5 slices
Oyster crackers	24
Popcorn (popped, no fat added)	3 cups
Pretzels	¾ oz.
Rye crisp, 2 in. × 3½ in.	4
Saltine-type crackers	6
Whole wheat crackers, no fat added (crisp breads, such as Finn®, Kavli®, Wasa®)	2–4 slices (¾ oz.)

Starch Foods Prepared with Fat

(Count as 1 starch/bread serving plus 1 fat serving)

Biscuit, 2½ in. across	1
Chow mein noodles	½ cup
Corn bread, 2 in. cube	1 (2 oz.)
Cracker, round butter type	6
French fried potatoes, 2 in. to 3½ in. long	10 (1½ oz.)
Muffin, plain, small	1
Pancake, 4 in. across	2
Stuffing, bread (prepared)	¼ cup
Taco shell, 6 in. across	2
Waffle, 4½ in. square	1
Whole wheat crackers, fat added (such as Triscuits®)	4–6 (1 oz.)

⚜ *3 grams or more of fiber per serving.*

Meat List

Each serving of meat and substitutes on this list contains about 7 grams of protein. The amount of fat and number of Calories varies depending on what kind of meat or substitute you choose. The list is divided into three parts based on the amount of fat and Calories: lean meat, medium-fat meat, and high-fat meat. One ounce (one meat exchange) of each of these includes

	Carbohydrate (grams)	Protein (grams)	Fat (grams)	Calories
Lean	0	7	3	55
Medium-fat	0	7	5	75
High-fat	0	7	8	100

You are encouraged to use more lean and medium-fat meat, poultry, and fish in your meal plan. This will help decrease your fat intake, which may help decrease your risk for heart disease. The items from the high-fat group are high in saturated fat, cholesterol, and Calories. You should limit your choices from the high-fat group to three times per week. Meat and substitutes do not contribute any fiber to your meal plan.

Tips

1. Bake, roast, broil, grill, or boil these foods rather than frying them with added fat.
2. Use a nonstick pan spray or a nonstick pan to brown or fry these foods.
3. Trim off visible fat before and after cooking.
4. Do not add flour, bread crumbs, coating mixes, or fat to foods when preparing them.
5. Weigh meat after removing bones and fat and after cooking. Three ounces of cooked meat is about equal to 4 ounces of raw meat. Some examples of meat portions are

   2 ounces meat (2 meat exchanges) =

   1 small chicken leg or thigh

   ½ cup cottage cheese or tuna

   3 ounces meat (3 meat exchanges) =

   1 medium pork chop

   1 small hamburger

   ½ of a whole chicken breast

   1 unbreaded fish fillet

   cooked meat, about the size of a deck of cards

6. Restaurants usually serve prime cuts of meat, which are high in fat and calories.

📍 *Meats and meat substitutes that have 400 milligrams or more of sodium per exchange are indicated with this symbol.*

Lean Meat and Substitutes

(One exchange is equal to any one of the following items.)

Beef:	USDA Good or Choice grades of lean beef, such as round, sirloin, and flank steak; tenderloin; chipped beef 🧂	1 oz.
Pork:	Lean pork, such as fresh ham; canned, cured, or boiled ham 🧂 Canadian bacon 🧂 tenderloin.	1 oz.
Veal:	All cuts are lean except for veal cutlets (ground or cubed). Examples of lean veal are chops and roasts.	1 oz.
Poultry:	Chicken, turkey, Cornish hen (without skin)	1 oz.
Fish:	All fresh and frozen fish	1 oz.
	Crab, lobster, scallops, shrimp, clams (fresh or canned in water 🧂)	2 oz.
	Oysters	6 medium
	Tuna 🧂 (canned in water)	¼ cup
	Herring (uncreamed or smoked)	1 oz.
	Sardines (canned)	2 medium
Wild game:	Venison, rabbit, squirrel	1 oz.
	Pheasant, duck, goose (without skin)	1 oz.
Cheese:	Any cottage cheese	¼ cup
	Grated parmesan	2 Tbsp.
	Diet cheese 🧂 (with fewer than 55 Calories per ounce)	1 oz.
Other:	95% fat-free luncheon meat	1 oz.
	Egg whites	3 whites
	Egg substitutes with fewer than 55 Calories per ¼ cup	¼ cup

🧂 *400 mg or more of sodium per exchange*

Medium-Fat Meat and Substitutes

(One exchange is equal to any one of the following items.)

Beef:	Most beef products fall into this category. Examples are all ground beef, roast (rib, chuck, rump), steak (cubed, Porterhouse, T-bone), and meatloaf.	1 oz.
Pork:	Most pork products fall into this category. Examples are chops, loin roast, Boston butt, cutlets.	1 oz.
Lamb:	Most lamb products fall into this category. Examples are chops, leg, and roast.	1 oz.
Veal:	Cutlet (ground or cubed, unbreaded)	1 oz.
Poultry:	Chicken (with skin), domestic duck or goose (well drained of fat), ground turkey.	1 oz.
Fish:	Tuna 🧂 (canned in oil and drained)	¼ cup
	Salmon 🧂 (canned)	¼ cup
Cheese:	Skim or part-skim milk cheeses, such as	
	Ricotta	¼ cup
	Mozzarella	1 oz.
	Diet cheeses 🧂 (with 56–80 Calories per ounce)	1 oz.
Other:	86% fat-free luncheon meat 🧂	1 oz.
	Egg (high in cholesterol, limit to three per week)	1
	Egg substitutes with 56–80 Calories per ¼ cup	¼ cup
	Tofu (2½ in. x 2¾ in. x 1 in.)	4 oz.
	Liver, heart, kidney, sweetbreads (high in cholesterol)	1 oz.

🧂 *400 mg or more of sodium per exchange*

High-Fat Meat and Substitutes

Remember, these items are high in saturated fat, cholesterol, and Calories and should be used only three times per week.

(One exchange is equal to any one of the following items.)

Beef:	Most USDA Prime cuts of beef, such as ribs, corned beef 🧂	1 oz.
Pork:	Spareribs, ground pork, pork sausage 🧂 (patty or link)	1 oz.
Lamb:	Patties (ground lamb)	1 oz.
Fish:	Any fried fish product	1 oz.
Cheese:	All regular cheeses 🧂 such as American, Blue, Cheddar, Monterey, Swiss	1 oz.
Other:	Luncheon meat 🧂 such as bologna, salami, pimento loaf	1 oz.
	Sausage 🧂 such as Polish, Italian	1 oz.
	Knockwurst, smoked	1 oz.
	Bratwurst 🧂	1 oz.
	Frankfurter 🧂 (turkey or chicken)	1 frank (10/lb.)
	Peanut butter (contains unsaturated fat)	1 tbsp.
	Count as one high-fat meat plus one fat exchange:	
	Frankfurter 🧂 (beef, pork, or combination)	1 frank (10/lb.)

🧂 *400 mg or more of sodium per exchange*

Vegetable List

Each vegetable serving on this list contains about 5 grams of carbohydrate, 2 grams of protein, and 25 Calories. Vegetables contain 2 to 3 grams of dietary fiber. Vegetables that contain 400 mg of sodium per serving are identified with a ▮ symbol.

Vegetables are a good source of vitamins and minerals. Fresh and frozen vegetables have more vitamins and less added salt. Rinsing canned vegetables will remove much of the salt.

Unless otherwise noted, the serving size for vegetables (one vegetable exchange) is

½ cup of cooked vegetables or vegetable juice
1 cup of raw vegetables

Artichoke (½ medium)	Mushrooms, cooked
Asparagus	Okra
Beans (green, wax, Italian)	Onions
Bean sprouts	Pea pods
Beets	Peppers (green)
Broccoli	Rutabaga
Brussels sprouts	Sauerkraut ▮
Cabbage, cooked	Spinach, cooked
Carrots	Summer squash (crookneck)
Cauliflower	Tomato (one large)
Eggplant	Tomato/vegetable juice ▮
Greens (collard, mustard, turnip)	Turnips
Kohlrabi	Water chestnuts
Leeks	Zucchini, cooked

▮ 400 mg or more of sodium per serving

Starchy vegetables such as corn, peas, and potatoes are found on the Starch/Bread list.

For free vegetables, see Free Food list on page 380.

Fruit List

Each item on this list contains about 15 grams of carbohydrate and 60 Calories. Fresh, frozen, and dry fruits have about 2 grams of fiber per serving. Fruits that have 3 or more grams of fiber per serving have a ᐷᐷᐴ symbol. Fruit juices contain very little dietary fiber.

The carbohydrate and Calorie content for a fruit serving are based on the usual serving of the most commonly eaten fruits. Use fresh fruits or fruits frozen or canned without sugar added. Whole fruit is more filling than fruit juice and may be a better choice for those who are trying to lose weight. Unless otherwise noted, the serving size for one fruit serving is

½ cup of fresh fruit or fruit juice
¼ cup of dried fruit

Fresh, Frozen, and Unsweetened Canned Fruit

Apple (raw, 2 in. across)	1 apple
Applesauce (unsweetened)	½ cup
Apricots (medium, raw)	4 apricots
Apricots (canned)	½ cup or 4 halves
Banana (9 in. long)	½ banana
ᐷᐷᐴ Blackberries (raw)	¾ cup
ᐷᐷᐴ Blueberries (raw)	¾ cup
Cantaloupe (5 in. across) (cubes)	⅓ melon / 1 cup
Cherries (large, raw)	12 cherries
Cherries (canned)	½ cup
Figs (raw, 2 in. across)	2 figs
Fruit cocktail (canned)	½ cup
Grapefruit (medium)	½ grapefruit
Grapefruit (segments)	¾ cup
Grapes (small)	15 grapes
Honeydew melon (medium) (cubes)	⅛ melon / 1 cup
Kiwi (large)	1 kiwi
Mandarin oranges	¾ cup
Mango (small)	½ mango
ᐷᐷᐴ Nectarine (1½ in. across)	1 nectarine
Orange (2½ in. across)	1 orange
Papaya	1 cup
Peach (2¾ in. across)	1 peach or ¾ cup
Peaches (canned)	½ cup or 2 halves
Pear	½ large or 1 small
Pears (canned)	½ cup or 2 halves
Persimmon (medium, native)	2 persimmons
Pineapple (raw)	¾ cup
Pineapple (canned)	⅓ cup
Plum (raw, 2 in. across)	2 plums
ᐷᐷᐴ Pomegranate	½ pomegranate
ᐷᐷᐴ Raspberries (raw)	1 cup
ᐷᐷᐴ Strawberries (raw, whole)	1¼ cup
Tangerine (2½ in. across)	2 tangerines
Watermelon (cubes)	1¼ cup

Dried Fruit

ᐷᐷᐴ Apples	4 rings
ᐷᐷᐴ Apricots	7 halves
ᐷᐷᐴ Dates	2½ medium
ᐷᐷᐴ Figs	1½
ᐷᐷᐴ Prunes	3 medium
Raisins	2 tbsp.

Fruit Juice

Apple juice/cider	½ cup
Cranberry juice cocktail	⅓ cup
Grapefruit juice	½ cup
Grape juice	⅓ cup
Orange juice	½ cup
Pineapple juice	½ cup
Prune juice	⅓ cup

ᐷᐷᐴ 3 or more grams of fiber per serving

Milk List

Each serving of milk or milk products on this list contains about 12 grams of carbohydrate and 8 grams of protein. The amount of fat in milk is measured in percent (%) of butterfat. The Calories vary depending on what kind of milk you choose. The list is divided into three parts based on the amount of fat and Calories: skim/very lowfat milk, lowfat milk, and whole milk. One serving (one milk exchange) of each of these includes the carbohydrate, protein, fat, and Calories listed in the table.

	Carbohydrate (grams)	Protein (grams)	Fat (grams)	Calories
Skim/very lowfat	12	8	trace	90
Lowfat	12	8	5	120
Whole	12	8	8	150

Milk is the body's main source of calcium, the mineral needed for growth and repair of bones. Yogurt is also a good source of calcium. Yogurt and many dry or powdered milk products have different amounts of fat. If you have questions about a particular item, read the label to find out the fat and Calorie content.

Milk is good to drink, but it can also be added to cereal and to other foods. Many tasty dishes such as sugar-free pudding are made with milk (see the Combination Foods list). Add life to plain yogurt by adding one of your fruit servings to it.

Skim and Very Lowfat Milk

Skim milk	1 cup
$\frac{1}{2}$% milk	1 cup
1% milk	1 cup
Lowfat buttermilk	1 cup
Evaporated skim milk	$\frac{1}{2}$ cup
Dry nonfat milk	$\frac{1}{3}$ cup
Plain nonfat yogurt	1 cup

Lowfat Milk

2% milk	1 cup
Plain lowfat yogurt (with added nonfat milk solids)	1 cup

Whole Milk

The whole milk group has much more fat per serving than the skim and lowfat groups. Whole milk has more than $3\frac{1}{4}$% butterfat. Try to limit your choices from the whole milk group as much as possible.

Whole milk	1 cup
Evaporated whole milk	$\frac{1}{2}$ cup
Whole plain yogurt	1 cup

Fat List

Each serving on the fat list contains about 5 grams of fat and 45 Calories.

The foods on the fat list contain mostly fat, although some items may also contain a small amount of protein. All fats are high in Calories and should be carefully measured. Everyone should modify fat intake by eating unsaturated fats instead of saturated fats. The sodium content of these foods varies widely. Check the label for sodium information.

Unsaturated Fats

Avocado	$\frac{1}{8}$ medium
Margarine	1 tsp.
*Margarine, diet	1 tbsp.
Mayonnaise	1 tsp.
*Mayonnaise, reduced Calorie	1 tbsp.
Nuts and Seeds:	
Almonds, dry roasted	6 whole
Cashews, dry roasted	1 tbsp.
Other nuts	1 tbsp.
Peanuts	20 small or 10 large
Pecans	2 whole
Pumpkin seeds	2 tsp.
Seeds, pine nuts, sunflower (without shells)	1 tbsp.
Walnuts	2 whole
Oil (corn, cottonseed, safflower, soybean, sunflower, olive, peanut)	1 tsp
*Olives	10 small or 5 large
*Salad dressing (all varieties)	1 tbsp.
Salad dressing, mayonnaise type	2 tsp.
Salad dressing, mayonnaise type, reduced Calorie	1 tbsp.
▮ Salad dressing, reduced Calorie	2 tbsp.

(Two tablespoons of low-Calorie salad dressing is a free food.)

Saturated Fats

*Bacon	1 slice
Butter	1 tsp.
Chitterlings	$\frac{1}{2}$ oz.
Coconut, shredded	2 tbsp.
Coffee whitener, liquid	2 tbsp.
Coffee whitener, powder	4 tsp.
Cream, sour	2 tbsp.
Cream (light, coffee, table)	2 tbsp.
Cream (heavy, whipping)	1 tbsp.
Cream cheese	1 tbsp.
*Salt pork	$\frac{1}{4}$ oz.

*If more than one or two servings are eaten, these foods have 400 mg or more of sodium.

▮ *400 mg or more of sodium per serving*

Free Foods

A free food is any food or drink that contains fewer than 20 Calories per serving. You can eat as much as you want of those items that have no serving size specified. You may eat two or three servings per day of those items that have a specific serving size. Be sure to spread them out through the day.

Drinks:

Bouillon, low-sodium

Bouillon 🜂 or broth
  without fat

Carbonated drinks, sugar
  free

Carbonated water

Club soda

Cocoa powder,
  unsweetened (1 tbsp.)

Coffee/Tea

Drink mixes, sugar free

Tonic water, sugar free

Nonstick pan spray

Fruit:

Cranberries, unsweetened
  (½ cup)

Rhubarb, unsweetened
  (½ cup)

Vegetables:

(raw, 1 cup)

Cabbage

Celery

Chinese cabbage ∿

Cucumber

Green onion

Hot peppers

Mushrooms

Radishes

Zucchini ∿

Salad greens:

Endive

Escarole

Lettuce

Romaine

Spinach

Seasonings can make food taste better. Be careful of how much sodium you use. Read the label, and choose those seasonings that do not contain sodium or salt.

Basil (fresh)

Celery seeds

Chili powder

Chives

Cinnamon

Curry

Dill

Flavoring extracts
  (vanilla, almond,
  walnut, peppermint,
  butter, lemon, etc.)

Garlic

Garlic powder

Herbs

Hot pepper sauce

Lemon

Lemon juice

Lemon pepper

Lime

Lime juice

Mint

Onion powder

Oregano

Paprika

Pepper

Pimento

Soy sauce 🜂

Soy sauce, low sodium
  ("lite")

Spices

Wine, used in cooking
  (¼ cup)

Worcestershire sauce

∿ *3 grams or more of fiber per serving*

🜂 *400 mg or more of sodium per serving*

Sweet Substitutes

Candy, hard, sugar free

Gelatin, sugar free

Gum, sugar free

Jam/Jelly, sugar free (2 tsp.)

Pancake syrup, sugar free (1–2 tbsp.)

Sugar substitutes (saccharin, aspartame)

Whipped topping (2 tbsp.)

Condiments:

Catsup (1 tbsp.)

Horseradish

Mustard

Pickles 🜂, dill, unsweetened

Salad dressing, low Calorie (2 tbsp.)

Taco sauce (1 tbsp.)

Vinegar

Combination Foods

Much of the food we eat is mixed together in various combinations. These combination foods do not fit into only one exchange list. It can be quite hard to tell what is in a certain casserole dish or baked food item. This is a list of average values for some typical combination foods. This list will help you fit these foods into your meal plan. Ask your dietitian for information about any other foods you'd like to eat. The *American Diabetes Association/American Dietetic Association Family Cookbooks* and the *American Diabetes Association Holiday Cookbook* have many recipes and further information about many foods, including combination foods. Check your library or local bookstore.

Food	Amount	Exchanges
Casseroles, homemade	1 cup (8 oz.)	2 starch, 2 medium-fat meat, 1 fat
Cheese pizza ▌ thin crust	¼ of 15 oz. or ¼ of 10"	2 starch, 1 medium-fat meat, 1 fat
Chili with beans ⋙ ▌ (commercial)	1 cup (8 oz.)	2 starch, 2 medium-fat meat, 2 fat
Chow mein ⋙ ▌ (without noodles or rice)	2 cups (16 oz.)	1 starch, 2 vegetable, 2 lean meat
Macaroni and cheese ▌	1 cup (8 oz.)	2 starch, 1 medium-fat meat, 2 fat
Soup:		
Bean ⋙ ▌	1 cup (8 oz.)	1 starch, 1 vegetable, 1 lean meat
Chunky, all varieties ▌	10 ¾ oz. can	1 starch, 1 vegetable, 1 medium-fat meat
Cream ▌ (made with water)	1 cup (8 oz.)	1 starch, 1 fat
Vegetable ▌ or broth ▌	1 cup (8 oz.)	1 starch
Spaghetti and meatballs ▌ (canned)	1 cup (8 oz.)	2 starch, 1 medium-fat meat, 1 fat
Sugar-free pudding (made with skim milk)	½ cup	1 starch
If beans are used as a meat substitute:		
Dried beans ⋙ peas ⋙ lentils ⋙	1 cup (cooked)	2 starch, 1 lean meat

⋙ *3 grams or more of fiber per serving*   ▌ *400 mg or more of sodium per serving*

Foods for Occasional Use

Moderate amounts of some foods can be used in your meal plan, in spite of their sugar or fat content, as long as you can maintain blood-glucose control. The following list includes average exchange values for some of these foods. Because they are concentrated sources of carbohydrate, you will notice that the portion sizes are very small. Check with your dietitian for advice on how often and when you can eat them.

Food	Amount	Exchanges
Angel food cake	1/12 cake	2 starch
Cake, no icing	1/12 cake or a 3" square	2 starch, 2 fat
Cookies	2 small (1¾" across)	1 starch, 1 fat
Frozen fruit yogurt	1/3 cup	1 starch
Gingersnaps	3	1 starch
Granola	¼ cup	1 starch, 1 fat
Granola bars	1 small	1 starch, 1 fat
Ice cream, any flavor	½ cup	1 starch, 2 fat
Ice milk, any flavor	½ cup	1 starch, 1 fat
Sherbet, any flavor	¼ cup	1 starch
Snack chips ▌ all varieties	1 oz.	1 starch, 2 fat
Vanilla wafers	6 small	1 starch, 1 fat

▌ *If more than one serving is eaten, these foods have 400 mg or more of sodium.*

The Exchange Lists are the basis of a meal planning system designed by a committee of the American Diabetes Association and the American Dietetic Association. While designed primarily for people with diabetes and others who must follow special diets, the Exchange Lists are based on principles of good nutrition that apply to everyone. © 1986 American Diabetes Association, Inc., American Dietetic Association.

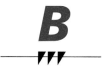

B

Scoring Tables for Cooper's Distance Tests of Aerobic Capacity

Table B.1 1.5-Mile Run Test
Time (Minutes)

Fitness Category		Age (Years)					
		13–19	*20–29*	*30–39*	*40–49*	*50–59*	*60+*
Very Poor	(Men)	>15:31*	>16:01	>16:31	>17:31	>19:01	>20:01
	(Women)	>18:31	>19:01	>19:31	>20:01	>20:31	>21:01
Poor	(Men)	12:11–15:30	14:01–16:00	14:44–16:30	15:36–17:30	17:01–19:00	19:01–20:00
	(Women)	18:30–16:55	19:00–18:31	19:30–19:01	20:00–19:31	20:30–20:01	21:00–21:30
Fair	(Men)	10:49–12:10	12:01–14:00	12:31–14:45	13:01–15:35	14:31–17:00	16:16–19:00
	(Women)	16:54–14:31	18:30–15:55	19:00–16:31	19:30–17:31	20:00–19:01	20:30–19:30
Good	(Men)	9:41–10:48	10:46–12:00	11:01–12:30	11:31–13:00	12:31–14:30	14:00–16:15
	(Women)	14:30–12:30	15:54–13:31	16:30–14:31	17:30–15:56	19:00–16:31	19:30–17:30
Excellent	(Men)	8:37–9:40	9:45–10:45	10:00–11:00	10:30–11:30	11:00–12:30	11:15–13:59
	(Women)	12:29–11:50	13:30–12:30	14:30–13:00	15:55–13:45	16:30–14:30	17:30–16:30
Superior	(Men)	<8:37	<9:45	<10:00	<10:30	<11:00	<11:15
	(Women)	<11:50	<12:30	<13:00	<13:45	<14:30	<16:30

*< Means "less than"; > means "more than."

Source: *From* The Aerobics Program for Total Well-Being *by Dr. Kenneth H. Cooper. Reprinted by permission of the publisher, M. Evans and Co., Inc., New York, N.Y. 10017.*

Table B.2 3-Mile Walking Test (No Running)
Time (Minutes)

Fitness Category		Age (Years)					
		13–19	*20–29*	*30–39*	*40–49*	*50–59*	*60+*
Very Poor	(Men)	> 45:00*	> 46:00	> 49:00	> 52:00	> 55:00	> 60:00
	(Women)	> 47:00	> 48:00	> 51:00	> 54:00	> 57:00	> 63:00
Poor	(Men)	41:01–45:00	42:01–46:00	44:31–49:00	47:01–52:00	50:01–55:00	54:01–60:00
	(Women)	43:01–47:00	44:01–48:00	46:31–51:00	49:01–54:00	52:01–57:00	57:01–63:00
Fair	(Men)	37:31–41:00	38:31–42:00	40:01–44:30	42:01–47:00	45:01–50:00	48:01–54:00
	(Women)	39:31–43:00	40:31–44:00	42:01–46:30	44:01–49:00	47:01–52:00	51:01–57:00
Good	(Men)	33:00–37:30	34:00–38:30	35:00–40:00	36:30–42:00	39:00–45:00	41:00–48:00
	(Women)	35:00–39:30	36:00–40:30	37:30–42:00	39:00–44:00	42:00–47:00	45:00–51:00
Excellent	(Men)	<33:00	<34:00	<35:00	<36:30	<39:00	<41:00
	(Women)	<35:00	<36:00	<37:30	<39:00	<42:00	<45:00

*< Means "less than"; > means "more than."

The walking test, covering 3 miles in the fastest time possible without running, can be done on a track or anywhere with an accurately measured distance.

Source: *From* The Aerobics Program for Total Well-Being *by Dr. Kenneth H. Cooper. Reprinted by permission of the publisher, M. Evans and Co., Inc., New York, N.Y. 10017.*

Table B.3 1.5-Mile Run Standards for Moderately Fit* College Students (D. Draper & G. Jones, 1990)

Fitness Category		Time: Age 17–25	Time: Age 26–35
1. Superior	(females)	<10:30	<11:30
	(males)	<8:30	<9:30
2. Excellent	(females)	10:30–11:49	11:30–12:49
	(males)	8:30–9:29	9:30–10:29
3. Good	(females)	11:50–13:09	12:50–14:29
	(males)	9:30–10:29	10:30–11:29
4. Moderate	(females)	13:10–14:29	14:10–15:29
	(males)	10:30–11:29	11:30–12:29
5. Fair	(females)	14:30–15:49	15:30–16:49
	(males)	11:30–12:29	12:30–13:29
6. Poor	(females)	>15:49	>16:49
	(males)	>12:29	>13:29

*"Moderately fit college students" are not athletes, but lay persons who engage in continuous aerobic activity lasting a minimum of 20 minutes, 3 times a week.

This article is reprinted with permission from the Journal of Physical Education and Dance, September, 1990, page 79. The Journal is a publication of the American Alliance for Health, Physical Education, Recreation and Dance, 1900 Association Drive, Reston, Va. 22091.

Table B.4 Predicted $\dot{V}O_2$ max (ml O_2/kg) on Basis of Cooper's Fitness Categories

Fitness Category		Age (Years)					
		13–19	20–29	30–39	40–49	50–59	60+
Very Poor	(Men)	<35.0	<33.0	<31.5	<30.2	<26.1	<20.5
	(Women)	<25.0	<23.6	<22.8	<21.0	<20.2	<17.5
Poor	(Men)	35.0–38.3	33.0–36.4	31.5–35.4	30.2–33.5	26.1–30.9	20.5–26.0
	(Women)	25.0–30.9	23.6–28.9	22.8–26.9	21.0–24.4	20.2–22.7	17.5–20.1
Fair	(Men)	38.4–45.1	36.5–42.4	35.5–40.9	33.6–38.9	31.0–35.7	26.1–32.2
	(Women)	31.0–34.9	29.0–32.9	27.0–31.4	24.5–28.9	22.8–26.9	20.2–24.4
Good	(Men)	45.2–50.9	42.5–46.4	41.0–44.9	39.0–43.7	35.8–40.9	32.2–36.4
	(Women)	35.0–38.9	33.0–36.9	31.5–35.6	29.0–32.8	27.0–31.4	24.5–30.2
Excellent	(Men)	51.0–55.9	46.5–52.4	45.0–49.4	43.8–48.0	41.0–45.3	36.5–44.2
	(Women)	39.0–41.9	37.0–40.9	35.7–40.0	32.9–36.9	31.5–35.7	30.3–31.4
Superior	(Men)	>56.0	>52.5	>49.5	>48.1	>45.4	>44.3
	(Women)	>42.0	>41.0	>40.1	>37.0	>35.8	>31.5

Source: From The Aerobics Way by Dr. Kenneth H. Cooper. Copyright © 1982 by Kenneth H. Cooper. Reprinted by permission of the publisher, M. Evans and Company, Inc., New York, N.Y. 10017.

C

*Approximate Caloric Expenditure per Minute for Various Physical Activities**

When using this appendix, keep the following points in mind:

1. The figures are approximate and include the resting metabolic rate. Thus, the total cost of the exercise includes not only the energy expended by the exercise itself, but also the amount you would have used anyway during the same period of time. Suppose you ran for 1 hour and the calculated energy cost was 800 Calories. During that same time at rest you may have expended 75 Calories, so the net cost of the exercise is 725 Calories.

2. The figures in the table are only for the time you are performing the activity. For example, in an hour of basketball, you may exercise strenuously for only 35 to 40 minutes, as you may take time-outs and may rest during foul shots. In general, record only the amount of time that you are actually moving during the activity.

3. The figures may give you some guidelines to total energy expenditure, but actual caloric costs may vary somewhat due to such factors as skill level, environmental factors (running against the wind or up hills), and so forth.

4. Not all body weights could be listed, but approximate by going to the closest weight listed.

5. There may be small differences between men and women, but not enough to make a marked difference in the total caloric value for most exercises.

*Note: The energy cost, in Calories, will vary for different physical activities in a given individual depending on several factors. For example, the caloric cost of bicycling will vary depending on the type of bicycle, going uphill or downhill, and wind resistance. Walking with hand weights or ankle weights will increase energy output. Thus, the values expressed here are approximations and may be increased or decreased depending upon factors that influence energy cost.

Body weight												
Kilograms	45	48	50	52	55	57	59	61	64	66	68	70
Pounds	100	105	110	115	120	125	130	135	140	145	150	155

Sedentary activities

	45	48	50	52	55	57	59	61	64	66	68	70
Lying quietly	.99	1.0	1.1	1.1	1.2	1.3	1.3	1.4	1.4	1.5	1.5	1.5
Sitting and writing, card playing, etc.	1.2	1.3	1.4	1.5	1.5	1.6	1.7	1.7	1.8	1.8	1.9	2.0
Standing with light work, cleaning, etc.	2.7	2.9	3.0	3.1	3.3	3.4	3.5	3.7	3.8	3.9	4.1	4.2

Physical activities

	45	48	50	52	55	57	59	61	64	66	68	70
Archery	3.1	3.3	3.5	3.6	3.8	4.0	4.1	4.3	4.5	4.6	4.8	4.9
Badminton												
Recreational singles	3.6	3.8	4.0	4.2	4.4	4.6	4.7	4.9	5.1	5.3	5.4	5.6
Social doubles	2.7	2.9	3.0	3.1	3.3	3.4	3.5	3.7	3.8	3.9	4.1	4.2
Competitive	5.9	6.1	6.4	6.7	7.0	7.3	7.6	7.9	8.2	8.5	8.8	9.1
Baseball												
Player	3.1	3.3	3.4	3.6	3.8	4.0	4.1	4.3	4.4	4.5	4.7	4.8
Pitcher	3.9	4.1	4.3	4.5	4.7	4.9	5.1	5.3	5.5	5.7	5.9	6.0
Basketball												
Half court	3.0	3.1	3.3	3.5	3.6	3.8	3.9	4.1	4.2	4.4	4.5	4.7
Recreational	4.9	5.2	5.5	5.7	6.0	6.2	6.5	6.7	7.0	7.2	7.5	7.7
Vigorous competition	6.5	6.8	7.2	7.5	7.8	8.2	8.5	8.8	9.2	9.5	9.9	10.2
Bicycling, level												
(mph) (min/mile)												
5 12:00	1.9	2.0	2.1	2.2	2.3	2.4	2.5	2.6	2.7	2.8	2.9	3.0
10 6:00	4.2	4.4	4.6	4.8	5.1	5.3	5.5	5.7	5.9	6.1	6.4	6.6
15 4:00	7.3	7.6	8.0	8.4	8.7	9.1	9.5	9.8	10.0	10.5	10.9	11.3
20 3:00	10.7	11.2	11.7	12.3	12.8	13.3	13.9	14.4	14.9	15.5	16.0	16.5
Bowling	2.7	2.8	3.0	3.1	3.3	3.4	3.5	3.7	3.8	3.9	4.1	4.2
Calisthenics												
Light type	3.4	3.6	3.8	4.0	4.1	4.3	4.5	4.7	4.8	5.0	5.2	5.4
Timed vigorous	9.7	10.1	10.6	11.1	11.6	12.1	12.6	13.1	13.6	14.1	14.6	15.1
Canoeing												
(mph) (min/mile)												
2.5 24	1.9	2.0	2.1	2.2	2.3	2.4	2.5	2.6	2.7	2.8	2.9	3.0
4.0 15	4.4	4.6	4.9	5.1	5.3	5.5	5.8	6.0	6.2	6.4	6.7	6.9
5.0 12	5.7	6.0	6.3	6.6	6.9	7.2	7.5	7.8	8.1	8.4	8.7	9.0
Dancing												
Moderately (waltz)	3.1	3.3	3.5	3.6	3.8	4.0	4.1	4.3	4.5	4.6	4.8	4.9
Active (square, disco)	4.5	4.7	5.0	5.2	5.4	5.6	5.9	6.1	6.3	6.6	6.8	7.0
Aerobic (vigorously)	6.0	6.3	6.7	7.0	7.3	7.6	7.9	8.2	8.5	8.8	9.1	9.4
Fencing												
Moderately	3.3	3.5	3.6	3.8	4.0	4.1	4.3	4.5	4.6	4.8	5.0	5.2
Vigorously	6.6	7.0	7.3	7.7	8.0	8.3	8.7	9.0	9.4	9.7	10.0	10.4
Football												
Moderate	3.3	3.5	3.6	3.8	4.0	4.1	4.3	4.5	4.6	4.8	5.0	5.2
Touch, vigorous	5.5	5.8	6.1	6.4	6.6	6.9	7.2	7.5	7.8	8.0	8.3	8.6
Golf												
Twosome (carry clubs)	3.6	3.8	4.0	4.2	4.4	4.6	4.7	4.9	5.1	5.3	5.4	5.6
Foursome (carry clubs)	2.7	2.9	3.0	3.1	3.3	3.4	3.5	3.7	3.8	3.9	4.1	4.2
Power-cart	1.9	2.0	2.1	2.2	2.3	2.4	2.5	2.6	2.7	2.8	2.9	3.0

| 73 | 75 | 77 | 80 | 82 | 84 | 86 | 89 | 91 | 93 | 95 | 98 | 100 |
160	165	170	175	180	185	190	195	200	205	210	215	220
1.6	1.6	1.7	1.7	1.8	1.8	1.9	1.9	2.0	2.0	2.1	2.1	2.2
2.0	2.1	2.2	2.2	2.3	2.4	2.4	2.5	2.5	2.6	2.7	2.7	2.8
4.4	4.5	4.6	4.8	4.9	5.0	5.2	5.3	5.4	5.6	5.7	5.9	6.0
5.1	5.3	5.4	5.6	5.7	5.9	6.0	6.2	6.4	6.5	6.7	6.9	7.0
5.8	6.0	6.2	6.4	6.6	6.7	6.9	7.1	7.3	7.4	7.6	7.8	8.0
4.4	4.5	4.6	4.8	4.9	5.0	5.2	5.3	5.4	5.6	5.7	5.9	6.0
9.4	9.7	10.0	10.3	10.6	10.9	11.2	11.5	11.8	12.1	12.4	12.7	13.0
5.0	5.2	5.3	5.5	5.6	5.8	5.9	6.1	6.3	6.4	6.6	6.8	6.9
6.3	6.5	6.7	6.9	7.1	7.3	7.4	7.7	7.9	8.0	8.2	8.5	8.6
4.8	5.0	5.1	5.3	5.4	5.6	5.7	5.9	6.0	6.2	6.4	6.5	6.7
8.0	8.2	8.5	8.7	9.0	9.2	9.5	9.7	10.0	10.2	10.5	10.7	11.0
10.5	10.9	11.2	11.5	11.9	12.2	12.5	12.9	13.2	13.5	13.8	14.2	14.5
3.1	3.2	3.3	3.4	3.5	3.6	3.7	3.8	3.9	4.0	4.1	4.2	4.3
6.8	7.0	7.2	7.4	7.6	7.9	8.1	8.3	8.5	8.7	8.9	9.1	9.4
11.6	12.0	12.4	12.7	13.1	13.4	13.8	14.2	14.5	14.9	15.3	15.6	16.0
17.1	17.6	18.1	18.7	19.2	19.7	20.3	20.8	21.3	21.9	22.4	22.9	23.5
4.4	4.5	4.6	4.8	4.9	5.0	5.2	5.3	5.5	5.6	5.7	5.9	6.0
5.5	5.7	5.9	6.1	6.3	6.4	6.6	6.8	7.0	7.1	7.3	7.5	7.7
15.6	16.1	16.6	17.1	17.6	18.1	18.6	19.1	19.6	20.0	20.5	21.0	21.5
3.1	3.2	3.3	3.4	3.5	3.6	3.7	3.8	3.9	4.0	4.1	4.2	4.3
7.1	7.4	7.6	7.8	8.0	8.2	8.5	8.7	8.9	9.1	9.4	9.6	9.8
9.3	9.5	9.8	10.1	10.4	10.7	11.0	11.3	11.6	11.9	12.2	12.5	12.8
5.1	5.3	5.4	5.6	5.7	5.9	6.0	6.2	6.4	6.5	6.7	6.9	7.0
7.3	7.5	7.7	7.9	8.2	8.4	8.6	8.9	9.1	9.3	9.5	9.8	10.0
9.7	10.0	10.3	10.6	10.9	11.2	11.5	11.8	12.1	12.4	12.7	13.0	13.3
5.3	5.5	5.7	5.8	6.0	6.2	6.3	6.5	6.7	6.8	7.0	7.1	7.3
10.7	11.0	11.4	11.7	12.1	12.4	12.7	13.1	13.4	13.8	14.1	14.4	14.8
5.3	5.5	5.7	5.8	6.0	6.2	6.3	6.5	6.7	6.8	7.0	7.1	7.3
8.9	9.2	9.4	9.7	10.0	10.3	10.6	10.8	11.1	11.4	11.7	12.0	12.2
5.8	6.0	6.2	6.4	6.6	6.7	6.9	7.1	7.3	7.4	7.6	7.8	8.0
4.4	4.5	4.6	4.8	4.9	5.0	5.2	5.3	5.4	5.6	5.7	5.9	6.0
3.1	3.2	3.3	3.4	3.5	3.6	3.7	3.8	3.9	4.0	4.1	4.2	4.3

Body weight

	Kilograms	45	48	50	52	55	57	59	61	64	66	68	70
	Pounds	100	105	110	115	120	125	130	135	140	145	150	155
Handball													
Moderate		6.5	6.8	7.2	7.5	7.8	8.2	8.5	8.8	9.2	9.5	9.9	10.2
Competitive		7.7	8.0	8.4	8.8	9.2	9.6	10.0	10.4	10.8	11.1	11.5	11.9
Hiking, pack (3 mph)		4.5	4.7	5.0	5.2	5.4	5.6	5.9	6.1	6.3	6.6	6.8	7.0
Hockey, field		5.0	6.3	6.7	7.0	7.3	7.6	7.9	8.2	8.5	8.8	9.1	9.4
Hockey, ice		6.6	7.0	7.3	7.7	8.0	8.3	8.7	9.0	9.4	9.7	10.0	10.4
Horseback riding													
Walk		1.9	2.0	2.1	2.2	2.3	2.4	2.5	2.6	2.7	2.8	2.9	3.0
Sitting to trot		2.7	2.9	3.0	3.1	3.3	3.4	3.5	3.7	3.8	3.9	4.1	4.2
Posting to trot		4.2	4.4	4.6	4.8	5.1	5.3	5.5	5.7	5.9	6.1	6.4	6.6
Gallop		5.7	6.0	6.3	6.6	6.9	7.2	7.5	7.8	8.1	8.4	8.7	9.0
Horseshoes		2.5	2.6	2.8	2.9	3.0	3.1	3.3	3.4	3.5	3.7	3.8	3.9
Jogging (see Running)													
Judo		8.5	8.9	9.3	9.8	10.2	10.6	11.0	11.5	11.9	12.3	12.8	13.2
Karate		8.5	8.9	9.3	9.8	10.2	10.6	11.0	11.5	11.9	12.3	12.8	13.2
Mountain climbing		6.5	6.8	7.2	7.5	7.8	8.2	8.5	8.8	9.2	9.5	9.8	10.2
Paddle ball		5.7	6.0	6.3	6.6	6.9	7.2	7.5	7.8	8.1	8.4	8.7	9.0
Pool (billiards)		1.5	1.6	1.6	1.7	1.8	1.9	1.9	2.0	2.1	2.2	2.2	2.3
Racketball		6.5	6.8	7.1	7.5	7.8	8.1	8.4	8.8	9.1	9.4	9.8	10.1
Roller skating (9 mph)		4.2	4.4	4.6	4.8	5.1	5.3	5.5	5.7	5.9	6.1	6.4	6.6
Running (steady state)													
(mph)	(min/mile)												
5.0	12:00	6.0	6.3	6.6	7.0	7.3	7.6	7.9	8.2	8.5	8.8	9.1	9.4
5.5	10:55	6.7	7.0	7.3	7.7	8.0	8.4	8.7	9.0	9.4	9.7	10.0	10.4
6.0	10:00	7.2	7.6	8.0	8.4	8.7	9.1	9.5	9.8	10.2	10.6	10.9	11.3
7.0	8:35	8.5	8.9	9.3	9.8	10.2	10.6	11.0	11.5	11.9	12.3	12.8	13.2
8.0	7:30	9.7	10.2	10.7	11.2	11.6	12.1	12.6	13.1	13.6	14.1	14.6	15.1
9.0	6:40	10.8	11.3	11.9	12.4	12.9	13.5	14.0	14.6	15.1	15.7	16.2	16.8
10.0	6:00	12.1	12.7	13.3	13.9	14.5	15.1	15.7	16.4	17.0	17.6	18.2	18.8
11.0	5:28	13.3	14.0	14.6	15.3	16.0	16.7	17.3	18.0	18.7	19.4	20.0	20.7
12.0	5:00	14.5	15.2	16.0	16.7	17.4	18.2	18.9	19.7	20.4	21.1	21.9	22.6
Sailing, small boat		2.7	2.9	3.0	3.1	3.3	3.4	3.5	3.7	3.8	3.9	4.1	4.2
Skating, ice (9 mph)		4.2	4.4	4.6	4.8	5.1	5.2	5.5	5.7	5.9	6.1	6.4	6.6
In-line skating (rollerblading)													
8 mph		3.3	3.5	3.7	4.0	4.2	4.4	4.6	4.9	5.1	5.3	5.6	5.8
9 mph		4.9	5.1	5.3	5.6	5.8	6.0	6.2	6.5	6.7	6.9	7.2	7.4
10 mph		6.5	6.7	6.9	7.2	7.4	7.6	7.8	8.1	8.3	8.5	8.7	9.0
11 mph		7.9	8.1	8.4	8.6	8.9	9.1	9.4	9.6	9.9	10.1	10.3	10.6
Skiing, cross country													
(mph)	(min/mile)												
2.5	24:00	5.0	5.2	5.5	5.7	6.0	6.2	6.5	6.7	7.0	7.2	7.5	7.8
4.0	15:00	6.5	6.8	7.2	7.5	7.8	8.2	8.5	8.8	9.2	9.5	9.9	10.2
5.0	12:00	7.7	8.0	8.4	8.8	9.2	9.6	10.0	10.4	10.8	11.1	11.5	11.9
Skiing, downhill		6.5	6.8	7.2	7.5	7.8	8.2	8.5	8.8	9.2	9.5	9.9	10.2
Soccer		5.9	6.2	6.6	6.9	7.2	7.5	7.8	8.1	8.4	8.7	9.0	9.3
Squash													
Normal		6.7	7.0	7.3	7.7	8.0	8.4	8.7	9.1	9.5	9.8	10.1	10.5
Competition		7.7	8.0	8.4	8.8	9.2	9.6	10.0	10.4	10.8	11.1	11.5	11.9

| 73 | 75 | 77 | 80 | 82 | 84 | 86 | 89 | 91 | 93 | 95 | 98 | 100 |
160	165	170	175	180	185	190	195	200	205	210	215	220
10.5	10.9	11.2	11.5	11.9	12.2	12.5	12.9	13.2	13.5	13.8	14.2	14.5
12.3	12.7	13.1	13.5	13.9	14.3	14.7	15.0	15.4	15.8	16.2	16.6	17.0
7.3	7.5	7.7	7.9	8.2	8.4	8.6	8.9	9.1	9.3	9.5	9.8	10.0
9.7	10.0	10.3	10.6	10.9	11.2	11.5	11.8	12.1	12.4	12.7	13.0	13.3
10.7	11.0	11.4	11.7	12.1	12.4	12.7	13.1	13.4	13.8	14.1	14.4	14.8
3.1	3.2	3.3	3.4	3.5	3.6	3.7	3.8	3.9	4.0	4.1	4.2	4.3
4.4	4.5	4.6	4.8	4.9	5.0	5.2	5.3	5.4	5.6	5.7	5.9	6.0
6.8	7.0	7.2	7.4	7.6	7.9	8.1	8.3	8.5	8.7	8.9	9.1	9.4
9.3	9.5	9.8	10.1	10.4	10.7	11.0	11.3	11.6	11.9	12.2	12.5	12.8
4.0	4.2	4.3	4.4	4.5	4.7	4.8	4.9	5.2	5.2	5.3	5.4	5.6
13.6	14.1	14.5	14.9	15.4	15.8	16.2	16.6	17.1	17.5	17.9	18.4	18.8
13.6	14.1	14.5	14.9	15.4	15.8	16.2	16.6	17.1	17.5	17.9	18.4	18.8
10.5	10.8	11.2	11.5	11.8	12.1	12.5	12.8	13.1	13.5	13.8	14.1	14.5
9.3	9.5	9.8	10.1	10.4	10.7	11.0	11.2	11.6	11.9	12.2	12.5	12.8
2.4	2.5	2.6	2.6	2.7	2.8	2.9	2.9	3.0	3.1	3.2	3.2	3.3
10.4	10.7	11.1	11.4	11.7	12.0	12.4	12.7	13.0	13.4	13.7	14.0	14.4
6.8	7.0	7.2	7.4	7.6	7.9	8.1	8.3	8.5	8.7	8.9	9.1	9.4
9.7	10.0	10.3	10.6	10.9	11.2	11.6	11.9	12.2	12.5	12.8	13.1	13.4
10.7	11.1	11.4	11.7	12.1	12.4	12.8	13.1	13.4	13.8	14.1	14.5	14.8
11.7	12.0	12.4	12.8	13.1	13.5	13.8	14.3	14.6	15.0	15.4	15.7	16.1
13.6	14.1	14.5	14.9	15.4	15.8	16.2	16.6	17.1	17.5	17.9	18.4	18.8
15.6	16.1	16.6	17.1	17.6	18.1	18.5	19.0	19.5	20.0	20.5	21.0	21.5
17.3	17.9	18.4	19.0	19.5	20.1	20.6	21.2	21.7	22.2	22.8	23.3	23.9
19.4	20.0	20.7	21.3	21.9	22.5	23.1	23.7	24.2	24.8	25.4	26.0	26.7
21.4	22.1	22.7	23.4	24.1	24.8	25.4	26.1	26.8	27.5	28.1	28.8	29.5
23.3	24.1	24.8	25.6	26.3	27.0	27.8	28.5	29.2	30.0	30.7	31.5	32.2
4.4	4.5	4.6	4.8	4.9	5.0	5.2	5.3	5.4	5.6	5.7	5.9	6.0
6.8	7.0	7.2	7.4	7.6	7.9	8.1	8.3	8.5	8.7	8.9	9.1	9.4
6.1	6.3	6.5	6.8	7.0	7.2	7.4	7.7	7.9	8.1	8.3	8.6	8.8
7.7	7.9	8.1	8.4	8.6	8.8	9.0	9.3	9.5	9.7	9.9	10.2	10.4
9.2	9.4	9.7	9.9	10.2	10.4	10.7	11.0	11.2	11.4	11.7	11.9	12.2
10.8	11.0	11.2	11.4	11.7	11.9	12.1	12.4	12.6	12.8	13.0	13.2	13.5
8.0	8.3	8.5	8.8	9.0	9.3	9.5	9.8	10.0	10.3	10.6	10.8	11.1
10.5	10.9	11.2	11.5	11.9	12.2	12.5	12.9	13.2	13.5	13.8	14.2	14.5
12.3	12.7	13.1	13.5	13.9	14.3	14.7	15.0	15.4	15.8	16.2	16.6	17.0
10.5	10.9	11.2	11.5	11.9	12.2	12.5	12.9	13.2	13.5	13.8	14.2	14.5
9.6	9.9	10.2	10.5	10.8	11.1	11.4	11.7	12.0	12.3	12.6	12.9	13.2
10.8	11.2	11.5	11.8	12.2	12.5	12.9	13.2	13.5	13.9	14.2	14.6	14.9
12.3	12.7	13.1	13.5	13.9	14.3	14.7	15.0	15.4	15.8	16.2	16.6	17.0

Body weight

	Kilograms	45	48	50	52	55	57	59	61	64	66	68	70
	Pounds	100	105	110	115	120	125	130	135	140	145	150	155

Swimming (yards/min)

		45	48	50	52	55	57	59	61	64	66	68	70
Backstroke													
25		2.5	2.6	2.8	2.9	3.0	3.1	3.3	3.4	3.5	3.7	3.8	3.9
30		3.5	3.7	3.9	4.1	4.2	4.4	4.6	4.8	4.9	5.1	5.3	5.5
35		4.5	4.7	5.0	5.2	5.4	5.6	5.9	6.1	6.3	6.6	6.8	7.0
40		5.5	5.8	6.1	6.4	6.6	6.9	7.2	7.5	7.8	8.0	8.3	8.6
Breaststroke													
20		3.1	3.3	3.5	3.6	3.8	4.0	4.1	4.3	4.5	4.6	4.8	4.9
30		4.7	5.0	5.2	5.4	5.7	5.9	6.2	6.4	6.7	6.9	7.1	7.4
40		6.3	6.7	7.0	7.3	7.6	8.0	8.3	8.6	8.9	9.3	9.6	9.9
Front crawl													
20		3.1	3.3	3.5	3.6	3.8	4.0	4.1	4.3	4.5	4.6	4.8	4.9
25		4.0	4.2	4.4	4.6	4.8	5.0	5.2	5.4	5.6	5.8	6.0	6.2
35		4.8	5.1	5.4	5.6	5.9	6.1	6.4	6.6	6.8	7.0	7.3	7.5
45		5.7	6.0	6.3	6.6	6.9	7.2	7.5	7.8	8.1	8.4	8.7	9.0
50		7.0	7.4	7.7	8.1	8.5	8.8	9.2	9.5	9.9	10.3	10.6	11.0
Table tennis		3.4	3.6	3.8	4.0	4.1	4.3	4.5	4.7	4.8	5.0	5.2	5.4
Tennis													
Singles, recreational		5.0	5.2	5.5	5.7	6.0	6.2	6.5	6.7	7.0	7.2	7.5	7.8
Doubles, recreational		3.4	3.6	3.8	4.0	4.1	4.3	4.5	4.7	4.8	5.0	5.2	5.4
Competition		6.4	6.7	7.1	7.4	7.7	8.1	8.4	8.7	9.1	9.4	9.8	10.1
Volleyball													
Moderate, recreational		2.9	3.0	3.2	3.3	3.5	3.6	3.8	3.9	4.1	4.2	4.4	4.5
Vigorous competition		6.5	6.8	7.1	7.5	7.8	8.1	8.4	8.8	9.1	9.4	9.8	10.1

Walking

(mph)	(min/mile)	45	48	50	52	55	57	59	61	64	66	68	70
1.0	60:00	1.5	1.6	1.7	1.8	1.8	1.9	2.0	2.1	2.2	2.2	2.3	2.4
2.0	30:00	2.1	2.2	2.3	2.4	2.5	2.6	2.8	2.9	3.0	3.1	3.2	3.3
2.3	26:00	2.3	2.4	2.5	2.7	2.8	2.9	3.0	3.1	3.2	3.4	3.5	3.6
3.0	20:00	2.7	2.9	3.0	3.1	3.3	3.4	3.5	3.7	3.8	3.9	4.1	4.2
3.2	18:45	3.1	3.3	3.4	3.6	3.8	4.0	4.1	4.3	4.4	4.5	4.7	4.8
3.5	17:10	3.3	3.5	3.7	3.9	4.0	4.2	4.4	4.6	4.7	4.9	5.1	5.3
4.0	15:00	4.2	4.4	4.6	4.8	5.1	5.3	5.5	5.7	5.9	6.1	6.4	6.6
4.5	13:20	4.7	5.0	5.2	5.4	5.7	5.9	6.2	6.4	6.7	6.9	7.1	7.4
5.0	12:00	5.4	5.7	6.0	6.3	6.5	6.8	7.1	7.4	7.7	7.9	8.2	8.4
5.4	11:10	6.2	6.6	6.9	7.2	7.5	7.9	8.2	8.5	8.8	9.2	9.5	9.8
5.8	10:20	7.7	8.0	8.4	8.8	9.2	9.6	10.0	10.4	10.8	11.1	11.5	11.9
Water skiing		5.0	5.2	5.5	5.7	6.0	6.2	6.5	6.7	7.0	7.2	7.5	7.8
Weight training		5.2	5.4	5.7	6.0	6.2	6.5	6.8	7.0	7.3	7.6	7.8	8.1
Wrestling		8.5	8.9	9.3	9.8	10.2	10.6	11.0	11.5	11.9	12.3	12.8	13.2

73	75	77	80	82	84	86	89	91	93	95	98	100
160	165	170	175	180	185	190	195	200	205	210	215	220
4.0	4.2	4.3	4.4	4.5	4.7	4.8	4.9	5.1	5.2	5.3	5.4	5.6
5.6	5.8	6.0	6.2	6.4	6.5	6.7	6.9	7.1	7.2	7.4	7.6	7.8
7.3	7.5	7.7	7.9	8.2	8.4	8.6	8.9	9.1	9.3	9.5	9.8	10.0
8.9	9.2	9.4	9.7	10.0	10.3	10.6	10.8	11.1	11.4	11.7	12.0	12.2
5.1	5.3	5.4	5.6	5.7	5.9	6.0	6.2	6.4	6.5	6.7	6.9	7.0
7.6	7.9	8.1	8.3	8.6	8.8	9.1	9.3	9.5	9.8	10.0	10.3	10.5
10.2	10.5	10.9	11.2	11.5	11.9	12.2	12.5	12.8	13.1	13.5	13.8	14.1
5.1	5.3	5.4	5.6	5.7	5.9	6.0	6.2	6.4	6.5	6.7	6.9	7.0
6.4	6.6	6.8	7.0	7.2	7.4	7.6	7.8	8.0	8.2	8.4	8.6	8.8
7.8	8.0	8.3	8.5	8.8	9.0	9.2	9.4	9.7	9.9	10.2	10.4	10.7
9.3	9.5	9.8	10.1	10.4	10.7	11.0	11.3	11.6	11.9	12.2	12.5	12.8
11.3	11.7	12.0	12.4	12.8	13.1	13.5	13.8	14.2	14.5	14.9	15.2	15.6
5.5	5.7	5.9	6.1	6.3	6.4	6.6	6.8	7.0	7.1	7.3	7.5	7.7
8.0	8.3	8.5	8.8	9.0	9.3	9.5	9.8	10.0	10.3	10.6	10.8	11.1
5.5	5.7	5.9	6.1	6.3	6.4	6.6	6.8	7.0	7.1	7.3	7.5	7.7
10.4	10.8	11.1	11.4	11.8	12.1	12.4	12.8	13.1	13.4	13.7	14.1	14.4
4.7	4.8	5.0	5.1	5.3	5.4	5.6	5.7	5.9	6.0	6.1	6.3	6.4
10.4	10.7	11.1	11.4	11.7	12.0	12.4	12.7	13.0	13.4	13.7	14.0	14.4
2.4	2.5	2.6	2.7	2.8	2.9	2.9	3.0	3.1	3.2	3.2	3.3	3.4
3.4	3.5	3.6	3.7	3.9	4.0	4.1	4.2	4.3	4.4	4.5	4.6	4.7
3.7	3.8	4.0	4.1	4.2	4.3	4.4	4.5	4.7	4.8	4.9	5.0	5.1
4.4	4.5	4.6	4.8	4.9	5.0	5.2	5.3	5.4	5.6	5.7	5.9	6.0
5.0	5.2	5.3	5.5	5.6	5.8	5.9	6.1	6.3	6.4	6.6	6.8	6.9
5.4	5.6	5.8	6.0	6.2	6.3	6.5	6.7	6.9	7.0	7.2	7.4	7.6
6.8	7.0	7.2	7.4	7.6	7.9	8.1	8.3	8.5	8.7	8.9	9.1	9.4
7.6	7.9	8.1	8.3	8.6	8.8	9.1	9.3	9.5	9.8	10.0	10.3	10.5
8.7	9.0	9.2	9.5	9.8	10.1	10.4	10.6	10.9	11.2	11.5	11.8	12.0
10.1	10.4	10.8	11.1	11.4	11.8	12.1	12.4	12.7	13.0	13.4	13.7	14.0
12.3	12.7	13.1	13.5	13.9	14.3	14.7	15.0	15.4	15.8	16.2	16.6	17.0
8.0	8.3	8.5	8.8	9.0	9.3	9.5	9.8	10.0	10.3	10.6	10.8	11.1
8.3	8.6	8.9	9.1	9.4	9.7	9.9	10.2	10.5	10.7	11.0	11.2	11.5
13.6	14.1	14.5	14.9	15.4	15.8	16.2	16.6	17.1	17.5	17.9	18.4	18.8

D

Calories, Percent Fat, and Cholesterol in Selected Fast-Food Restaurant Products*

	Calories	% Fat Calories	Cholesterol (milligrams)
Arby's			
Regular roast beef	383	43	43
Chicken breast fillet	445	45	45
Potato cakes	204	48	0
Turkey sub	533	43	56
Garden salad	117	40	12
Burger King			
Dutch apple pie	308	43	0
Double cheeseburger	450	50	90
Double whopper with cheese	950	59	195
Onion rings	339	50	0
Vanilla milk shake (medium)	310	17	20
Croissan'wich with bacon/egg/cheese	353	58	230
Salad dressing, thousand island	145	80	18
Salad dressing, reduced calorie Italian	5	60	0
Domino's Pizza			
Cheese, 2 slices	376	24	18
Pepperoni, 2 slices	460	34	28
Veggie, 2 slices	498	33	36
Double cheese/pepperoni 2 slices	545	42	48
Hardee's			
Steak biscuit	580	50	30
Hamburger, regular	260	31	20
Bacon cheeseburger	600	54	50
Big country breakfast (sausage)	930	59	340
Chef salad	200	50	45
Chicken fillet	400	32	55
Fisherman's fillet	500	40	60
Fried chicken, breast	370	36	75

*All fast food restaurants have pamphlets available describing the nutrient content of all foods they serve, in many cases including whole sandwiches and meals, but also individual components such as bread, meat, vegetables, condiments, etc. Fast food offerings change often, so use these free publications to assess the quality of their products. Just ask for a copy at the counter.

	Calories	% Fat Calories	Cholesterol (milligrams)
KFC			
BBQ baked beans	132	14	3
Cole slaw	114	47	4
Mashed potatoes with gravy	70	13	4
Side breast (original recipe)	245	55	78
Side breast (extra tasty)	400	61	75
Chicken sandwich	482	50	47
Long John Silver's			
Baked fish	120	6	110
Baked shrimp-scampi	120	15	205
Baked chicken	140	26	70
Fish with batter, 1 piece	202	50	31
Hush puppies, 2 pieces	145	43	1
McDonald's			
Hamburger	255	31	35
McLean Deluxe	320	28	75
Big Mac	500	47	100
McChicken sandwich	470	48	60
Chicken McNuggets (6 pieces)	270	50	55
French Fries	320	48	0
Hotcakes with margarine and syrup	435	25	10
Egg McMuffin	280	35	235
Breakfast burrito	280	55	135
Sausage biscuit	420	60	45
Apple bran muffin	180	0	0
Chunky chicken salad	150	24	80
Pizza Hut			
Pan pizza, cheese, 2 slices	492	33	34
Handtossed, cheese, 2 slices	518	35	55
Personal pan pizza, supreme (whole pizza)	647	39	49
Taco Bell			
Bean burrito	381	33	9
Beef burrito	431	44	57
Taco, beef	183	54	32
Soft taco, beef	225	48	32
Light taco, beef	140	36	20
Nachos Supreme	367	66	18
Taco salad	905	61	80
Wendy's			
Big classic hamburger	480	43	75
Fish fillet sandwich	460	49	55
Grilled chicken sandwich	290	22	60
Plain potato, baked	300	1	0
Potato with broccoli and cheese	450	28	15
Chicken nuggets	280	64	50

E

Approximate Metabolic Cost of Various Occupational and Recreational Activities in METS*

METS	Occupation	Exercise or Recreational Activity
1–2	Desk work Light housework Sewing, knitting Light office work	Strolling, 1 mile/hour Standing Playing cards
2–3	Light janitorial work Auto repair Bartending Woodworking, light Bakery work, general	Walking, 2 miles/hour Golf, motor cart Horseback riding (walk) Easy canoeing
3–4	Moderate housework, cleaning windows Yard work, power mower Electrical work Machine tooling	Walking, 3 miles/hour Cycling, 6 miles/hour Golf, pull cart Horseback riding (trot) Badminton (doubles)
4–5	Light carpentry Painting, masonry work Raking leaves Hoeing garden	Walking, 3.5 miles/hour Cycling, 8 miles/hour Golf, carrying clubs Tennis, doubles Dancing
5–6	Moderate gardening, shoveling Farming, general	Walking, 4 miles/hour Cycling, 10 miles/hour
6–7	Heavy shoveling Splitting wood Snow shoveling Lawn mowing, hand mower Forestry, general	Walking, 5 miles/hour Cycling, 11 miles/hour Tennis, singles Folk dancing
7–8	Digging ditches Sawing wood, lumber work	Jogging, 5 miles/hour Cycling, 12 miles/hour Horseback riding, gallop Basketball Climbing hills
8–9		Running, 5.5 miles/hour Cycling, 13 miles/hour Cross-country skiing, 4 miles/hour Squash, handball
10+		Running, over 6 miles/hour Cycling, over 14 miles/hour Cross-country skiing, over 5 miles/hour Competitive squash and handball

Source: Modified from Fox, S.; Naughton, J.; and Gorman, P. "Physical Activity and Cardiovascular Health. III. The Exercise Prescription; Frequency and Type of Activity." Modern Concepts of Cardiovascular Disease 41:25 (1972). Reprinted by permission of the American Heart Association.

One MET is defined as 3.5 ml of oxygen per kilogram body weight per minute, which is the resting metabolic rate.

Glossary

A

abdominal and low back-hamstring musculoskeletal function   The concept that optimal strength and flexibility of the abdominal muscles, the muscles in the low back area, and the hamstring muscles will help prevent the low back pain syndrome.

abdominal:gluteal ratio   *See* waist:hip ratio.

acclimatization   The ability of the body to undergo physiological adaptations so that the stress of a given environment, such as high environmental temperature, is less severe.

accommodating resistance   An automatic change in resistance associated with the isokinetic technique of weight training; designed to match resistance with strength at all points in the range of motion.

acetaldehyde   An intermediate breakdown product of alcohol.

acetyl CoA   The major fuel for the oxidative processes in the body. It is derived from the breakdown of glucose and fatty acids.

Achilles tendinitis   An inflammation in the Achilles tendon in the lower back portion of the leg.

acquired immunodeficiency syndrome   *See* AIDS.

ACSM   American College of Sports Medicine.

acute muscular soreness   The muscle soreness or pain that may occur during a very strenuous exercise bout. It is usually temporary. Compare to delayed muscle soreness.

addiction   A chronic, compulsive use of some substance, usually drugs. Cessation of use is usually associated with both psychological and physical or physiological withdrawal symptoms.

additives   Substances added to food to improve color, texture, stability, or other similar purposes.

adenosinetriphosphate   *See* ATP.

ADH   The antidiuretic hormone secreted by the pituitary gland; its major action is to conserve body water by decreasing urine formation.

adherence   In relation to a Positive Health Life-style, the ability to stay with a program, such as exercise, for a lifetime.

adrenalin   A hormone secreted by the adrenal medulla gland; it is a stimulant and prepares the body for "fight or flight."

adult-onset obesity   Obesity that occurs during adulthood, usually hypertrophy-type obesity. *See also* creeping obesity.

aerobic   Relating to energy processes that occur in the presence of oxygen.

aerobic capacity   The capacity of the individual to utilize oxygen to produce energy. *See also* $\dot{V}O_2$ max.

aerobic dancing   A wide variety of aerobic and flexibility exercises set to music.

aerobic exercise   The term coined by Dr. Kenneth Cooper to mean those exercise activities that use the oxygen system to improve the health of the cardiovascular-respiratory system.

aerobic fitness   Synonymous with cardiovascular fitness or cardiovascular endurance; the ability to sustain prolonged endurance activities that use the oxygen energy system.

aerobic walking   Rapid walking designed to elevate the HR so a training effect would occur; more strenuous than ordinary leisure walking.

AIDS   acquired immunodeficiency syndrome; caused by the human immunodeficiency virus (HIV), ultimately leading to deterioration of the immune system.

alanine   A nonessential amino acid.

alcohol   A colorless liquid with depressant effects; ethyl alcohol (or ethanol) is the alcohol designed for human consumption.

alcoholism   A rather undefined term used to refer to individuals who abuse the effect of alcohol; an addiction or habituation that may result in physical and/or psychological withdrawal effects.

aldosterone   The main electrolyte-regulating hormone secreted by the adrenal cortex; primarily controls sodium and potassium balance.

alpha-linolenic fatty acid   An essential fatty acid.

alpha-tocopherol   The most biologically active alcohol in vitamin E.

alveoli   The tiny air sacs in the lungs where the exchange of gases between the blood and the lungs takes place.

amenorrhea   Cessation or abnormal stoppage of normal menstrual blood flow.

amino acids   The chief structural material of protein, consisting of an amino group (NH_2), an acid group (COOH), and other components.

amino group   The nitrogen-containing component of amino acids (NH_2).

aminostatic theory   A theory suggesting that hunger is controlled by the presence or absence of amino acids in the blood acting upon a receptor in the hypothalamus.

anabolic steroids   Drugs designed to mimic the actions of testosterone to build muscle tissue (anabolism) while minimizing the androgenic effects (masculinization).

anabolism   Constructive metabolism; the process whereby simple body compounds are formed into more complex ones.

anaerobic   Relating to energy processes that occur in the absence of oxygen.

anaerobic threshold   The intensity level of exercise at which the metabolism begins to shift to increased dependence upon anaerobic sources of energy such as the lactic acid energy system.

android:gynoid ratio   *See* waist:hip ratio.

android-type obesity   Characterized by accumulation in the abdominal region, particularly the intraabdominal region, of deep, visceral fat, but also subcutaneous fat. Often referred to as the apple-shape obesity.

anemia   Below normal levels of circulating RBCs and hemoglobin; there are many different types of anemia.

angina   The pain experienced under the breastbone or other areas of the upper body when the heart is deprived of oxygen.

anorexia athletica   A term used in conjunction with athletes who demonstrate some symptoms of anorexia nervosa; usually a temporary condition observed among competitive athletes, such as gymnasts or distance runners, when excessive stress is put on body weight control.

anorexia nervosa   A serious eating disorder, particularly among teenage girls and young women, marked by a loss of appetite and leading to various degrees of emaciation.

antidiuretic hormone   *See* ADH.

antioxidant   Compounds, such as vitamins C and E, that block the oxidation of various body cells, such as the membranes of RBC.

antipromoters   Compounds that block the actions of promoters, agents associated with the development of certain diseases such as cancer.

apoplexy   *See* stroke.

apoprotein   The protein component of a lipoprotein, usually classified as alpha or beta apoproteins.

appetite   A pleasant desire for food for the purpose of enjoyment developed through previous experience; controlled in humans by an appetite center, or appestat, in the hypothalamus.

arrhythmia   An irregularity in the normal heart rate rhythm.

arteriosclerosis   Hardening of the arteries. *See also* atherosclerosis.

artery   The major blood vessels that transport blood away from the heart to various parts of the body.

arthritis   An inflammation in the joints between bones.

ascorbic acid   Vitamin C.

assertiveness   The quality of being assertive and positive, of expressing your feelings honestly and openly to others.

atherosclerosis   A specific form of arteriosclerosis characterized by the formation of plaque on the inner layers of the arterial wall.

athletic amenorrhea   The cessation of menstruation seen in female athletes, in particular those involved in prolonged endurance activities.

ATP   Adenosinetriphosphate, a high-energy phosphate compound found in the body; one of the major forms of energy available for immediate use in the body.

ATP-PC system   The energy system for fast, powerful muscle contractions; uses ATP as the immediate energy source, the spent ATP being quickly regenerated by breakdown of the PC. ATP and PC are high-energy phosphates in the muscle cell.

autogenic relaxation   A technique to induce relaxation in which you attempt to relax specific body parts in a set sequence, such as starting with the muscles in the head and progressing to the feet.

B

BAC   Blood alcohol content; the concentration of alcohol in the blood.

backward pelvic tilt   Backward rotation of the pelvic bone, usually caused by contracting the abdominal muscles; flattens out the lumbar curve.

ballistic   A rapid motion, often used in conjunction with flexibility exercises, in which the muscle is stretched rapidly.

ballistic stretching exercises   Flexibility exercises that involve rapid stretching or bouncing type movements.

basal metabolic rate   *See* BMR.

Basic Four Food Groups   Grouping of foods into four categories that can be used as a means to educate individuals on how to obtain essential nutrients. The four groups are meat, milk, bread-cereals, and fruit-vegetable.

behavior modification   Relative to weight-control methods, the modification of personal behavioral patterns to help achieve weight loss.

benefit-risk ratio   Relative to a Positive Health Life-style, the relationship of the health benefits to be received versus the risks associated with certain behaviors.

Benson's relaxation response   A meditation technique used for relaxation purposes; similar to Transcendental Meditation.

beta-carotene   A precursor of vitamin A found in plant foods such as yellow-orange fruits and vegetables.

BIA   Bioelectrical impedance analysis, a technique to evaluate body composition by measuring resistance to electric current in the body.

bile   A fluid that aids in the breakdown process of fats; secreted into the intestine by the liver or gall bladder.

binge-purge syndrome   A symptom seen in bulimia in which the individual will consume large amounts of food followed by self-induced regurgitation.

Bioelectrical Impedance Analysis   *See* BIA.

biotin   A component of the B complex.

blood alcohol content   *See* BAC.

blood glucose   Blood sugar; the means by which carbohydrate is carried in the blood; normal range is 70 to 120 mg/ml.

blood pressure   The pressure of the blood in the various blood vessels; usually means arterial blood pressure. *See also* systolic blood pressure and diastolic blood pressure.

BMI   Body Mass Index; the ratio of weight to height, expressed as $Kg/(M)^2$.

BMR   The basal metabolic rate; measurement of energy expenditure in the body under resting, post-absorptive conditions; indicative of the energy needed to maintain life under these basal conditions.

body building   A sport designed to increase muscle size and definition for aesthetic competition; weight training is the primary mode of training.

body composition   The analysis of the body into two primary components, body fat and lean body mass. Lean body mass is primarily muscle and bone tissue.

body image   The image or impression the individual has of his or her body. A poor body image may lead to personality problems.

Body Mass Index   *See* BMI.

brown fat   A type of fat that is very active metabolically and that is found in very small amounts in the body; may burn Calories without producing ATP.

bulimarexia   Condition in which symptoms of both bulimia and anorexia nervosa are present.

bulimia   Excessive hunger; often associated with the binge-purge syndrome.

bulimia nervosa   *See* bulimia.

C

CAD   Coronary artery disease; atherosclerosis in the coronary arteries.

caffeine   A stimulant drug found in many food products such as coffee, tea, and colas; stimulates the central nervous system.

calciferol   A synthetic form of vitamin D, vitamin D_2.

calcium   A silver-white metallic element essential to human nutrition.

caloric concept of weight control   The concept that Calories are the basis of weight control. Excess Calories will add body weight; caloric deficiencies will contribute to weight loss.

Calorie   A measure of heat energy. A small calorie represents the amount of heat needed to raise one gram of water one degree Celsius. A large Calorie (kilocalorie, KC, or C) is 1,000 small calories.

calorie free   Less than 5 Calories per serving.

calorimeter   A device used to measure the calorie value of a given food or to measure heat production of animals or man.

cancer   A disease characterized by unregulated and disorganized growth of body cells.

capillary   The smallest blood vessels in the body where nutrients, gases, and waste products are exchanged between the blood and the tissues.

carbohydrate   A group of compounds containing carbon, hydrogen, and oxygen. Glucose, glycogen, sugar, starches, fiber, cellulose, and the various saccharides are all carbohydrates.

carbohydrate loading   A dietary method utilized by endurance-oriented athletes to help increase the carbohydrate (glycogen) levels in their muscles and livers.

carbon monoxide   A tasteless, odorless, poisonous gas resulting from incomplete oxidation of carbon fuels.

carcinogens   Substances that contribute to the development of cancer, either as initiators or promoters.

cardiac output   The amount of blood pumped by the heart per minute.

cardiovascular endurance   The ability of the cardiovascular system to provide sufficient energy to sustain aerobic exercise for prolonged periods of time. *See also* aerobic exercise.

catabolism   Destructive metabolism whereby complex chemical compounds in the body are degraded to simpler compounds.

ceftriaxone   An antibiotic drug for use with several sexually transmitted diseases.

cellulite   A name given to the lumpy fat that often appears in the thigh and hip regions of women. It is simply normal fat in small compartments formed by connective tissue, but it may also contain glycoproteins, substances that hold water.

cellulose   The fibrous carbohydrate that provides the structural backbone for plants; plant fiber.

central circulation   The role of the heart, or center, in pumping blood to the periphery. *See also* peripheral circulation.

cerebral thrombosis   A blood clot in a cerebral artery. *See also* stroke.

cerebral vascular accident   *See* CVA.

CHD   Coronary heart disease; a degenerative disease of the heart caused primarily by arteriosclerosis or atherosclerosis of the coronary vessels of the heart.

chlamydia   A sexually transmitted disease caused by a bacterium, Chlamydia trachomatis.

chloride   A compound of chlorine present in a salt form carrying a negative charge; Cl^-.

cholesterol   A fatlike pearly substance, an alcohol, found in all animal fats and oils; a main constituent of some body tissues and body compounds.

cholesterol free   Less than 2 milligrams per serving.

cholesterol reduced   In nutritional labeling, decreased cholesterol content by 75 percent or more compared to the original product.

chondromalacia   A softness in cartilage; may result in pain around the involved joints.

chromium   A whitish metal essential to human nutrition; it is involved in carbohydrate metabolism via its role with insulin.

chronic diseases   Diseases that develop over prolonged periods of time, such as coronary heart disease and lung cancer. A Positive Health Life-style may help retard their development.

chronic obstructive pulmonary disease   *See* COPD.

chronic training effect   Repeated bouts of exercise will elicit physiological changes in the body that will help make the body more efficient during exercise.

chronological age   Actual age of an individual; compare to functional age.

circuit aerobics   A combination of aerobic and weight-training exercises in order to derive the specific benefits of each type of exercise.

circuit weight training   Weight-training exercises organized in a specific sequence or circuit.

cirrhosis   A degenerative disease of the liver; one cause is excessive consumption of alcohol.

cis fatty acids   An arrangement of hydrogen ions in the carbon chain of a fatty acid in which hydrogen ions attached to a carbon at a double bond are both on the same side. Compare to trans fatty acids.

claudication   Symptoms of pain in the calf muscle, intermittent in nature, often observed with peripheral vascular disease.

cobalamin   The cobalt-containing complex common to all members of the vitamin B_{12} group; often used to designate cyanocobalamin.

cobalt   A gray, hard metal that is a component of vitamin B_{12}.

cocaine   An alkaloid derivative from the coca plant, Erythroxylon coca. An addictive drug.

coenzyme   An activator of an enzyme; many vitamins are coenzymes.

collateral circulation   A secondary or accessory blood vessel, such as a small side branch that may develop from a primary vessel.

complex carbohydrates   A term used to describe foods high in starch (bread, cereals, fruits, and vegetables).

Computed Tomography   *See* CT.

conduction   In relation to body temperature, the transfer of heat from one substance to another by direct contact.

congenital heart disease   Certain heart defects present at birth.

contributory risk factor   A risk factor that may predispose an individual to a particular disease; the strength of the association to the disease is not as significant as a major risk factor.

convection   In relation to body temperature, the transfer of heat via currents in either the air or water.

COPD   Chronic obstructive pulmonary disease. A condition, such as emphysema, that makes breathing very difficult, even during mild physical exertion.

copper   A reddish metallic element essential to human nutrition; it functions with iron in the formation of hemoglobin and cytochromes.

core temperature   The temperature of the deep tissues of the body; usually measured orally or rectally.

coronary arteries   The arteries that supply blood to the heart muscle.

coronary artery disease   *See* CAD.

coronary heart disease   *See* CHD.

coronary occlusion   A blockage of blood supply in a coronary artery.

coronary risk factors   The behaviors (smoking) or body properties (cholesterol levels) that may predispose an individual to coronary heart disease.

coronary thrombosis   A clot in a coronary artery that may lead to a coronary occlusion.

crack   A potent form of cocaine, usually smoked for an instant effect.

creeping obesity   A gradual accumulation of body fat, possibly over several years, that leads to obesity. *See also* adult-onset obesity.

cross training   Exercise training programs consisting of several physical activities that stress different muscle groups, such as running, cycling, and swimming.

cruciferous vegetables   Vegetables in the cabbage family, such as broccoli, cauliflower, kale, and all cabbages.

CT   Computed tomography, an X-ray scanning technique to image body tissues; may be used to measure body composition.

curl-up   An abdominal exercise similar to a sit-up; the individual sits up only about 30 degrees from the floor.

CVA   Cerebral vascular accident; impaired blood supply in the brain resulting in impaired oxygen delivery; a stroke.

cyanocobalamin   Vitamin B_{12}.

D

Daily Reference Value   *See* DRV.

Daily Value   *See* DV.

dehydration   A reduction of the body water to below the normal level of hydration; water output exceeds water intake.

delayed muscle soreness   Muscle soreness or pain that develops a day or two after a severe exercise bout that usually involves eccentric muscle contractions.

delta-9-tetrahydrocannabinol   *See* THC.

densitometry   An underwater weighing technique to evaluate body composition.

diabetes mellitus   A disorder of carbohydrate metabolism due to inadequate production of insulin; results in high blood glucose levels and loss of sugar in the urine.

diastolic blood pressure   The blood pressure in the arteries when the heart is at rest between beats.

diet   The food consumed to obtain essential nutrients. A balanced diet will provide adequate nutrition. Adjectives may be used to describe specific diets, e.g., low-Calorie diet, diabetic diet, etc.

dietary fiber   Fiber in plant foods that cannot be hydrolyzed by digestive enzymes.

Dietary Induced Thermogenesis   *See* DIT.

distressor   A stressor characterized by negative life events, such as death in the family; compare to eustressor.

disuse phenomena   The degeneration that may occur in various body tissues or systems when they are not used; lack of exercise may result in certain pathological effects in some body tissues.

DIT   Dietary induced thermogenesis; the increased heat production associated with the metabolism of food following a meal.

DNA   Deoxyribonucleic acid; a complex protein found in chromosomes that is the carrier of genetic information and the basis of heredity.

domains of health   The concept that total health is dependent on various health components, including emotional, intellectual, physical, social, and spiritual health.

Doxycycline   Antibiotic drugs used in treating some sexually transmitted diseases.

drug abuse   A rather unstandardized term used to indicate the abuse or misuse of drugs to the extent that they cause personal or social problems.

DRV   Daily reference value, a term used in food labeling; recommended daily intakes for the major nutrients (carbohydrate, fat, and protein) as well as for cholesterol, sodium, and potassium. On a food label, the DRV is based on a 2,000 Calorie diet.

duration concept   One of the major concepts of aerobic exercise; the amount of time spent exercising during each bout.

DV   Daily value, a term used in food labeling; the DV is based on a daily energy intake of 2,000 Calories and for the food labeled presents the percentage of the RDI and the DRV recommended for healthy Americans. *See also* RDI and DRV.

dynamic flexibility   Flexibility exercises that involve rapid, bouncing movements to stretch a particular muscle group.

dysmenorrhea   Painful cramps during the menstrual flow period.

E

early-onset obesity   Obesity that develops early in life, as early as the first year of life or even at puberty. May often be a hyperplasia-type obesity.

eating disorder   Gross disturbance in eating behavior, such as bulimia.

eccentric muscle contraction   A lengthening muscle contraction in which the muscle is trying to shorten, but the outside force is causing the muscle to lengthen.

ECG   The electrocardiogram; a measure of the electrical activity of the heart.

eicosanoids   Derivatives of fatty acid oxidation in the body, including prostaglandins, thromboxanes, and leukotrienes.

elastic fibers   Protein fibers found in soft tissues, such as muscles and tendons, that are capable of elongating or shortening.

electrolytes   A solution that contains ions and can conduct electricity; often the ions of salts such as sodium and chloride are called electrolytes. *See also* ions.

embolus   A blood clot that travels freely in the bloodstream.

emphysema A chronic pulmonary disease characterized by excessive distention of the alveoli and impaired respiration.

EMR Exercise metabolic rate; an increased metabolic rate due to the need for increased energy production during exercise; the BMR may be increased more than twenty-fold. *See also* Thermic Effect of Exercise.

endometrium The mucus membrane lining the inner surface of the uterus.

endorphins Naturally occurring chemicals produced in the brain that resemble narcotic drugs and may help reduce pain.

energy The ability to do work; energy exists in various forms, notably mechanical, heat, and chemical forms in the human body.

energy balance The concept that weight control is a measure of energy, or caloric, balance. *See also* positive and negative energy balance.

enriched In nutritional labeling, thiamin, riboflavin, niacin, and iron are added after the milling process.

enzyme A complex protein in the body that serves as a catalyst, facilitating reactions between various substances without being changed itself.

epidemiological research Research investigating the relationship between various health risks and the prevalence of disease in a given population.

epidemiology A science that investigates the relationship between various factors and the prevalence of a disease or other physiological condition in a given population.

essential amino acids Those amino acids that must be obtained in the diet and cannot be synthesized in the body.

essential fat Fat in the body that is an essential part of the tissues, such as cell membrane structure, nerve coverings, and the brain. *See also* storage fat.

essential fatty acids The unsaturated fatty acids that may not be synthesized in the body and must be obtained in the diet; linoleic fatty acid and alpha-linolenic acids.

essential hypertension High blood pressure without any detected underlying cause.

essential nutrients Those nutrients found to be essential to human life and optimal functioning.

estrogen The female sex hormones responsible for the development of secondary sexual characteristics and the various phases of the menstrual cycle; also essential for bone formation.

ethanol Alcohol; ethyl alcohol.

ethyl alcohol Alcohol; ethanol.

eumenorrhea A normal menstrual cycle.

eustressor A stressor characterized by positive life events, such as marriage; compared to distressor.

evaporation The energy consuming conversion of a liquid to a vapor; evaporation of sweat cools the body by using body heat as the energy source.

exercise A form of structured physical activity generally designed to enhance physical fitness; exercise usually refers to strenuous physical activity.

exercise adherence Starting and staying with an exercise program for a lifetime.

exercise duration The amount of time of an exercise session; the American College of Sports Medicine recommends a duration of 20 to 60 minutes as a sound guideline for aerobic exercise.

exercise ECG stress test An exercise test usually administered on a treadmill. The ECG is recorded to determine if any pathological condition is present in the heart, to derive information for an exercise prescription, and to determine present fitness level.

exercise frequency In an aerobic exercise program, the number of times per week that an individual exercises.

exercise intensity The tempo, speed, or resistance of an exercise. Intensity can be increased by working faster, doing more work in a given amount of time.

exercise metabolic rate *See* EMR.

exercise mode The type of exercise an individual performs, such as walking, running, swimming, bicycling, resistance training, etc.

experimental research Research investigating a cause-and-effect relationship between two or more variables; an independent variable, such as dietary cholesterol, is manipulated in order to evaluate the effect on a dependent variable, such as blood cholesterol.

extra lean In nutritional labeling, fewer than 5 grams of fat, 2 grams of saturated fat, or 95 milligrams of cholesterol per 100 grams.

F

fasting Starvation; abstinence from eating that may be partial or complete.

fast twitch, glycolytic fiber The type IIb muscle fiber, or white fast twitch fiber, that depends primarily upon the lactic acid energy system, or anaerobic glycolysis, for energy production.

fast twitch, oxidative, glycolytic fiber The type IIa muscle fiber, or red fast twitch fiber, that produces ATP anaerobically via the lactic acid system (anaerobic glycolysis) or aerobically via the oxygen system.

fat free Less than 0.5 grams of fat per serving.

fatigue A generalized or specific feeling of tiredness that may have a multitude of causes; may be mental or physical.

fat patterning Localization of body fat stores in specific areas of the body, such as the abdominal area or the gluteal-femoral area.

fats Triglycerides; a combination, or ester, of three fatty acids and glycerol.

fatty acids Any one of a number of aliphatic acids containing only carbon, oxygen, and hydrogen; may be saturated or unsaturated.

feeding center A collection of nerve cells in the hypothalamus involved in the control of feeding reflexes.

Fetal Alcohol Effects (FAE) Symptoms noted in children born to women who consumed alcohol during pregnancy. Not as severe as the fetal alcohol syndrome.

Fetal Alcohol Syndrome (FAS) A syndrome of effects seen in children born to women who consumed alcohol while pregnant.

FFA Free fatty acids; formed by the hydrolysis of triglycerides.

fiber The indigestible carbohydrate in plants that forms the structural network. *See also* cellulose.

fibrin A protein, formed in the blood, that is involved in the blood clotting process.

flexibility A measure of the range of motion of a given joint in the body; usually a measure of the flexibility or elasticity of soft tissues such as muscles and tendons.

fluoride A salt of hydrofluoric acid; a compound of fluorine that may be helpful in the prevention of dental decay.

folacin Folic acid.

folic acid A water-soluble vitamin that appears to be essential in preventing birth defects and certain types of anemia.

food additives *See* additives.

Food Exchange Lists A grouping of foods into six different exchange lists; foods in each list are similar in caloric value and in carbohydrate, fat, and protein content.

food guide pyramid A food group approach to healthful nutrition, containing five food groups.

fortified In nutritional labeling, nutrients are added above amounts normally contained in the food.

free fatty acids *See* FFA.

free radicals An atom or group of atoms that have an unpaired electron. Formed in a variety of chemical reactions in the body.

fructose A monosaccharide known also as levulose or fruit sugar; found in all sweet fruits.

functional age The physiological age of an individual.

G

genetics The science or study of heredity and the differences or similarities among organisms.

genital herpes A sexually transmitted disease caused by the type 2 strain of the herpes simplex virus; characterized by small, painful, itching sores.

genital warts Venereal warts; caused by the human papilloma virus (HPV); small elevations on the skin.

glucose A monosaccharide; a thick, sweet, syrupy liquid.

glucose intolerance Inability to metabolize glucose properly; usually determined by a glucose tolerance test.

glucostatic theory The theory of hunger based upon the levels of glucose in the blood.

glycerol A sweet alcohol that is a by-product of fat metabolism; glycerol plus three fatty acids yields a triglyceride.

glycogen A polysaccharide that is the chief storage form of carbohydrate in animals; stored primarily in the liver and muscles.

glycogen sparing effect The theory that certain dietary techniques, such as the utilization of caffeine, may facilitate the oxidation of fatty acids for energy and thus spare the utilization of glycogen.

glycolysis The degradation of sugars into smaller compounds; the main quantitative anaerobic energy process in muscle tissue.

gonorrhea An inflammatory sexually transmitted disease caused by the Neisseria gonorrhoeae bacterium.

gynoid-type obesity Characterized by accumulation of fat in the gluteal-femoral region—the hips, buttocks, and thighs. Often referred to as the pear-shape obesity.

H

habituation A term associated with addiction to a substance, usually a drug; withdrawal involves only psychological symptoms, not physical or physiological ones.

hamstrings The three muscles in the posterior portion of the thigh.

HDL *See* high density lipoprotein.

HDL cholesterol High density lipoprotein cholesterol; one mechanism whereby cholesterol is transported in the blood. High HDL levels are somewhat protective against CHD.

health promotion practices The concept of maximizing one's health status by adopting life-style behaviors consistent with good health.

health promotion services Environmental or regulatory measures that confer protection to large segments of the population, such as water fluoridation for prevention of tooth decay.

health related fitness Those components of physical fitness whose improvement have health benefits, such as cardiovascular fitness, body composition, flexibility, and muscular strength and endurance.

Health Risk Appraisal *See* HRA.

health risk management Practicing prudent health behaviors so as to reduce health risks to a level compatible with good health.

heat cramps Painful muscular cramps or tetanus following prolonged exercise in a hot environment without water or salt replacement.

heat exhaustion Weakness or dizziness from overexertion in a hot environment.

heat stroke Elevated body temperature of 106° F or greater caused by exposure to excessive heat gains or production and diminished heat loss.

heat syncope Fainting caused by excessive heat exposure.

height and weight charts Charts that use combinations of height and weight to determine if an individual is overweight or underweight.

hemoglobin The protein-iron pigment in red blood cells that transports oxygen.

hernia The protrusion of some body tissue through a weakened wall of the cavity within which it is normally contained.

HGH Human growth hormone, also known as somatotropin. A hormone secreted by the pituitary gland that stimulates bone growth and other physiological processes.

hidden fat The unobservable fat contained in foods. Cheese contains over 70 percent of its Calories as fat.

high blood pressure *See* hypertension.

high density lipoprotein A protein-lipid complex in the blood that facilitates the transport of triglycerides, cholesterol, and phospholipids. *See* HDL cholesterol.

hip flexion Bending over at the waist or raising the thigh forward.

histidine An essential amino acid.

HIV Human immunodeficiency virus; the cause of acquired immunodeficiency syndrome.

homeostasis A term used to describe a condition of normalcy in the internal body environment.

hormone A chemical substance produced by specific body cells and secreted into the blood; acts on specific target tissues.

HPV Human papilloma virus; the cause of genital warts.

HRA Health risk appraisal; an inventory of health status and behaviors that generates a profile of an individual relative to the risk of developing certain diseases or health problems.

HR$_{MAX}$ The normal maximal heart rate of an individual during exercise.

human growth hormone *See* HGH.

human immunodeficiency virus *See* HIV.

human papilloma virus *See* HPV.

hunger A basic physiological desire to eat, normally caused by a lack of food; may be accompanied by stomach contractions.

hydrogenated fats Fats to which hydrogen has been added, usually causing them to be saturated.

hydrogen peroxide A free oxygen radical in the body.

hypercholesteremia Elevated blood cholesterol levels.

hyperglycemia Elevated blood glucose levels.

hyperplasia An increased number of cells.

hyperplastic obesity Obesity associated with an increased number of fat cells.

hypertension A condition with various causes whereby the blood pressure is higher than normal.

hypertriglyceridemia Elevated blood levels of triglycerides.

hypertrophic obesity Obesity associated with an increased size of fat cells.

hypertrophy An enlargement of cells.

hypoglycemia A low blood sugar level.

hypohydration Dehydration; a state of decreased water content in the body.

hypothalamus The part of the brain involved in the control of involuntary activity in the body; contains many centers for neural control, such as temperature, hunger, appetite, and thirst.

I

ice A clear, crystal form of methamphetamine.

iliotibial band injury An inflammation or irritation of the iliotibial band on the lateral aspect of the knee; often seen in joggers and runners.

imagery A relaxation technique to help reduce stress whereby a relaxing image is created in the mind.

imitation In nutritional labeling, nutritionally inferior to the original product.

in-line skating Rollerblading; exercise with skates that have one line of wheels.

insensible perspiration Perspiration on the skin not detectable by ordinary senses.

insulin A hormone secreted by the pancreas involved in carbohydrate metabolism.

insulin-dependent diabetes Diabetes in which insulin is required to help control it; most common in juvenile-onset diabetes.

insulin reaction Excessive concentration of insulin in the body that results in hypoglycemia; usually seen in diabetics who overdose or who exercise a muscle that has been injected with insulin.

insulin response Blood insulin levels rise following the ingestion of sugar and the resultant hyperglycemia; the insulin causes the sugar to be taken up by the fat cells, muscles and liver, possibly creating a reactive hypoglycemia.

interferon A protein formed by the body cells, usually through exposure to a virus, that protects healthy body cells from exposure to the virus.

interleukin-2 A protein formed in the white blood cells that is believed to act as an antipromoter, possibly helping in the prevention of cancer.

International Unit *See* IU.

interval training A form of training that involves repeated bouts of exercise with intervals of rest between each repetition.

inverted-U hypothesis The hypothesis that both too much and too little anxiety lead to inferior performance levels.

iodine A nonmetallic element necessary for the proper development and functioning of the thyroid gland.

ions Particles with an electrical charge; anions are negative and cations are positive.

iron A metallic element essential for the development of several chemical compounds in the body, notably hemoglobin.

iron-deficiency anemia Anemia caused by inadequate intake or absorption of iron that results in impaired hemoglobin formation.

ischemia Lack of blood supply.

isokinetic Same speed.

isokinetic contraction A muscle contraction in which the speed of movement is controlled.

isoleucine An essential amino acid.

isometric Same length.

isometric contraction A muscle contraction in which very little or no movement occurs.

isotonic Same tension.

isotonic concentric contraction A shortening muscle contraction.

isotonic contraction A muscle contraction in which the same tension is developed through a range of motion.

isotonic eccentric contraction A lengthening muscle contraction. Actually the muscle is trying to shorten, but since the external force, usually gravity, is greater, the muscle lengthens.

IU International Unit; a method of expressing the quantity of some substance (such as vitamins) that is an internationally developed and accepted standard.

J

jogging A term used to designate slow running; the distinction between running and jogging is relative to the individual involved; a common value used for jogging is a 9-minute mile or slower.

joule A measure of work or energy equivalent to one newton meter; one joule also equals 0.00024 Calorie.

juvenile-onset diabetes   Diabetes that occurs at a young age; now known as insulin-dependent diabetes.

K

KC   Kilocalorie or KCAL. *See also* Calorie.

key nutrient concept   The concept that if certain key nutrients are adequately supplied by the diet, the other essential nutrients will be present in adequate amounts.

kilocalorie   A large Calorie. *See also* Calorie.

kilogram   A unit of mass in the metric system; in ordinary terms, 1 kilogram is the equivalent of 2.2 pounds.

kilojoule   A measure of work or energy; one thousand joules, or the energy equivalent of 0.24 Calorie.

Krebs cycle   The main oxidative reaction sequence in the body that removes hydrogen ions in order to generate ATP; also known as the citric acid or tricarboxylic acid cycle.

kyphosis   An abnormal forward curvature in the upper region of the back, giving rise to a condition commonly known as hunchback.

L

lactic acid   The anaerobic end product of glycolysis; it has been implicated as a causative factor in the etiology of fatigue.

lactic acid system   The energy system that produces ATP anaerobically by the breakdown of glycogen to lactic acid; used primarily in events that require maximal effort for one to two minutes.

lactovegetarian   A vegetarian who includes milk products in the diet as a form of high-quality protein.

LDL   *See* low density lipoprotein.

LDL cholesterol   Low density lipoprotein cholesterol; a mechanism whereby cholesterol is transported in the blood. High blood levels are associated with increased incidence of CHD; *see also* oxidized LDL cholesterol.

lean   In nutritional labeling, meat with less than 10 grams of fat, 4 grams of saturated fat, and 95 milligrams of cholesterol per 100 grams.

lean body mass   Body weight minus body fat; composed primarily of muscle, bone, and other nonfat tissue.

legume   The fruit or pod of vegetables, including soybeans, kidney beans, lima beans, garden peas, black-eyed peas, and lentils; high in protein.

leucine   An essential amino acid.

life expectancy   The number of years of life expected from birth for a given individual in the population. The median for men in the United States is seventy-one years; for women, seventy-six years.

life span   The biological limit to length of life; the potential median life span age is eighty-five.

light   Term used in food labeling; if a food normally derives 50 percent or more of its Calories from fat, it can be labeled light or lite if it is reduced in fat by 50 percent.

lipids   A group of fats or fatlike substances, including triglycerides, phospholipids, and cholesterol.

lipoprotein   A combination of lipid and protein possessing the general properties of proteins. Practically all the lipids of plasma are present in this form.

lipostatic theory   The theory that hunger and satiety are controlled by the blood lipid level.

liquid protein diets   Protein in a liquid form; a common form consists of predigested protein into simple amino acids.

local muscular endurance   The ability of a small muscle group to perform prolonged exercise, such as sit-ups that focus on the abdominal muscles.

long-haul concept   Relative to weight control, the idea that weight loss via exercise should be gradual; the individual should not expect to lose large amounts of weight in a short period of time.

lordosis   An increased forward curvature, or hyperextension, of natural curves in the spine; *see also* lumbar lordosis.

low back pain syndrome   Pain (usually of the dull, aching type) that persistently occurs in the lumbar region of the lower back.

low calorie   In nutritional labeling, no more than 40 Calories per serving, or 0.4 Calories per gram.

low cholesterol   In nutritional labeling, less than 20 milligrams of cholesterol per serving.

low density lipoprotein   A protein-lipid complex in the blood that facilitates the transport of triglycerides, cholesterol, and phospholipids. *See also* LDL cholesterol.

low fat   In nutritional labeling, no more than 3 grams of fat per serving.

low sodium   In nutritional labeling, 40 milligrams or less of sodium per serving.

lumbar lordosis   An increased forward curve in the lower (lumbar) region of the back.

lysine   An essential amino acid.

M

macrophage   A phagocytic tissue cell derived from monocytes (white blood cells) that protects the body from infection.

magnesium   A white, metallic mineral element essential in human nutrition.

Magnetic Resonance Imaging   *See* MRI.

major minerals   Those minerals essential to human nutrition with an RDA in excess of 100 mg/day: calcium, magnesium, phosphorus, sodium, potassium, chloride.

major risk factor   A risk factor that has a highly significant relationship to the development of a particular disease, such as cigarette smoking and lung cancer.

malnutrition   Poor nutrition that may be due to inadequate amounts of essential nutrients. Too many Calories leading to obesity is also a form of malnutrition.

mantra   A secret word or phrase used as part of the relaxation technique in Transcendental Meditation (TM).

marijuana   The shredded, dried leaves, flowers, and stems from the plant Cannabis sativa.

maturity-onset diabetes   Diabetes that occurs later in life, usually after age forty. It is usually the noninsulin-dependent type.

maximal heart rate   *See* HR$_{MAX}$.

maximal heart rate reserve   The difference between the maximal HR and resting HR. A percentage of this reserve, usually 50 to 85 percent, is added to the resting HR to get the target HR for aerobic training programs.

maximal oxygen uptake   *See* $\dot{V}O_{2\,MAX}$.

megadose   In vitamin and mineral nutrition, a dose that is usually significantly greater than the RDA. The amount may vary depending upon the specific vitamin or mineral.

megajoule   A measure of energy; a million joules; one megajoule is the equivalent of about 240 Calories; 1,000 Calories equals 4.2 MJ.

menarche   The first menses, usually between the ages of nine and sixteen.

menopause   The period that marks the end of menstrual activity, usually between the ages of thirty-five and fifty-five.

menses   The monthly flow of blood from the uterine lining.

menstrual cycle   The periodic series of changes in the reproductive system of the female; various phases include the follicular, luteal, premenstrual, and menstrual periods.

metabolic aftereffects of exercise   The theory that the aftereffects of exercise cause the metabolic rate to be elevated for a period of time, thus expending Calories and contributing to weight loss.

metabolic disorders   Diseases of human metabolism; a common one is diabetes.

metabolic rate   The energy expended in order to maintain all physical and chemical changes occurring in the body.

metabolic specificity   A concept of physical training in which certain exercises activate specific energy systems in the body. These specific energy systems adapt and improve through training.

metabolic syndrome   The syndrome of symptoms often seen with android-type obesity, or abdominal obesity, particularly hyperinsulinemia, insulin resistance, hypertriglyceridemia, and hypertension.

metabolic water   The water that is a by-product of the oxidation of carbohydrate, fat, and protein in the body.

metabolism   The sum total of all physical and chemical processes occurring in the body.

metastasis   Spreading of cells, particularly cancer cells, from one part of the body to another.

methamphetamine   Methamphetamine hydrochloride, a powerful form of amphetamine.

methionine   An essential amino acid.

METS   A measurement unit of energy expenditure; one MET equals approximately 3.5 ml O_2/kg body weight per minute.

mineral   An inorganic element occurring in nature.

mitochondria   Structures within the cells that serve as the location for aerobic production of ATP.

mode of exercise   The means by which a person exercises, such as running, swimming, or bicycling.

modified LDL cholesterol   *See* oxidized LDL cholesterol.

molybdenum A hard, heavy, silvery-white metallic element.

monosaccharides Simple sugars (glucose, fructose, and galactose) that cannot be broken down by hydrolysis.

monounsaturated fatty acids Fats that have one free bond remaining for hydrogenation; olive oils are rich in monounsaturated fatty acids.

morbid obesity Obesity that significantly increases health risks; usually being 100 pounds overweight or having a BMI of 40 or greater.

MRI Magnetic resonance imaging, a technique to image body tissues; may be used to evaluate body composition.

muscle endurance Endurance usually specific to a small muscle group.

muscle fiber A muscle cell. A common method of classifying muscle fibers is by their speed of contraction (either fast twitch or slow twitch).

muscle fiber splitting A theory that muscle cells can increase in number by splitting and forming two cells.

muscle glycogen The form in which carbohydrate is stored in the muscle.

muscle hyperplasia The increase in muscle size caused by an increase in the number of muscle cells.

muscle strength The ability of a muscle to develop force; usually measured by tension devices and machines or the one repetition-maximum technique (1RM).

muscular hypertrophy An increase in the size of a muscle.

mutagens Compounds or agents that cause genetic mutations; includes agents such as chemicals or ultraviolet rays.

myocardial infarct Death of part of the heart muscle, the myocardium.

myofibrils A protein substructure in the muscle fiber. Many myofibrils make up a single muscle fiber.

myoglobin An iron-containing compound, similar to hemoglobin, found in the muscle tissues; myoglobin binds oxygen in the muscle cells.

N

natural In nutritional labeling, the term has no meaning except for meat products; meat products with no artificial or synthetic flavors, colors, or additives.

natural, organic foods Foods that are grown without use of man-made chemicals such as pesticides and artificial fertilizers.

Nautilus® A brand of exercise equipment designed for strength training programs; uses weight-training principles to provide optimal resistance throughout the full range of motion.

negative addiction A term coined by Dr. William Morgan to indicate the excessive devotion some individuals have to running, to the extent that they disregard other important facets of their lives.

negative energy balance A condition whereby the caloric output exceeds the caloric intake, thus contributing to a weight loss.

neoplasm New tissue; abnormal tissue growth that has no useful function and results in the formation of tumors.

neuromuscular specificity Training muscle groups through movement patterns specific to the desired skill to be learned.

NHLBI National Heart, Lung, and Blood Institute.

niacin Nicotinamide; nicotinic acid; part of the B complex and an important part of several coenzymes involved in aerobic energy processes in the cells.

nicotinamide An amide of nicotinic acid; niacin.

nicotine A poisonous compound found primarily in the leaves of tobacco plants.

nicotinic acid Niacin.

nitrogen A colorless, tasteless, odorless gas composing about 80 percent of atmospheric gas; an essential component of protein formed in plants during their developmental process.

nonessential amino acids Amino acids formed in the body that do not need to be obtained in the diet. *See also* essential amino acids.

noninsulin-dependent diabetes Diabetes that may be controlled by diet, exercise, and possibly other medication besides insulin; usually associated with adult-onset diabetes.

nonshivering thermogenesis Heat production by brown fat in response to a cold environment, but without shivering.

nulliparity Having never given birth to a child.

nutraceutical A nutrient that may function as a pharmaceutical when taken in certain quantities.

nutrient Substances found in food that provide energy, promote growth and repair of body tissues, or regulate metabolic processes.

nutrient density The degree of nutrient concentration in a given food.

nutrition The science of food and its interactions in the body; involves intake, digestion, assimilation, and metabolism.

nutritional labeling A listing of selected key nutrients and Calories on the label of commercially prepared food products.

O

obesity An excessive accumulation of body fat; usually reserved for individuals who are 20 to 30 percent or more above the average weight for their size.

oligomenorrhea Infrequent or scanty menstrual blood flow.

omega-3 fatty acids Polyunsaturated fatty acids that have a double bond between the third and fourth carbon from the terminal, or omega, carbon; found in fish oils; theorized to help in the prevention of coronary heart disease.

organic In nutritional labeling, a meaningless term; no legal definition.

osteoarthritis A chronic disease of the joints characterized by destruction of articular cartilage and decreased function.

osteoporosis Increased porosity or softening of the bone.

overload principle The major concept of physical training whereby the individual imposes a stress greater than that normally imposed upon a particular body system.

overtraining Excessive exercise training that may lead to impaired health.

overweight Body weight greater than that which is considered normal. *See also* obesity.

ovolactovegetarian A vegetarian who consumes eggs and milk products as a source of high-quality animal protein.

ovovegetarian A vegetarian who includes eggs in the diet to obtain adequate amounts of protein.

oxalates Salts of oxalic acid; found in green leafy vegetables such as spinach and beet greens.

oxidized LDL cholesterol An oxidized form of LDL cholesterol believed to be associated with the development of atherosclerosis.

oxygen A gas essential for human cell metabolism and the production of energy in the body.

oxygen consumption The total amount of oxygen utilized in the body for the production of energy; directly related to the metabolic rate.

oxygen debt The amount of oxygen consumed in the recovery period immediately after exercise beyond that which would be normally consumed during rest.

oxygen system The energy system that produces ATP via the oxidation of various foodstuffs, primarily fats and carbohydrates.

P

pancreas A gland that produces many hormones (including insulin) associated with digestion and metabolism.

pantothenic acid A vitamin of the B complex.

parasympathetic nervous system A part of the autonomic nervous system that helps maintain homeostasis.

passive smoking The inhalation of sidestream smoke or exhaled smoke from the cigarette of another individual.

PC Phosphocreatine; a high energy phosphate compound found in the body cells; part of the ATP-PC energy system.

peak bone mass Development of optimal bone mass, within genetic limitations, prior to age twenty-five.

pelvic inflammatory disease *See* PID.

pelvic tilt A movement of the pelvic girdle in an anterior, posterior, or lateral direction. An anterior tilt will increase lumbar lordosis; a backward tilt will decrease it.

peripheral circulation The vessels that carry blood to and from the various body tissues. (Compare to central circulation.)

peripheral vascular disease Arteriosclerosis in peripheral blood vessels other than the coronary and cerebral arteries.

peripheral vascular resistance The resistance to blood flow provided by the peripheral blood vessels.

personal choice The concept that most of the health decisions made are based upon personal freedom and free choice.

phenylalanine An essential amino acid.

phosphocreatine Creatine phosphate, a high energy compound stored naturally in the body. *See also* PC.

phospholipids A lipid containing phosphorus that, in hydrolysis, yields fatty acids, glycerin, and a nitrogenous compound. Lecithin is an example.

phosphorus   A nonmetallic element essential to human nutrition.

phosphorus-calcium ratio   The ratio of calcium to phosphorus intake in the diet; the normal ratio is 1:1.

photosynthesis   The process whereby nature harnesses the energy from the sun to produce plant food.

phylloquinone   Vitamin K; essential in the blood-clotting process.

physical activity   Any activity that involves human movement; in relation to health and physical fitness, physical activity is often classified as structured and unstructured.

physical fitness   A general term to denote the ability to do certain activities characteristic of specific types of fitness.

phytates   Salts of phytic acid; produced in the body during the digestion of certain grain products; can combine with some minerals, such as iron, and possibly decrease their absorption.

phytochemicals   Chemicals found in plants that may affect metabolic and physiological processes in the human body.

PID   A generalized inflammation within the pelvic region; may lead to sterility.

pituitary gland   An endocrine gland located in the brain that produces a wide variety of hormones that may eventually affect almost all tissues in the body. Often called the master gland.

plantar fascitis   An inflammation of the plantar fascia, a tough fibrous membrane on the bottom of the foot.

plaque   The material that forms in the inner layer of the artery and contributes to atherosclerosis. It contains cholesterol, lipids, and other debris.

PMS   Premenstrual syndrome; a condition associated with a wide variety of symptoms during the time prior to menses.

PNF   Proprioceptive neuromuscular facilitation; a technique used by physical therapists and athletic trainers to help improve flexibility and strength; several varieties are available.

polyunsaturated fatty acids   Fats that contain two or more double bonds; open to hydrogenation.

positive addiction   Formation of a habit that has positive, not negative, effects on health status.

positive energy balance   A condition whereby caloric intake exceeds caloric output; the resultant effect is a weight gain.

Positive Health Life-style   A life-style characterized by health behaviors designed to promote health and longevity by helping to prevent many of the chronic diseases afflicting modern society.

potassium   A metallic element essential in human nutrition; it is the principal cation present in the intracellular fluids.

power   Work divided by time; the ability to produce work in a given period of time.

power-endurance continuum   In relation to strength training, the concept that power or strength is developed by high resistance and few repetitions and that endurance is developed by low resistance and many repetitions.

power lifting   A competitive sport involving three types of lifts: the bench press, the dead lift, and the squat.

PRE   Progressive resistive exercise.

predisposing risk factor   See contributory risk factor.

premenstrual syndrome   See PMS.

preventive medicine   The concept that certain health behaviors may prevent chronic diseases such as coronary heart disease.

preventive services   The use of screening tests to detect the early onset of disease processes so that appropriate health behaviors may be initiated to minimize health risks.

principle of disuse   In relation to exercise, lack of use of a given energy system will lead to atrophy and decreased efficiency of that system.

principle of progression   Principle in the design of exercise programs that the increase of exercise intensity involves a gradual progression.

principle of recuperation   The principle in exercise training that rest between workouts is essential in order for the muscle tissue to develop properly.

principle of reversibility   Fitness gains made following the principle of use are reversed if not used; the principle of disuse results in atrophy.

principle of specificity   The principle that training should be specific to the energy system and the activity that the individual desires to improve.

principle of use   The principle that if a body system is not used, it will lose its potential to perform optimally.

Pritikin program   A dietary program developed by Nathan Pritikin that severely restricts the intake of certain foods (like fats and cholesterol) and greatly increases the consumption of complex carbohydrates.

progressive relaxation   A form of relaxation training in which various muscle groups are contracted and then consciously relaxed, progressively covering all major muscle groups in the body.

progressive resistive exercise (PRE)   The concept that as one gets stronger through a weight-training program, the resistance needs to be increased progressively to continue to gain strength.

promoters   Substances or agents necessary to support or promote the development of a disease once it is initiated.

proof   A term used to express the percentage of alcohol in a solution; the proof value is double the percentage—an 80 proof bottle of whiskey is 40 percent alcohol.

proprioceptive neuromuscular facilitation   See PNF.

prostaglandins   Eicosanoids that possess hormone-like activity in numerous cells in the body.

protein   Any one of a group of complex organic compounds containing nitrogen; formed from various combinations of amino acids.

protein complementarity   The practice among vegetarians of eating foods from two or more different food groups together (usually legumes, nuts, or beans with grain products) in order to ensure a balanced intake of essential amino acids.

protein sparing effect   An adequate intake of energy Calories, as from carbohydrates, will decrease somewhat the rate of protein catabolism in the body and hence spare protein.

prudent health behavior   Although many of the health behaviors of the Positive Health Life-style have not been proven to increase longevity, they are prudent health behaviors because there is a very strong possibility they can increase longevity by preventing many chronic diseases.

psoas major   One of the main muscles involved in hip flexion; it may increase lumbar lordosis in the lower spine when a sit-up is done improperly.

pyridoxine   A component of the vitamin B complex, vitamin B_6.

Q

quality calories   The concept of nutrient density, the presence of significant amounts of nutrients in foods with low Calorie content.

R

radiation   Electromagnetic waves given off by an object; the body radiates heat to a cool environment.

ratings of perceived exertion   See RPE.

RDA   Recommended dietary allowances; the levels of intake of essential nutrients considered to be adequate to meet the known nutritional needs of practically all healthy persons.

RDI   Reference daily intake, a term used in food labeling; the recommended daily intake for protein and selected vitamins and minerals. It replaces the old USRDA (United States Recommended Daily Allowance).

recommended dietary allowances   See RDA.

recommended dietary goals   Dietary goals for Americans established by a United States Senate subcommittee on nutrition; goals stress dietary reduction of fat, cholesterol, salt, and sugar and an increased intake of complex carbohydrates.

rectus abdominis   One of the main muscles involved in doing a curl-up. Strength of this muscle is important in prevention of low back pain.

rectus femoris   One of the main muscles for hip flexion and knee extension; may be involved in creating lumbar lordosis in some improperly performed exercises.

reduced   In nutritional labeling, at least 25 percent fewer Calories or nutrients than the standard product.

REE   See RMR.

Reference Daily Intake   See RDI.

regional fat patterning   Deposition of fat in different regions of the body; fat deposited in the abdominal region appears to pose a greater risk for development of coronary heart disease.

relapse   As related to health behavior changes, slipping back into unhealthy habits.

relative humidity   The percentage of moisture in the air compared with the amount of moisture needed to cause saturation (which is taken as 100).

relative risk A term used in epidemiology to evaluate the increased or decreased risk of disease associated with some variable; a relative risk of 3.0 means some variable, such as smoking, may increase the risk of a disease threefold.

repetition maximum In resistance training, the amount of weight that can be lifted for a specific number of repetitions.

repetitions In relation to resistance training or interval training, the number of times an exercise is done.

resistance In weight training, the amount of weight to be lifted.

resistance training Training programs using various forms of resistance, such as free weights or exercise machines like the Nautilus, with the primary purpose of increasing muscle mass and muscular strength and endurance.

resting energy expenditure *See* RMR.

resting metabolic rate *See* RMR.

retinol Vitamin A.

rheumatoid arthritis A form of arthritis characterized by joint inflammation, swelling, stiffness, and pain.

RHR Resting heart rate.

riboflavin Vitamin B$_2$, a member of the B complex.

risk factor A health behavior or condition that predisposes an individual to a disease statistically related to that behavior or condition.

RMR Resting metabolic rate; the energy required to drive all physiological processes while in a state of rest. *See also* BMR and EMR.

RNA Ribonucleic acid; a cellular component involved in the formation of cell proteins.

round shoulders A postural condition in which the shoulders are inclined forward and inward.

routine In resistance training, a number of different types of exercises.

RPE A subjective rating, on a numerical scale, used to express the perceived difficulty of a given work task.

running Although the distinction between running and jogging is relative to the individual involved, a common value used for running is 9 minutes/mile or faster.

S

sacroiliac The immovable joint in the lower back region where the sacrum of the spine meets the ilium, part of the hip bone.

SAD Seasonal affective disorder; anxiety or depression associated with changes in the seasons, particularly during dark, grey winters in the northern part of the northern hemisphere.

salt free In nutritional labeling, no salt added.

salt or sodium sensitive A characteristic of certain individuals whose blood pressure becomes elevated when they consume excess amounts of salt, or sodium.

satiety center A group of nerve cells in the hypothalamus that responds to certain stimuli in the blood and provides a sensation of satiety.

saturated fat free Less than 0.5 grams per serving.

saturated fatty acids Fats that have all chemical bonds filled.

Seasonal Affective Disorder *See* SAD.

secondary amenorrhea A cessation of normal menstrual flow after it has once been established at puberty; with primary amenorrhea, menstruation never appears in the first place.

selenium A nonmetallic element resembling sulfur; poisonous to some animals.

self-actualization One of the highest levels in Maslow's hierarchy of development; an individual exhibits characteristics of a well-adjusted personality.

self-concept The feelings individuals have about their worth or value as an individual; their self-esteem.

self-efficacy Belief in oneself to accomplish self-determined goals and objectives.

self-empowerment Giving power and control to yourself; comparable to self-efficacy, the belief that you may control your behavior.

self-esteem An objective respect and favorable impression of oneself.

semivegetarians A class of vegetarians, sometimes called new vegetarians, who eat most foods, but who usually restrict their consumption of meat to white meats, such as fish and poultry.

serum cholesterol The level of cholesterol in the blood serum.

serum lipid level The concentration of lipids in the blood serum.

set In resistance training, a certain number of repetitions; for example, a lifter may do three sets of six repetitions in each set.

set point theory The weight-control theory that postulates that each individual has an established normal body weight (set point). Any deviation from this set point will lead to changes in body metabolism to return the individual to the normal weight.

sexually transmitted diseases *See* STDs.

shin splints A painful condition in the shin area of the lower leg that often develops in joggers or runners who run on hard surfaces such as concrete.

short chain fatty acids Fatty acids with chains less than six carbons.

silicon A nonmetallic element.

simple carbohydrates Usually refers to table sugar, or sucrose (a disaccharide); may also refer to other disaccharides and monosaccharides.

skinfold technique A technique used to compute an individual's percentage of body fat; various skinfolds are measured, and a regression formula is then used to compute the body fat.

slow-twitch, oxidative fibers Red muscle fibers that have a slow contraction speed; designed for aerobic activity.

snuff A powdered form of smokeless tobacco.

sodium A soft, metallic element; combines with chloride to form salt; the major extracellular cation in the human body.

sodium free Less than 5 milligrams per serving.

soft tissues In relation to flexibility, the muscles and tendons that can be stretched due to their content of elastic fibers.

somatotype A classification system for body types; for example, endomorphs are round and fat, mesomorphs are muscular, and ectomorphs are thin.

specific dynamic action (SDA) Often used to represent the increased energy cost observed during the metabolism of protein in the body. *See also* TEF.

spinal flexion A forward, bending movement of the spine.

sports anemia A temporary condition of low hemoglobin levels often observed in athletes during the early stages of training.

spot reducing The theory that exercising a specific body part, such as the thighs, will facilitate the loss of body fat from that spot.

standard error of measurement A measure of the error normally found with most measurement techniques. One standard error above and below a score will provide the range in which the actual score may be, with about a 70 percent chance of probability.

standardized exercise An exercise task that conforms to a specific standardized protocol.

state anxiety A transient period of anxiety caused by a temporary stressor; state anxiety disappears when the stressor is removed.

static flexibility Flexibility as measured by a slow, steady movement to the limit of the range of motion. Static flexibility exercises are done slowly. (Compare with dynamic flexibility.)

STDs Sexually transmitted diseases; infectious diseases caused almost exclusively via sexual contact.

steady state A level of metabolism, usually during exercise, when the oxygen consumption satisfies the energy expenditure and an individual is performing in an aerobic state.

steady-state threshold The intensity level of exercise above which the production of energy appears to shift rapidly to an anaerobic mechanism, such as a rapid rise in lactic acid. The oxygen system will still supply a major portion of the energy, but the lactic acid system begins to contribute an increasing share.

stimulus period In exercise programs, the time period over which the stimulus is applied, such as an HR of 150 for 15 minutes.

storage fat Fat that accumulates and is stored in the adipose tissue. *See also* essential fat.

strength The ability of a muscle to exert maximal force during one contraction.

strength-endurance continuum *See* power-endurance continuum.

stress The physiological response the body makes to any stressor. *See also* stress response.

stress fracture A fracture in the outer layer of the bone; may be involved in shin splints.

stress management Procedures or treatments designed to decrease the potential harmful effects of stress on an individual.

stressor Anything that will elicit a stress response in a given individual.

stress response The characteristic physiological responses that the human body makes when confronted by a stressor.

stroke Common term used to describe the results of a cerebral vascular accident or a ruptured blood vessel in the brain.

stroke volume The amount of blood pumped by the heart during each beat.

structured physical activity A planned program of physical activities usually designed to enhance physical fitness; structured physical activity is often referred to as exercise.

subcutaneous fat Adipose cell storage of fat directly under the skin.

substance abuse Excessive reliance on drugs, such as alcohol or tobacco, to cope with society.

sucrose Table sugar, a disaccharide; yields glucose and fructose upon hydrolysis.

sugar free Less than 0.5 grams per serving.

sulforaphane A phytochemical found in plants such as broccoli.

sulfur A pale yellow nonmetallic element essential in human nutrition; a component of the sulfur-containing amino acids.

superoxide An oxygen free radical in the body.

superoxide dismutase An enzyme that may neutralize superoxide radicals.

syndrome A group of signs and symptoms that may characterize a particular disease or disorder.

Syndrome X *See* metabolic syndrome.

synovial fluid The fluid in the joint capsule that aids in lubrication; decreases friction during movement.

syphilis A sexually transmitted disease caused by the spiral-shaped bacterium, Treponema pallidum.

systolic blood pressure The blood pressure in the arteries when the heart is contracting and pumping blood.

T

tar Chemicals and other substances in cigarette tobacco that form when exposed to the high temperature in a lighted cigarette.

target heart rate In an aerobic exercise program, the heart rate level that will provide the stimulus for a beneficial training effect.

target heart rate range (target HR) The range of heart rate response during exercise necessary to achieve a beneficial training effect from the exercise.

TEE The elevation in metabolism and body temperature associated with increased levels of physical activity.

TEF Thermic effect of food; the increase in heat production seen following the consumption of food. *See also* DIT.

tendon The connective tissue in the muscle that merges with and connects the muscle to the bone.

teratogens Substances that cause abnormal development of the embryo and result in a deformed fetus.

test anxiety An increase in tension or anxiety associated with preparation for and taking of an examination.

testosterone The male sex hormone produced by the testes.

THC Tetrahydrocannabinol (delta-9-tetrahydrocannabinol), the psychoactive ingredient in marijuana.

Thermic Effect of Exercise (TEE) The elevation in metabolism and body temperature associated with increased levels of physical activity.

thermic effect of food *See* TEF.

thiamin Vitamin B$_1$.

threonine An essential amino acid.

threshold stimulus In exercise, the intensity level necessary to elicit a beneficial training effect, such as a target heart rate.

thrombus A blood clot that does not move.

tocopherol Generic name for an alcohol that has the activity of vitamin E.

total body fat The sum total of the body's storage and essential fat stores.

trace elements Those minerals essential to human nutrition that have an RDA less than 100 mg daily.

trait anxiety A more enduring anxiety level that appears to be characteristic of a given individual. (Compare to state anxiety.)

Transcendental Meditation (TM) A passive relaxation technique characterized by quiet meditation.

trans fatty acids An alteration in the arrangement of the hydrogen ions to the carbon chain of the fatty acid during the hydrogenation process of vegetable oils; a hydrogen ion is translocated to the opposite side of the carbon. (Compare to cis fatty acids.)

triglycerides One of the many fats formed by the union of glycerol and fatty acids.

tryptophan An essential amino acid.

type A personality A personality trait of an individual characterized by constant anxiety or time urgency.

U

underwater weighing A technique for measuring the percentage of body fat in humans.

United States recommended daily allowances *See* U.S. RDA.

Universal Gym® A brand name for exercise equipment, particularly weights, for strength development.

unsaturated fatty acids Fatty acids that contain double or triple bonds and can add hydrogen atoms.

unstructured physical activity Many of the normal daily physical activities that are generally not planned as exercise, such as walking to work, climbing stairs, gardening, domestic activities, and games and other childhood pursuits.

urethritis An inflammation of the urethra.

U.S. RDA The United States recommended daily allowances; the RDA figures used on labels representing the percentage of the RDA for a given nutrient contained in a serving of the food. Now called RDI.

V

vaginitis An inflammation of the vagina.

validity The degree to which a test accurately measures what it is designed to measure.

valine An essential amino acid.

Valsalva phenomenon A condition in which a forceful exhalation is attempted against a closed epiglottis and no air escapes; such a straining may cause the person to faint or black out due to an eventual lack of blood to the brain.

variable resistance An automatic change in resistance associated with the isokinetic technique and other forms of weight training; designed to match resistance with strength at all points in the range of motion.

vegan An extreme vegetarian who eats no animal protein.

vegetarian An individual whose food is of vegetable or plant origin. *See also* semivegetarian, lactovegetarian, ovovegetarian, ovolactovegetarian, and vegan.

veins The blood vessels that carry blood back to the heart.

very low calorie diets *See* VLCD.

very low density lipoprotein *See* VLDL.

visceral fat Fat located deep in the abdominal, or visceral, region of the body.

vitamin, natural Often referred to as a vitamin derived from natural sources, i.e., foods in nature. (Contrast with vitamin, synthetic.)

vitamin, synthetic A man-made vitamin commercially produced from the separate components of the vitamin.

vitamin A An unsaturated aliphatic alcohol that is fat soluble.

vitamin B$_1$ Thiamin; the antineuritic vitamin.

vitamin B$_2$ Riboflavin.

vitamin B$_6$ Pyridoxine and related compounds.

vitamin B$_{12}$ Cyanocobalamin.

vitamin B$_{15}$ Not a vitamin but marketed as one; usual composition is calcium gluconate and dimethylglycine (DMG).

vitamin C Ascorbic acid; the antiscorbutic vitamin.

vitamin D Any one of related sterols that have antirachitic properties; fat soluble.

vitamin deficiency Subnormal body vitamin levels due to inadequate intake or absorption; specific disorders occur depending on the deficient vitamin.

vitamin E Alpha-tocopherol (one of three tocopherols); fat soluble.

vitamin K The antihemorrhagic (or clotting) vitamin; fat soluble.

vitamins A general term for a number of substances deemed essential for the normal metabolic functioning of the body.

VLCD Diets containing fewer than 800 Calories, most commonly about 400–500 Calories.

VLDL Very low density lipoproteins; a protein-lipid complex in the blood that transports triglycerides, cholesterol, and phospholipids and has a very low density. *See also* HDL and LDL cholesterol.

V̇O$_{2MAX}$ Maximal oxygen uptake; measured during exercise, the maximal amount of oxygen consumed reflects the body's ability to utilize oxygen for energy production; equals the maximal cardiac output times the maximal arterio-venous oxygen difference.

W

waist:hip ratio A measure of regional fat distribution in which the waist girth is divided by the hip girth; also known as the abdominal:gluteal ratio or the android:gynoid ratio.

warm-down A gradual tapering period after the stimulus period of an exercise bout in which the individual exercises mildly. Also known as a cool-down period.

warm-up Low level exercises used to increase the muscle temperature and/or stretch the muscles before a strenuous exercise bout.

water A tasteless, colorless, odorless fluid essential to life; composed of two parts hydrogen and one part oxygen (H_2O).

water depletion heat exhaustion Weakness caused by excessive loss of body fluids, such as through exercise-induced dehydration in a hot or warm environment.

water-insoluble fiber Dietary fiber that is not soluble in water.

water-soluble fiber Dietary fiber that is soluble in water, such as the gums and pectins found in plants.

weight cycling Repeated bouts of weight gain and weight loss; also referred to as the yo-yo diet.

weight lifting A competitive sport; the two most common lifts are the clean-and-jerk and the snatch.

weight training A conditioning method with heavy weights; designed to increase strength, power, and muscle size.

wellness clinics Educational seminars designed to help individuals develop health behaviors characteristic of a Positive Health Life-style.

wheat In nutritional labeling, not necessarily whole wheat unless whole wheat is listed as the first ingredient.

work Effort expended to accomplish something; in terms of physics, force times distance.

Y

yo-yo diet Diets, usually seen in the obese, that are characterized by repeated bouts of weight loss followed by weight gain; such diets usually alternate periods of very low intake with normal or above average intake.

Z

zinc A blue-white crystalline metallic element essential to human nutrition.

Credits

Chapter 1

Chapter Opener Digital Stock Photo CD.

Chapter 2

Chapter Opener © Kevin Syms/David Frazier PhotoLibrary CD.

Chapter 3

Chapter Opener David Frazier PhotoLibrary CD.
Figure 3.7 From J. Daniels, R. Fitts, and G. Sheehan, *Conditioning for Long Distance Running.* Copyright © 1978 by John Wiley & Sons, Inc., New York, NY. Reprinted by permission.
Figure 3.15 Courtesy Randal™ Sports Medical Products, Inc. Stairmaster Exercise Systems.

Chapter 4

Chapter Opener © Kevin Syms/David Frazier PhotoLibrary CD.
Figure 4.1 From John W. Hole, Jr. *Human Anatomy and Physiology,* 6th edition. Copyright © 1993 Wm. C. Brown Communications, Inc. Reprinted by permission of Times Mirror Higher Education Group, Inc., Dubuque, Iowa. All Rights Reserved.

Chapter 5

Chapter Opener David Frazier PhotoLibrary CD.

Chapter 6

Chapter Opener Corel Photo CD.
Figure 6.12 1–6 © Arnold and Brown Photographers, Peoria, IL.
Figures 6.15 and 6.16 © Bob Coyle.

Chapter 7

Chapter Opener © Kevin Syms/David Frazier PhotoLibrary CD.
Figure 7.3 Reprinted by permission of the American Alliance for Health, Physical Education, Recreation and Dance, 1900 Association Drive, Reston, VA 22091.

Chapter 8

Chapter Opener Digital Stock Photo CD.
Figure 8.6 From M. S. Bahrki and W. P. Morgan, "Anxiety Reduction Following Exercise and Meditation" in *Cognitive Therapy and Research,* 2:323. Copyright © 1978 Plenum Publishing Corporation. Reprinted by permission.

Chapter 9

Chapter Opener David Frazier PhotoLibrary CD.
Figure 9.1 From Charles R. Carroll, *Drugs in Modern Society,* 2nd edition. Copyright © 1989 Wm. C. Brown Communications, Inc. Reprinted by permission of Times Mirror Higher Education Group, Inc., Dubuque, Iowa. All Rights Reserved.
Figure 9.4 From Harry Avis, *Drugs & Life.* Copyright © 1990 Wm. C. Brown Communications, Inc. Reprinted by permission of Times Mirror Higher Education Group, Inc., Dubuque, Iowa. All Rights Reserved.
Figure 9.7a, b, and c Drug Enforcement Administration.
Figure 9.8 From *Beyond Training* (fig 4.2, p. 98) by Melvin H. Williams, 1989, Champaign, IL: Leisure Press. Copyright 1989 by Melvin H. Williams. Reprinted by permission.
Figures 9.9, 9.11, 9.12, and 9.13 From Curtis O. Byer and Louis W. Shainberg, *Dimensions of Human Sexuality,* 3rd edition. Copyright © 1991 Wm. C. Brown Communications, Inc. Reprinted by permission of Times Mirror Higher Education Group, Inc., Dubuque, Iowa. All Rights Reserved.
Figure 9.14a, b, and c © Bob Coyle.
Figure 9.14d Wisconsin Pharmacal Company.

Chapter 10

Chapter Opener © Kevin Syms/David Frazier PhotoLibrary CD.

Chapter 11

Chapter Opener David Frazier PhotoLibrary CD.
Figure 11.2 Courtesy Ward's Natural Science, Inc., Rochester, NY.

Figure 11.3 (left) From Stuart I. Fox, *Human Physiology.* Copyright © 1984 Wm. C. Brown Communications, Inc., Reprinted by permission of Times Mirror Higher Education Group, Inc., Dubuque, Iowa. All Rights Reserved.

Figure 11.3 (right) © Carroll Weiss, 1973. All Rights Reserved.

Figure 11.6 Reproduced with permission. © American Heart Association.

Figure 11.7 Reprinted by permission from *What About Blood Pressure* by Daniel E. James, copyright 1981 by Carolina Biological Supply Company.

Figures 11.10 and 11.11 From Curtis O. Byer and Louis W. Shainberg, *Dimensions of Human Sexuality,* 3rd edition. Copyright © 1991 Wm. C. Brown Communications, Inc. Reprinted by permission of Times Mirror Higher Education Group, Inc., Dubuque, Iowa. All Rights Reserved.

Figure 11.12 From John W. Hole, Jr. *Human Anatomy and Physiology,* 3rd edition. Copyright © 1984 Wm. C. Brown Communications, Inc. Reprinted by permission of Times Mirror Higher Education Group, Inc., Dubuque, Iowa. All Rights Reserved.

Chapter 12

Chapter Opener David Frazier PhotoLibrary CD.

Laboratory Inventories

Laboratory Inventory 3.5 © (1990) The Rockport Company, Inc. All Rights Reserved. Reprinted by permission of The Rockport Company, Inc.

Laboratory Inventory 8.2 From Girdano and Everly, *Controlling Stress and Tension,* Copyright © Prentice-Hall, Inc., Englewood Cliffs, N.J.

Index

Morgan, W. M., 16
Mortality rates, and physical activity, 48
Motivation, and hierarchy of needs, 177
Motor-skill related fitness, 14, 15
Muscle
  endurance, 61
  function of, 59–60
  hypertrophy, 61
  strength, 60–61
  structure of, 58–59
  See also Resistance training
Muscle contraction
  isokinetic contraction, 67
  isometric contraction, 66
  isotonic concentric contraction, 66–67
  isotonic eccentric contraction, 67
Muscle fibers, 58, 60, 89
Muscle soreness
  acute soreness, 49
  delayed soreness, 49
  relief of, 49
Muscle strength tests
  abdominal muscle strength, 309
  lower body strength, 307
  upper body strength, 305–306
Musculoskeletal disorders, 257–265
  arthritis, 263–265
  low back pain, 257–262
  osteoporosis, 262–263
Myocardial infarct, 242
Myofibrils, 58

N

National Cholesterol Education Program, 111,
    244, 245
Nautilus machines, 68, 89, 91
Neck, flexibility exercises for, 94, 97, 98
Negative addiction, 187
Negative energy balance, 145
Negative muscle contraction, 67
Neoplasm, 253
Neuromuscular specificity, and exercise
    program, 21
Neutron activation analysis, body composition
    measure, 142
Niacin, to decrease LDL cholesterol, 247
Nicotine, 200–201
  physiological effects, 200–201
Noise, as stressor, 182
Noninsulin-dependent diabetes, 252
No-pain/no-gain concept, 273
Nulliparity, 227
Nutraceuticals, 104
Nutrient density, low-calorie/high-nutrient
    foods, 151
Nutrients
  carbohydrates, 106–108
  fat, 108–112
  functions of, 105–106
  minerals, 117
  protein, 112–113
  vitamins, 113–117
  water, 117–119
Nutrition
  definition of, 104
  diet planning, basics of, 119–120
  Food Exchange System, 122–123
  Food Guide Pyramid, 121–123
  food labels, 123–126
  guidelines for healthy eating, 127–131
  and healthy life-style, 7
  How's Your Diet questionnaire, 323–326
  key nutrient concept, 120
  major reports on, 105, 127
  nutrient density, 120–121

Recommended Dietary Allowances
    (RDA), 120
  vegetarianism, 131–133
Nutrition Facts, food labels, 124, 126
Nutrition Labeling and Education Act, 123

O

Obesity, 250–251
  android-(male) type obesity, 143, 144, 251
  cancer link, 254
  and coronary heart disease, 246
  creeping obesity, 139, 140
  definition of, 139
  dietary fat, role in, 151
  gynoid-(female) type obesity, 143, 144
  health effects, 251
  morbid obesity, 139, 251
  and psychological problems, 251
  treatment of, 251
  See also Weight control
Oligomenorrhea, 227
Omega-3 fatty acids, 108
Optimist's Creed, 182
Oral contraceptives, and coronary heart disease,
    246, 247
Orioli, E., 181
Ornish, Dean, 247
Osteoarthritis, 263–264
Osteoporosis, 262–263
  and amenorrhea, 227
  and bone fractures, 262
  and calcium, 117, 262–263
  causes of, 227, 262
  and estrogen replacement therapy, 227, 263
  treatment of, 227, 263–264
  and weight-bearing exercise, 228, 263
Overcrowding, as stressor, 182
Overload principle, 20–21, 39, 46
  duration in, 20
  frequency of training in, 20
  intensity in, 20
  resistance training, 61–62
Overtraining, negative effects of, 187
Ovolactovegetarians, 131
Ovovegetarians, 131
Oxygen system
  and calories, 28–29
  human energy system, 27, 28
  maximal oxygen consumption ($\dot{V}O_{2MAX}$),
    30–31, 33
  measurements of aerobic system, 32–34
  oxygen debt, 32
  programs for development of, 21
  and resistance training, 66
  steady-state threshold, 31–32
Oxygen uptake, physiological processes in, 30

P

Paffenbarger, Ralph, 16, 48
Paige, Leroy (Satchel), 265
Pap smear, 254
Passive smoking, 201, 202–203
PC (phosphocreatine), in human energy
    system, 27
Peale, Norman Vincent, 182
Pelvic inflammatory disease (PID), 213
Peripheral vascular disease, 250
Personal choice, and health behaviors, 9
Phosphorus, facts about, 118
Photosynthesis, 26
Physical activity
  structured, 14
  unstructured, 14

Physical fitness
  and aerobic fitness, 30
  health-related components, 15
  meaning of, 14
  motor-skill related fitness, 14, 15
Physical fitness program
  adherence to program, 19–20
  benefit/risk ratio, 18–19
  design of, 17
  equipment for, 19
  evaluation of progress, 20
  medical clearance for, 18
  needs assessment for, 17
  planning questions, 17–18
  skills for, 19
  starting program, 18
Phytochemicals, 104
Pi-Suyner, F. Xavier, 151
Pituitary gland, regulation of, 177–178
Plaque, in atherosclerosis, 242, 243, 244
Polyunsaturated fatty acids, 108
Portions, for weight loss diet, 152
Positive addiction, 273
Positive energy balance, 145
Positive health life-style, 2, 3
  adherence to, 272
  and attitude, 272–273
  and behavior modification, 9–10
  behaviors related to, 7
  benefits of, 8
  goal-setting in, 273–274
  goals of, 3
  and health/fitness club, 275
  primary goal of, 5
  relapse prevention, 274
  reward system in, 274
  and self-efficacy, 273
  and self-esteem, 273
  and social environment, 274
Posture problems
  flexibility exercises for, 87, 94
  kyphosis, 87, 89
Potassium, facts about, 118
Pregnancy, 230–233
  and alcohol use, 197
  and cocaine use, 209
  exercise in, 231–233
  and genital herpes, 213
  high-risk women, 233
  nutrition in, 230–231
  recommended weight gain, 230
  teratogens in, 230
  vitamins in, 116
Premenstrual syndrome (PMS), 228–230
  cause of, 229
  inventory for assessment of, 365
  symptoms of, 228
  treatment approaches, 229–230
Preventive services, scope of, 2
Principle of disuse, meaning of, 20
Principle of progression
  meaning of, 20
  and planning of program, 20
Principle of recuperation, importance of, 22
Principle of specificity, and training, 21
Principle of use, meaning of, 20
Progesterone, 223
Progressive relaxation, 185–186
  steps in, 185–186
Progressive resistance exercise (PRE), 21, 62
Project PACE, 18, 283
  exercise program implementation inventory,
    283–288
Promoters, of disease, 104
Proof, of alcohol, 193